introduction to
aural rehabilitation

a volume in the perspectives in audiology series

introduction to aural rehabilitation

SECOND EDITION

RONALD L. SCHOW

MICHAEL A. NERBONNE

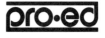

8700 Shoal Creek Boulevard
Austin, Texas 78758

Perspectives in Audiology Series

Series Editor
Lyle L. Lloyd

Copyright ©1989 by PRO-ED, Inc.

Printed in the United States of America

Library of Congress Cataloging-in-Publication Data

Introduction to aural rehabilitation / edited by Ronald L. Schow and Michael A. Nerbonne. — 2nd ed.
    p.   cm. — (perspectives in audiology series)
    Bibliography: p.
    Includes index.
    ISBN 0-89079-172-4
    1. Deaf—Rehabilitation. 2. Audiology. I. Schow, Ronald L.
II. Nerbonne, Michael A. III. Series
RF297.I57 1989
617.8′9—dc19   87-34808
                                          CIP

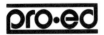

8700 Shoal Creek Boulevard
Austin, Texas 78758

10 9 8 7 6 5 4 3 2 1   88 89 90 91 92

To our students—past, present, and future—
for the many contributions they make to us
professionally and personally.

contents

partthree: implementing aural rehabilitation: case studies and resource materials

foreword

The first book I read in audiology was the 1947 edition of *Hearing and Deafness* by Silverman and Davis. In the foreword to that book, Louise Tracy, founder of the John Tracy Clinic, began by saying that although the "first handicap of deafness lies in communication, a close second might be the attitude of hearing people toward it and that the former would be considerably lessened if we could do something to improve the latter." It is now over forty years since these words were written. We have learned so much about the impact of a hearing loss upon the affected individual and the measures that must be undertaken to ensure effective habilitation and rehabilitation. This book is ample evidence of how far we have come. Yet, as I view the current scene in aural rehabilitation (AR), Mrs. Tracy's forty-year-old words still resonate with a valid insight.

Hearing loss is still a vastly underestimated impairment. Most children with hearing losses look perfectly normal, even "cute;" the awesome effect of impaired hearing upon auditory-based speech and language skills is still imperfectly realized by most people. Those with lesser losses, whose behavior is often inconsistent, unpredictable, and troublesome, are frequently accused of willfully misbehaving when they fail to respond appropriately. Remediation measures are often half-hearted and superficial, not from malignant design, but because of insufficient understanding of both the heterogeneity of the effects of hearing loss and the various treatment and educational options that must be available.

One does not "cure" hearing loss simply by providing amplification (although this is a prerequisite measure for most hearing-impaired children) and then expecting normal responses. Underlying all our efforts with young hearing-impaired children must be a sense of urgency, a realization of the time-limited restrictions inherent in many of our remediation measures; everything must be done "yesterday" if we are to realize the full benefits of such measures today.

The key to unlock the door of effective treatment continues to be the commonly held feelings toward hearing loss reflecting a lack of information and empathy. One of the major challenges currently facing our profession, therefore, is to change these attitudes through public education. An underestimated and misunderstood condition will not receive the treatment priorities it deserves and requires. But before we can engage in informed public education, our own colleagues and future generations of professionals must acquire a solid grounding in both the handicapping consequences of the impairment and the most effective rehabilitation procedures for hearing-handicapped individuals. The authors of this book have presented to us the current state of our knowledge in these areas.

My own professional background has mainly involved children; recently, however, I have had the opportunity to be more involved with hearing-impaired adults as well. Revisiting AR after all this time has been both a heartening and a discouraging experience. On the one hand, hearing aids have been significantly improved, an entire array of useful assistive devices have been developed, sensitive clinical self-assessment tools are now available, and defensible models of AR are being practiced. This book is evidence that effective AR is perfectly feasible, but— and this is the caveat—only to those who take advantage of our services.

It is apparent that the overwhelming majority of hearing-impaired adults never avail themselves of many of our rehabilitation services— partly because it is uneconomical under current models of hearing aid dispensing, partly because many professionals remain unconvinced of the need and efficacy of time-consuming AR programs, but mainly because, even when available, too many of our clients deny the necessity of AR. However, the results of studies employing self-assessment scales are clear evidence of the frequency and extent of the handicapping effects of a hearing loss. There is no doubt that a hearing loss leads to many secondary problems; what is also undeniable is that, for many, such problems remain unresolved in spite of the consequences this has upon their overall quality of life. A lot of people seem to find it difficult to come to terms with the reality of their own condition. In this, they both reflect current attitudes and are its victims.

The feelings surrounding hearing loss can, perhaps, best be appreciated by considering the typical response of an adventitiously hearing-impaired adult. After years of difficulty, of accusing others of mumbling, of heightened tensions within the family and restriction in their personal and social life, only a minority (approximately 20%) finally accept the need for an amplification device. And even then, most seem to be looking for a device that is virtually invisible. What is this but a continual denial of their own condition? Hearing loss is simply not an acceptable condition for people in our society to admit to. I do not know the reasons why so many view a hearing loss with shame, as some kind of personal stigma, which must be disguised and denied at almost all costs. I suspect that we will find there are many reasons, but one conclusion seems inescapable—their attitudes are not just personal, but reflect widespread societal values. The logical consequence of this conclusion is that, in the long term, we can be most effective if society's attitudes toward hearing loss can be made more rational and more accepting.

Unfortunately, in the marketing of hearing aids, many professionals and hearing aid manufacturers, by focusing primarily on the cosmetics, are continually reinforcing the sense of stigma associated with hearing aid usage. If a hearing loss and the necessity of wearing a hearing aid were nothing to be ashamed of, why the emphasis on size, on invisibility of the aid? The message, unintended I am sure, is that the more a hearing aid can be disguised, the better. In my opinion, for every person who succumbs to a purely cosmetic appeal, many other potential candidates are being driven further away from the acceptance of their own condition. What they "hear" is the underlying deprecation in society toward hearing loss. Is it any wonder, therefore, that they are reluctant to accept this derogatory judgment for themselves? Certainly, we must respond to people who will only wear a cosmetically acceptable hearing aid, even if another device offers them more assistance. However, we also have a concurrent responsibility, and that is to eliminate the attitudes in our society which preclude effective AR for those who need it.

Hearing aids, while most often a necessary component of AR, are not always sufficient in themselves. For many people, much more is needed. But before we can convince others of the necessity of AR, we must truly believe in its efficacy ourselves. In spite of both clinical and experimental evidence of the value of AR, there is an ongoing need for sustained research on the topic. There has to be a continued series of publications on the various aspects of AR. We need to convince a skeptical profession and public of its benefits and then stimulate the development of service delivery models in which AR can be economically viable. Perhaps because I myself was the recipient of an exemplary AR program 37 years ago at Walter Reed Army Medical Center, I have never doubted the value or necessity of AR. In retrospect, it is disheartening to contemplate how little has changed since then in terms of the availability of first-class AR programs. In other respects, however, changes are being made. This book is visible evidence in that regard and testifies to the increased maturation of our profession.

For many years, the emphasis in the field has been upon the impairment, how to measure it, and the diagnostic implications of these measurements. We see now an increased concern with the resulting handicap of the impairment, and the nonmedical rehabilitation steps which can be employed. I would argue that it is *only* through rehabilitation that we can acquire complete professional autonomy and practice our skills in a fully realized fashion. It is *only* in the area of aural rehabilitation that we can diagnose and attempt to remediate the consequences of a hearing loss. Although we provide valuable diagnostic information when we deal with the impairment of hearing loss, this information, technically sophisticated as it may be, is designed for our medical colleagues to use in their diagnosis and treatment. The converse, in my judgment, is also true; it is our profession which bears the greater responsibility in regard to aural rehabilitation. If this simple distinction were accepted, we could have prevented some of the interprofessional disputes which have arisen over the years.

The challenge, then, that we face is neither short-term nor trivial. We are frequently reminded of the increased proportion of the elderly in our country. We know the high incidence of hearing loss among this group and the debilitating personal impact a hearing loss can have. It will be from among the readers of this book that the leadership must emerge to first help people accept the reality of a hearing loss, and then to offer them the kind of informed assistance that is so ably presented in the pages that follow.

Mark Ross, PhD
Consultant, Research and Training
New York League for the Hard of Hearing

Adjunct Professor
City University of New York

preface

It has now been nearly nine years since the first edition of INTRODUC-
TION TO AURAL REHABILITATION was published. In that period aural
rehabilitation has shown a vitality and resurgence that is most encouraging. Among the developments which have occurred in this time we would
include the emergence of cochlear implants and assistive listening devices
as major rehabilitative tools, the use of real-ear measures in hearing aid
fitting, increased use of hearing self-assessment measures, expanded
efforts in counseling for the hearing impaired, computer software inno-
vations in aural rehabilitation, new approaches to language and speech
remediation for the deaf including the use of ''tracking'' as a rehabilitation procedure, not to mention new improved models to more clearly
define the aural rehabilitation process. This edition has been designed
to provide appropriate emphasis on all these new developments.

This book was originally developed for use as an introductory text
at the undergraduate level. That is still the major intent. We regularly
teach undergraduate students the fundamentals of aural rehabilitation
and feel the need to give them a broad overview without overwhelming
them with too much advanced material. At the same time, we have used
this text to supplement our graduate courses, precisely because the fundamental issues are all treated in a way that provides a framework for
advanced study.

We have selected the authors of the various chapters again with care.
They are professionals with proven credentials in aural rehabilitation
who have published and presented widely. To the returning authors
from the first edition (Ken Berger, Joe Millin, Nick Hipskind, John Hutchinson, Linda Smith, McCay Vernon, Paula Ottinger, Julia and Don
Moores, Susan Watkins, Jerry Alpiner, and Curt Tannahill), we have
added several other well-known persons including Dean Garstecki, Jim
Maurer, Mary Pat Moeller, Tom Giolas, Gwenyth Vaughn, Robert Lightfoot, Adrienne Karp, Debbie Noall Seyfried, Thayne Smedley and Carole
Flevaris-Phillips.

The framework of the book remains very similar to the first edition.
There are seven chapters on fundamental issues, followed by three chapters dealing with the major client populations: children, adults, and elderly

adults. The final three chapters consist of two with case studies and one which lists rich resource material.

Special emphasis has been placed on new developments in amplification in Chapter 2, on self-assessment procedures which are highlighted in Chapter 9, and on counseling techniques in Chapter 10. Chapter 13, the resource chapter, includes important lists of materials with addresses and publication details, as well as information on sample rehabilitation outlines, enrichment information on assistive listening devices and on the visually impaired. In addition, the official ASHA statement on definitions and competencies in aural rehabilitation is contained in that chapter.

It is our intent that this new edition be harmonious with the upbeat mood in aural rehabilitation which has been emerging these past few years. Hopefully, it will inspire the beginning student to see the possibilities and the bright future in this most important audiological endeavor.

acknowledgments

We express gratitude to the fine authors who worked with us on this project. They have cheerfully responded to our many requests. Thanks also to Steve Mathews at PRO-ED and Kirsten McBride, our copy editor, for having faith in us and for expert assistance.

Our university colleagues have been generously helpful, and we appreciate their encouragement. Especially we note the administrative support of Tom Longhurst, Bob McLauchlin, and Ed Poynor and the technical suggestions of Frank Cirrin, Bob Pehrrson, Paul Deputy, and Jerry Church. We express thanks to Nancy O'Brien, Jill Hauck, Linda Poole, and Lucille MacKay for the superb job they did in typing portions of the manuscript.

We also thank Dodie Stein and Lyle Lloyd who reviewed the entire project at the beginning and offered many helpful recommendations.

Our wives, Adonna and Nancy, have rendered much appreciated moral support, technical assistance, and patience when we delayed other domestic and family projects. To them and our children, Leann, Mindy, Blake, Bart, Cammy/Nick, Brian, Jennifer, and Christina we tender heartfelt thanks. Also, since they already have a book (the first edition) dedicated in their honor, we dedicate to them something more tangible—any proceeds that may trickle in our direction.

contributors

Jerome G. Alpiner, PhD
  Chief, Audiology Section
  Veterans Administration
    Medical Center
  Adjunct Professor
  Department of
    Biocommunication
    School of Dentistry &
    Medicine
  University of Alabama
  Birmingham, AL 35233

Kenneth W. Berger, PhD
  Professor Emeritus of
    Audiology
  School of Speech
  Kent State University
  Kent, OH 44242

Carole Flevaris-Phillips, PhD
  24315 Hoover Court
  Farmington Hills, MI 48331

Dean C. Garstecki, PhD
  Professor and Program Head
  Audiology and Hearing
    Impairment
  Northwestern University
  Evanston, IL 60201

Thomas G. Giolas, PhD
  Dean of the Graduate School
    and Director of the
    Research Foundation
  Professor of Communication
    Sciences
  University of Connecticut
  Storrs, CT 06268

Nicholas M. Hipskind, PhD
  Associate Professor and
    Director of Clinical
    Audiology
  Department of Speech and
    Hearing Sciences
  Indiana University
  Bloomington, IN 47401

John M. Hutchinson, PhD
  Academic Vice-President
  Professor of Speech-Language
    Pathology
  Idaho State University
  Pocatello, ID 83209

Adrienne Karp, MA
  Audiologist
  New York Association for
    the Blind
  111 East 59th Street
  New York, NY 10022

Robert K. Lightfoot, MS
  Rehabilitative Audiologist
  Birmingham Veterans
    Administration Medical
    Center
  Birmingham, AL 35216

James F. Maurer, PhD
  Professor of Audiology
  Speech and Hearing
    Sciences
  Portland State University
  Portland, OR 97207

Joseph P. Millin, PhD
  Professor of Audiology
  School of Speech
  Kent State University
  Kent, OH 44242

contributors

Mary Pat Moeller, MS
Aural Rehabilitation
  Specialist
Boys Town National Institute
Omaha, NE 68181

Donald F. Moores, PhD
Director, Center for Studies
  in Education and Human
  Development
Gallaudet Research Institute
Gallaudet College
Washington, DC 20002

Julia Maestas Y. Moores, MS
Policy Analyst
U.S. Department of Health &
  Human Services
Washington, DC 20202

Michael A. Nerbonne, PhD
Professor and Director of
  Audiology
Department of
  Communication Disorders
Central Michigan University
Mt. Pleasant, MI 48859

Paula J. Ottinger, MA
Coordinator of Services for
  the Handicapped
Montgomery County
  Community College
Montgomery County, MD

Ronald L. Schow, PhD
Professor of Audiology
Department of Speech
  Pathology and Audiology
Idaho State University
Pocatello, ID 83209

Deborah Noall Seyfried, MS
Department of Speech
  Pathology and Audiology
University of Iowa
Iowa City, IA 52242

Thayne C. Smedley, PhD
Assistant Professor of
  Audiology
Department of Speech
  Pathology and Audiology
Idaho State University
Pocatello, ID 83209

Linda Lou Smith, PhD
Assistant Dean, College of
  Communication Arts and
  Sciences
Michigan State University
East Lansing, MI 48824

J. Curtis Tannahill, PhD
Professor of Audiology
Department of Speech
  Pathology and Audiology
Illinois State University
Normal, IL 61761

Gwenyth R. Vaughn, PhD
Chief, Audiology-Speech
  Pathology Service
Birmingham Veterans
  Administration Medical
  Center
Professor
Department of
  Biocommunication
University of Alabama
Birmingham, AL 35216

contributors

McCay Vernon, PhD
Professor
Department of Psychology
Western Maryland College
Westminster, MD 21157

Susan Watkins, EdD
SKI-HI Institute
Department of
   Communicative Disorders
Utah State University
Logan; UT 84321-9605

.

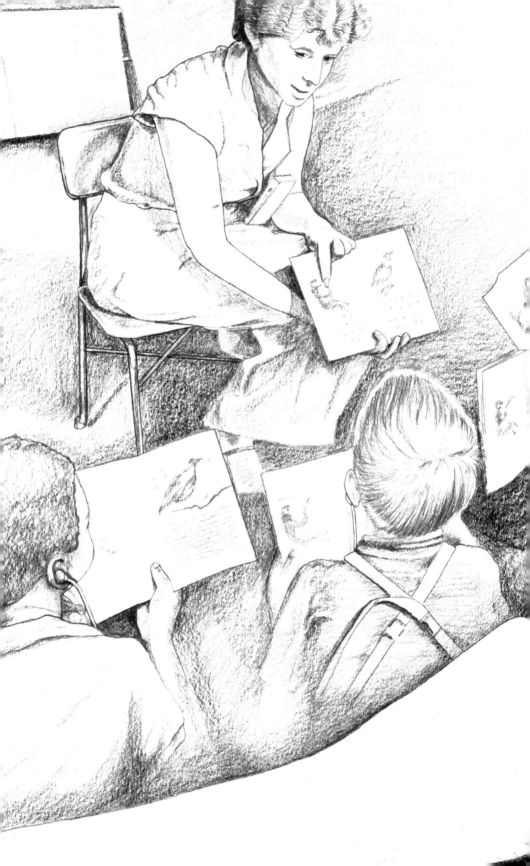

partone

fundamental aspects of aural rehabilitation

The impact of hearing loss on an individual can be extensive. In addition to creating difficulties associated with basic receptive communication, a hearing impairment often produces difficulties in other significant areas such as psychosocial adjustment, educational placement, and expressive communication. To be successful in the management of the hearing impaired, a professsional must understand the fundamentals associated with the effects of hearing loss. This section provides this vital foundation.

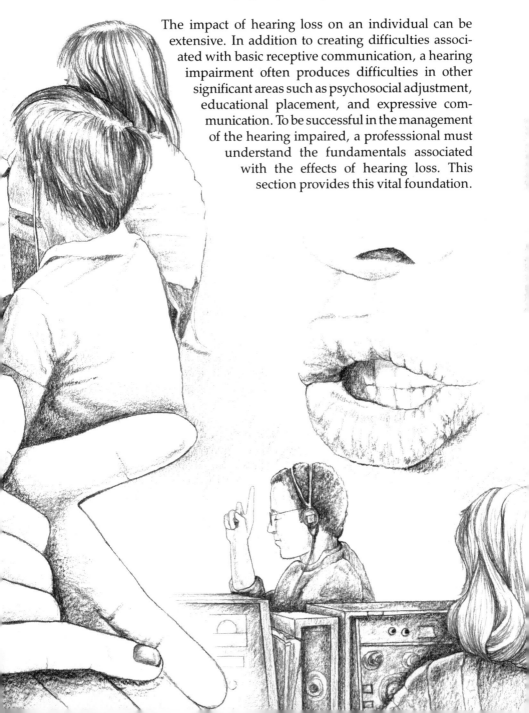

chapterone

OVERVIEW OF AURAL REHABILITATION

RONALD L. SCHOW

MICHAEL A. NERBONNE

contents

introduction

Most of us have had occasion to converse with someone who has a hearing problem. Unless the person had received proper help for the hearing difficulties it probably was a frustrating experience for both parties. When the person with hearing loss is a family member or close friend we become aware that the emotional and social ramifications of this communication barrier can be substantial. Providing help to remedy these hearing problems is the focus of this book. Help is possible, but often not utilized. This chapter overviews a process that is crucial for the welfare of persons who suffer from hearing impairment and in turn, for those who communicate with them.

definitions—synonyms

Simply stated, we may define *aural habilitation/rehabilitation* as those professional efforts designed to help a person with hearing loss. This includes services and procedures for lessening or compensating for a hearing impairment and specifically involves facilitating adequate receptive and expressive communication (ASHA, 1984). A key element in this rehabilitation process involves assisting the hearing-impaired person in attaining full potential by using personal resources to overcome difficulties resulting from the hearing loss. Two kinds of service that are closely related but distinct from the aural habilitation/rehabilitation process are *medical intervention* and *formal education of the hearing impaired.*

Several terms have been used to describe this helping process. *Aural habilitation* refers to remedial efforts with children having a hearing loss at birth, since technically it is not possible to restore (*re*habilitate) something that has never existed. *Aural rehabilitation,* then, refers to efforts designed to restore a lost state or function. In the interest of simplicity, the terms *habilitation* and *rehabilitation* are used interchangeably in this text, technicalities notwithstanding. Variations of the aural rehabilitation term include *auditory* and *audiologic rehabilitation, hearing rehabilitation,* and *rehabilitative audiology.* Terms used to refer to habilitative efforts with the very young child include *parent advising/counseling/tutoring* and *pediatric auditory habilitation. Educational* or *school audiology* are sometimes used to refer to auditory habilitative efforts in the school setting.

providers of aural rehabilitation

Aural rehabilitation (AR), then, is referred to by different names, and is performed in a number of different settings. All aspects of assisting the client in the aural rehabilitation process are not performed by one person. In fact, professionals from several different disciplines are often involved, including educators, psychologists, social workers, and rehabilitation counselors. Nevertheless, the audiologist in particular, in some circumstances the speech-language pathologist or the educator of the hearing impaired, will assume a major AR role. These professionals provide overall coordination of the process or act as advocates for the hearing-impaired person. Aural rehabilitation is not something we *do* to a person. It is a process designed to help hearing-impaired persons actualize their own resources in order to meet their unique life situations. This text has been written with the hope of orienting and preparing such ''team managers'' or ''advocates for the hearing impaired.''

education needs of providers

To successfully perform an AR advocacy role a person must possess an understanding of and familiarity with several aspects, including (a) hearing impairment, (b) effect of hearing loss on persons, and (c) competencies needed for rehabilitation (see ASHA, 1984, Definition of and Competencies for AR Position Statement, Chapter 13). For purposes of the present treatment, it is assumed that previous coursework or study has brought the reader familiarity with the various forms of hearing impairment, as well as procedures used in the measurement of hearing loss. These procedures, referred to as *diagnostic audiology*, serve as a preliminary step towards rehabilitative audiology. The task at hand, then, is to briefly review some characteristics of hearing loss, to explore the major consequences of hearing impairment, and finally to discuss the methods used to cope with this disability.

hearing-loss characteristics

Important characteristics of hearing loss as they relate to aural rehabilitation include (a) degree of impairment, (b) time of onset, (c) type of loss, and (d) auditory speech identification ability.

degree of impairment

One major aspect of hearing impairment or loss is the person's hearing sensitivity or degree of loss (see Table 1.1). The category of hearing impairment includes both the hard of hearing and the deaf. Persons with limited amounts of hearing loss are referred to as being *hard of hearing*. Those with an extensive loss of hearing are considered *deaf*. Generally, when hearing losses, measured by pure tone average (PTA) or speech recognition threshold (SRT), are poorer than 80-90 dB HL a person is considered to be *audiometrically deaf*. However, deafness generally can be described as the inability to use hearing for the ordinary purposes of life, especially for verbal communication.

The prevalence of hearing impairment may be considered for all persons combined and for children and adults separately. In the United States the prevalence of hearing impairment is estimated to be from 14 to 40 million depending on whether conservative or liberal figures are used (Goldstein, 1984). These estimates vary depending on the defini-

TABLE 1.1
Hearing Impairment Degree
Descriptions Based on Pure-Tone Findings[a]

Hearing Impairment Degrees	PTA in dB based on .5, 1, 2, 4 K[b] Hz	
	Children	Adults
Slight to mild	21-40	26-40
Mild to moderate	----------41-55 ----------	
Moderate	----------56-70 ----------	
Severe	----------71-90 ----------	
Profound	----------91 plus---------	

[a] Based on levels advocated by the Committee on Hearing of the American Academy of Ophthalmology and Otolaryngology (adapted from AAOO, 1965).
[b] K = 1,000.

tion of loss; loss may involve a hearing level cutoff as low as 15 dB, but usually cutoffs are higher, most commonly 20-25 dB. Authorities have suggested that a different definition of loss should be applied for children because the consequences are greater for the same amount of loss in a younger person (Roeser & Price, 1988). The prevalence of loss also varies depending on whether the conventional pure-tone average (500, 1,000, 2,000 Hz) is used or whether some additional upper frequencies (like 3,000 and 4,000 Hz) are included. In this book we are recommending that different pure-tone average cutoffs be used for children and adults at the "slight-to-mild" degree of loss level, although the degree designation is similar at most levels. In addition, we recommend that either 3,000 or 4,000 Hz be used in evaluating loss. Table 1.1 indicates that a hearing loss is found in children at a lower (better) dB level than in adults; this is consistent with ASHA screening levels for school children that define normal hearing up to and including 20 dB (ASHA, 1985). A reasonable estimate until further clarification is available would be that at least 10% of the population have permanent, significant hearing impairment (22 million). Approximately 1% of the population are deaf (about 2 million), leaving the remaining 20 million in the hard-of-hearing group.

Children form a subpopulation of the total group of 22 million hearing-impaired individuals. It is estimated that about 3 million children in the United States are hearing impaired, and even more fit in this category if high-frequency and conductive losses are included (Rand Report, 1974;

Shepherd, Davis, Gorga, & Stelmachowicz, 1981; see Chapter 8). Of this total 3 million, about 50,000 school-age youngsters are classified as deaf (American Annals of the Deaf, 1987; Schein & Delk, 1974). As with children, most hearing-impaired adults are considered to be hard of hearing and only a small minority are deaf (Glorig & Roberts, 1965; Ries, 1982; Singer, Tomberlin, Smith, & Schrier, 1982).

Degree (sensitivity), however, is only one of several important dimensions of a hearing loss. Knauf (1978) made the following observation about the degree of loss:

> The hearing threshold level is perhaps the primary variable for estimating the impact of a child's (or adult's) hearing impairment and it frequently is the first measurement available. It is not surprising then that judgments and classifications of the hearing impaired are sometimes based only on this criterion. While classifications based on hearing level are valuable, there are many exceptions. Some unusual children with profound losses of 90 dB perform better in language and academic skills compared to other children with average intelligence and . . . losses of 70 dB. Similar individual variations will be found along the entire continuum of hearing levels. (p. 550)

Table 1.2 contains a description of deafness and hard-of-hearing categories in terms of typical hearing aspects, use of hearing, use of vision, language development, use of language, speech, and educational needs. Prevalence estimates are also shown.

time of onset

The time when a hearing loss is acquired will determine, in part, the extent to which normal speech and language will be present. Most hard-of-hearing youngsters are thought to have the loss from their earliest years, although prevalence data on young children are scarce (Shepherd et al., 1981). Severe hearing impairment may be divided into three categories (*prelingual, postlingual, deafened*) depending on the person's age when the loss occurs (Department of Labor, 1971; see Tables 1.2 and 1.3). *Prelingual deafness* refers to impairment which is present at birth or shortly thereafter. The longer a person has normal hearing during the crucial language development years (up to age five), the less chance there is that language development will be profoundly affected. *Postlingual deafness* means the loss occurs after about age five; it is generally less serious. However, even though language may be less affected, speech and education will be affected substantially (see Chapters 5 and 6). *Deafened* persons are those who lose hearing after their schooling is completed (i.e., sometime in their late teen years or thereafter). Normal

TABLE 1.2

Categories and Characteristics of Hearing Impairment

Characteristic	Hard of Hearing (20,000,000)[a]	Category of Deafness		
		Prelingual (220,000)[a]	Postlingual (440,000)[a]	Deafened (1,300,000)[a]
Hearing impairment	*Sensitivity:* mild, moderate, or severe; *Identification:* fair to good (70%-90%)	*Sensitivity:* severe or profound degree of loss; *Identification:* fair to very poor		
Use (level) of hearing	Functional speech understanding (lead sense)	Functional signal-warning/environmental awareness (hearing minimized)		
Use of vision	Increased dependence	Increased dependence		
Language and speech development	Dependent on rehabilitation measures (e.g., amplification)	Dependent on amplification and early intervention	Dependent on amplification and school rehabilitation	Normal
Use of language	May be affected	Almost always affected	May be affected	Usually not affected
Use of speech	May be affected	Always affected	Usually affected	May be affected
Educational needs	Some special education	Considerable special education	Some special education	Education complete

[a] United States prevalence data for these categories, based on Schein and Delk (1974) and Goldstein (1984) incidence figures.

speech, language, and education can be acquired by these individuals, but difficulty in verbal communication and other social, emotional, and vocational problems will occur (see Table 1.3).

type of loss

The type of loss may be *conductive* (damage in the outer or middle ear), *sensorineural* (impairment in the inner ear or nerve of hearing), or *mixed* (a combination of conductive and sensorineural). Generally, conductive

---

TABLE 1.3
Definitions of Hearing Impairment

Persons with hearing disabilities have been divided into the following groups:

Prelingually Deaf persons were either born without hearing (congenitally deaf) or lost hearing before the age of 5 years (adventitiously deaf). Both speech and language are affected to varying degrees and—because they usually are acquired formally instead of naturally—may be stilted, mechanical, and difficult to understand. The pre-lingually deaf person communicates primarily through fingerspelling, signs, and writing, but may possess enough speech and speech(lip)reading ability for basic social expression.

Postlingually Deaf persons are those who became profoundly deaf after the age of 5 years and, although possessing no hearing for practical purposes, had normal hearing long enough to establish fairly well developed speech and language patterns. While speech generally is affected, communication may be through speech, signs, fingerspelling and writing. Once the counselor becomes accustomed to their speech, it may be quite understandable. Speech-reading, however, may be more haphazard and not always dependable.

Deafened refers to those people who suffer hearing loss *after* completing their education—generally in their late teens or early twenties and upward. Such people usually have fairly comprehensible, nearly normal speech and language, but they need instruction to acquire useful speechreading. Quite frequently they face problems of adjustment because of the late onset of their hearing loss.

Hard-of-Hearing persons may have been born thus or subsequently experienced a partial loss of hearing. While they have acquired speech normally through hearing and communicate by speaking, speech may be affected to some extent; for example, the voice may be too soft or too loud. They understand others by speechreading, by using a hearing aid, or by asking the speaker to raise his voice or to enunciate more distinctly.

From *Interviewing Guides* (pp. 1–2) by U.S. Dept. of Labor, 1971, Washington, DC: Author.

losses are amenable to medical intervention whereas sensorineural losses are primarily aided through aural rehabilitation. Other less common types of loss are possible as well, such as *functional* (nonorganic) problems and *central auditory language processing disorders* (which arise from the processing centers in the brainstem or the brain). In the latter type of loss the symptoms may be very subtle. Usually in cases of sensorineural loss, the auditory speech identification or hearing clarity is affected. This is also the case in difficult listening situations for those with auditory language processing problems.

auditory speech identification ability

Auditory speech identification or recognition ability (clarity of hearing) is another important dimension of hearing loss. The terms *speech identification, speech recognition,* and *speech discrimination* will be used interchangeably throughout this text, and all are included under the general category of speech perception or comprehension (see Chapter 3). Speech discrimination has been used for many years to describe clarity of hearing as measured in typical word intelligibility tests, but speech identification and recognition have, of late, begun to replace discrimination since they more precisely describe what is being measured. Discrimination technically implies only the ability involved in a same-different judgment whereas identification and recognition indicate an ability to repeat or identify the stimulus. Recognition is commonly used by diagnostic audiologists, but identification meshes nicely with the nomenclature of aural rehabilitation procedures as discussed further in Chapter 3. All three terms will at times be used due to historical precedents and evolving nomenclature.

The speech identification ability in a hard-of-hearing individual typically is better than in a deaf person. The deaf are generally considered unable to comprehend conversational speech whereas the hard-of-hearing can use their hearing to some extent for speech perception. As Ramsdell (1978) pointed out, however, some minimal auditory identification may be present in the deaf even if verbal speech reception is limited, since a person may use hearing for signal-warning purposes or simply to maintain contact with the auditory environment (see Table 1.2). Nevertheless, auditory identification ability and degree of loss are somewhat independent.

In a person of advanced age, a mild degree of loss may be accompanied by very poor speech identification. This is referred to as *phonemic regression* and is not unusual in hearing losses among elderly persons who evidence some degree of central degeneration. Disparity in degree of loss and speech-identification ability is also possible in young hearing-impaired persons. For example, a child may be considered deaf in terms of sensitivity but not in terms of auditory identification or educational placement. Some children with a degree of loss classified as audiometrically deaf (e.g., PTA = 90 + dB) may have unexpectedly good speech identification. Thus, speech identification is an important variable in describing a hearing loss.

consequences of hearing loss: disability/handicap

communication consequences

The most devastating effect of hearing loss is its impact on verbal communication. Children with severe to profound hearing loss do not generally develop speech and language normally because they are not exposed to the sounds of language in daily living. In instances of a lesser degree of loss or if the loss occurs in adults, the influence on speech and language expression tends to be less severe. Nevertheless, affected individuals still experience varying degrees of difficulty in receiving the auditory speech and environmental stimuli which allow us to communicate and interact with other humans and with our environment. For children, the choice of a communication (educational) system relates directly to this area of concern. If the educational setting and methods are chosen and implemented appropriately, according to the abilities of the child, the negative impact of the loss can be minimized. Other serious consequences and side effects of hearing loss include vocational, social, and psychological implications (see chapters 4 and 7 for a discussion of communication systems and psychosocial implications).

variable hearing disability/handicap

Disability and *handicap* are terms which refer to the *effect* of a hearing loss as opposed to the characteristics of the loss as measured by the degree of loss and speech identification ability. While disability and handicap may be thought of as equivalent in some ways since they both concern the effect of the loss, some choose to make fine and generally useful distinctions between the two terms. Due to the lack of unanimity in this area, we shall avoid the technicalities by using them interchangeably and refer the reader elsewhere for a discussion of this topic (see ASHA, 1981; Davis, 1983).

A useful method for measuring the impact of hearing loss is through self-assessment of hearing, wherein persons make personal estimates about the degree of their hearing difficulties. This procedure has been applied with children and adults. Both the hearing-impaired person and other significant individuals can respond on questionnaires to provide a more complete picture of the communication, psychosocial, and other effects from the loss (see Chapter 9; Schow & Smedley, in press; Weinstein, 1984).

In preparing to deal with the broad consequences of hearing loss, we must recognize that the impact of a hearing impairment will vary considerably depending on a number of factors. Several of the most important of these factors are presented in Table 1.2. Although not included there, other variables are also important. For example, certain basic characteristics of the individual may have considerable impact on how much handicap results from a hearing loss. The presence of other serious handicaps like blindness, physical disability, or mental retardation will complicate the situation. A person's native intelligence can also have a tremendous impact in conjunction with a hearing loss. Naturally, basic intelligence will vary from person to person regardless of whether or not he/she is hearing impaired. However, Goetzinger (1978) reported that, as a group, persons with hereditary deafness demonstrate a normal range of IQs as measured by performance scales. Whatever the native intellectual ability, it will influence the resultant handicap/disability.

rehabilitative alternatives

Little can be done to change basic, innate IQ or native abilities. Nevertheless, a number of AR procedures may have a profound effect on a person's overall handicap resulting from a hearing loss. For example, it is estimated that 90% of Americans who are potentially successful hearing-aid users are not using amplification (Goldstein, 1984). In addition, there are: babies and young children who have hearing loss requiring amplification, but whose losses have not been identified; hearing-impaired school children whose aids are not in good condition (Bess, 1977; Robinson & Sterling, 1980); teenagers and young adults who, because of vanity or unfortunate experiences with hearing aids, are not getting the necessary help; adults and elderly individuals who have not acquired aids because of pride or ignorance; and others whose aids are not properly fitted or oriented to regular hearing aid use. Adults also have been found to be using many poorly functioning hearing aids (Schow, Maxwell, & Crookston, 1980). All of these cases represent a need for aural rehabilitation. Identifying those who need amplification, persuading them to obtain and use hearing aids, orienting the new user to the instrument, and adjusting it for maximum benefit are all tasks in the province of aural rehabilitation—tasks that may reduce the negative effects of a hearing loss.

Aural rehabilitation also includes efforts to improve communication as well as addressing a variety of other concerns for the hearing-impaired person. Before discussing procedures and the current status of aural rehabilitation, however, a brief review of the history of AR is in order.

historical background

Although aural rehabilitative procedures are common today, they have not always been utilized for individuals with hearing loss. For many years it was assumed that prelingual deafness and the resultant language development delay and inability to learn were inevitable aspects of the impairment. The deaf were thought to be retarded, so for many years, no efforts were made to try to teach them. The first known teacher of the deaf was Ponce de Leon of Spain, who in the mid-to-late 1500s demonstrated that the deaf could be taught to speak and were capable of learning. Other teachers and methods were promoted in the 1600s, including the work of Bonet and de Carrion in Spain and Bulwer in England. During the 1700s Pereira (Pereire) introduced education of the deaf to France, and a school was started there by the Abbe de L'Epée. Schools were also established by Thomas Braidwood in Great Britain and by Heinicke in Germany. De L'Epée employed fingerspelling and sign language in addition to speechreading, whereas Heinicke and Braidwood stressed oral speech and speechreading. Beginning in 1813, John Braidwood, a grandson of Thomas Braidwood, tried to establish this oral method in America, but he was unsuccessful because of his own ineptness and poor health. Thomas Gallaudet went to England in 1815 to learn the Braidwood oral method, but was refused help because it was feared that he would interfere with John Braidwood's efforts. Consequently, Gallaudet learned the manual method of de L'Epée in Paris through contact with Sicard and Laurent Clerc. He returned to the United States and opened his own successful school. (See additional detail in Chapter 7; and in Berger, 1972; DeLand, 1968; Moores, 1987.)

The manual approach to teaching the deaf remained the major force in America until the mid-1800s, when speechreading and oral methods were promoted and popularized by Horace Mann, Alexander Graham Bell, and others. The stress on residual hearing had been suggested earlier, but it began to receive strong emphasis with the oral methods used during the 1700s and 1800s. Until electric amplification was developed in the early 1900s, the use of residual hearing required ear trumpets and ad concham (speaking directly in the ear) stimulation. More vigorous efforts in the use of hearing followed the introduction of electronic hearing aids in the 1920s (Berger, 1988).

Also in the early 1900s, between 1900 and 1930, several schools of lipreading were started and became quite prominent. Although these institutions were directed principally toward teaching hearing-impaired adults (Berger, 1972), considerable public recognition was gained for this method of rehabilitating the hearing impaired. (Speechreading and lipreading will be used interchangeably in this text although speechreading is the more technically accurate term; see Chapter 4 for details.)

Birth of Audiology. During World War II, the need to rehabilitate hearing-impaired servicemen resulted in the birth of audiology. The cumulative effect of electronic amplification developments, adult lipreading courses, and the World War II hearing rehabilitation efforts gradually led to recognition of aural rehabilitation as separate from education for the hearing impaired. Eventually, audiologists were recognized as the professionals responsible for providing such services to adults, and soon it was also realized that audiologists could provide crucial help to hearing-impaired youngsters.

In the army rehabilitation centers a number of methods were developed to help the hearing impaired, including procedures for selecting hearing aids (Carhart, 1946). Hearing-aid orientation methods requiring up to 3 months of coursework were developed. Considerable emphasis was also placed on speechreading and auditory training (Albrite & Shutts, 1955; Northern, Ciliax, Roth, & Johnson, 1969).

In the late 1940s and 1950s as audiology moved into the private sector, the approach to hearing aids changed. Whereas hearing aids were freely dispensed in government facilities, in civilian life people bought amplification from hearing aid dealers. Methods evolved wherein audiologists would perform tests and recommend aids, but dealers would sell and service the instruments. The American Speech-Language-Hearing Association (ASHA) maintained that audiologists could not sell hearing aids because this would compromise their professional objectivity. Thus, strict rules were written into the ASHA Code of Ethics, and, except in military facilities, audiologists were excluded from hearing aid sales and follow-up (ASHA, 1967).

In aural rehabilitation, audiologists performed preliminary hearing aid work (hearing aid evaluations), concentrating on speechreading and auditory training. These two methods were promoted and used extensively. For example, speech and hearing centers often set up speechreading and auditory training classes, and adult community education programs using these methods were sponsored (Mussen, 1977). With newer and better hearing aids, however, the magic and motivation of the lipreading schools dissipated, and the ideas worked out in the leisurely 3-month military rehabilitation programs were found to be economically unfeasible in the "real world." In one center it was reported that everything had been tried to attract clients for aural rehabilitation therapy except "dancing girls" (Alpiner, 1973).

Recognition of Aural Rehabilitation Needs. Because of these setbacks, the 1960s and 1970s were years of examination and reflection for audiologists. Such self-examination revealed that the potential clientele for auditory rehabilitation is large and most are not receiving help.

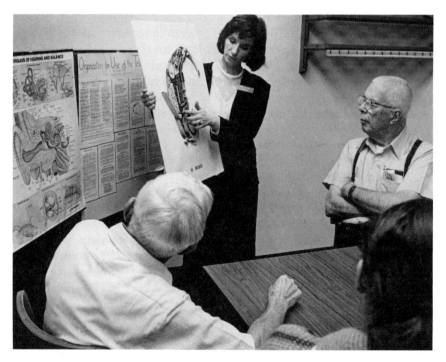

Figure 1.1. Orienting adults about how a hearing aid functions.

Infants. Beginning in the 1960s many audiologists recognized the need for early identification of hearing loss so that remediation could be initiated during the critical language development years (Downs & Sterrit, 1964). The incidence of hearing loss in newborns was found to be about 1 per 1,000 children, a higher prevalence than for other disabilities screened routinely in the newborn. Identification methods were subsequently developed and recommended (Cunningham, 1971; Mencher, 1974), and programs evolved to provide early auditory rehabilitation (Clark, Watkins, Reese, & Berg, 1975; Horton, 1972; Northcott, 1972; John Tracy Clinic Correspondence Course, 1983).

Children. Hearing-impaired school-age youngsters also were found to be in need of remedial help. Many hard-of-hearing children were (and still are) educated in the regular schools. Several studies indicated that these children were not receiving the help they needed (Quigley, 1970). Compared to normal-hearing youngsters, children with 15 to 45 dB losses showed delays of 15 to 19 months in reading skills and arithmetic (Ling, 1972). In addition, educational lags of 1-2 years were common, and many such children repeated grades (Kodman, 1963). Even children with mild temporary losses from otitis media showed serious delays in academic progress (Holm & Kunze, 1969). As of 1972-73 it was estimated that only 21% of the 440,000 hard-of-hearing school-age youngsters (40-90 dB) in the United States received any of the special education assistance they needed (Marge, 1977). Recent reports indicate these children are still being underserved (Bess, 1986; Blair, Peterson, & Viehweg, 1985). Although hearing-aid procurement for these children is now better, it is still in need of improvement since an estimated 15-75% (depending on degree of loss) of hearing-impaired children do not use hearing aids (Matkin, 1984; Shepherd et al., 1981). Rehabilitation for school-age children has become an important priority and clearly an area where the rehabilitative or educational audiologist is needed.

Adults. Among adults, the needs for hearing rehabilitation are also apparent. Thus, Glorig and Roberts' (1965) data revealed that from 25 to 34 years of age hearing loss is present in 13.5 per 1,000 individuals. This figure rises dramatically with age so that for 75–79 years, it is 480 per 1,000. It is estimated that there are almost 4 million hearing-aid users in this country, but conservative estimates suggest that another 10-15 million should be using hearing aids (Goldstein, 1984; Mahon, 1986). Further, about 1/4 of the aids being used by adults have been shown to be in poor working condition (Schow et al., 1980).

Difficulties in Acceptance of Aural Rehabilitation. When audiologists reflected on the limited acceptance of aural rehabilitation, it became apparent that, despite its importance, many in the profession lacked interest.

Students typically are attracted to audiology because of the diagnostic process, whereas those who find therapy more appealing often pursue speech-language pathology instead. In 1966, the Academy of Rehabilitative Audiology was organized to help audiologists with rehabilitative interests direct their efforts toward reversing these trends (Oyer, 1983). This organization and its members have had an important influence on ASHA.

One reason for the noted neglect of rehabilitation is the hearing aid situation in the past. Primarily because of the success of aggressive sales practices by hearing aid dealers and the ASHA policy which prevented heavy audiologic involvement, 70-90% of all hearing aids in this country were for many years being sold without active involvement of medical or audiological consultants (DHEW, 1975; Stutz, 1969). Because audiologists have not, until recently, dispensed hearing aids, they have been deprived of close contact with clients during the post-fitting period (ASHA, 1972). In contrast, the dealers have been intimately involved in the most crucial rehabilitation process. This situation began to change in the mid-to-late 1970s because of relaxation in the ASHA policy. Finally, due to a Supreme Court decision, ASHA removed its restrictions on allowing audiologists to dispense in 1979 (ASHA, 1978, 1979). (Also in 1979 the official name of ASHA was changed from the American Speech and Hearing Association to the American Speech-Language-Hearing Association. However, the acronym–ASHA–remains the same, ASHA, 1979.)

current status

Fortunately, audiologists generally have begun to recognize the opportunities for rehabilitation through early intervention and the provision of services in schools and in neglected adult and geriatric settings. This awareness has been reflected within ASHA, as evidenced in 1972, 1974, and 1984 policy statements on rehabilitative audiology issued by special ASHA subcommittees (ASHA, 1972, 1974, 1984).

In the last few years, a number of alternate aural rehabilitation approaches have been suggested. For example, Alpiner (1971) described what he called "progressive rehabilitative audiology" which focuses on counseling and improving communication ability rather than on only teaching speechreading and auditory training. Similarly, Fleming (1972) recommended a "communication therapy program" which emphasizes learning to become a more effective communicator. Tannahill (1973) described a group hearing-aid adjustment program designed to help persons understand their hearing losses and hearing aids better. Hardick

(1977) and Giolas (1982) outlined similar programs in which the major focus is on hearing-aid fitting and orientation. The programs revolve around amplification and/or modifying the communication environment.

A common factor in all these new approaches is the recognition that hearing-aid adjustment, orientation, and general communication help are the central issues in most aural rehabilitation. In most cases, the focus in AR is on amplification whereas extensive speechreading and auditory training have become occasional, ancillary procedures. Heavy emphasis on these methods is needed only in certain instances (Goldstein & Stephens, 1981).

The 1980s have seen the emergence of a new breed of audiologists, more aware of the millions of children and adults in need of aural rehabilitation. Results of several surveys conducted in the 1980s showed that approximately 50% of all ASHA audiologists are involved in direct dispensing of hearing aids (Margolis, 1987). According to one survey conducted in 1980, 80-83% of all audiologists are involved in hearing-aid evaluation, hearing-aid orientation, and rehabilitation counseling. A smaller number (40%) reported being involved in communication rehabilitation, including speechreading and auditory training (Whitcomb, 1982).

procedures in aural rehabilitation: an AR model

This section will describe important procedures and elements of aural rehabilitation in order to provide a framework for the remainder of this text.

The aural rehabilitation model used in this text has been slightly revised from the first edition based on the work of Goldstein and Stephens (1981), and is in harmony with the most recent statement from the ASHA Committee on Rehabilitative Audiology (ASHA, 1984). The model is intended to encompass all types and degrees of hearing impairment as well as all age groups.

Entry and discharge are considered peripheral to the central aspects of the model. The model consists of two major components: evaluation and remediation. Each component has four divisions and associated subsections. The model is shown in Table 1.4.

Rehabilitation-Evaluation Procedures. Following the initial auditory diagnostic tests that indicate the need for aural rehabilitation, it is necessary to perform more indepth workups that determine the feasibility of various forms of aural rehabilitation. These evaluation procedures should focus on communication status, associated variables, related conditions, and attitude (CARA).

TABLE 1.4
Aural Rehabilitation Model as Used in This Text

	(Enter through Diagnostic-Identification Process)		
Evaluation (CARA)	Communication Status	(I-A,B)	Auditory Visual Language Manual Prev. Rehabilitation Overall
	Associated Variables	(II-B)	Psychological Sociological Vocational Educational
	Related Conditions		Mobility Upper Limb Aural Pathology
	Attitude	(II-D)	Type I Type II Type III Type IV
Remediation (PACO)	Psychosocial	(II-A,B,D)	Interpretation Information Counseling/Guidance Acceptance Understanding Expectation
	Amplification (Instrumental)	(I-C)	Hearing Aid Fitting Alert Warning Other Assistive Devices Instruction/Orientation Adjustment
	Communication Training Strategy	(II-B,C; III-A,V)	Goals Philosophy Tactics Skill Building
	Overall Coordination (Ancillary)	(II-B,C,E; III-C,IV)	Vocational Educational Social Work Medicine
	(Discharge)		

Note: This model is consistent with the Goldstein/Stephens (1981) model and the ASHA position statement on definitions and competencies in aural rehabilitation (ASHA, 1984). The numbers and letters in parentheses refer to the ASHA statement related to the procedures listed.

Communication status. Within the area of communication status both traditional audiometric tests and questionnaires may be used to assess auditory abilities and handicaps. Visual abilities assessment should include a simple screening and measurement of speechreading abilities. Any evaluation of communication must also consider language, since it is at the heart of verbal communication. If the patient understands a manual/gesture system this needs to be evaluated as does any prior treatment. Included in *overall communication* are combined sensory abilities as in audiovisual and tactile-kinesthetic capacities. Expressive and receptive communication skills should both be considered.

Associated variables. Included in this area are psychological, sociological, vocational, and educational factors. Personality and intelligence are major psychological factors, along with motivation, emotional stability, conformity, and assertiveness. Sociological factors such as family and significant others, social class, and lifestyle are also relevant according to the Goldstein and Stephens model. The vocational domain includes position, responsibility, and competence. In addition, the patient's level and form of education must be considered.

Related conditions. In this area, physical conditions like visual acuity and physical mobility are evaluated, along with upper-limb movement, sensation, and control due to their bearing on hearing-aid use. In addition, symptoms of tinnitus, vertigo, pressure, and otitis media should be considered. Finally, the acoustic environmental conditions confronted by the hearing-impaired person should be evaluated.

Attitude. The person's attitude is considered a crucial aspect of remediation. Goldstein and Stephens (1981) suggested that rehabilitation candidates can be categorized into four types according to attitude. Type I candidates have a strongly positive attitude toward remediation and are thought to comprise 2/3 or 3/4 of all patients. Most of the remaining candidates fit into Type II; their expectations are essentially positive, but slight complications are present such as hearing loss which is difficult to fit with amplification. Persons with Type III attitudes are negative about rehabilitation, but show some willingness to cooperate, while those in Type IV reject hearing aids and the rehabilitation process altogether. In the latter two categories remediation cannot proceed in the usual fashion until some modification of attitude is achieved. For these reasons, we consider it important to evaluate attitude *prior* to remediation; Goldstein and Stephens include it as the first phase in the remediation process, however.

Remediation Procedures. Once a thorough, rehabilitation-oriented evaluation has been completed, remediation efforts should be initiated. These may take the form of short- or long-term therapy, and may involve individual or group sessions. The four aspects of remediation included here are those detailed in the previous edition of this book. They are also prominently featured in the Goldstein/Stephens model as well as in the ASHA position statement (ASHA, 1984). These include (a) psychosocial and counseling aspects, (b) amplification aspects, (c) communication remediation, and (d) overall coordinative functions (PACO).

Though all four remediation components are listed sequentially, they may occur simultaneously or in a duplicative and interactive fashion. Many actions in one phase may be duplicated, in part, in other phases. For example, information about communication is generally introduced early in the counseling phase. However, additional information on how we hear, basics of speech acoustics, visible dimensions of speech, and how to maximize conversation may be further emphasized in the communication remediation phase.

Psychosocial/counseling. Psychosocial/counseling includes interpretation of audiologic findings to the client and other significant persons. In addition, pertinent information, counseling, and guidance is needed to help these individuals understand the educational, psychosocial, and communicative effects of hearing impairment. Considerable understanding and support are necessary in dealing with hearing-impaired children, their parents, hearing-handicapped adults of all ages, and their families. Hopefully, this process will bring acceptance and understanding of the conditions along with appropriate expectations for remediation. It is at this stage that good attitude—Type I and II—patients can be moved into amplification whereas clients with poor attitudes (Types III and IV), if not modified toward acceptance and understanding, may need ideas for modifying communicative behavior, attitudes and strategies rather than being confronted with amplification fitting which they may resist.

Amplification/assistive devices.

• Amplification fitting. This phase is sometimes referred to as *hearing-aid evaluation*, but it needs to be broader in scope. Here we must consider all forms of amplification, not just hearing aids. For example, signal warning devices and other assistive devices like telephone amplifiers should be considered in this phase. In many cases, accurate fitting of these devices will go a long way toward resolution of the hearing problem.

• Amplification orientation. Individuals need to learn about the purpose, function, and maintenance of hearing aids and other assistive devices used by themselves or their child/significant other to avoid misunderstandings and misuses of hearing aids. Amplification units are relatively complex and often require that this instruction be given more emphasis than a 5-minute explanation or a pamphlet. (This is referred to as *instruction* by Goldstein and Stephens.)

• Amplification adjustment. In most cases, the fitting of hearing devices should be followed by adjustment, modification, and alteration of the basic controls and coupler arrangement until satisfactory amplification is achieved. Effort should be made to insure that no other amplification arrangements are substantially superior to the ones being used. (This is called *instrumental II* by Goldstein and Stephens.)

Communication training. As previously indicated, the major impact of hearing loss lies in the area of communication. Communication deficits often manifest themselves in educational difficulties for children and in vocational difficulties for adults. While, in most cases, amplification is considered the most important tool, communication training and related strategies still remain central to aural rehabilitation.

The first phase here consists of developing overall plans, goals, and tactics that suit the patient's lifestyle, philosophy, and attitudes. As Goldstein and Stephens suggested (1981), assertiveness may be a good tactic for overcoming hearing impairment unless it is contrary to the patient's personality. With children the educational philosophy will help dictate the methods and tactics used.

Skill building involves helping the patient acquire skills which facilitate effective communication. Speechreading and improvement of auditory listening strategies are included here as are related speech- and language-remediation efforts. Specific communication difficulties are identified in this phase of therapy, and then strategies are developed to cope with these problems.

Overall coordination: referral and evaluation (ancillary). This refers to referral and coordination rather than direct service. While referrals in all areas are not always necessary they should be considered. Liaison between client, family, and other agencies is included as are reevaluation and modification of the intervention program.

The team manager is a useful concept in aural rehabilitation. Particularly in the case of the hearing-impaired youngster, many persons may work with or need to work with the child. The parents are important assets in the rehabilitative process. Also, physicians, social workers, hearing-aid dispensers, teachers, school psychologists, and other school personnel need to be coordinated to assist the child and family. For adults, much depends on the particular setting in which the rehabilitation occurs. Sometimes physicians, psychologists or social workers function in the same clinical setting. In these cases, involvement of another professional may occur naturally and easily. In other situations, the therapist can make referrals, when indicated, and encourage the adult to follow up. Sometimes persons are resistant to obtaining medical care or seeing a rehabilitation counselor. Often patients resist social services, psychiatric assistance, or hearing-aid devices. When a client refuses to accept advice, the audiologist must provide whatever insight and help he can, based on his background and training. Nevertheless, the aural rehabilitation process demands that referrals be made when indicated, and overall coordination and evaluation of progress are important dimensions which should not be neglected.

Additional clarification and details on this AR model can be found in Goldstein and Stephens (1981). Furthermore, computer software to support the use of the model is commercially available (Traynor & Smaldino, 1986).

settings for aural rehabilitation

Aural rehabilitation may be conducted with both deaf and hard-of-hearing persons in a variety of settings. Clients may be children, adults, or elderly persons. A review of these settings may help to demonstrate the many applications of aural rehabilitation (see Table 1.5).

Children. Very young hearing-impaired children and their parents may be recipients of early intervention efforts through home visits or clinic programs. Parent groups are also an important rehabilitation option. As children enter preschool and other school settings, aural rehabilitation takes on a supportive, coordinative function with teachers of normal or hearing-impaired youngsters managing the classroom learning. Specifically, children in resource rooms, in residential deaf school classrooms,

TABLE 1.5
Summary of Aural Rehabilitation Settings
for Children, Adults, and Elderly Persons

Children	Adults	Adult Elderly
Early Intervention	University and Technical	Most settings listed
Preschool	Schools	under Adults
Parent Groups	Vocational Rehabilitation	Community Programs
Regular Classrooms	Military–Related Facilities	Nursing Homes/
School Conservation	ENT Clinic–Private	Long-Term Care
Program Followup	Practice	Facilities
School Resource Rooms	Community, Hospital and	
Residential School	University Hearing	
Classrooms	Clinics	
	Hearing Aid Specialists/	
	Dispensers	

and in regular classrooms can be helped with amplification (both group and individual), communication therapy, and academic subjects. Important help and insights can also be given to the child's parents and teachers, and other professionals may be involved as needed. Hearing conservation followup for youngsters who fail traditional school screenings represents another type of rehabilitative work carried out with children.

Adults. Adult AR services are needed for individuals with long-standing hearing loss as well as for persons who acquire loss during adulthood. Such traumatic or progressive hearing disorders may be brought on by accident, heredity, disease, or noise.

Adults may be served in university or technical school settings, through vocational rehabilitation programs, in military-related facilities, in the office of an ear specialist, or in the private practice of an audiologist. In addition, many adults are served in community, hospital, or university hearing clinics or through hearing aid dealers/dispensers. A variety of rehabilitative services may be provided in all of these settings.

Adult Elderly. The vast majority of elderly clients are served through the conventional programs previously described for adults. A substantial proportion of clients seen in these settings for hearing-aid evaluations and related services are 65 years or older.

The full array of hearing aid and communication rehabilitation services may be provided for the elderly in these clinics, including hearing aid evaluation, orientation, and group and individual therapy. Aside from conventional clinical service, rehabilitation may be provided to the elderly in community screening and rehabilitation programs in well elderly clinics, retirement apartment houses, senior citizen centers, churches, and a variety of other places where senior citizens congregate. Nursing homes or long-term care facilities also provide opportunities for aural rehabilitation since so many residents in these settings have substantial hearing loss (Hull, 1977; Schow & Nerbonne, 1980). Nevertheless, rehabilitation personnel should expect somewhat limited success with the elderly who are residents in health care facilities (Schow, 1982).

summary

Auditory habilitation/rehabilitation involves a variety of evaluation and remedial efforts for the hearing-impaired person, coordinated by a professional with audiologic training. Audiologic commitment to this endeavor has waxed and waned during the past 40 years, but recently a resurgence of interest has been spurred by a variety of factors.

A model of rehabilitation was presented here to provide a framework for evaluation and remediation procedures in aural rehabilitation. Professionals who intend to engage in AR must be familiar with the ramifications of hearing loss if they are to perform effective rehabilitation evaluations. They also need to be aware of AR remediation procedures rendered through amplification, communication rehabilitation, counseling, and other ancillary services such as the educational alternatives available for the hearing impaired. The ASHA position statement on aural rehabilitation lists a number of minimal competencies required by those involved (ASHA, 1984; see Chapter 13). Consistent with this model and the ASHA guidelines, the present text is designed to introduce basic information pertaining to amplification (Chapter 2), communication (Chapters 3, 4, 5), psychosocial aspects (Chapter 6), and educational alternatives (Chapter 7). These chapters are followed by a thorough discussion of aural rehabilitation for children (Chapter 8), adults (Chapter 9), and the elderly (Chapter 10). The next two chapters (11, 12) contain case examples, while Chapter 13 includes resource options to assist readers as they carry out their efforts in aural rehabilitation.

recommended readings

Alpiner, J.G., & McCarthy, P.A. (1987). *Rehabilitative audiology: children and adults.* Baltimore: Williams & Wilkins.

Berg, F.S., Blair, J.C., Viehweg, S.H., & Wilson-Vlotman, A. (1986). *Educational audiology for the hard of hearing child.* New York: Grune and Stratton.

Giolas, T.G. (1986). *Aural rehabilitation.* Austin, TX: Pro-Ed.

Katz, J. (Ed.). (1985). *Handbook of clinical audiology* (3rd ed., pp. 769-1056). Baltimore: Williams & Wilkins.

Mueller, H. G., & Geoffrey, V. C. (1987). *Communication disorders in aging: Advances in assessment and management.* Washington, DC: Gallaudet University Press.

Ross, M. (1986). *Aural habilitation.* Austin, TX: Pro-Ed.

references

Albrite, J.P., & Shutts, E. (1955). Audiology in the Army. *Hearing News* (Reprint No. 290).

Alpiner, J.G. (1971). Planning a strategy of aural rehabilitation for the adult. *Hearing and Speech News, 39,* 21-26.

Alpiner, J.G. (1973). The hearing aid in rehabilitation planning for adults. *Journal of the Academy of Rehabilitative Audiology, 6,* 55-57.

American Academy of Ophthalmology and Otolaryngology (AAOO). (1965). *Guide for the classification and evaluation of hearing handicap.* Committee on Conservation for Hearing. Transact, *AAOO, 69,* 740-751.

American Annals of the Deaf. (1987). Educational programs and services. *American Annals of the Deaf, 120*(2), 124.

ASHA-American Speech and Hearing Association. (1967). *A conference on hearing aid evaluation procedures. ASHA Report, 7*(2), 57-66.

ASHA-American Speech and Hearing Association. (1972). *Comprehensive audiologic services for the public. Asha, 14,* 204-206.

ASHA-American Speech and Hearing Association. (1974). The audiologist: Responsibilities in the habilitation of the auditorily handicapped. *Asha, 16,* 68-70.

ASHA-American Speech and Hearing Association. (1978). Board moves to change dispensing rules. *Asha, 16,* 68-70.

ASHA-American Speech-Language-Hearing Association. (1979). Legislative council changes ASHA's name, ratifies ERA motion, adopts code changes. *Asha, 21,* 33-35.

ASHA-American Speech-Language-Hearing Association. (1981). On the definition of hearing handicap: A report of the American Speech-Language-Hearing Association task force. *Asha, 23,* 293-297.

ASHA-American Speech-Language-Hearing Association. (1984). Definition of and competencies for aural rehabilitation. A report from the committee on rehabilitative audiology. *Asha, 26,* 37-41.

ASHA-American Speech-Language-Hearing Association. (1985). Guidelines for identification audiometry. *Asha, 27,* 49-52.

Berger, K.W. (1972). *Speechreading: Principles and methods.* Baltimore: National Educational Press, Inc.

Berger, K.W. (1988). History and development of hearing aids. In M.C. Pollack (Ed.), *Amplification for the hearing-impaired* (3rd ed., pp. 1-20). New York: Grune & Stratton.

Bess, F.H. (1977). Condition of hearing aids worn by children in a public school setting. In *The condition of hearing aids worn by children in a public school program.* DHEW Publication N. (OE) 7705002. Washington, DC: U.S. Printing Office.

Bess, F.H. (1986). Unilateral sensorineural hearing loss in children. Special issue. *Ear and Hearing, 7*(1), 3-54.

Blair, J.C., Peterson, M., & Viehweg, S.H. (1985). The effects of mild hearing loss on academic performance among school-age children. *The Volta Review,* 87-94.

Carhart, R. (1946). Selection of hearing aids. *Archives of Otolaryngology, 44,* 10-18.

Clark, T.C., Watkins, S., Reese, R., & Berg, F. (1975). *A state-wide program for identification and language facilitation for hearing handicapped children through home management.* Unpublished progress performance report for Handicapped Children's Early Education Program. Washington, DC: DHEW Office of Education, Bureau of Education for the Handicapped.

Cunningham, G.C. (1971). *Conference on newborn hearing screening.* Berkeley: California Department of Public Health. Rockville, MD: Public Health Service, DHEW.

Davis, A. (1983) Hearing disorders in the population. First phase findings of the MRC national study of hearing. In M. Lutman & M. Haggard (Eds.), *Hearing science and hearing disorders.* London: Academic Press.

DeLand, F. (1968). *The story of lip-reading.* Washington, DC: Alexander Graham Bell Association for the Deaf.

Department of Health Education and Welfare (DHEW). (1975). *Final report to the secretary on hearing aid health care.* Springfield, VA: U.S. Department of Commerce.

Department of Labor. (1971). *Interviewing guides.* Washington, DC: Department of Labor.

Downs, M.P., & Sterrit, G.M. (1964). Identification audiometry for neonates: A preliminary report. *Journal of Auditory Research, 4,* 69-80.

Fleming, M. (1972). A total approach to communication therapy. *Journal of the Academy of Rehabilitative Audiology, 5,* 28-31.

Giolas, T.G. (1982). *Hearing-handicapped adults.* Englewood Cliffs, NJ: Prentice-Hall, Inc.

Glorig, A., & Roberts, J. (1965). *Hearing level of adults by age and sex: United States (1960-62).* National Center for Health Statistics, Series 11, No. 11. Washington, DC: U.S. Department of Health, Education and Welfare.

Goetzinger, C.F. (1978). The psychology of hearing impairment. In J. Katz (Ed.), *Handbook of clinical audiology* (2nd ed. pp. 447-463). Baltimore: The Williams & Wilkins Co.

Goldstein, D.P. (1984). Hearing impairment, hearing aids, and audiology. *Asha, 25*(9), 24-38.

Goldstein, D.P., & Stephens, S.D.G. (1981). Audiological rehabilitation: Management Model I. *Audiology, 20,* 432-452.

Hardick, E.G. (1977). Aural rehabilitational programs for the aged can be successful. *Journal of the Academy of Rehabilitative Audiology, 10,* 51-66.

Holm, V.A., & Kunze, L.H. (1969). Effect of chronic otitis media on language and speech development. *Pediatrics, 43,* 833-839.

Horton, K.B. (1972). Early amplification and language learning-Or sounds should be heard and not seen. *Journal of the Academy of Rehabilitative Audiology, 5,* 15-23.

Hull, R.H. (1977). *Hearing impairment among aging persons.* Lincoln, NE: Cliff Notes.

John Tracy Clinic Correspondence Course. (1983). *For parents of young deaf children. Part A and B.* John Tracy Clinic, 806 West Adams Blvd., Los Angeles, CA 90007.

Knauf, V.H. (1978). Language and speech training. In J. Katz (Ed.), *Handbook of clinical audiology* (2nd ed., pp. 549-564). Baltimore: The Williams & Wilkins Co.

Kodman, F., Jr. (1963). Educational status of hard-of-hearing children in the classroom. *Journal of Speech and Hearing Disorders, 28,* 297-299.

Ling, D. (1972). Rehabilitation of cases with deafness secondary to otitis media. In A. Glorig & K.S. Gerwin (Eds.), *Otitis media* (pp. 249-253). Springfield, IL: Charles C. Thomas Publisher.

Mahon, W.J. (1986). Expanding the hearing aid market: Hearing Journal Roundtable. *The Hearing Journal, 39*(1), 7-17.

Marge, M. (1977). The current status of service delivery systems for the hearing impaired. *Asha, 19,* 403-409.

Margolis, R. (1987). Hearing instrument dispensing in university clinics. *Hearing Instruments, 38*(10), 38-39, 67.

Matkin, N.D. (1984). Wearable amplification. A litany of persisting problems. In J. Jerger (Ed.), *Pediatric audiology: Current trends* (pp. 125-145). San Diego, CA: College Hill Press.

Mencher, G.T. (1974). Infant hearing screening: The state of the art. *Maico Audiological Library Series, 12,* 7.

Moores, D. (1987). *Educating the deaf: psychology, principles, practices* (3rd ed.). Boston: Houghton Mifflin.

Mussen, E.F. (1977). Problems of rehabilitative audiology in the retirement community setting. *Journal of the Academy of Rehabilitative Audiology, 10,* 68-70.

Northcott, W.H. (Ed.). (1972). *Curriculum guide: Hearing impaired children–birth to three years–and their parents.* Washington, DC: Alexander Graham Bell, Association for the Deaf

Northern, J.L., Ciliax, D.R., Roth, D., & Johnson, R. (1969). Military patient attitudes toward aural rehabilitation. *Asha, 11,* 391-395.

Oyer, H.J. (1983). Founding philosophy of the Academy of Rehabilitative Audiology. *Journal of Academy of Rehabilitative Audiology, 16,* 9-11.

Quigley, S.F. (1970). *Some effects of impairment upon school performance.* Manuscript prepared for the Division of Special Education Services. Springfield, IL: Office of the Superintendent of Public Instruction for the State of Illinois.

Ramsdell, D. (1978). The psychology of the hard-of-hearing and the deafened adult. In H. Davis & R. Silverman (Eds.), *Hearing and deafness* (4th ed., pp. 499-510). New York: Holt, Rinehart & Winston.

Rand Report. (1974). *Improving services to handicapped children.* Santa Monica, CA: The Rand Corporation.

Ries, P.W. (1982) *Hearing ability of persons by sociodemographic and health characteristics: United States.* (Vital and Health Statistics, Series 10, No. 140, DHHS Publication No. (PHS) 82-1568). Washington, DC: U.S. Government Printing Office.

Robinson, D.O., & Sterling, G.R. (1980). Hearing aids and children in school: A follow-up study. *The Volta Review, 82,* 229-235.

Roeser, R., & Price, D. (1981). Audiometric and impedance measures: Principles and interpretation. In R. Roeser & M. Downs (Eds.), *Auditory disorders in school children.* New York: Thieme-Stratton, Inc.

Schein, J., & Delk, M. (1974). *The deaf population of the United States.* Silver Spring, MD: National Association of the Deaf.

Schow, R.L. (1982). Success of hearing aid fitting in nursing home residents. *Ear and Hearing, 3*(3), 173-177.

Schow, R.L., Christensen, J.M., Hutchinson, J.J., & Nerbonne, M.A. (1978). *Communication disorders of the aged*. Baltimore: University Park Press.

Schow, R.L., Maxwell, S., & Crookston, G. (1980). *Status of hearing aids used by adults*. American Speech-Language-Hearing Association Convention, Detroit.

Schow, R.L., & Nerbonne, M.A. (1980). Hearing levels in elderly nursing home residents. *Journal of Speech and Hearing Disorders, 45*(1), 124-132.

Schow, R.L., & Smedley, T.C. (Eds.). (in press). Self-assessment of hearing. *Special Supplement. Ear and Hearing*.

Shepherd, N., Davis, J., Gorga, M., & Stelmachowicz, P. (1981). Characteristics of hearing impaired children in the public schools: Part I—Demographic data. *Journal of Speech and Hearing Disorders, 46*, 123-129.

Singer, J.D., Tomberlin, T.J., Smith, J.M., & Schrier, A.J. (1982). *Hearing status in the United States and the auditory and non-auditory correlates of occupational noise exposure*. Washington, DC: Environmental Protection Agency.

Stutz, R. (1969). The American hearing aid user. *Asha, 11*, 459-461.

Tannahill, J.C. (1973). Hearing aids: Trial and adjustment by new users. *Audecibel, 22*, 90-97.

Traynor, V., & Smaldino, V. (1986). Computerized adult aural rehabilitation. Software Disk. San Diego, CA: College Hill Press.

Weinstein, B.E. (1984). A review of hearing handicap scales. *Audiology, 9*, 91-109.

Weinstein, B.E. (1986). Validity of a screening protocol for identifying elderly people with hearing problems. *Asha, 28*, 41-46.

Whitcomb, C.J. (1982). *A survey of aural rehabilitation services among ASHA audiologists*. Unpublished master's thesis, Idaho State University.

chaptertwo

AMPLIFICATION/ASSISTIVE DEVICES FOR THE HEARING IMPAIRED

KENNETH W. BERGER

JOSEPH P. MILLIN

contents

introduction

Hearing aids and auditory trainers are electronic amplifiers, specifically designed to assist those with impaired hearing. Although these forms of amplification are the most commonly used, a variety of other assistive listening devices are also available, designed, like the conventional systems, to modify incoming acoustic signals and convey them to the hearing-impaired individual. Ideally, the modification and efficient delivery of these signals will enable the wearer to achieve better receptive communication. (Assistive listening devices [ALDs] collectively represent one of several types of assistive devices for the hearing impaired. ALDs are designed to enhance the speech signal, while other types of assistive devices serve as warning/wake-up systems.)

Professionals working with the hearing impaired, including educators of the hearing impaired, speech-language pathologists, and audiologists, are confronted with an almost endless number of options. For example, the number of commercial hearing aids and modifications of hearing aids currently available is astounding. It is not surprising, therefore, that newly trained professionals may find themselves overwhelmed by the dramatic differences that can be found among the various hearing aids and other assistive devices used by the adults or children whom they serve. Furthermore, each of these professionals will have a different responsibility with respect to the selection, maintenance, and use of the aids.

Regarding hearing aids the major responsibility of educators of the hearing impaired is to ensure that instruments are functioning properly. At times, however, they should also question whether the hearing aid used by a particular child or adult is appropriate. Speech-language pathologists frequently work with hearing-impaired children in the classroom. Like educators of the hearing impaired, they should be able to determine whether a hearing aid is functioning properly. However, these professionals usually do not need to concern themselves directly with the selection process; nor do they modify the aid or formally assess the client's amplification needs. In addition to the aspects already mentioned, audiologists also are responsible for evaluating the client's changing amplification needs, determining when a modification of hearing aid or auditory trainer is necessary, or when a new instrument of a different design is advisable. Obviously, the audiologist must also be able to evaluate the client's hearing capability initially, and to recommend the appropriate hearing aid for clients who have never used amplification.

In our judgment it is impossible for any of these three professional groups to have too much information about hearing aids and other assistive devices, and it is our hope that an increased sophistication in the understanding of these instruments will take place among all these persons. Therefore, a major purpose of this chapter is to provide in one source the technical and applied information about amplification and other assistive devices that hearing professionals need to know about to function effectively.

types of hearing aids

Electronic hearing aids are devices in which a *microphone* picks up auditory signals that are then routed to an *amplifier*. The amplifier boosts the energy of the signal and sends it to the *receiver*, which acts as a miniature speaker to transform the signal from electrical to acoustical energy for presentation to the listener. These three basic components are powered by a battery and controlled by a variety of switches and adjustment knobs. The components are available in a number of specialized cosmetic enclosures. In the past the most common was the *body instrument*, which was enclosed in a simple box-like case made of metal or plastic. It is also called a *pocket aid* since it is often carried in a shirt or blouse pocket. Beginning in the 1950s, the invention of transistors allowed hearing aids to be built into specially designed *eyeglass* temples, or worn *behind the ear* in a curved enclosure. As amplifier miniaturization continued, the hearing aid could be built small enough to be placed in the concha of the ear. This *in-the-ear* instrument, which is built into a custom earmold shell, is the most popular type at the present time.

body aid

Many years ago, individuals with more than moderate hearing loss could benefit only from a body hearing aid, since this was the only type with sufficient power. Figure 2.1 shows a typical contemporary body-type hearing aid with microphone, amplifier, and battery in a plastic case. A cord connects the case to an external receiver, and in use an earmold would be connected to the nub of the receiver for insertion into the ear.

The body hearing aid, because of its size and the availability of space for a larger battery, can provide slightly more acoustic power than other hearing aid types. It also usually permits inclusion of extra circuitry and controls. For example, many body aids, in addition to a volume-control dial or knob, have a switch that permits the wearer to alter the input from microphone to telephone coil, and usually also to a combined microphone-telecoil position. The body type is also likely to have a tone control, and in addition, since the receiver is external, the audiologist

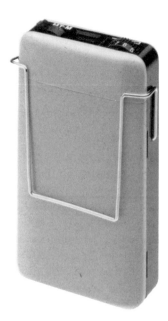

Figure 2.1. Body hearing aid. (Courtesy of Beltone Electronics Corporation.)

may consider using various receivers with different frequency response and output characteristics.

Most users of body hearing aids are fitted monaurally; that is, they use a hearing aid fitted to one ear only. It is possible also to wear two body hearing aids in a binaural fitting. If the two aids are separated by at least a few inches the wearer will be able to localize sound reasonably well. In addition to the single cord leading to a receiver, there is a variation called a *Y-cord fitting*, in which the single cord divides and leads to two receivers, one worn at each ear. The Y-cord permits bilateral stimulation but not true binaural hearing since there is only one microphone and amplifer. Most clinicians believe that the Y-cord is of little use, except on a temporary basis for a very young child from whom only limited audiometric test data can be obtained. In such instances, the child's two ears, or at least the better ear, will be sure to receive sound with a Y-cord. Later, when accurate audiometric test data can be obtained, the instrument can be changed to either a monaural or a true binaural fitting as needed.

As a result of microminiaturization, amplifiers with high power can fit into an extremely small space. Individuals with severe hearing loss rarely choose to use more than 55 dB of gain; therefore, most of the hearing-aid types can be built to provide adequate power. However, as we shall see later in this chapter, problems of acoustic feedback can dictate the use of body aids. Thus, body aids are still in use to a limited extent, but sometimes for reasons related to feedback rather than gain.

behind-the-ear aid

Figure 2.2 shows a behind-the-ear (BTE) hearing aid. It rests behind and over the pinna, and has a plastic earhook attached at one end near the receiver. A short piece of plastic tubing connects the earhook to an earmold. Since the receiver is inside the hearing aid plastic case it is referred to as an *internal receiver* type.

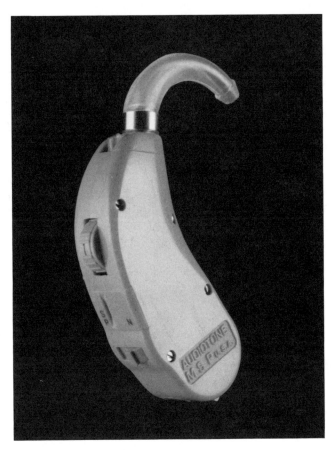

Figure 2.2. Behind-the-ear hearing aid. (Courtesy of Audiotone Corp.)

The behind-the-ear hearing aid, as illustrated in Figure 2.2, has a serrated volume-control wheel which also serves as an on/off switch. The switch located near the bottom of the hearing aid, just above the battery switch, activates a noise-suppression circuit. The battery drawer hinges outward from the bottom for easy insertion of the tiny battery. The microphone port on BTE hearing aids is typically at the front or top, next to the earhook. This places it just above the front of the pinna, when worn, making the sound pickup fairly natural. Behind-the-ear hearing aids come in several colors to match the hair or skin color of the wearer.

eyeglass aid

Another type that was popular many years ago, but now accounts for a very small percentage of total hearing aid sales, is the eyeglass hearing aid (see Figure 2.3). The microphone, amplifier, and receiver are built into the temple portion of an eyeglass. In Figure 2.3 the hearing aid is located in the right temple.

Figure 2.3 shows a metal nubbin which is connected by plastic tubing to an earmold. Just in front of the nubbin is the volume-control wheel. The microphone port is located on the underside of the temple, just in front of the volume control. Some hearing aid manufacturers make behind-the-ear and eyeglass models with identical circuits and, thus, identical electroacoustic characteristics so that the client may choose either type for a particular hearing loss.

Figure 2.4 shows both behind-the-ear and eyeglass hearing aids with the outer half of the plastic case removed. The illustration clearly shows the position of the microphone port, the receiver and its nubbin, the volume control, and the amplifier. The battery is inserted in the open space near the back of these hearing aid styles.

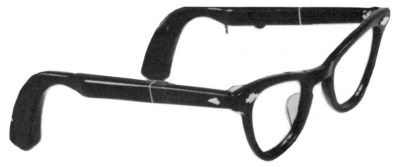

Figure 2.3. Eyeglass hearing aid. (Courtesy of Dahlberg Inc.)

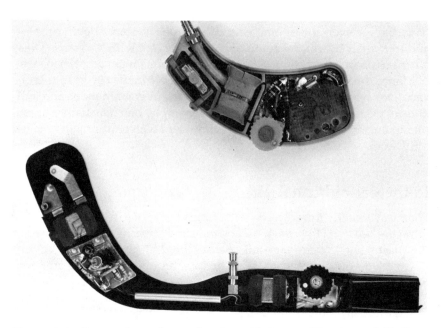

Figure 2.4. Inner view of two hearing aid types. (Courtesy of Radioear Corporation.)

As mentioned previously, current technology permits building ear-level (i.e., eyeglass or behind-the-ear or in-the-ear) hearing aids with considerable gain. However, because the microphone and receiver in such models are close together, acoustic feedback may occur with moderate or higher gain settings. Acoustic feedback is the result of amplified sound leaking from the receiver or earmold back to the microphone where it is re-amplified, causing a whistling or high-pitched sound. One method of overcoming this problem is to separate the microphone and receiver as much as possible. Historically, this has been one advantage of a body aid. However, improved technology and snugly fitted earmolds generally prevent feedback when ear-level aids are properly fitted and the user's gain requirements are not too great.

Feedback can also be controlled with an across-the-head arrangement which, in its basic form, is referred to as CROS (contralateral routing of signals). CROS aids are generally used to provide amplification for a person with an unaidable ear. In these cases, sound is picked up by a microphone near the poor ear and the signal, after amplification, is routed to the good ear.

A convenient CROS arrangement is provided with the eyeglass-type aid wherein the microphone is in one temple, with internal wiring leading forward and behind the glass rims to the other temple, which contains the receiver and tubing/earmold coupler system. Behind-the-ear and in-the-ear hearing aids are also available in CROS versions. These are usually wireless versions which use an FM transmitter/receiver system.

Since the introduction of the CROS principle in the 1960s, numerous variations have been spawned, involving various combinations and locations of microphones and receivers. For example, one may have a microphone on each side of the head leading to a receiver at one ear, called a BICROS.

in-the-ear aid/canal aid

The most recently introduced style of conventional ear-level hearing aid is the in-the-ear (ITE) type, whereby the entire hearing aid is built within the plastic shell of an earmold (see Figure 2.5). Sales of this kind of hearing aid now approach 80% of the total number of hearing aids sold in the U.S. (Mahon, 1987).

An advantage of the in-the-ear aid is that the microphone is located in a natural position, at the concha. The pinna effect, although relatively small, adds some preamplification for the important high frequencies. As mentioned previously, technology now permits high gain in a small package, so the power of in-the-ear hearing aids can be relatively great. However, the microphone and receiver are extremely close together, thereby often making acoustic feedback problems a concern.

For many individuals, the choice of a hearing aid is based on a cosmetic or personal preference. Others are restricted to one type because, for example, they do not regularly wear eyeglasses, or their concha is too small to permit an in-the-ear hearing aid. Greater miniaturization has recently allowed the entire hearing aid to be placed into the external auditory canal. These are referred to as *canal* or *in-the-canal* (ITC) aids. ITC instruments comprised 17% of total ITE sales in 1987 (Mahon, 1987).

Because of body baffle effects, the location of the hearing aid microphone on the body has a significant effect on the instrument's frequency response. For this reason, plus some of the considerations mentioned previously, the clinician must recognize the physical characteristics as well as the acoustic effects of the various hearing aid types. Only then can the client be counseled appropriately and the correct fitting be obtained.

An advantage of behind-the-ear, eyeglass, and in-the-ear types is that they can readily be fitted to each ear, thereby providing aided binaural hearing in appropriate cases. Ample experimental evidence suggests that under most environmental conditions two normal ears are better than

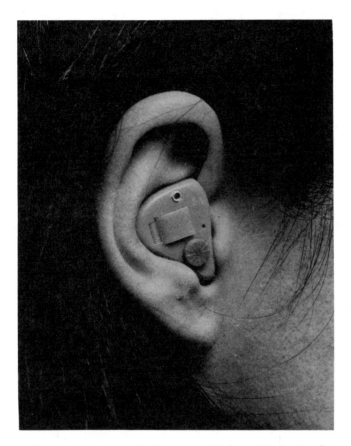

Figure 2.5. In-the-ear hearing aid. (Courtesy of Beltone Electronics Corporation.)

one. Therefore, there is considerable support for binaural fitting of hearing aids, especially for children (Ross, 1977). Unfortunately, no universally acceptable tests can objectively show the advantages or disadvantages of monaurally versus binaurally aided hearing. Consequently, client preference and the use of a trial period are important in making decisions concerning binaural fittings. It is suggested that clinicians recommend binaural amplification more frequently.

bone conduction amplification

Nearly all the hearing aids used by the hearing impaired are of the *air conduction* variety described above; however, sometimes another type, the *bone conduction* hearing aid, is more appropriate. Rather than directing acoustical energy down the ear canal, a bone conduction unit makes use of a vibrator placed on the mastoid process of the temporal bone. Mechanical vibrations from the side of the vibrator's outer case are transmitted directly to the inner ear through the skull. Thus, the amplified signal reaches the inner ear without being routed through the outer or middle ears. This form of hearing aid can be advantageous in certain cases, as with a person who has chronic middle ear drainage or absent ear canals and/or malformed pinnas. For effective use, inner ear function must be normal or near normal.

The earliest form of bone conduction systems made use of a conventional body aid. Instead of the external air conduction receiver, a small bone vibrator attached to a headband was used. Later, eyeglass hearing aids were modified for use as a bone conduction aid by building a bone vibrator into the frame of the glasses. Both of these modifications are still used.

Recently, two other approaches to bone conduction amplification have been developed. Hakansson, Tjellstrom, and Rosehall (1984) reported on a clinical study of what the developers termed a bone-anchored hearing aid. A titanium screw is surgically inserted into the temporal bone and attached to a permanently skin-penetrating titanium abutment; this, in turn, is attached to a unique bone conduction hearing aid.

Another system, the Audiant Bone Conductor, was introduced by Hough et al. (1986). A small external processor, looking somewhat like a conventional BTE hearing aid, is worn over the ear. A microphone in the processor picks up the sound and transduces it into electrical energy. This is then routed to the processor, which amplifies the signal and transmits it via an output induction coil to a surgically implanted internal magnetic disc imbedded directly under the skin in the temporal bone. The internal magnetic disc vibrates, and these vibrations are carried via the temporal bone to the inner ear, creating hearing. The processor is held in place by the magnetic attraction between a magnet inside its case and the implanted magnetic disc. Potential advantages of such a system compared to previous bone conduction aids include (a) direct stimulation of the temporal bone, (b) more stationary, anchored apparatus, and (c) more appealing and cosmetically acceptable appearance.

Although use of the new system presently is limited, it shows great promise and is likely to be used more frequently in the near future by individuals requiring permanent use of a bone conduction hearing aid system. For example, persons having had radical mastoidectomy or fenestration operations, where the ossicles and other outer/middle ear structures are removed or modified surgically, generally profit a great deal from the newer bone conduction system.

amplification components

basic components

The basic components of a conventional hearing aid or an auditory trainer are the *microphone, amplifier,* and *receiver*. For these elements to function, there must also be a power supply. With all wearable hearing aids and certain auditory trainers, the power supply is a battery. For some auditory trainer units the power supply comes from the regular alternating current from a wall plug.

Figure 2.6 shows, in diagrammatic form, the basic components of a hearing aid. Here we see sound waves being received by the microphone and transduced (changed to electrical energy), and then coupled to the first (or input) stage of the hearing aid amplifier. Commonly, three or more amplification stages are coupled together to provide the requisite gain and stability. At each stage the energy of the signal, as represented in Figure 2.6 by a sine wave, is increased. At the output stage (often called the *power amplifier*), the electrical energy, now amplified, is coupled to the receiver where it is transduced back to acoustic energy. The receiver is coupled to an earmold to efficiently direct the amplified sound into the ear canal and the tympanic membrane.

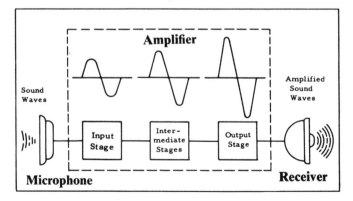

Figure 2.6. Basic diagram of a hearing aid. (Adapted by permission, Zenith Hearing Instrument Corp., 1968.)

DEVICES FOR THE HEARING IMPAIRED

The amplifier portion of hearing aids is not unlike that of any other audio amplifier, such as those found in a radio, television set, or an audiometer. The analogy often made between a hearing aid and a personal miniature public address system is reasonably accurate.

The transducers and amplifier may be enclosed in a single external plastic case. The input transducer is the microphone, the output transducer the receiver. The receiver is sometimes referred to as an *earphone* or miniature earphone, and in Europe the external receiver is called a *telephone*. The purpose of a transducer is to change energy from one form to another. Inasmuch as acoustic energy is extremely weak and cannot be amplified directly, the hearing aid's microphone is of great importance. If the microphone does not faithfully respond to sound, it will be amplified in a distorted manner. The microphone diaphragm responds to acoustic energy (varying atmospheric air pressure) and transforms (transduces) it into an electrical signal, analogous to the sound-pressure changes.

Throughout the early history of transistor hearing aids the magnetic microphone was used. Figure 2.7 shows a diagram of a magnetic microphone. Here we see a permanent magnet (1), the pole shoes (2-5), the magnetic armature, which is a tongue surrounded by a wire coil (6), and the flattened, cone-shaped diaphragm (7), made of thin aluminum foil. Part of the diaphragm has been omitted to show the rest of the parts. The diaphragm is connected to the coil arrangement by a small rod. As the diaphragm moves in and out, the rod pushes or pulls on the tongue, which has a coil of wire around it that is not shown. As the tongue and coil move alternately toward the north (4) or the south (5) poles, a voltage and current with corresponding waveform are induced in the coil. The resultant signal has the same waveform as the input sound-pressure wave. The signal from the microphone is coupled to the amplifier.

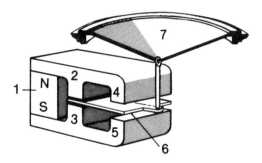

Figure 2.7. Diagram of a magnetic microphone.

In the 1960s the ceramic microphone was used in some hearing aids. More recently, the electret microphone has replaced both the magnetic and the ceramic microphone in most hearing aid models. An *electret* is a piece of material that is electrically polarized permanently. The technically correct term for a microphone employing an electret is *electret condenser microphone*. It is a specialized version of a conventional condensor microphone (which is too large and bulky for hearing aid use) having all the superior performance characteristics of the condensor microphone.

Visually, the electret microphone resembles the magnetic or ceramic microphones, but its operation is substantially different (see Figure 2.8). Like conventional condenser microphones, electret microphones have a wide, flat frequency response, high resistance to damage by dropping or shock, and much lower sensitivity to vibration than previously used microphones. Therefore, the microphone is, for the most part, eliminated as a source of significant signal distortion (Berger, 1984).

The amplifier of the hearing aid, as its name suggests, increases the magnitude of the electrical signal and conducts it to the receiver. Depending on the gain of the amplifier it may increase the signal by varying amounts. The receiver, essentially a microphone in reverse, transduces the amplified electrical signal back to acoustic energy. A receiver may be connected directly to an earmold (the external receiver), thereby coupling the amplified signal to the wearer's external auditory canal. If the receiver is inside the case with the amplifier (an internal receiver), the amplified acoustic signal goes through an earhook and then tubing, to an earmold.

controls

In addition to these basic elements, a hearing aid may include other controls or circuits. For example, there may be a *telephone coil* that the

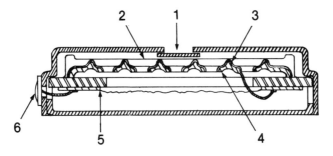

Figure 2.8. Diagram of an electret microphone.

wearer can use when telephoning. Special circuitry housed in the hearing aid picks up an electromagnetic signal from the receiver of the telephone and this is amplified and transduced to acoustic energy and routed to the ear. While this accessory has proven to be helpful to many hearing-impaired persons, variability in the performance of the hearing aid's telephone coil systems and in telephone receivers makes it necessary to monitor its use carefully.

Many hearing aids also have an external or internal *tone control*. With this control the user, or the dispenser of the instrument, can make an adjustment so that there is greater or lesser amplification in certain frequency regions. Another device is an *output limiting control,* commonly using a compression circuit called *automatic gain control* (AGC). AGC circuits compress the amplified sound so that in those cases where the wearer has a small dynamic range (i.e., the distance in dB between the auditory threshold and the uncomfortable loudness level) loud sounds will not be uncomfortable while soft sounds can still be heard. Another form of output-limiting procedure is termed *peak clipping*. While easier to accomplish electronically, this is a less popular option for controlling the hearing aid's output when the dynamic range of the user is restricted sharply.

earmolds

The earmold is not an electronic part of a hearing aid, yet it is no less important than the other components. It alters the amplified signal and can be deliberately modified to improve the signal for the wearer. The earmold must be comfortable, seal sufficiently to prevent acoustic feedback, and be cosmetically acceptable.

Earmolds are made of several different materials. A popular material is a hard clear plastic, but several softer materials are also used. The earmold may cover the entire concha or be reduced in varying degrees down to no more than an eartip that fits in the outer portion of the external auditory canal. In general, the greater the hearing loss, the more material is needed in the earmold to reduce acoustic feedback problems.

Earmolds come in assorted types or styles. The three most common types are the receiver mold (also termed *standard* or *regular*), the tube-type mold, and the mold used with in-the-ear hearing aids. The receiver earmold is used almost exclusively with body-type hearing aids. The tube-type mold comes in a variety of forms and is employed with behind-the-ear and eyeglass hearing aids. Tube-type earmolds include shell, skeleton, canal, and open varieties. Some of these earmold types are shown in Figure 2-9. The mold used with in-the-ear hearing aids houses the electronic circuitry in its base (see Figure 2.5).

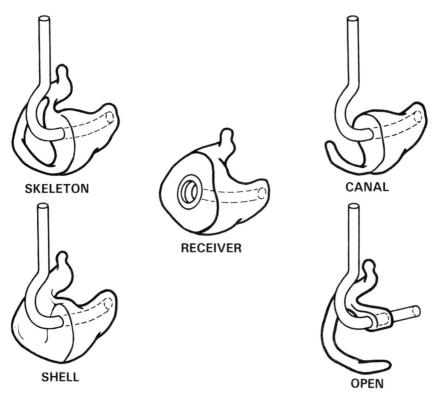

Figure 2.9. Basic types of earmolds. (From *Custom Earmold Manual*, 1983, Microsonic, Inc.)

The receiver or regular earmold snaps directly onto an external receiver (the "button"), and sound exiting the receiver is directed through the earmold to the external auditory canal. The tube-type earmolds connect to the earhook of the hearing aid by means of a short piece of clear tubing; sound exits the receiver of the hearing aid, through the earhook and tubing, and through the earmold to the ear canal. Both of these earmold types have a hole (the bore) through the canal portion of the earmold for sound to be efficiently directed to the external auditory canal.

The skeleton mold, as depicted in Figure 2.9, is one of the most popular of the tube-type molds. The canal mold, also popular, consists of the canal portion plus a small additional bend for retention purposes. Also in Figure 2.9 is a shell mold, usually the one of choice in cases of a severe or profound hearing loss when an ear-level hearing aid is employed.

Significant changes in the spectral composition of the signal can be accomplished by venting the earmold. With venting, an additional small hole is drilled in the canal portion of the earmold. Further modifications can occur with the use of an open earmold where most of the canal and much of the concha portion are removed.

Children's ears outgrow earmolds. Therefore, with small children, a new earmold may be needed several times a year (see Chapter 8, Table 8.2). With upper-elementary school-age children a new mold will probably not be required more often than every two or three years.

A detailed description of the electronic components in the hearing aid is not given here. Instead, the interested reader is referred to other sources where this subject is discussed in greater detail (Berger, 1983; Millin, 1978; Staab, 1978).

electroacoustic characteristics of hearing aids

We have described briefly some of the physical characteristics of hearing aids and their components. From the standpoint of hearing aid fitting, the most important characteristics of hearing aids are electroacoustic. The two primary electroacoustic characteristics are *gain* and *saturation sound pressure level* (SSPL). We might also add frequency response, which is gain as a function of frequency. Gain has little meaning unless frequency is also specified, so gain and frequency response are, for most purposes, considered together. In addition, hearing aids can be described in terms of their internal noise, telephone coil sensitivity, distortion properties, and other parameters.

gain

Gain refers to the increase, in decibels, of the output sound pressure from the receiver over the input sound pressure to the microphone. Obviously, the greater the hearing loss, the greater the gain needs to be. Persons with sensorineural hearing loss will, on the average, choose to use operating gain amounting to one-half or slightly more of their hearing threshold level (Brooks, 1973; McCandless & Miller, 1972; Millin, 1965). For example, a person with a hearing threshold level averaging about 60 dB will require and choose a gain setting somewhere around

30-33 dB. It is not desirable for the hearing aid to be worn at the full-on gain control position. Rather, about 10 dB of reserve gain is usually recommended. A hearing aid with about 43 dB of gain is, therefore, recommended. In summary, maximum gain – reserve gain = operating gain.

However, as noted above, gain cannot be separated from frequency. We may not want, for example, high gain at very low frequencies because that would amplify low-frequency background noise and contribute masking to the hearing mechanism. On the other hand, the greater the hearing loss, the more gain that is needed. It follows that the gain by frequency is related, but imperfectly, to the hearing loss pattern by frequency.

Under a Food and Drug Administration (FDA) regulation the hearing aid gain is measured and described in a particular manner. The ANSI S3.22-1987 standard is the official document that explains how gain and other performance parameters of the hearing aid are measured and described. Unfortunately, the acquisition of electroacoustic information based on this regulation requires a complicated series of procedures, some of which will be foreign to the beginning student. Since all persons dealing with amplification need to have a general orientation to specification sheets derived from these procedures, the details are reviewed here to provide some understanding of the process. Keep in mind, however, that ordinarily the audiologist is responsible for making these measurements and for understanding the intricacies of the process.

According to the FDA regulation the manufacturer or audiologist places a particular model in a hearing aid test unit (like the ones shown in Figure 2.10; Pollack [1988] described the function of this equipment). With the gain control of the aid set to full-on, the output of the hearing aid is measured with a given input, which may be 50 or 60 dB SPL. The difference between the input and output, as already mentioned, is the gain of that instrument. For example, assume that with an input of 60 dB SPL the output is 125 dB SPL; the gain is 125 – 60 = 65 dB. The ANSI standard calls for reporting an average gain, which is obtained by averaging the individual gain values at 1,000, 1,600, and 2,500 Hz. While these are the routine frequencies used, with certain aids having extreme low- or high-frequency emphasis, the manufacturer may select the three frequencies to be used in computing gain and SSPL 90 values.

frequency response

The ANSI S3.22-1987 standard specifies that a frequency response be measured and described. Unlike the gain measures just described, this is a graph of gain across the complete frequency range, rather than at only three discrete frequencies. Thus, it gives a visual indication of the

DEVICES FOR THE HEARING IMPAIRED

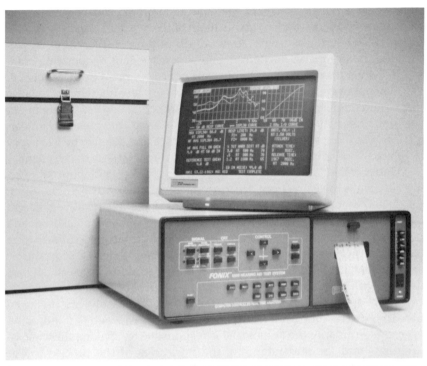

A

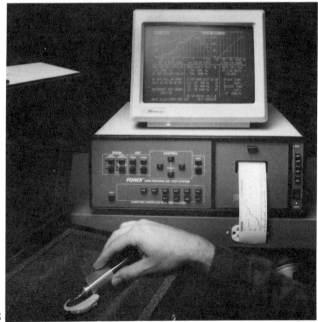

B

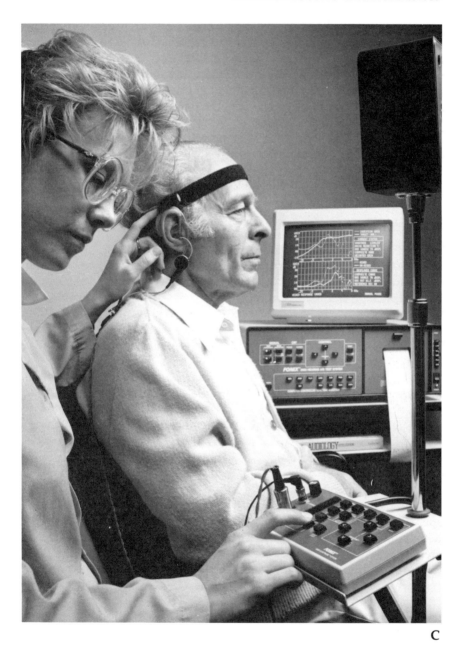

C

Figure 2.10. Components of an electroacoustic hearing aid analyzer are shown in *A* and *B*. As shown in *C*, this particular system can also be used to obtain real-ear probe microphone information about hearing aids. (Courtesy of Fry Electronics.)

variation in gain with frequency, suggesting how the instrument modifies the speech spectrum as well as other sounds. This information cannot be derived from average gain data. Furthermore, in the measurement of the frequency response the gain is adjusted to a level so as to minimize the possibility that the instrument is in partial or total saturation, a condition that may dramatically alter the frequency response. Presumably, this curve specifies the input-output relationship under typical conditions of use. Under the ANSI standard, the frequency response is obtained with gain control set so that the average coupler sound-pressure levels at 1,000, 1,6000, and 2,500 Hz, with a pure-tone input SPL of 60 dB, is 17 dB less than the high-frequency average SSPL90.

saturation sound-pressure level

The SSPL90 measurement is the average of the output at 1,000, 1,600, and 2,500 Hz, made with an input of 90 dB SPL and with the gain set at maximum. For the gain and SSPL90 measurements the full title includes the prefix "high-frequency-average"; this is designed to avoid confusion with the older ANSI S3.8-1967 and Hearing Aid Industry Conference (1961) standards, which employed 500, 1,000, and 2,000 Hz in the averages. Inasmuch as the newer standard involves the average of somewhat higher frequencies, and since more individuals need emphasis in the high than in the low frequencies, the newer standard seems to be more nearly representative of client needs. In the 1967 standard the SSPL was referred to as *output*, and many writers use the term *maximum power output* although that term appears in no standard and is technically incorrect inasmuch as all measures are pressure measurements and power (in watts) is not measured.

ANSI S3.22-1987 also includes some reference to tolerances. That is, the manufacturer must make certain that the HF-average SSPL90, the HF-average full-on gain, and the frequency response are within a specified number of decibels from that shown on the specification sheets describing the hearing aid models. The tolerances for gain and for SSPL90 are for the average of three frequencies, so, although it is a step in the right direction to include tolerances, they really are not very stringent. As an extreme example, assume that the HF-average full-on gain for a given instrument at 1,000, 1,600, and 2,500 Hz is quoted as 40 dB; the gain at these frequencies could be 40, 40, and 40 dB; or 20, 40, and 60 dB; or 60, 40, and 20 dB. Although each would be within the prescribed tolerance average, the gain by frequency would not satisfy the needs of a given client.

The standards published by ANSI (S3.3-1960; S3.8-1967; S3.22-1976; S3.22-1987) and those published in 1961 by the Hearing Industries Association (then called Hearing Aid Industry Conference) were designed primarily for comparing hearing aid performance from laboratory to laboratory rather than for assisting in the fitting of hearing aids. Therefore, some of the data required to be published in specification sheets are not necessarily directly applicable to hearing aid fitting. Nonetheless, until more realistic in-use descriptions of the electroacoustic characteristics for the purposes of hearing aid fitting are available, these standards are the best we have and we should use them to the best of our ability.

hearing aid specification sheets

A hearing aid specification sheet is provided by the hearing aid manufacturer for each model. It is a graphic description of how a particular hearing aid or auditory trainer is designed to operate. The specification sheet will, in large measure, consist of electroacoustic data such as those described previously. The audiologist makes frequent reference to specification sheets when selecting a hearing aid for a particular client or determining if a hearing aid is operating as it did when it left the manufacturer. The teacher of the hearing impaired and the speech-language pathologist also should be able to read and interpret basic information from specification sheets to recognize the capabilities and limitations of a particular hearing aid. All hearing aids sold are accompanied by specification data, which may need to be explained to the client or the client's parents.

Figure 2.11 shows a portion of a hearing aid specification sheet. The manufacturer has provided performance data for four different combinations of frequency response and AGC settings. With a frequency response of "L" and the AGC set at 75, this behind-the-ear hearing aid has a high-frequency average full-on gain of 42 dB. The HF-average SSPL90 is 116 dB. As illustrated in the SSPL90 graph, at 1,000 Hz the SSPL90 is 113 dB, at 1,600 Hz it is 120 dB, and at 2,500 Hz it is 116 dB, an average of 116 dB.

Again, with "L" tone and 75 AGC settings, this hearing aid has a reference-test gain of 38 dB. The lower and upper limits of the frequency response are also provided for each of the tone-AGC combinations. As shown, the "L" tone setting results in slightly more amplification for lower frequencies and less for higher frequencies than the "H" setting. In addition to gain, SSPL90, and frequency response, the specification sheet also contains a statement of total harmonic distortion and, since this is an automatic gain control instrument, the attack and release times of the compression are given, as well as its input-output characteristics. Important information about batteries is also provided.

Audiotone Performance Data

A-54 SR

A-54 SR Sensori-Neural Response Automatic Signal Processor (ASP) hearing aid

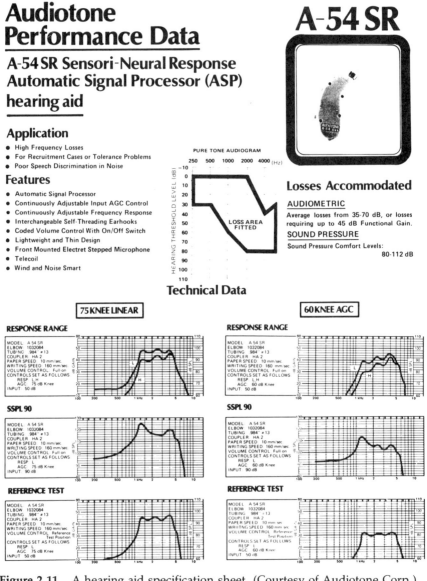

Application
- High Frequency Losses
- For Recruitment Cases or Tolerance Problems
- Poor Speech Discrimination in Noise

Features
- Automatic Signal Processor
- Continuously Adjustable Input AGC Control
- Continuously Adjustable Frequency Response
- Interchangeable Self-Threading Earhooks
- Coded Volume Control With On/Off Switch
- Lightweight and Thin Design
- Front Mounted Electret Stepped Microphone
- Telecoil
- Wind and Noise Smart

Losses Accommodated

AUDIOMETRIC
Average losses from 35-70 dB, or losses requiring up to 45 dB Functional Gain.

SOUND PRESSURE
Sound Pressure Comfort Levels:
80-112 dB

Figure 2.11. A hearing aid specification sheet. (Courtesy of Audiotone Corp.)

The specification sheets, or technical data sheets, are useful in clinics where a hearing aid test apparatus is available. If there is a question of whether a hearing aid is operating normally, the clinician can make the same measurements as the manufacturer and compare them with

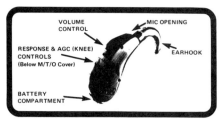

A-54 SR Fitting Information

ADJUSTMENTS

The FREQUENCY RESPONSE and AGC (KNEE CONTROL) are continuously adjustable. To set, position the red dot or arrow of the control to the desired setting. Examples:

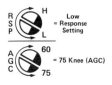

R H Low
S = Response
P L Setting

A 60
G = 75 Knee (AGC)
C 75

ANSI S3.22-1982 (ASA) 7-1982

75 KNEE LINEAR

Resp.	HF-avg. Full-on Gain	HF-avg. SSPL90 (dB)	Max. Gain (dB)	Ref.Test Gain (dB)	Max. SSPL90 (dB)	Freq. Range (Hz)
L	42	116	49	38	125	700-7000
H	34.5	115	45	34	125	900-7500

Total Harmonic Distortion	500 Hz	800 Hz	1600 Hz	ATTACK	4 ms
Typical	N/A	N/A	1%	RELEASE	25 ms
Max.			2%		

60 KNEE AGC

Resp.	HF-avg. Full-on Gain	HF-avg. SSPL90 (dB)	Max. Gain (dB)	Ref.Test Gain (dB)	Max. SSPL90 (dB)	Freq. Range (Hz)
L	35	105	46	25	114	700-7000
H	27	105	43	24	113	800-7000

Total Harmonic Distortion	500 Hz	800 Hz	1600 Hz	ATTACK	8 ms
Typical	N/A	N/A	1%	RELEASE	36 ms
Max.			2%		

INPUT-OUTPUT CHARACTERISTICS

L_n	
Typical	27 dB
Max.	29 dB

Induction Coil Sensitivity
83 dB @ 1000 Hz
105 dB @ Max.

Battery Information		
Type	Mercury	Zinc-Air
Drain	1.7 mA Max.	1.7 mA Max.
Est. Battery Life	130 hrs.	250 hrs.
Recommended Batteries	M675	A675

How To Order

1. Specify Model A-54 SR.
2. Specify Beige or Mink Brown Color.

COLORS . . . Beige, Mink Brown
CASE . . . Non-allergic Tenite II
WEIGHT . . 0.12 oz (4 Grams)

Zwislocki Coupler Performance-75 and 60 KNEE

KEMAR-Practical Effects Of Tube Fitting

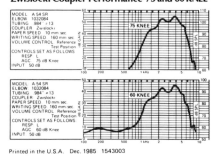

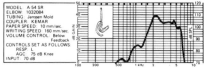

AUDIOTONE®
A DIVISION OF LEAR SIEGLER, INC.
P.O. BOX 2905 • PHOENIX, ARIZONA 85062
(800) 528-5424 • (800) 528-4068 • (602) 254-5886
TWX 910-950-0197

Printed in the U.S.A. Dec. 1985 1543003

Figure 2.11. (Continued)

those on the specification sheet. In this way it can readily be determined if a particular hearing aid meets the manufacturer's specifications. If not, it can be sent back for repair.

candidates for amplification

The question of who should have a hearing aid might seem an easy one. Many might argue that anyone who thinks he needs a hearing aid should have one, but experience shows this to be invalid. Surely, the professional involved with hearing and hearing aids is qualified to help make the decision along with the person who will wear the aid. However, many persons mistake poor listening habits for hearing loss and think they or their child need a hearing aid. On the other hand, countless individuals who cannot easily hear normal conversation because of a hearing loss do not believe they need a hearing aid. At least they say so. Thus, in our judgment the decision as to who should have a hearing aid first involves ruling out a medically remediable hearing loss; then it is based primarily on audiometric test results. The audiologist, rather than the speech-language pathologist or teacher of the hearing impaired, will be directly involved in choosing the hearing aid candidate and selecting a hearing aid. Nonetheless, the speech-language pathologist and teacher of the hearing impaired should be familiar with potential problems and divergent philosophies in this area.

Some might also argue that anyone with a significant hearing loss should be fitted with a hearing aid. This argument is only partially valid, since we must first define *significant* hearing loss. The person with average hearing no better than 30 dB (ANSI, 1969) at 1,000 and 2,000 Hz in the better ear is, in our opinion, a potential candidate for a hearing aid. We consider 30 dB hearing level (HL) the borderline in most instances. However, some persons with slightly less hearing loss may profit from a hearing aid if their circumstances require excellent receptive communication. Others, who are typically less active, probably will not profit from a hearing aid unless their losses are slightly greater. The milder the hearing loss, the less likely individuals are to consider themselves handicapped, and the less likely they will accept a hearing aid recommendation. The rationale for choosing an average of 30 dB HL as the point of first considering a hearing aid is that the next lower HL (25 dB) equals 33 dB SPL (or 30 dB SPL if the two ears are identical); that is, under this circumstance the hearing sensitivity readily permits understanding moderate and loud speech sounds. Some weak speech sounds (such as /θ/, /s/, and /f/) may be missed from soft female speech.

At the other extreme, the more profound the hearing loss, the less likely it is that the individual can tolerate the requisite gain and SSPL. In spite of arguments to the contrary, in our experience, unless the individual has some measurable hearing at 500 and 1,000 Hz, he is unlikely to accept a hearing aid and wear it. If the individual responds to test stimuli at frequencies no higher than 500 Hz, we suspect that the response is more often tactile than auditory. Although tactile stimulation has a decided place in auditory rehabilitation, this is not usually the purpose of conventional hearing aids. Between these two extremes, minimal and virtually total hearing loss, we believe that all individuals will profit from a hearing aid once any psychologic barrier to its use is overcome.

It is sometimes said that a person with very poor unaided speech discrimination is a poor candidate for a hearing aid. In general, this argument is fallacious (Millin, 1988). If a client's optimum-word discrimination score (which is called PB-MAX) is only 30% but he can understand nothing at ordinary conversational levels without amplification, it is likely that amplification will be of great benefit. Even if this person can only achieve 20% discrimination with an aid, he will likely prefer this to nothing. No maximum or minimum discrimination score will predict precisely hearing aid candidacy. Indeed, if one ear has good discrimination and the other poor discrimination, the ear to be aided—other things being equal (although they seldom are)—should be the one with the best discrimination.

For profound hearing losses, the hearing aid may enable the wearer to detect only the presence and absence of sound, or perhaps rhythm cues. With such a loss the individual may not be able to depend upon audition alone for receptive communication. However, countless studies have shown that whatever auditory information an amplifier provides will assist tremendously in speechreading precision. A little auditory stimulation seems to be more important than a lot of anything else!

Occasionally, professionals argue whether aided word discrimination can be better than unaided. We suggest that speech *discrimination* (recognition) is an innate ability. That ability may be enhanced by auditory training, for example, and it may be worsened as a result of disease or injury to the hearing mechanism; but at any given time, it is relatively fixed.

On the other hand, the *intelligibility* of speech is, in large part, a property of the speech signal itself and the effects of the acoustic environment. A hearing aid that filters out low frequencies could, therefore, reduce the upward masking effect of environmental noise, resulting in better intelligibility than that produced by the speech audiometer, with which the unaided score was obtained. The audiometer has no such filtering. Likewise, the frequency shaping deliberately introduced into the hearing aid to compensate for the client's abnormal hearing contour could produce better speech intelligibility than that obtained with the flat response of the speech audiometer. Thus, the hearing aid can sometimes provide a more intelligible signal than the audiometer, and, in turn, result in higher word-discrimination scores.

hearing aid evaluation

When, or before, a hearing aid is recommended for a client it may be evaluated by a number of persons. Certainly, the wearer will evaluate it informally in a number of respects, under assorted environmental conditions, perhaps in comparison with other hearing aids or amplifying devices or in comparison with remembered unimpaired hearing. The dispenser of the hearing aid is also likely to evaluate the hearing aid and obtain opinions from the wearer. In addition, the manufacturer has already, by Food and Drug Administration regulation, evaluated the hearing aid electroacoustically on a number of parameters.

We know a great deal about how the hearing mechanism is constructed and how it operates. A large number of audiometric tests enable the clinician to measure degree and type of hearing loss. Also, we know a great deal about amplification devices. Hearing aids can be measured and described electroacoustically from a large number of aspects, as we saw earlier. However, there is considerable variation on what constitutes an appropriate hearing aid evaluation. These differences encompass determination of hearing aid candidacy, what test signals should be employed for unaided and aided testing, what electroacoustic factors are most appropriate for a given hearing loss, the criteria for an appropriate hearing aid fitting, and the method whereby a specific hearing aid is chosen for a particular hearing impairment.

selective amplification

The wearable electronic (vacuum tube) hearing aid made its appearance in the late 1930s and efforts to scientifically fit hearing aids rarely appeared before that time. Around 1940 a flurry of activity centered on more objective fitting of hearing aids. One of the ideas brought forth at that time was selective amplification. In its pure form *selective amplification* meant amplifying sound to produce aided thresholds that were the same as the unaided thresholds of normal-hearing listeners, the so-called *mirror fitting of the audiogram*.

Pure selective amplification was not successful, partly because it led to too much amplification in the low frequencies and, because of the severity of the loss in the high frequencies, amplification had to be so great in many sensorineural losses that it added distortion to the already distorted hearing mechanism. Several other versions of selective amplificaton have been suggested.

In 1940 Watson and Knudsen published their hearing aid fitting scheme. They had their clients balance the loudness of various frequencies to a 1,000-Hz tone and, based upon those results, they attempted to fit a hearing aid so that it amplified frequencies to the user's most comfortable loudness level (MCL). The procedure was an acceptable psychophysical procedure, but it was rather difficult for unsophisticated listeners and it was also time-consuming. The use of MCL in fitting hearing aids remains popular, however, and Victoreen (1960) introduced a modification of the Watson and Knudsen procedure.

Fitting a hearing aid to the client's MCL is one of the more commonly used procedures among audiologists today. Weaknesses include the fact that (a) MCL appears to be more a range than a level, (b) test-retest reliability is not as high as desirable, and (c) maximum discrimination is not typically obtained at MCL (Posner & Ventry, 1977; Schmitz, 1969). Furthermore, the MCL is affected by the duration and type of stimulus used to determine it, instructions given to the listener, and the level of background noise. Despite these weaknesses, fitting to MCL seems to provide a fairly good first-order approximation of appropriate gain.

comparative evaluation

At the close of World War II a large number of hearing-impaired military personnel needed assistance. Several hospitals in the United States were designated for the purpose of rehabilitating these veterans. Raymond Carhart (1946), at that time a captain in the army, is credited with refining a rationale and procedure for evaluating hearing aids in this military program. His rationale and procedure are now often referred to as the "traditional hearing aid evaluation" or "comparative approach." Carhart's procedure consisted of a thorough otologic and audiologic evaluation. If a hearing aid seemed warranted, the individual was tested with three or four preselected instruments.

The aided tests included speech reception threshold (SRT), word discrimination, and usually speech audiometry in noise—all accomplished with the hearing aid gain control set by the client to a comfort level while listening to cold running speech in free field at 40 dB HL. After a number of instruments had been tested, the clinician compared the various aided and unaided audiometric scores. The aid or aids that produced the best scores were then loaned to the client for trial use around the hospital for a day or more for evaluation under various environmental conditions. Finally, one hearing aid was selected and another of the same brand and model was issued to the client.

Assumptions related to this form of hearing aid evaluation are (a) that the instrument that produces the best speech audiometric scores in the quiet nonreverberant test room will also be the best instrument under normal everyday conditions, (b) that the purchased hearing aid will have electroacoustic characteristics like those of the trial instrument of the same brand and model, and (c) that speech audiometry is sufficiently sensitive and reliable to reveal differences between trial hearing aids.

The first serious criticism of hearing aid comparison procedures was published by Shore, Bilger, and Hirsh (1960), who presented evidence that the reliability of the procedures was poor. They did not condemn the concept of hearing aid evaluations, but pointed out that word-discrimination scores are insensitive to differences between the preselected hearing aids used in the comparisons. Others have reached the same conclusion (Beattie & Edgerton, 1976; Jerger, 1967; Resnick & Becker, 1963; Thompson & Lassman, 1969; Walden et al., 1983). More sensitive and reliable speech-discrimination tests have not appeared, although many efforts in this direction have been made.

Since speech-discrimination tests appear to be the culprit in the low reliability of comparative procedures, one solution would be to improve the tests. This can be done to some extent. For example, instead of using 50-word test lists for each condition, 200 words could be used to improve test reliability, as shown by Pascoe (1975). However, such long word lists increase the testing time and seem impractical. In fact, the trend among audiologists is to use 25-word test lists in an effort to save clinician time as well as client endurance.

Despite the limitations inherent in the comparative form of hearing aid evaluation, it remains popular, especially in audiology clinics. Surveys (Smaldino & Hoene, 1981; Whitcomb, 1982) indicate that many audiologists continue to use this approach in some form.

the harvard report

Almost at the same time as Carhart was first using the hearing aid comparison procedures credited to him, a group at the Psycho-Acoustic Laboratory at Harvard University was completing an involved study on amplification characteristics and their effect on hearing impairment (Davis et al., 1947). The resulting document, now usually referred to as the

Harvard Report, took strong exception to the need for laborious hearing aid comparison procedures and to selective amplification fitting. Its authors were critical of "pure" selective amplification or complete compensation; instead, they recommended, in essence, to limit the number of frequency responses available for use. The Harvard Report, thus, recommended a slightly rising frequency response or a flat response for most clients. In other words, the researchers at Harvard did not find sufficient evidence to warrant meticulous tailoring of hearing aid responses to individual hearing losses. Similar results were published in England at about the same time by the Medical Research Council.

The Harvard Report may be the most quoted and least read of all audiologic literature. While the most comprehensive such study published up to that date, and more complete than most studies on the subject done since, its experimental design, lack of counterbalancing, choice of speech audiometric materials, subject selection, and other factors leave much to be desired by current standards. Thus, the conclusions of the Harvard Report are not necessarily appropriate for today's hearing-impaired population and today's hearing aid technology.

the master hearing aid

A number of modifications of the traditional or modified hearing aid evaluation have appeared, ranging from an extended trial with two or three hearing aids to the use of a so-called *master hearing aid,* also called a *pressure measuring instrument.* It is intended to permit simulation of an assortment of electroacoustic factors, such as gain, output, and frequency response. With the master hearing aid the clinician can focus rather quickly on some broad combination of electroacoustic factors that seems best for the client, or compare several combinations of electroacoustic factors in much the same manner as trial hearing aids in the traditional comparative procedure. With the master hearing aid, the number of loaner hearing aids can be reduced or removed entirely from the clinic (Berger, 1980).

An advantage of the use of a master hearing aid is that it saves time by not having to place successive instruments on the client. Instead, a comfort level with one set of factors can be achieved, and the factors can be manipulated after each group of tests under speech audiometry. Disadvantages of the master hearing aid include (a) the data obtained may only be applicable to the manufacturer of a particular instrument, (b) the device may not be typical of current hearing aids, and (c) the microphone position on the master hearing aid may not be where it would be in typical use.

prescriptive fitting methods

A number of formulas or prescriptions have been developed for hearing aid fittings. Despite some criticism of the word *prescription*, the term has gradually gained popularity for certain types of hearing aid fitting protocols. We use the term when, as a minimum, it encompasses the specification of an explicit set of electroacoustic characteristics for a particular hearing loss on a deductive basis. A number of procedures meet this definition (Berger, Hagberg, & Rane, 1984; Brooks & Tonnison, 1976; Cox, 1988; Kee, 1972; Libby, 1986; Lybarger, 1953; McCandless & Lyregaard, 1983; Pascoe, 1975, 1978; Shapiro, 1975, 1976; and Victoreen, 1973). A short review of most of these methods was presented by Byrne (1987).

In our prescription procedures we follow a set of guidelines to first determine whether a hearing aid is appropriate, and if so, whether the individual should be fitted by air conduction or bone conduction, and whether the person should be fitted in the right, the left, or both ears. Once these decisions are made, the electroacoustic characteristics of the instrument are prescribed (Berger et al., 1984). These include the gain-frequency response and the saturation sound pressure level.

Our formula for the gain-frequency response is based on overlaying upon the hearing threshold level an incomplete mirroring of the speech spectrum. This formula is used to predict the individual's desired aided threshold. Modifications of the formula take into account alterations of the hearing aid's response depending upon where the microphone is located, and whether there is a sizable air-bone gap.

The SSPL is prescribed so as to prevent uncomfortably loud sounds from reaching the ear; this level is chosen on the basis of testing for the uncomfortable loudness level (UCL). Many client failures with hearing aids are due to excessive SSPL. However, in our clinical experience, earmold problems account for more initial client dissatisfacton than all other problems combined. That is, the earmold may feel too rough, too loose, too tight, or it may rub the pinna. Earmold problems such as these can usually be easily corrected. A secondary complaint is that the amplified sound is too loud. It is not always clear whether this complaint results from too much gain in the low frequencies, from an SSPL setting higher than the client's UCL, or from a combination of the two.

The many details of our gain-frequency response and SSPL formulas are not discussed here. Suffice it to say that our prescription method, and those of others, was designed to add objectivity to hearing aid fitting and provide a method for checking how nearly the prescribed hearing instrument has attained the aided performance predicted from the formula. This is accomplished by using warbled or pulsed pure tones, or narrow band noise, for both the unaided and the aided threshold conditions. The difference between these two conditions reveals what the *functional gain* of the instrument is. During the past few years, this information has also been obtained with real-ear/probe-tube microphone measures. From this comparison one can also visualize how closely the obtained instrument has reached the specified values. Group data accumulated on over 1,000 consecutive clients strongly indicate that the closer we can get to the predicted aided threshold, the better will be the client's word-discrimination scores.

real-ear/probe-tube microphone evaluation

Until recently, the only way to assess the electroacoustic performance of hearing aids on individual users was to measure "functional gain." As stated earlier, functional gain is the difference between a patient's aided and unaided thresholds for warble tones or narrow band noises measured in a sound field. These were perhaps the first of the "real-ear" hearing aid evaluation procedures, so called because they measure hearing aid performance on the ear of the user. Because the determination of functional gain requires behavioral responses, the procedure can be time consuming and unreliable, and errors can result from inherent problems in establishing stable sound levels in the field. Furthermore, the procedure provides data at only a few test frequencies and may not reveal unwanted peaks and valleys in the intensity-frequency response of a hearing aid. Functional gain measurement, nonetheless, has important clinical usefulness and is an integral part of some hearing aid evaluation or prescriptive procedures. There is the additional advantage that the procedure for obtaining functional gain does not require expensive special equipment.

Another way to estimate hearing aid performance on a listener is to remove the aid from a patient and evaluate it in a test box system. These systems, however, were designed to test hearing aids electroacoustically in the absence of listeners so that aids could be tested by manufacturers before sale to individuals. Their usefulness for evaluating the performance of hearing aids as worn is limited because the couplers (types HA-1 and HA-2) which must be used in the test box are poor simulations of real ears. Although they closely simulate the average adult ear, the acoustical properties of the ears of actual hearing aid wearers often vary greatly from the median. Furthermore, in recent years, a number of new methods for coupling hearing aids to the ear have been developed, including vented earmolds and the open earmolds used in CROS and BICROS fittings. Standard couplers and test boxes are often inappropriate for evaluating hearing aids using these coupling methods.

In recent years, real-ear probe-tube systems have been developed employing objective procedures which do not require behavioral responses. A very slim probe-tube microphone is inserted into the ear canal to measure sound pressure levels (SPL) near the eardrum. Tones of known sound level are generated in the field and canal pressure levels are measured at many points across the frequency range. These measurements are made with and without a hearing aid in the ear. As the tones sweep through the frequency range, the system automatically subtracts SPL values obtained unaided from the aided SPL values and plots a curve of insertion gain, either on a video monitor or a graph. *Insertion gain* refers to the difference in the unaided and aided SPL measured in the ear canal. Some systems not only provide gain curves, but can plot aided canal pressure levels and graphs of the difference between canal pressures among different hearing aids or different internal tone settings of the same hearing aid. It is also possible to plot the desired canal pressures predicted by various prescriptive procedures and use the probe system to determine if these values have been attained.

The advantages of probe-tube microphone measurement of hearing aid performances are numerous. Measures can be obtained quickly and many frequencies are sampled, revealing any peaks or valleys in hearing aid response. Numerous comparisons of different hearing aid fittings are possible, and the effects produced by altering hearing aid frequency response or modifying earmolds can be assessed quickly and accurately. The effects of ear canal resonance can also be taken into account. Finally, since no behavioral response from the listener is necessary, the performance of hearing aids on most difficult-to-test patients can be easily accomplished (see Figure 2.10).

There has long been a gap between advances in technology and clinical application. At present, it is safe to say that probe systems provide many useful measurement options for audiologists to use in hearing aid fitting. Even though the cost of the instrumentation is high, the potential value of probe-tube microphone systems is so great that more and more audiologists are incorporating them into routine use for hearing aid evaluation and fitting (Pollack, 1988).

combined approach

Even though the methods described above constitute the major ones, a number of professionals do not use any of them in a pure form. Rather, they combine key elements from one or more. This has been discussed by Harford (1979), who referred to this practice as the *combined approach*.

One form is exemplified by a concept introduced in the 1960s, *hearing aid consultation* (Resnick & Becker, 1963; Shore & Kramer, 1963). This method essentially represents a de-emphasis on extensive prefitting tests with an increased concentration on post-fitting adjustment and orientation to the hearing aid.

computer applications

In recent years efforts have been made to incorporate computerization into the hearing aid selection process, particularly in conjunction with prescription approaches. Software packages are now available which rank order the appropriateness of available hearing aids for a given hearing loss pattern. This selection is based on a number of key factors associated with the functional and electroacoustic characteristics of instruments available to the clinician, as well as key features of the person's hearing loss. Software of this type has been described based on work at several facilities (Berger, 1983; Craig & Siegenthaler, 1980; Hertzano, Levitt, & Slosberg, 1979; Katz, 1984; Popelka, 1982). (See Chapter 13, Adult List of Resources and Materials.)

hearing aid adjustment and orientation

No matter how a hearing aid is evaluated, whether by comparative procedures, prescription, or client preference, there is need for client orientation to the hearing aid when initially fitted and after a specified period of adjustment. Many new hearing aid users require considerable help in adjusting to their hearing problem as well as orientation in hearing aid use. For instance, they need to know what a hearing aid will and will not do, how to care for it, how to use the batteries, and how to troubleshoot minor repairs. The individual also needs to know about the limitations of amplification and some of the myths surrounding hearing aids. If, for example, the client believes that a hearing aid will restore hearing to normal or "cure" the hearing loss, this assumption must be corrected. (The client wearing eyeglasses may naively expect a hearing aid to correct hearing as eyeglasses correct seeing.) Counseling is also needed to make certain that the client understands that the hearing aid is unlikely to make the hearing worse if the aid is fitted correctly (Berger & Millin, 1978).

An analogy is often drawn between hearing aids and eyeglasses. Like many analogies, it has serious shortcomings. Although it is true that hearing aids alter the acoustic signal and eyeglasses modify the visual image, the vast majority of visual problems for which eyeglasses are appropriate result from the inability of the lens of the eye to focus the image on the retina. Thus, the purpose of the eyeglasses is not to magnify (amplify) the image, but to refocus it on the retina. "Amplification," as in hearing loss, is not necessary since the sensitivity of the eye is normal. Hearing aids, on the other hand, primarily amplify the signal, since in both conductive and sensorineural losses sensitivity is reduced. Although visual and auditory problems share common features, these fundamental differences dictate that we do not push the analogy too far.

Most important in the orientation, especially for parents of children, is to make clear that the hearing aid will not enable the individual to process linguistically what is heard. Rather, along with auditory habilitation, the hearing aid may be necessary to develop this skill. Nonetheless, the hearing aid is a vital, and often first, link in the rehabilitative process because it enables the client to use the auditory sense to its fullest. The hearing aid thus becomes a means to an end.

Once the hearing aid is fitted, the response to amplified sound for some persons is immediately positive, and little further counseling is needed. For many others, however, adjustment to the amplified sound takes time and patience. For example, one often has to experiment with the gain control setting in several acoustic environments and also learn the best place to sit in a concert hall or at church when using the hearing aid.

hearing aid maintenance

Hearing aids require the usual care that should be taken with any sophisticated electronic device. Naturally, care should be taken not to drop the instrument, and it should not be stored in a very warm location. Since moisture is an enemy of the microphone and receiver, precautions should be taken to avoid their being damaged by perspiration or rain. Earmolds occasionally need washing with soapy water or with one of the antiseptic solutions available through hearing aid supply companies or dispensers. When cleaned with a liquid, the earmold must be dried thoroughly before being reattached to the receiver or to the earhook.

Wearing an earmold may, of itself, encourage cerumen production. Therefore, it may be necessary to periodically clean cerumen from the earmold. Cerumen can be removed easily by pushing a pipe cleaner through the bore of the mold, but only after the earmold has been removed from the receiver or earhook. The plastic tubing on ear-level hearing aids ultimately becomes stiff and may crack, and consequently must be replaced. Similarly, the cord on body aids is likely to become frayed from rubbing against clothing or bent from continuous wear, and likewise will need replacement.

Reports from audiologists and hearing aid dealers indicate that most hearing aid failures and problems stem from the battery and the battery compartment. The use of an incorrect-size battery can damage the instrument case or battery connections. The battery is sometimes placed in the aid backward, and an exhausted battery sometimes continues to be used because a peak of energy is still heard, leading the listener to believe it is still good.

A number of reports have shown that as many as 50% of the hearing aids worn by hard-of-hearing and deaf children in various classroom placements are not functioning adequately or appropriately (see Chapter 8 and Zink, 1972). It behooves the teacher of the deaf or the person otherwise involved with auditory rehabilitation to check each child's hearing aid or auditory trainer at the beginning of each school day or therapy period to make certain that it is functioning within prescribed limits. Monitoring of the amplification device should include a visual check of the instrument as well as a quick auditory check. If any malfunction is suspected, a more detailed electroacoustic check should be made.

The teacher or therapist ought to have a battery tester available to test for exhausted batteries. Since batteries are often the culprit in malfunctioning hearing aids, the child should be encouraged to keep a spare battery on hand, or leave a spare with the teacher. Nonfunctioning or intermittently functioning cords can be tested informally by listening to the hearing aid while slowly and gradually twisting the cord. (A cord tester is available through hearing aid supply houses.)

Those working with children who are wearing hearing aids or using auditory trainers might well take a lesson from those who teach instrumental music groups. The music teacher knows that for the lesson or rehearsal to be profitable, the instruments must be in proper working order and tuned. Therefore, at the beginning of the music lesson or class a brief period is spent in tuning the instruments. So too will the teacher or therapist find it helpful and time saving to "tune" amplification units, so to speak, by checking them for possible malfunction. The child with a malfunctioning amplification device is unlikely to profit from the class lesson or therapy session.

The following is a partial list of hearing aid problems and some of their causes:

Problem	Cause
Hearing aid dead	Bad battery, battery in backward, dirty cord contacts, broken cord, loose cord plug, earmold plugged with cerumen, switch turned to TEL
Hearing aid weak	Bad battery, earmold partially plugged with cerumen, microphone opening plugged with dirt or foreign object
Intermittency	Dirty cord contacts, broken cord, loose cord plug, plastic tube collapsed
Accoustic feedback	Earmold not inserted correctly, child has outgrown earmold, earmold loose from receiver nubbin, microphone too close to receiver, volume control too high, microphone housing loose, crack in plastic tubing, ear canal blocked with cerumen
Distorted sound	Weak battery, earmold partially plugged with cerumen, amplifier no longer working correctly
Noice in the sound	Dirty or frayed cord, loose receiver cap, loose microphone housing, volume control worn

Some of these problems can be handled on the spot, but others require that the hearing aid be returned to the manufacturer for repair. The school or the hearing aid dispenser should have on hand a supply of loaner instruments for use until the original unit has been replaced and returned. Although the loaner instrument may have different electroacoustic factors, at least the client will have some amplification available until the personal hearing aid is again usable.

auditory trainers

Hearing aids and auditory trainers operate on many of the same electronic principles, and both are used in the rehabilitation of hearing-impaired clients. In many respects, auditory trainers are not readily differentiated from hearing aids. The major components and principles related to operation of auditory trainers are much like those of hearing aids; however, there are some variations in auditory trainers that are not available in a wearable hearing aid.

A primary difference between hearing aids and auditory trainers is the purpose for which they are used. Most often, auditory trainers serve not as a hearing device in everyday listening, but as a training device to be used in the classroom or other special sites. Since they are used primarily in the classroom, their size and cosmetic appearance are not crucial. Therefore, large microphones and earphones with better fidelity than those found in hearing aids may be used and the amplifier can be made large enough to include specialized circuitry that increases the flexibility of the device. For example, some auditory trainers have a user-adjustable output limiter control, which permits the listener to select quickly any maximum output pressure level found to be comfortable or desirable. They typically also offer several readily adjustable frequency-response choices. Still other auditory trainers permit change from monaural to binaural reception and have independently adjustable controls that permit the listener to balance the sensation levels between ears.

There are four basic types of auditory trainers: portable desk models, hardwire units, induction loop units, and FM radio frequency units. The latter three are considered group auditory training systems. While FM systems have been utilized almost exclusively in recent years in the classroom, some treatment is included here of desk, hardwire, and induction loop systems for historical reasons, and because some of these units are still being utilized on a limited scale. Discussion of these older systems should not be construed as an endorsement of their use with school-age children, however. Extensive improvements of FM systems have resulted in a situation where most professionals advocate the use of FM systems exclusively (Ross, 1982b), particularly for educational purposes.

Systems that utilize infrared transmissions are used in group auditory systems, but typically not for auditory training purposes. (See Chapter 13 for further details about infrared.)

desk trainers

Desk trainers are built in a small metal case, which is generally positioned on the student's desk. The microphone, amplifier, and battery supply are mounted inside the case. Flexible cords lead from the enclosure to hearing aid receivers or to large earphones in cushions. The desk model has a gain control, and some also have frequency-response and output controls, which can be adjusted by the teacher or student. The device is portable, so the child can carry it around the room, to the blackboard, or to the teacher's desk. Figure 2.12 shows a binaural desk trainer: the earphones are not shown.

Desk trainers are handy when the therapist or the teacher is working with one child. They are also convenient in case a child's hearing aid malfunctions. A disadvantage of the desk auditory trainer is that if the teacher or the therapist is some distance from the child, the signal to noise (S/N) ratio is poor. *Signal-to-noise* ratio refers to the difference in intensity between a wanted signal and distracting noise. In this circumstance the unit amplifies environmental noise near the user; the speech at the microphone weakens as the distance between the speaker and auditory trainer increases. Thus, one may expect S/N ratios to be poorer when the speaker is farther away. Reducing the distance between speaker and child minimizes this problem. Desk trainers are usually not the desired auditory trainer for classes of hearing-impaired children, but are useful for auditory training sessions with one child.

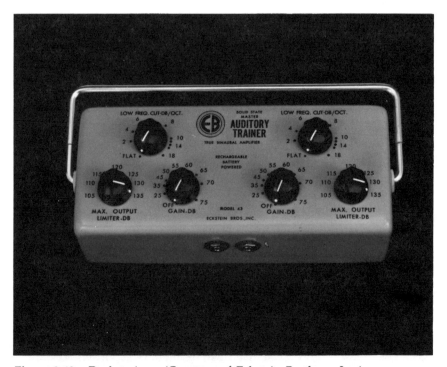

Figure 2.12. Desk trainer. (Courtesy of Eckstein Brothers, Inc.)

group hardwire units

Using the hardwire unit the teacher speaks into a microphone, and the amplified signal is led to any number of units placed at the children's desks. Each child typically has an individual volume control. Some units, however, have only a master volume control, which is generally adjusted by the teacher. Connected to the child's amplifier are the same type of cords with receiver or earphone as used in the desk-type units. Since the teacher is speaking directly into a microphone, the S/N ratio with these units is good. The disadvantages of hardwire units are that the teacher must remain in a fixed location, or move only in a limited area; similarly, the child's movement is limited to the length of the cords leading to the receiver or earphone. A wireless teacher's microphone is available with some hardwire units, permitting greater mobility for the teacher.

induction loop system

The induction loop system was popular in the 1960s in classrooms for the hearing impaired. The system involves a wire loop around the room—attached to the wall, under the outer edge of a carpet, or permanently mounted under a tile floor. A heavy current of electromagnetic energy runs through the wire loop which is altered by audio input from the teacher's microphone. This results in a magnetic field around the loop, which fills the room if it is not too large. The child wears a personal hearing aid set to the TEL (telephone) position for input. The telephone coil in the hearing aid will pick up the electromagnetic signal, convert it into an audio signal, and present it to the ear as if it were picked up by the microphone. The S/N ratio is excellent since only noises near the teacher's microphone will be transmitted to the child's hearing aid. Noises near the child, no matter what his position, will not reach his hearing aid when the aid is set on the TEL position.

The loop system is flexible inasmuch as the child can move anywhere within the room and still pick up a good signal. It is also possible to use other inputs in addition to the teacher's microphone, such as a phonograph, tape recorder, radio, or television set. Initially, one disadvantage of the loop system was that, although the child could hear the teacher, the child could not hear himself or other children in the class through the hearing aid. However, hearing aids became available with a combination microphone-telecoil switch so that both the signal within the loop and the signal picked up by the microphone are amplified and delivered to the child's ear.

Greater teacher and student mobility is possible with the loop system than with the desk auditory trainer or the hardwire system. However, the child and teacher are restricted to the area within the loop. Another disadvantage of this system is that it is susceptible to outside electrical interference, such as a ballast in a fluorescent light. Also, loop system energy spills over somewhat to adjacent areas although the energy beyond the loop gradually lessens. Thus, two adjacent classrooms sometimes cannot use a simple loop system due to spillover of energy from one room to the other. A number of unique solutions for the spillover problem have minimized this concern.

Use of induction loops is not necessarily confined to the educational setting; they can be used elsewhere—in the home environment or an auditorium. In some cases, loops are used to provide an ideal listening arrangement for TV or radio.

fm radio frequency units

The most recent development in auditory trainer systems is the FM radio frequency unit. Introduced several years ago, these wireless units are now used widely in classrooms as well as in churches, public auditoriums, and homes. With no outside wires and no installation of any sort, the FM system is flexible inasmuch as the teacher and children can be in a classroom, move outdoors, or go as a group to the lunchroom while still maintaining continuous reception. If two nearby classroom are using FM systems, they are merely placed on different broadcasting frequencies. With some FM systems one of several broadcast frequencies can be selected by a mere change of an external switch. With other systems frequency can only be changed by means of an internal control.

A serious problem for all sensorineural hearing losses while employing amplification is the possibility of an unfavorable signal-to-noise ratio. That is, as the primary signal is located farther and farther from the amplifier, the noise in the environment becomes a greater portion of the amplification received. Generally, the signal-to-noise ratio can be kept high by placing the speaker near the microphone of any hearing aid or auditory trainer; however, the FM auditory trainer system has an inherently good signal-to-noise ratio capability. Often the signal-to-noise ratio is underestimated, or not considered at all. However, considerable clinical evidence suggests that for the deaf child it is one of the most important aspects of amplification (Ross, 1982a).

An FM wireless system consists of a microphone-transmitter worn by the teacher and an FM receiver-plus-hearing-aid worn by the child (see Figure 2.13). The teacher's transmitter broadcasts by FM directly

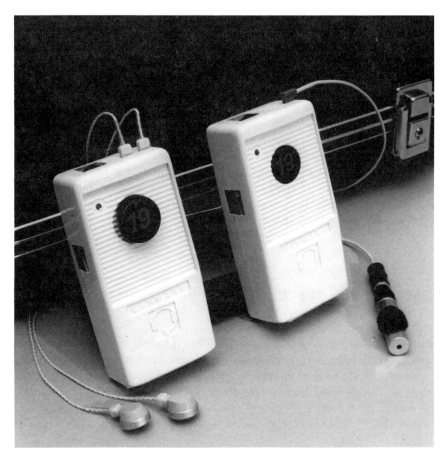

Figure 2.13. FM auditory trainer system. (Courtesy of Earmark, Inc.)

to the child's wearable unit on a frequency-modulated radio carrier wave. Inasmuch as the teacher's microphone is worn typically by means of a light-weight collar around the neck (lavalier microphone), with the microphone close to the mouth, the result is a good signal-to-noise ratio. Unlike that of the wired loop system, the power of the teacher's transmitter is sufficient to be picked up in even large classrooms or outdoors.

The students' wearable FM receiver units are typically powered by rechargeable batteries. Manufacturers make the battery rechargers so that a number of receiver units can be recharged at the same time. Required recharging time varies from one hour to overnight. With some systems a small light on the receiver goes on when the battery voltage is low.

The microphone of the FM receiver may also be activated, allowing receiver units to function as monaural or binaural body-type hearing aids at the same time that the FM signal is being received from the teacher. In this manner, the children can hear their own speech and that of others in the classroom. This is important since self-monitoring of speech is a critical element in auditory habilitation.

In summary, FM auditory trainer systems are the most popular and effective classroom amplification system in use. In this regard, Ross (1987) recently stated:

> In my judgement, the advent of the FM Auditory Training System has been the most significant educational tool for the average hearing-impaired child since the initial appearance of modern hearing aids. Indeed, historically, they may be the most powerful such tool we've ever had. (p. 4)

assistive devices

In addition to hearing aids and auditory trainers, a number of other devices have been designed for assisting those with hearing impairment. Several of these devices are briefly described in this section; further information is contained in Chapter 13.

for the deaf

Cochlear Implants. In the late 1950s and early 1960s, experimental work started on cochlear implant devices for profoundly hearing-impaired or deaf persons whose hearing was too poor to benefit from hearing aids. Experimental systems were first surgically implanted in patients in 1970. The device was approved for general use in 1984, and improved models are now being used in over 125 medical centers nationwide (Bebout, 1986).

The basic system employs an externally worn microphone and a signal processor about the size of a large body-type hearing aid, which processes incoming signals and transmits them by way of a magnetic induction device worn on the mastoid to a receiver which is surgically implanted in the mastoid. A microelectrode extends from the receiver into the cochlea, where it is inserted into the scala tympani.

The earliest devices employed a single processing channel and a single electrode, but multichannel, multi-electrode devices with 22 channels are now being implanted, which selectively distribute stimulation along much of the length of the cochlea. Early hopes were that cochlear implants would enable the profoundly deaf at least to perceive basic temporal, intensity, and frequency patterns of speech, but with the development of the more sophisticated systems, it is now evident that a portion of implanted patients can also identify a significant number of words; some can even engage in simple conversation without the help of visual clues. In addition, speechreading skills are routinely enhanced as a result of the increased information provided by the cochlear implant. Research on cochlear implantation devices is continuing at a rapid pace, and the general conviction is that increasingly more effective systems will be developed. At the present time, implants are being used exclusively with persons having profound hearing loss for whom hearing aids do not provide any significant improvements in hearing. (Chapter 12 contains a case study of an adult cochlear implant recipient.)

Vibrotactile Devices. The vibrotactile sense is limited somewhat in its ability to differentiate the intensity and frequency cues contained in sound. Nonetheless, in cases of profound deafness the perception of vibrotactile cues can be important by permitting, at a minimum, recognition of the presence or absence of sound, as well as useful information regarding the spectral, durational and rhythmic features of speech. Vibrotactile aids are employed in the educational setting, as well as in routine daily activities. They primarily are intended to supplement audition and vision rather than replace them in receptive communication, and may serve as a viable alternative to the cochlear implant for some deaf individuals.

Vibrotactile devices typically consist of a powerful body-type amplifier with small vibrator(s) attached by a harness or a velcro strip to the client's wrist or chest. It is anticipated that the use of these systems will increase as their design and efficiency improves.

Alarm and Signal Systems. A number of alarm and signal systems are available to the deaf. For example, a microphone may be placed next to or connected to the doorbell, which in turn sends a signal through a unit which activates a vibrator or turns on a signal light. Similarly, such a system can be programmed to flash a light when the telephone rings. Also, vibrating alarm clocks have an attachment to the bed springs or to a vibrator under the pillow; in this manner, when the alarm clock is set the person can be awakened.

Telecommunication Devices. Often the person with severe hearing impairment has to rely on a normally hearing individual for telephone communications. One solution to this problem is telecommunication devices for the deaf (TDD). The first TDDs employed teletypewriters, one at the location being called, the other at the caller's location. The caller would dial the number of the person having compatible equipment, place the telephone receiver in a special coupler (modem), and wait for the other party to answer the telephone. That person placed the receiver in a similar coupler and typed out a message. In this manner, the two individuals could communicate by typing out messages. TDD equipment now is available in portable versions only slightly larger than a telephone. These units can be found at many large businesses, government offices, and libraries, as well as the homes of the deaf. With the growing popularity of home computers the TDD speed and flexibility have been considerably improved.

for the hard of hearing

Telephone Devices. In addition to hearing aids with built-in telephone coils, mentioned earlier in this chapter, the person needing help during telephone usage has several other options. For example, telephone amplifiers are available which permit the telephone to be used as a regular instrument or, with a quick change of a dial, presents an amplified signal to the listener. Still another telephone device is a small, flat unit which slips over the telephone receiver and amplifies the incoming acoustic signal.

With some of the newer telephone models, the telephone coil cannot be used. However, a small device is now available which fastens over the telephone earpiece, making the telephone induction coil of the hearing aid compatible with the telephone.

Direct-Input Microphones. Some hearing aids are available with direct input (or audio input) capability. For these models a boot or shoe connects to the hearing aid. Connected to the boot is a wire, and at the other end a connector which may be attached to a television set, radio, tape recorder, or microphone. In this manner the wearer receives the input with a good signal-to-noise ratio. The boot can be quickly removed for regular hearing aid usage.

TV. A variety of options are available for the hard-of-hearing to provide improved reception of the audio signal during television viewing. These include the use of hardwire units, FM transmitter-receiver systems, and infrared transmitter-receiver systems. Each type of assistive device provides an enhanced audio signal, generally much improved over that received with a conventional hearing aid.

Theater/Church Devices.   FM and infrared transmitter-receiver systems are also available for use in many theaters, auditoriums and churches throughout the country. The growth in the number of facilities equipped with one of these assistive listening systems during the 1980s has been substantial, with several hundred currently operational. Their availability has made it possible for thousands of hearing-impaired person to more fully experience cultural and religious functions.

Tinnitus Maskers.   *Tinnitus,* a frequent accompaniment of sensorineural hearing loss, can be defined basically as ''noises in the head.'' The noise may be much like a pure tone, a roar, a buzz, or sound like surf. Often the tinnitus is more bothersome than the hearing loss itself. For some tinnitus sufferers, an external noise which masks the tinnitus lessens the problem. Some hearing aid manufacturers make devices called *tinnitus maskers* housed in plastic, ear-level hearing aid cases. The intent of these devices is not to amplify external sounds, as would a hearing aid, but to create an auditory signal that masks the tinnitus. This signal is directed into the canal of the ear having tinnitus. Success in treating excessive tinnitus with these units has varied considerably.

consumer information

A majority of states have laws regulating the sales and fitting of hearing aids. Persons with questions about sales practices or complaints about their hearing aid purchase may contact the state hearing aid licensing board, or the state consumer protection board if one is available.

In addition, the Food and Drug Administration (FDA) published a regulation, effective August 1977, covering certain aspects of hearing aid manufacture and fitting. All hearing aid models are required to be accompanied by specified technical data and warranty information. One of the provisions of the FDA regulation is that individuals with hearing loss shall have a medical evaluation by a licensed physician within 6 months preceding the sale of the hearing aid. Fully informed adults may request that the medical evaluation be waived, however. Hearing aid dispensers are prohibited from actively encouraging individuals to exercise the waiver option.

The FDA regulations also require that instructional brochures describing the hearing aid be provided to prospective purchasers, and that the dispenser retain certain documentation relating to the hearing aid fitting and sale.

---

summary

During the past five decades the technology of hearing aids has improved dramatically. Today, hearing aids are smaller, less expensive to operate, cost less in reference to the buying power of the dollar, have better fidelity, and permit greater flexibility of electroacoustic manipulation than those available in the past. The scientific fitting of hearing aids has made slower progress than the technological aspects. Nonetheless, the hearing aid is more important in auditory habilitation and rehabilitation than ever before. Hearing aid fitting constitutes a first and critical step in habilitation or rehabilitation. In addition to conventional hearing aids, technology has also permitted the development of a large assortment of related assistive devices for the hearing impaired which can be helpful as well.

One of the most promising developments in hearing aid design in recent times is the digital hearing aid. This device transforms speech signals into a series of digital values which are processed by special logic circuits before being presented to the listener. The processor can alter the signal in many desirable ways. Precise control of hearing aid frequency response is possible, including adaptive filtering, in which a hearing aid automatically alters its response to changes in the wearer's listening environment. Another very important advantage is the ability to detect and reduce background noise to enhance the intelligibility of speech.

The digital conversion, modification, and reconversion of the signal for playback takes time, but this time must be made very short so that it will not be discerned by the listener. Such super-fast processing has been accomplished in the laboratory, but the required complex circuitry is too bulky at the present time for widespread public acceptance in wearable amplification. It is likely, however, that the problems will be solved rapidly and that wearable digital hearing aids will be available in the near future (Schmier, 1987; Staab, 1985).

The improvements in conventional hearing aids, the introduction of probe-tube microphone measures, the development of cochlear implants, vibrotactile devices, and digital hearing aids, and the application of assistive devices all are significant advancements. The new technology provides professionals with an increased opportunity to meet the complex needs of the hearing impaired.

recommended readings

ASHA-American Speech-Language-Hearing Association. (1986). Cochlear implants. Report of the Ad Hoc Committee on Cochlear Implants. *Asha, 28*(4), 29-52.

Berger, K.W. (1984). *The hearing aid: Its operation and development* (3rd ed.). Livonia, MI: National Hearing Aid Society.

Hodgson, W.R. (Ed.). (1986). *Hearing aid assessment and use in audiologic habilitation* (3rd ed.). Baltimore: The Williams & Wilkins Co.

Pollack, M.C. (Ed.). (1988). *Amplification for the hearing-impaired* (3rd ed.). New York: Grune & Stratton.

Skinner, M. (1988). *Hearing aid evaluation.* Englewood Cliffs, NJ: Prentice-Hall.

Staab, W.J. (1978). *Hearing aid handbook.* Blue Ridge Summit, PA: Tab Books.

references

American National Standards Institute. (1960). *Methods for measurement of electroacoustical characteristics of hearing aids. ANSI S3 3-1960.* New York: American National Standards Institute.

American National Standards Institute. (1967). *Method of expressing hearing aid performance. ANSI S3,* 8. New York: American National Standards Institute.

American National Standards Institute. (1969). *American national standard specifications for audiometers. ANSI, S3.* New York: American National Standards Institute.

American National Standards Institute. (1976). *Specifications for hearing aid.* New York: American National Standards Institute.

American National Standards Institute. (1987). *Standard for specification of hearing aid characteristics. ANSI S3,* 22. New York: American National Standards Institute.

ASHA-American Speech-Language-Hearing Association. (1985). FDA approves cochlear implant. *Asha, 27,* 9.

Beattie, R.C., & Edgerton, B.J. (1976). Reliability of monosyllabic discrimination tests in white noise for differentiating among hearing aids. *Journal of Speech and Hearing Disorders, 41,* 464-476.

Bebout, J. (1986). Update: Cochlear implants. *Hearing Journal, 39*(8), 7-14.

Berger, K.W. (1980). The search for a master hearing aid. In M. Pollack (Ed.), *Amplification for the hearing impaired* (2nd ed., pp. 325-380). New York: Grune & Stratton.

Berger, K.W. (1983). *Berger hearing aid prescription computer program in BASIC and in FORTRAN.* Kent, OH: Speech and Hearing Clinic, Kent State University.

Berger, K.W. (1984). *The hearing aid: Its operation and development* (3rd ed.). Livonia, MI: National Hearing Aid Society.

Berger, K.W., & Millin, J.P. (1978). Hearing aids. In E.E. Rose (Ed.), *Audiological assessment* (2nd ed., pp. 495-538). Englewood Cliffs, NJ: Prentice-Hall.

Brooks, D. (1973). Gain requirements of hearing aid users. *Scandinavian Audiology, 2,* 199-305.

Brooks, D., Tonnison, W. (1976). Selecting the gain of hearing aids for persons with sensorineural hearing impairments. *Scandinavian Audiology, 5,* 51-59.

Byrne, D. (1987). Hearing aid selection formulae: Same or different? *Hearing Instruments, 38,* 511.

Carhart, R. (1946). Selection of hearing aids. *Archives of Otolaryngology, 14,* 1-18.

Carlson, E.V. (1973). A subminiature condenser microphone. *Hearing Instruments, 24,* 12-13.

Castle, D.L. (1981). Telecommunication and the hearing impaired. *Volta Review, 83,* 5, 275-284.

Cox, R. (1988). The MSU hearing instrument prescription procedure. *Hearing Instruments, 39*(1), 6-10.

Craig, C., Siegenthaler, B. (1980, November). *Preliminary hearing aid selection (PHASS) by computer.* Paper presented at Annual Convention of the American Speech-Language-Hearing Association, Detroit.

Davis, H., & Silverman, S.R. (Eds.). (1978). *Hearing and deafness* (4th ed.). New York: Holt, Rinehart & Winston.

Davis, H., Steven, S.S., Nichols, Jr., R.H., Hudgins, C.V., Marquis, R.J., Peterson, G.E., & Ross, D.A. (1947). *Hearing aids: An experimental study of design objectives.* Cambridge, MA: Harvard University Press.

Hakansson, B., Tjellstrom, A., Rosehall, U. (1984). Hearing thresholds with direct bone conduction versus conventional bone conduction. *Scandinavian Audiology, 13,* 1-13.

Harford, E. (1979). Hearing aid amplification for adults. *Monographs in Contemporary Audiology, 13,* 1-37.

Hearing aid industry conference standard method of expressing hearing aid performance. (1961). New York: Hearing Aid Industry Conference.

Hertzano, T., Levitt, H., & Slosberg, R. (1979). *Computer-assisted hearing-aid selection.* Paper presented at 97th meeting of the Acoustical Society of America.

Hough, J., Vernon, J., Johnson, B., Dormer, K., & Himelik, T. (1986). Experiences with implantable hearing devices and a presentation of a new device. *Annals of Otology, Rhinology and Laryngology, 95*(1), 60-65.

Jerger, J.F. (1967). Behavioral correlates of hearing-aid performance. *Bulletin of Prosthetic Research, 7,* 62-75.

Katz, K. (1984). *Computer assisted hearing aid fitting sales program.* Tucson, AZ: Katz Computer Software.

Kee, W.R. (1972). Use of pure tone measurement in hearing aid fittings. *Audecibel, 21,* 9-15.

Keith, R.W., & Sininger, L. (1978). "New ideas"? in hearing aid selection. *Hearing Instruments, 29,* 6-8, 34.

Libby, E. (1986). The 1/2 – 2/3 insertion gain hearing and selection guide. *Hearing Instruments, 3,* 27-28.

Lybarger, S.F. (1953). *Simplified fitting system for hearing aids* (rev. ed.). Canonsburg, PA: Radioear Corp.

Mahon, W. (1987). U.S. hearing aid sales summary. *The Hearing Journal, 40,* 9-14.

McCandless, G., & Lyregaard, P. (1983). Prescription of gain/output (POGO) for hearing aids. *Hearing Instruments, 1,* 16-21.

McCandless, G.A., & Miller, D.L. (1972). Loudness discomfort and hearing aids. *National Hearing Aid Journal, 25,* 7, 28, 32.

Millin, J.P. (1965). *Speech discrimination as a function of hearing aid gain: Implications in hearing-aid evaluation.* Unpublished master's thesis, Case Western Reserve University, Cleveland.

Millin, J.P. (1978). Basic hearing aid electronics. In L. Bradford (Ed.), *The audio journal.* New York: Grune & Stratton.

Millin, J.P. (1988). Practical and philosophical considerations. In M. Pollack (Ed.), *Amplification for the hearing impaired* (3rd ed., pp. 145-174). New York: Grune & Stratton.

Pascoe, D.P. (1975). Frequency responses of hearing aids and their effect on the speech perception of hearing impaired subjects. *Annals of Otology, Rhinology and Laryngology, 84* (Suppl. 23), 1-40.

Pascoe, D.P. (1978). An approach to hearing aid selection. *Hearing Instruments, 29,* 12-16, 36.

Pollack, M.C. (1988). Electroacoustic characteristics. In M. Pollack (Ed.), *Amplification for the hearing impaired* (3rd ed., pp. 21-104). New York: Grune & Stratton.

Popelka, G. (1982). *Hearing aid selection and evaluation program.* St. Louis: Central Institute for the Deaf.

Posner, J., & Ventry, I.M. (1977). Relationships between comfortable loudness levels for speech and speech discrimination in sensorineural hearing loss. *Journal of Speech and Hearing Disorders, 42,* 370-375.

Reddell, R.C., & Calvert, D.R. (1966). Selecting a hearing-aid by interpreting audiologic data. *Journal of Audiology Research, 6,* 445-452.

Resnick, D., & Becker, M. (1963). Hearing aid evaluation—A new approach. *Asha, 5,* 695-699.

Ross, M. (1977). Binaural vs. monaural hearing aid amplification for hearing impaired individuals. In F.H. Bess (Ed.), *Childhood deafness: Causes, assessment, and management* (pp. 235-249). New York: Grune & Stratton.

Ross, M. (1982a). Communication access. In G.A. Studebaker & F.H. Bess (Eds.), *The Vanderbilt hearing aid report.* Upper Darby, PA: *Monographs in Contemporary Audiology.*

Ross, M. (1982b). *Hard of hearing children in regular schools.* Englewood Cliffs, NJ: Prentice-Hall.

Ross, M. (1987). FM auditory training systems as an educational tool. *Hearing Rehabilitation Quarterly, 12*(4), 4-6.

Schmitz, H. (1969). Loudness discomfort level modifications. *Journal of Speech and Hearing Research, 12,* 807-817.

Schnier, W. (1987). Digital technology: The market impact. *Hearing Instruments,* *38*, 814.

Shapiro, I. (1975). Prediction of most comfortable loudness levels in hearing aid evaluation. *Journal of Speech and Hearing Disorders, 40,* 434-438.

Shapiro, I. (1976). Hearing aid fitting by prescription. *Audiology, 15,* 163-170.

Shore, I., Bilger, R.C., & Hirsh, I.J. (1960). Hearing aid evaluation: Reliability of repeated practices. *Journal of Speech and Hearing Disorders, 28,* 159-170.

Smaldino, J., & Hoene, J. (1981). Part I: A view of the state of hearing aid fitting practices. *Hearing Instruments, 32,* 1.

Sprung, A.K., & Miller, M.H. (1956). *A study of the variability of discrimination scores as a result of exposure to amplification and training.* Paper presented at the annual convention of the American Speech and Hearing Association, Chicago.

Staab, W. (1978). *Hearing aid handbook.* Blue Ridge Summit, PA: Tab Books.

Staab, W. (1985). Digital hearing aids. *Hearing Instruments, 11,* 14-24.

Thompson, G., & Lassman, F. (1969). Relationship of auditory distortion test results to speech discrimination through flat versus selective amplifying systems. *Journal of Speech and Hearing Research, 12,* 594-606.

Tonnison, W. (1975). Measuring in-the-ear gain of hearing aids by the acoustic reflex method. *Journal of Speech and Hearing Research, 18,* 17-30.

Vaughn, G.R., Lightfoot, R.K., & Gibbs, S.D. (1983). Assistive listening devices. Part III: SPACE. *Asha, 25,* 33-46.

Victoreen, J.A. (1960). *Hearing enhancement.* Springfield, IL: Charles C. Thomas Publisher.

Walden, B., Schwartz, D., Williams, D., Holum-Hardegen, L., & Crawley, J. Test of the assumptions underlying comparative hearing aid evaluations. *Journal of Speech and Hearing Disorders, 48,* 264-273.

Watson, N.A., & Knudsen, V.O. (1940). Selective amplification in hearing aids. *Journal of the Society of America, 11,* 406-419.

Whitcomb, C. (1982). *A survey of aural rehabilitation services among ASHA audiologists.* Unpublished master's thesis, Idaho State University.

Winchester, R.A. (1960). Modern concepts of aural rehabilitation. *Audecibel, 9,* 10-11.

Zenith Hearing Instrument Corporation. (1968). *Hearing aids and their components.* Chicago: Zenith Hearing Instrument Corp.

Zerlin, S. (1962). A new approach to hearing-aid selection. *Journal of Speech and Hearing Research, 5,* 370-376.

Zink, J. (1972). Hearing aids children wear: A longitudinal study of performance. *Volta Review, 74,* 41-51.

chapterthree

AUDITORY STIMULI IN COMMUNICATION

MICHAEL A. NERBONNE

RONALD L. SCHOW

contents

introduction

Traditionally, the ability to communicate meaningfully has been considered an important factor in differentiating humans from other forms of life. A human act of communication can take a variety of forms, involving the conveyance of various stimuli to one or more of our sensory modalities. However, the form most often used to express oneself involves utilization of speech. This results in extraordinary dependence on the sense of hearing to adequately receive and perceive the complex network of auditory stimuli which comprise oral communication. Audition, therefore, can be considered our most important sense.

The onset of a significant auditory impairment in an individual can seriously impede the ability to communicate. Although a hearing loss may trigger other difficulties of a psychosocial, educational, or vocational nature, it often is the hearing-impaired person's inability to communicate normally which causes these other problems.

Based on the critical role of audition in communication, aural rehabilitation represents an extremely important process whereby an individual's diminished ability to communicate as the result of a hearing loss can hopefully be sharpened and improved. One of the areas of aural rehabilitation which has traditionally been included in this process is *auditory training*. This procedure generally involves an attempt to assist the hearing-impaired child or adult in maximizing the use of whatever residual hearing remains.

This chapter will provide information regarding auditory training with the hearing impaired, including objectives and applications, assessment of auditory skills prior to therapy, past and present approaches to auditory training, and trends related to future use of this facet of aural rehabilitation. Because of the conviction that the professional providing auditory training must be familiar with the basic aspects of oral communication, information is also provided about the oral communication process. This includes the introduction of a communication model, information regarding auditory perception and the acoustics of speech, and a discussion of the possible effects of hearing loss on speech perception.

a communication model

Although a portion of the communication which normally takes place between individuals is nonverbal, we remain heavily dependent upon our ability to receive and interpret auditory stimuli presented during oral communication. Successful communication involves a number of key components which deserve elaboration so that the reader may gain an appreciation of the basic oral communication process.

All oral communication must originate with a source or *speaker* who has (a) a purpose for engaging in communication and (b) the ability to properly encode and articulate the thought to be conveyed. The actual thought to be expressed is termed the *message*. The message is made up of auditory stimuli which are organized in meaningful linguistic units. Visual cues are also provided in conjunction with the production of the auditory message. A critical component of the encoding process is the *feedback mechanism*, made up primarily of the auditory system of the speaker, which makes it possible to monitor, and if need be, correct the accuracy of the intended message. The communication situation in which the message is conveyed is referred to as the *environment*. Factors associated with the environment, such as the presence of competing background noise, can drastically alter the amount and quality of the communication which takes place. The final major component of the communication process is the receiver or *listener*, who is charged with the responsibility of receiving and properly decoding and interpreting the speaker's intended thought.

These basic components of the oral communication process and their sequence are found in Figure 3.1. All the major components are equally important in accomplishing the desired end—communication. Disruption or elimination of any one part may result in partial or complete failure of the communication process. Proper application of the communication model concerns us in this chapter and throughout the book.

auditory perception

Our ability to communicate verbally with others depends to a great extent on the quality of our auditory perception of the various *segmental* (individual speech sounds) and *suprasegmental* (rate, rhythm, intonation)

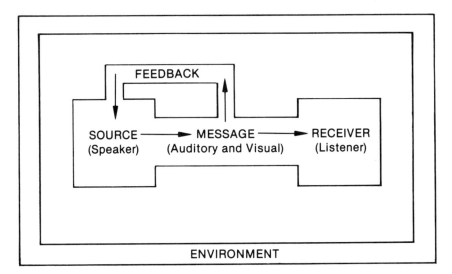

Figure 3.1. Simple model of normal communication process.

elements that comprise speech. The following sections will focus on the auditory perception of nonspeech stimuli, the intensity, frequency, and duration components of speech, as well as transitional cues. The impact of hearing loss is also discussed.

development of auditory skills

Substantial evidence indicates that the newborn infant possesses a functional auditory system, which allows the child to perceive auditory stimuli several weeks prior to birth (Bench, 1968; Eisenberg, 1965a, 1965b; Eisenberg, Griffin, Coursin, & Hunter, 1964; Johansson, Wedenberg, & Westin, 1964; Schulman, 1970). Rapid development and refinement in the neonate's auditory processing skills in the days and weeks immediately following birth have been demonstrated by Eisenberg (1970). Her findings indicate that the newborn infant is capable not only of detecting auditory stimuli, but also of making gross discriminations between various auditory signals on the basis of frequency and intensity parameters. This process of selective listening is extended to phonemic signals within a few weeks following birth (Eimas, 1975; Eisenberg, 1976; Moffitt, 1971). The rather rapid emergence of auditory skills, as described by Northern and Downs (1984), is crucial for the development of speech and language in the infant. Without the benefit of ample auditory stimulation, however, the development of language will be seriously effected. Although the basic auditory skills necessary for the normal acquisition of language and speech are present to some degree at birth or shortly thereafter, these skills are sharpened during the early years of an individual's life.

perception of nonspeech stimuli

Although the human auditory system has sophisticated perceptual capabilities, it is limited, to some extent, in terms of the signals it can process. Optimally, the normal human ear is capable of perceiving auditory signals comprised of frequencies ranging from about 20-20,000 Hz. Stimuli made up entirely of frequencies below and above these limits cannot be detected. Intensity limits, as shown in Figure 3.2, vary as a function of the frequency of the auditory stimulus. The maximum range of intensity we are capable of processing occurs at 3,000-4,000 Hz, and varies from about 0-140 dB SPL. Signals with less intensity than 0 dB SPL are generally not perceived; in contrast, signals in excess of 140 dB SPL produce the sensation of pain rather than hearing.

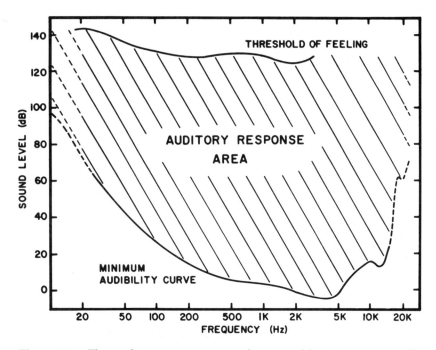

Figure 3.2. The auditory response area for normal-hearing persons. (From Durrant & Lovrinic, 1984, Baltimore, MD: Williams & Wilkins Co. Reprinted by permission.)

In addition to the detection of acoustic signals, the human ear is also able to discriminate different stimuli on the basis of only minor differences in their acoustical properties. The study of our ability to discriminate differences in auditory signals has centered around three parameters of sound, namely, frequency, intensity, and duration. Results of such investigations have revealed a complex interaction between these variables. Thus, our ability to discriminate changes in the frequency, intensity, or duration of a signal is influenced by the magnitude of each of the other factors. Stevens and Davis (1938) estimated that the normal ear is capable of perceiving approximately 340,000 distinguishable tones within the audible range of hearing. This total number was based on only frequency and intensity variations, and it suggests that our auditory system possesses amazing discrimination powers.

acoustics of speech

Knowledge about the acoustical properties of speech is important for understanding how speech is perceived. Therefore, basic information relevant to this process will be covered in the following sections.

Intensity Parameters of Speech. The human ear is capable of processing signals with an intensity approaching 130-140 dB SPL; however, the range of intensity normally found in speech is relatively small. When measured at a distance of approximately 1 meter from the speaker, Fletcher (1953) reported that the average intensity of connected speech approximates 65 dB SPL. This corresponds to a value of 45 dB HL when expressed audiometrically. The average shout will approach 85 dB SPL (65 dB HL), while faint speech occurs at about 45 dB SPL (25 dB HL). Thus, a range of about 40 dB typifies the softest to the loudest connected speech we are exposed to in common communication situations. Factors such as distance between speaker and listener can influence the intensity levels for a given communication situation.

Considerable variability exists in the acoustical energy associated with individual speech sounds. Table 3.1 lists the relative phonetic powers of the phonemes, as reported by Fletcher (1953). As illustrated, the most powerful phoneme, /ɔ/, possesses an average of about 680 times as much energy as the weakest phoneme, /θ/, representing an average overall difference in intensity between the two speech sounds of approximately 28 dB. Since a considerable amount of variability exists in the intensity of individual voices, Fletcher estimated that, collectively, different speakers may produce variations in the intensity of these two phonemes

TABLE 3.1
Relative Phonetic Power of Speech Sounds
as Produced by an Average Speaker

ɔ	680	l	100	t	15
ɑ	600	ʃ	80	g	15
ʌ	510	ŋ	73	k	13
æ	490	m	52	v	12
ʊ	460	tʃ	42	ð	11
ɛ	350	n	36	b	7
u	310	dʒ	23	d	7
ɪ	260	ʒ	20	p	6
i	220	z	16	f	5
r	210	s	16	θ	1

From *Speech and Hearing in Communication* by H. Fletcher, 1953, Princeton: D. VanNostrand.

as great as 56 dB. The relative power of vowels, according to Fletcher, is significantly greater than that of consonants, with the weakest vowel, /i/, having more energy than the most powerful consonant or semivowel, /ɜ/. Further, male speakers produce speech of an overall intensity about 3 dB greater than do females.

Frequency Parameters of Speech. The longtime average spectrum of speech, as seen in Figure 3.3, is composed of acoustical energy from approximately 50-10,000 Hz (Denes & Pinson, 1973). Closer examination of this figure also reveals that the greatest amount of energy in connected discourse occurs in the vicinity of 100-800 Hz. Above this frequency region, the energy of speech decreases at about a 9 dB/octave rate. The concentration of energy in the lower frequencies can be largely attributed to the fundamental frequency of the adult human voice (males - 130 Hz, females-260 Hz; Zemlin, 1981) and the high intensity and spectral characteristics associated with the production of vowels. It should be noted that the fundamental frequency of children is substantially higher than that of adults, around 450 Hz (McGlone, 1966). As a result, the major energy concentration for this age group occurs higher on the frequency scale than for adults.

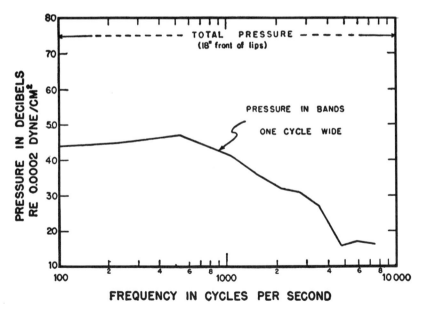

Figure 3.3. Long-interval acoustic spectrum of male voices. Measurement made with microphone 17 inches from speaker's lips (Miller, 1951).

The vowels in our language are comprised almost entirely of low-frequency energy and, as indicated earlier, contribute most of the acoustic power in speech. Specifically, the frequency spectrum of each vowel contains at least two or three areas of energy concentration which result from the resonances which occur in the vocal tract during phonation. These points of peak amplitude are referred to as *formants*, and their location on the frequency continuum varies for each vowel. Figure 3.4 illustrates the approximate location of the major formants associated with

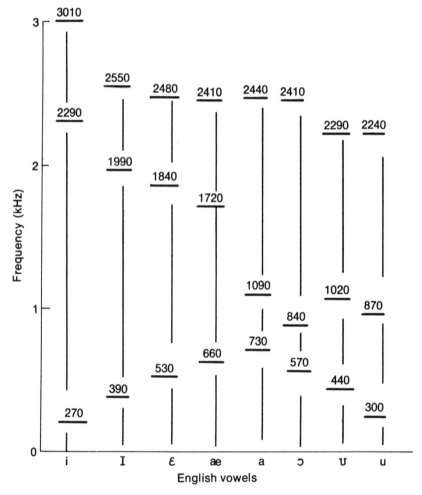

Figure 3.4. Mean values of formant frequencies for adult males of vowels of American English. (From "Control Methods Used in the Study of the Vowels" by G. E. Peterson & H. L. Barney, 1952, *Journal of the Acoustical Society of America, 32*, pp. 693–703.)

the vowels, as spoken by adult males. Even though vowels generally have several formants, we need only hear the first two or three to be able to accurately perceive the vowel spoken (Peterson & Barney, 1952).

The consonants in our language display a broader high-frequency spectral composition, with much more high-frequency energy than vowels. This is particularly true for those consonants for which voicing is not utilized and whose production involves substantial constriction of the articulators. Although they contain relatively little overall energy when compared with vowels, consonants are extremely important in determining the intelligibility of words and phrases in speech. Consequently, accurate perception of consonants is vital.

Figure 3.5 contains estimates of the combined intensity and frequency values associated with the speech sounds in our language. Specifically,

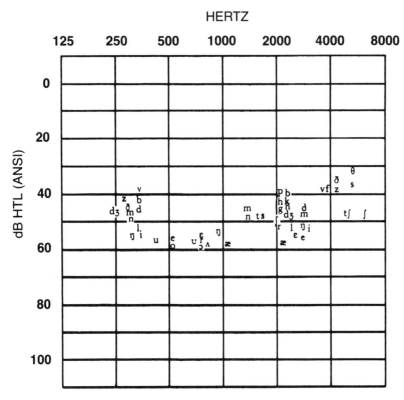

Figure 3.5. Intensity and frequency distribution of speech sounds in the English language. The values given should only be considered as approximations, and are based on data reported by Fletcher (1953) and Ling and Ling (1978). Sounds with more than one major component appear in the figure in more than one location.

the vertical axis presents the intensity levels in dB HL of the major components of each sound (if a particular sound has more than one major frequency component, each is noted by the same phonetic symbol), while the horizontal axis expresses the general frequency region for each speech sound. A close inspection of this figure discloses, as indicated earlier, that the vowels can generally be characterized as having considerable acoustic energy, for the most part confined to the low- and mid-frequency range. On the other hand, the consonants demonstrate decidedly less intensity overall and a much more diffuse frequency spectrum as a group. The voiced consonants generally possess a greater amount of low- and mid-frequency energy, while the unvoiced consonants are made up of mid and high frequencies. All consonants appear in the upper portion of the figure, reflecting their weaker intensity values.

In addition to the spectral properties associated with each of the consonants, it is important to identify the frequency characteristics associated with the distinctive features of these phonemes. Miller and Nicely's (1955) classification system includes five features: *voicing, nasality, affrication, duration,* and *place of articulation.* According to Boothroyd (1978), the voiced/voiceless distinction, as well as cues for nasality and affrication, are primarily carried by low-frequency energy. Information about place of articulation, on the other hand, is contained in the higher frequencies. Table 3.2 categorizes each consonant phoneme by its place and manner features and voicing.

TABLE 3.2
Categorizing Consonants on the Basis of
Manner and Place of Articulation and Voicing

Manner of Articulation	Place of Articulation						
	Bilabial	Labiodental	Linguadental	Alveolar	Palatal	Velar	Glottal
Plosives or Stops	p b			t d		k g	
Fricatives		f v	θ ð	s z	ʃ 3		h
Affricate					tʃ d_3		
Nasal	m			n		ŋ	
Liquid				l,r			
Glide	w				j		

Note: Voiceless consonants are listed first, with voiced consonants underneath.

Finally, as indicated by Ling (1978), the important suprasegmental aspects of speech (e.g., intonation, rhythm, pitch, stress) are conveyed primarily by the low-frequency components of speech.

Temporal Parameters of Speech. The duration of individual speech sounds in our language covers a range from about 30 to about 300 msec (Lehiste, 1976). A number of factors can significantly influence the duration of a given phoneme, making the direct comparison of duration among phonemes difficult. Yet, the research of Crandall (1925), as cited by Fletcher (1953) and Lisker (1957), suggests that vowels generally have a longer duration than consonants. Fletcher considered vowels to have average durations of between 130-360 msec, while the duration of consonants ranges from 20-150 msec. In spite of variations in the absolute durational properties of individual phonemes, duration does contribute toward speech perception. For instance, Minifie (1973) pointed out that the duration of stop consonants (examples: /p/ and /b/) varies systematically in a vowel-consonant-vowel context, with correct perception of the speech sound being dependent, to a degree, on the durational property of the phoneme produced.

The research of Goldman-Eisler, as discussed by Lehiste (1970), served to establish the average rates of speech during connected discourse. Thus, investigation showed that the speed of the articulatory movements associated with the production of speech sounds ranges from 4.4 to 5.9 syllables per second. The normal rate of speech, as expressed in phoneme output, will result in the production of as many as 15 phonemes per second (Orr, Friedman, & Williams, 1965). Thus, the articulatory process is swift and capable of producing a flood of speech sounds which must be processed as effectively by the receiver as they were produced by the speaker.

Transitional Cues. The acoustic properties of a given phoneme spoken in isolation are altered significantly when produced in connected discourse. In connected discourse the dynamic movements of the articulators in the production of adjacent phonemes produce acoustical biproducts, termed *transitional cues.* These cues make up a large portion of the total speech signal and are utilized extensively in the perception of speech, since they contain valuable information related to individual phoneme perception.

For example, the second and third formants of vowels often contain transitions in frequency that signal the presence of particular consonants that immediately follow. These formant transitions occur as the vocal resonances shift during articulation of vowels and consonants which are combined in speech. Likewise, the durational aspects of vowels in connected speech can be altered to convey information regarding the phoneme to follow. For example, a voiced consonant in the final position is often accompanied by increased duration of the vowel immediately before it. The prolonged vowel duration contributes to our perception of voicing in the consonant which precedes it. Consequently, transitional cues are an important part of speech perception.

speech perception/comprehension

Our discussion has emphasized the segmental and suprasegmental aspects that comprise speech. The organization and production of these crucial elements into a meaningful oral message by the speaker and the accurate reception of this dynamic signal by the listener represent a highly complex, sophisticated process. However, mere reception of the speech stimuli by a listener does not result in proper perception of the message. Perception of speech implies understanding and comprehension, and the reception of speech signals by the auditory mechanism is only a first step in its perception.

Although somewhat simplistic, the perception/comprehension of speech may be thought of as involving a number of components. Among these are:

Detection—This aspect of perception involves experiencing the awareness of sound. Our ability to detect speech is influenced by our hearing acuity and the intensity level of the speech signal.

Discrimination—Speech discrimination refers to the ability to distinguish between the individual speech stimuli (phonemes, syllables, etc.) of our language. How accurately we perceive the individual elements of speech is of relevance.

Identification—The ability to identify or label what one has heard by repeating, pointing to, or writing a word or sentence.

Attention—A fundamental ingredient in the perception of speech relates to attending to the speaker and the message being conveyed. The degree and quality of the listener's attention will influence how well speech is perceived.

Memory—A key component in speech perception is the ability to retain or store verbal information for relatively brief periods of time or, in some instances, for extended lengths of time. Memory is also fundamental to other components of speech perception and enables us to combine individual speech units for the purpose of deriving meaning from an entire verbal message, rather than from each individual unit of the message.

Closure—The speech elements which are received, properly discriminated, and retained for further processing must be brought together into a meaningful whole. This is a difficult task at best, but when we do not adequately receive all the contents of a verbal message, as with a hearing loss, closure can still occur through a process wherein missing information is deduced on the basis of the available context.

Each of these components combine to enable us to comprehend or perceive the meaning of verbal expressions. At the present time we understand very little about how this occurs. However, a number of theories have been proposed concerning the process of speech perception. McKay (1956) classified the many theories which have been offered to explain how speech is perceived into one of two categories. *Active theories* of speech perception share the view that decoding of speech stimuli involves a close neurological association with the production of speech. Consistent with this is the belief that the perception of speech is influenced by the articulatory patterns that are associated with the production of speech. *Passive theories*, on the other hand, are based largely on the notion that the neural structures of the auditory system are capable of achieving perception as a direct result of the decoding of the complex physical properties contained in speech. The mediating role of phonation is not considered in the passive theories as contributing to the perception process.

Recent attempts to describe the speech-perception process tend to center around a blending of some of the features of already existing theories (Perkins, 1971; Sanders, 1977). Thus, many of the individuals responsible for synthesizing the active and passive models of speech perception have begun to recognize that no one approach is capable of entirely explaining the speech perception process. For example, Denes (1967) stated: ''just as with many other kinds of human activity, there is probably more than one method by which speech perception can be achieved and normally we may well use several different methods simultaneously'' (p. 312).

Our task in aural rehabilitation should be to take into consideration what is currently known concerning speech perception as we work with individuals with hearing impairments.

speech perception and hearing loss

Our success in processing speech stimuli is closely related to our ability to receive the coded acoustical information which comprises the signal. Hence hearing impairment may have grave implications for proper speech perception. In the following section, we shall consider the effects of physical properties of speech and redundancy and constraints on speech perception.

Physical Properties. Information concerning the physical properties of speech is most relevant when considering the relationship between the perception of speech and hearing loss, for the degree of our success in processing speech stimuli appears closely related to our ability to receive the coded acoustical information which comprises the signal.

The normal ear is well equipped to receive and process speech. Speech is normally presented at intensity levels well within the sensitivity limits of the human ear. Also, although we are capable of hearing auditory signals ranging in frequency from about 20-20,000 Hz, only a portion of the entire range is required for the reception of speech, since it contains energy from roughly 50-10,000 Hz. Consequently, in most listening conditions, the normal-hearing will have no difficulty in adequately receiving the speech sounds of our language.

The same does not hold true for the hard of hearing. No longer are the intensity and frequency ranges of the ear always sufficient to provide total perception of speech. One or both of these stimulus parameters may be limited such that it becomes difficult to hear specific speech sounds adequately enough for identification purposes. The information in Figure 3.5 regarding the relative frequency and intensity characteristics of individual speech sounds is significant in explaining why this occurs.

While factors such as type of hearing loss and test materials can influence the outcome of investigations concerning hearing loss and speech discrimination of phonemes, some general patterns of speech discrimination difficulties have been observed for persons with hearing loss. For instance, most hearing-impaired listeners experience only minimal difficulty in vowel perception (Owens, Benedict, & Schubert, 1971). Specifically, in their research the vowel phonemes /ɛ/ and /o/ were found to have the highest probability of error. Only when the degree of impairment is severe to profound does the perception of vowels become significantly altered (Erber, 1979). Consonant perception, however, presents a far more difficult listening task for the hearing impaired. Owens (1978) found phonemes such as /s/, /p/, /k/, /d/, and /θ/ to be among the most frequently missed by adults with sensorineural hearing loss. He also found discrimination errors to be more frequent for phonemes in the final position of words than in the initial position. The most common errors in consonant phoneme discrimination occur with the place of articulation feature (Boothroyd, 1978; Byers, 1973; Owens, 1978), followed by manner of articulation. Errors in the perception of nasality and voice among consonants are generally far less frequent.

Owens and his colleagues have conducted a series of investigations regarding speech discrimination of consonants. In one such study Owens et al. (1972) examined the relationship between the configuration of the audiogram and the specific consonant errors made by a group of hearing-impaired individuals. The /s/, /ʃ/, /tʃ/, /dʒ/ in initial and final word positions, and the /t/ and /θ/ in the initial position only, were found to be difficult for listeners with sloping configurations. The authors noted that these phonemes became increasingly difficult to accurately hear as the steepness of the sloping high-frequency hearing loss increased. Correct recognition of /s/ and the initial /t/ and /θ/ was found to be closely related to hearing sensitivity above 2,000 Hz, while perception of /ʃ/, /tʃ/, and /dʒ/ was very dependent on sensitivity between 1,000-2,000 Hz. These findings point out the crucial role which hearing in this frequency region plays in the perception of several consonant phonemes. A similar study by Sher and Owens (1974) with listeners having high-frequency impairments confirmed that individuals with normal hearing to 2,000 Hz and a sharp sloping sensitivity loss above that experience difficulty in adequately hearing a number of consonant phonemes. These authors pointed out that information concerning phoneme errors is useful in establishing aural rehabilitation strategies for persons with hearing losses of this type.

The actual handicap imposed on an individual is closely related to the intensity and frequency features of the hearing loss. It can also be influenced by other related variables, to be discussed elsewhere in this chapter and throughout the text. Therefore, although research by Walden and Montgomery (1975) and Bilger and Wang (1976) supports the notion that the audiogram is our most useful single predictor of speech perception, predictions made only on the basis of pure-tone audiometry must be done with caution as they are prone to some degree of error (Sher & Owens, 1974).

Redundancy and Constraints. Another factor of importance in speech perception relates to what is termed *redundancy*, an aspect of speech which allows the listener to predict accurately those portions of a spoken message which were not heard clearly. Fortunately, redundancy normally is high and closely linked with certain constraints in our communication.

Three major types of constraints generally are associated with redundancy in speech: (a) structural, (b) semantic, and (c) situational. Structural constraints relate to the manner in which linguistic units are chained together in English. Selection and use of phonemes and words in an utterance are strongly influenced by the linguistic material that precedes them. For example, producing the phoneme /b/ in the initial position of a word will automatically eliminate the use of certain phonemes immediately following /b/, such as /h/ or /dʒ/. Likewise, the use of the word "the" as the first word in a sentence automatically eliminates the probability that the word "the" will occur as the second word in the sentence. Rather, we expect certain linguistic forms, such as a noun or adjective, to follow. Consequently, structural constraints produce considerable redundancy in speeech. This is invaluable to the hearing-impaired listener attempting to determine what was said after having heard only a portion of the message (closure).

Such syntactic clues can be used in conjunction with another factor related to redundancy, namely, semantic constraints, which allow the listener to predict the type of vocabulary and expressions to be used based on the semantic context. When the topic of conversation is food, for example, one can expect to hear a restricted range of vocabulary peculiar to that topic. Vocabulary that is specific to other topics, such as automobiles or the stock market, would in all probability not be used at that particular time. The semantic context, therefore, makes the predictability of what was being said high.

Situational constraints also result in high redundancy. When speaking to children in an elementary-school classroom about a particular topic, such as electricity, one would utilize a different vocabulary than if engaging in a similar conversation with an electrician. Thus, who we are communicating with, our relationship with that individual, and other related situational factors will influence the content of our communication.

All of these factors, then, contribute toward our being able to interpret (achieve closure on) portions of a communication which we did not adequately perceive. The use of these linguistic constraints, together with variables such as a person's ability to utilize visual information available during oral communication or the amount of competing background noise, plays a part in determining the perception of speech. Ultimately, therefore, audiometric results, plus these other factors, all interact to determine the degree of hearing handicap for speech which a hearing-impaired person experiences in a given situation.

auditory training and the hearing impaired

Traditionally, auditory training has been considered a major component of the aural rehabilitation process. Thus, its potential in assisting those with hearing loss has been expressed in major textbooks within the field of audiology, both past (Davis & Silverman, 1960; Newby, 1958; Oyer, 1966) and present (Alpiner & McCarthy, 1987; Boothroyd, 1982; Davis & Hardick, 1981; Sanders, 1982). Yet, even though auditory training is considered by many to constitute an integral part of aural rehabilitation, its actual benefits for the hearing impaired have rarely been fully assessed (Oyer, 1966; Rodel, 1985). This lack of validation, in part, serves to explain why classical auditory training procedures are not utilized more frequently.

The intent of the next major section of this chapter is to familiarize the reader with both the traditional and the current forms of auditory training and how they fit into the entire aural rehabilitation process.

definition/application of auditory training

Numerous attempts have been made to define auditory training in the past. Though similar in some respects, these definitions vary considerably due to the orientation of the definer and special considerations dictated by degree of hearing loss and time of onset.

Goldstein (1939), for example, felt that auditory training involved a development and/or improvement in the ability to discriminate various properties of speech and nonspeech signals. These properties include loudness, pitch, rhythm, and inflection. Goldstein's approach was directed toward facilitating the perception of speech, and included the use of a variety of verbal and nonverbal stimuli.

Probably the most common definition of auditory training is attributed to Carhart (1960), who considered auditory training a process of teaching the hearing-impaired child or adult to take full advantage of available auditory clues. As a result, Carhart recommended an emphasis on the awareness of sound, gross discrimination of nonverbal stimuli, and gross and fine discrimination of speech.

More recently, in discussing the use of auditory training with children, Erber (1982) described it as

the creation of special communication conditions in which teachers and audiologists help hearing-impaired children acquire many of the auditory speech-perception abilities that normally hearing children acquire naturally without their intervention. (p. 1)

Erber stated further that:

Our intent is to help the hearing-impaired child apply his or her impaired auditory sense to the fullest capacity in language communication, regardless of the degree of damage to the auditory system. Usually progress is achieved through careful application of amplification devices and through special teaching techniques. (p. 29)

When considering auditory training for adults, two general objectives are usually relevant: (a) learning to maximize the use of acoustic cues available for the perception of speech, and (b) adjustment and orientation to the use of amplification.

Inherent in the various views of auditory training, as well as those of other professionals in aural rehabilitation, is the notion that the hearing impaired can be trained to maximize the use of whatever degree of hearing they possess. The ultimate aim of auditory training is, therefore, to achieve maximum communication potential by developing the auditory sensory channel to its fullest. Although the primary goal of auditory training is to maximize communication abilities, it is important to point out that achieving this basic goal can result in other important achievements, including acquisition of more proficient speech and language skills, educational and vocational advancement, and successful psychosocial adjustment. As indicated earlier, if the communication skills of the hearing impaired can be improved, other areas of concern, such as educational progress, will be facilitated as well.

historical overview

The earliest efforts in auditory training date back to the 18th century. Goldstein (1939) stated that in 1761 Ernaud demonstrated to the Academy of Sciences in Paris that individuals with severe hearing loss could, with the benefit of a form of auditory training, accurately perceive certain aspects of speech auditorily. Others in Europe used auditory-training methods with the hearing impaired throughout the 1800s, including Itard of France, Beck in Germany, and Toynbee in England.

Interest in auditory training also spread to Vienna, where in 1893 Urbantschitsch demonstrated that systematic auditory training could produce considerable speech perception in persons otherwise considered deaf. Impressed with Urbantschitsch's accomplishments, Goldstein introduced a similar approach to auditory training in the United States in the late 1890s and early 1900s. Known as the Acoustic Method, this approach centered around systematic stimulation with individual speech sounds, syllables, words, and sentences to improve speech perception and to aid deaf persons in their own speech production. The Acoustic Method was utilized in a number of facilities throughout the country, including the Central Institute for the Deaf in St. Louis, Missouri, which Goldstein founded. Goldstein has exerted a significant influence on the thinking of many professionals over the years regarding the potential of auditory training with the hearing impaired.

Early applications of auditory training were directed almost exclusively toward individuals with severe to profound hearing loss in a deaf education setting. In recent times, however, use of auditory training has been expanded to include those with less severe impairments. Equally significant has been the inclusion of auditory-training activities in the management of hard-of-hearing adults and children. Thus, auditory training has become more widespread, in part, as a result of significant improvements in hearing aids and the development of other amplification systems for the hearing impaired, which have made it possible for more persons to use their hearing effectively for communication. Growth in the use of auditory training can also be associated with the emergence of audiology as a profession following World War II and the interest shown by audiologists in maximizing the use of residual hearing in persons with varying degrees of hearing loss. Thus, what was once perceived as a procedure to be used only with deaf children has become a more widely utilized aspect of aural rehabilitation for persons of varying ages and degrees of hearing impairment.

the auditory training process

As indicated, the definition and goals of auditory training have varied over the years, due, in part, to (a) the environment in which auditory training takes place (educational or clinical), (b) the age of the individual receiving services (child or adult), and (c) the degree of hearing loss involved (mild-moderate or severe-profound). These issues, as well as other related factors, including the need for speech/language development and adjustment to a new hearing aid, have been responsible for the many diversified approaches to auditory training which have evolved. The next section on implementation of auditory training will include a summary of the procedures commonly utilized to evaluate the auditory abilities of the hearing impaired, as well as a review of the key features of selected traditional and more current approaches to auditory training.

assessment of auditory skills

An integral part of any auditory-training program is the assessment of the client's performance. Before, during, and at the conclusion of auditory training the clinician should attempt to ascertain the hearing-impaired person's ability to discriminate speech accurately. Information of this nature is of utmost importance for several reasons, including

1. Determining whether or not auditory training appears warranted.

2. Providing a basis for comparison with performance following a period of therapy to assess the amount of improvement in speech perception, if any, that has occurred.

3. Identifying specific areas of speech perception difficulties to be concentrated on in future auditory training.

The nature of the auditory testing that takes place will vary considerably depending upon a number of variables, such as the age of the client, his or her language skills, and the type and degree of the hearing loss. The clinician must exercise care in selecting test materials for the person being tested, particularly with regard to the language levels required for a given test. This requires that a variety of tests of speech perception, both formal and informal, be available for assessment purposes so that the particular needs of each client can be met adequately.

Evaluating Children. Both the degree and the sophistication of testing appropriate for young children are limited by their physical and cognitive development. Therefore, informal testing and observation are relied upon heavily with this age group. For the infant the goal of assessment for auditory training purposes may not center on speech perception. Rather, an effort may be made to identify the extent to which auditory skills have emerged, such as gross discrimination and localization of a variety of stimuli. Once this information is known, a specific program for developing auditory skills, such as that described in Chapter 8, can be implemented in conjunction with therapy related to development of speech and language.

For older children more formal, indepth assessment of speech perception generally is possible. Specifically, materials have been developed for evaluating speech discrimination in children that require the child to respond in a prescribed manner to individual words or phonemes presented at a comfortable listening level. Formal tests designed for use with hearing-impaired children include:

1. *Word Intelligibility by Picture Identification* (WIPI) by Ross and Lerman (1970). The authors of the WIPI modified an existing speech discrimination test for children (Myatt & Landes, 1963) so as only to include vocabulary appropriate for hearing-impaired children. The WIPI requires a picture-pointing response in a closed-set format; according to the authors it is suitable for use with hearing-handicapped children with limited receptive and expressive language abilities.

2. *Northwestern University Children's Perception of Speech* (NU-CHIPS) by Katz and Elliott (1978). This test consists of 50 monosyllabic nouns which have been scrambled to form four individual lists. Like the WIPI, the NU-CHIPS uses a response format which requires that the child point to the one picture from four options which best represents the test items. Because of the vocabulary included and the response format, use of the NU-CHIPS with many children with hearing loss appears appropriate.

3. *Five Sound Test* by Ling (1976). Five isolated phonemes (/a/, /u/, /i/, /s/, and /ʃ/) are spoken to the child at a normal conversational level. Those with usable residual hearing up to 1,000 Hz should be able to detect the vowels. Children with some residual hearing up to 2,000 Hz should detect /ʃ/, and those with residual hearing up to 4,000 Hz (not worse than 90 dB HL at 4,000 Hz) should detect /s/.

Additional test batteries are designed to assess other aspects of auditory perception in addition to speech discrimination ability. Examples include:

1. *Test of Auditory Comprehension* (TAC), developed by the Audiologic Services of the Los Angeles County Schools (Tramwell & Owens, 1977). Designed for children ages 4-12 years with moderate to profound hearing losses, the TAC constitutes the evaluation part of a comprehensive auditory skills instructional plan. The instrument assesses several areas of auditory perception, including speech discrimination, memory sequencing, figure-ground discrimination, and story comprehension. Results of TAC subtests are used to establish baseline performance and direction for the companion auditory training curriculum.

2. *Glendonald Auditory Screening Procedure* (GASP), developed at the Glendonald Auditory School for the Deaf in Australia (Erber, 1982). GASP is based on a model of auditory perception described in the next section of this chapter (see Figure 3.6) and consists of three subtests: (a) phoneme detection, (b) word identification, and (c) sentence comprehension.

The GASP phoneme detection subtest is similar in format to the *Five Sound Test* developed by Ling (1976). According to Erber, the results from GASP can aid in planning auditory training because the child's performance on the subtests is predictive of other, related auditory tasks.

3. *Pediatric Speech Intelligibility Test* (PSI) by Jerger and colleagues (1980). It consists of 20 monosyllabic words and 20 sentences presented in quiet and with competing sentence messages at varying message-to-competition ratios (MCRs). The child points to the one picture from

SPEECH STIMULUS

		SPEECH ELEMENTS	SYLLABLES	WORDS	PHRASES	SENTENCES	CONNECTED DISCOURSE
RESPONSE TASK	DETECTION	1					
	DISCRIMINATION						
	IDENTIFICATION			2			
	COMPREHENSION					3	

Figure 3.6.   An auditory stimulus-response matrix showing the relative positions of the three GASP subtests: Phoneme Detection (1), Word Identification (2), and Sentence (Question) Comprehension (3). (From *Auditory Training* by N. Erber, 1982, Washington, DC: Alexander Graham Bell Association for the Deaf. Reprinted by permission.)

five options which corresponds to the word or sentence heard. Investigations of PSI results (Jerger, Jerger, & Abrams, 1983) suggest that in addition to the test's utility in assessing speech intelligibility with children having peripheral hearing impairments, it shows promise for detecting central auditory dysfunction.

These tests all attempt to take into account the limitations of hearing-impaired youngsters' receptive vocabulary level and their ability to respond orally. However, the variability observed in the receptive and expressive communication skills of these children makes it unwise to draw any firm generalizations about the specific age range of children for whom any of these tests are suited.

Evaluating Adults.   A number of formal speech-discrimination tests are available for use with adults. Any of the traditional monosyllabic word lists, such as the CID W-22s (Hirsh, Davis, Silverman, Reynolds, Eldert, & Bensen, 1952) or the *Northwestern University Auditory Test No. 6* (Tillman & Carhart, 1966), may be employed to evaluate overall speech-discrimination abilities.

Other tests allow for more indepth assessment of the discrimination of consonants, which can be especially difficult for hearing-impaired persons to perceive accurately. One example, the *Nonsense Syllable Test* (Levitt & Resnick, 1978; Resnick, Dubno, Howie, Hoffnung, Freeman, & Slosberg, 1976), consists of seven subtests, each having 7 to 9 nonsense syllables, as shown in Figure 3.7. Test items were selected in an effort to include those consonants known to present difficulty to hearing-impaired adults. Each subtest uses a closed-set response format, with the foils consisting of all the syllables within the subtest. Edgerton and Danhauer (1979) developed another discrimination test made up of nonsense syllables which appears appropriate for use with both adults and children (Danhauer, Lewis, & Edgerton, 1985).

Owens and Schubert (1977) developed a 100-item, multiple-choice consonant-discrimination test called the *California Consonant Test* (CCTs). Thirty-six of the test items assess consonant identification in the initial word position, while 64 items test recognition in the final position. Research by Schwartz and Surr (1979) demonstrated that, compared to the NU-6s, the CCTs are more sensitive to the speech-recognition difficulties experienced by individuals with high-frequency hearing loss. Consequently, the utility of the CCTs in assessing the speech-recognition abilities of many clinical patients has become well established.

Tests which employ a sentence format also can be informative. Kalikow, Stevens, and Elliott (1977) developed a test called *Speech Perception in Noise*, or SPIN. This test is unique in that it attempts to assess

1	2	3	4	5	6	7
af	uθ	iʃ	ab	fa	la	na
aʃ	up	if	að	ta	ba	va
at	us	it	ad	pa	da	ma
ak	uk	ik	am	ha	ga	za
as	ut	is	az	θa	ra	ga
ap	uf	iθ	ag	tʃa	ja	ba
aθ	uʃ	ip	an	sa	dʒa	ða
			aŋ	ʃa	wa	da
			av	ka		

Figure 3.7. Test items comprising the NST. Each column represents a subtest of the NST. (From *Phoneme Identification on a Closed-Response Syllable Test* by S. Resnick et al., 1976, Houston, TX. Reprinted by permission.)

a listener's utilization of both linguistic and situational cues in the perception of speech. Sentence material is presented against a background of speech babble, with the listener's task being to identify the final word in the sentence. Ten 50-item forms of SPIN have been generated, each version containing sentences with either high or low predictability relative to the final word in each sentence. Bilger, Rzcezkowski, Nuetzel, and Rabinowitz (1979) have revised the forms to make them more equivalent. The SPIN test shows promise by providing important information concerning how effectively a given listener makes use of contextual information in the perception of speech, in addition to providing insight regarding how the listener perceives the acoustical properties of speech.

The *Central Institute for the Deaf (CID) Everyday Speech Sentences* (Davis & Silverman, 1978) have been used extensively to evaluate a listener's ability to perceive connected discourse. They consist of ten 10-sentence sets that vary in length and form; the sentences possess several characteristics which are associated with typical conversation.

Results of these tests, as well as others, such as the *Modified Rhyme Test* (House, Williams, Hacker, & Kryter, 1965) and the *Multiple Choice Discrimination Test* (MCDT) (Schultz & Schubert, 1969), should provide the clinician with specific information concerning a client's consonant-sound discrimination and other speech-perception difficulties. Although not as commonly confused, vowel discrimination in the hearing impaired should also be evaluated, particularly if a severe hearing loss is present. This can be accomplished by utilizing a multiple-choice format and generating lists of monosyllabic words that systematically vary either the vowel or the diphthong while keeping the consonant environment consistent. The following list is an example of this type of material:

hat	hit	hot	hate
ball	bell	bull	bowl
nut	not	neat	night
tool	tall	tell	tale
see	sew	saw	Sue

Additional information about perception can be gained by introducing competing noise to the test situation and varying the degree of redundancy in the test material. Also, addition of visual cues during administration of these tests in a bisensory condition can provide evidence regarding a person's overall integrative skills (Garstecki, 1980; see Chapter 9).

Owens, Kessler, Telleen, and Schubert (1981) developed a comprehensive set of tests, the *Minimal Auditory Capabilities (MAC) Battery* for assessing auditory and visual skills with the severe to profoundly hearing impaired. The level of difficulty of the MAC is suitable for individuals for whom conventional speech tests are too challenging. Included in the MAC battery are the following 14 subtests: Question/Statement, Accent, Noise/Voice, Spondee Same/Different, Vowels, Initial Consonants, Final Consonants, Four-Choice Spondee, Environmental Sounds, Spondee Words, CID Everyday Sentences, Words in Context, Monosyllabic Words, and Visual Enhancement (lipreading). The battery has been slightly revised (Owens, Kessler, Raggio, & Schubert, 1985), and presently is being used widely in the evaluation of cases considered for a cochlear implant (see Chapter 12).

traditional auditory training methods

Wedenberg. An example of an early approach to auditory training used with severe and profoundly deaf children was that proposed by Wedenberg (1951, 1954). It was Wedenberg's view that auditory training systematically and individually serves to exploit whatever residual hearing remains. Wedenberg's approach was eventually labeled *unisensory*, since he advocated that lipreading not be consciously emphasized until the child developed a proper listening attitude. The preliminary efforts in Wedenberg's auditory training program were, therefore, directed toward generating attention to sound by the child. Both environmental and speech sounds were used in the early stages, with what Wedenberg referred to as *ad concham amplification*. This involved speaking directly into the child's ear at a close range (1-2 inches) rather than having the child use a hearing aid. Training also included exercises which helped the child become aware of and attend to sound at increasing distances. All these activities were intended to make the client more auditorily oriented. Vowels and voiced consonants whose formants were thought to be within the hearing-impaired child's audible range were presented in isolation. Syllables were used in a variety of formal therapeutic activities, as well as informal settings at home. Combining individual vowels and consonants learned in isolation resulted in perception of a limited number of words. At this point Wedenberg advocated part-time use of a hearing aid. Later, training progressed to short sentences formed by words already recognized by the child acoustically. Although not a direct focus, speechreading could be utilized by the child to supplement the information derived through the auditory channel. Wedenberg was convinced that children with a strong auditory orientation would eventually become as proficient at speechreading as those receiving intensive speechreading instruction early in life. In fact, he believed that his students' increased auditory vocabulary made them better able to utilize visual information than children with a background of multisensory training. An excellent example of the principles involved in Wedenberg's approach is contained in a summary of the work done with Staffan, a profoundly deaf son of the Wedenbergs (Wedenberg & Wedenberg, 1970).

Wedenberg's method, then, was directed toward development of speech and language skills in children with either a congenital or prelingual hearing loss of severe to profound proportions. In these respects it was similar to other auditory training methods proposed by Goldstein (1939), Whitehurst (1955, 1966), Watson (1961), and others. However, features such as his emphasis on unisensory management of the deaf child made Wedenberg's rehabilitative methods unique.

Until World War II the primary focus of auditory training was on profoundly deaf children in an effort to facilitate speech and language acquisition and increase their educational potential. However, the activities which occurred at VA audiology centers during World War II served to demonstrate on a mass basis that adults with mild to severe hearing impairments could profit from auditory training as well.

Carhart. Expansion of auditory training to encompass both children and adults continued after World War II. The thinking at that time concerning auditory training is perhaps best manifested in the approach to its use with both young and older individuals described by Carhart (1960). Carhart made one of the first extensive attempts to describe the role of auditory training in the aural rehabilitation process within an audiological context, and his theories were to have a significant and enduring impact on the profession.

Carhart's auditory training program for children was based on his belief that since listening skills are learned early in life, the child with a serious hearing loss at birth or soon after will not move through the normal developmental stages of these skills. Likewise, when a hearing loss occurs in later childhood or in adulthood, the person's auditory discrimination skills are usually impaired even though they were intact prior to the onset of the hearing loss. In each instance, Carhart believed that auditory training was warranted.

Childhood procedures. Carhart outlined four major steps involved in auditory training for children with congenital or prelingual deafness. These are:

1. Development of awareness of sound

2. Development of gross discriminations

3. Development of broad discriminations among simple speech patterns

4. Development of finer discriminations for speech

Development of awareness of auditory stimuli involves having the child acknowledge the presence of sound and its importance in his/her world. The development of gross discrimination initially involves demonstrating with various noisemakers that sounds differ. Once the child demonstrates discrimination of these, he/she is exposed to finer types of discrimination tasks which include variation in the frequency, intensity, and durational properties of sound. When the child is able to recognize the presence of sound and can recognize gross differences with nonverbal stimuli, Carhart's approach calls for the introduction of activities directed toward learning gross discrimination for speech signals. The final phase consists of training the child to make fine discriminations of speech stimuli and integrating an increased vocabulary to enable him/her to follow connected speech in a more rapid and accurate fashion.

Adult procedures. Because adults who acquire a hearing loss retain a portion of their original auditory skills, Carhart recommended that auditory training with adults focus on re-educating a skill diminished as a consequence of the hearing impairment. Initially, Carhart felt that it was important to establish "an attitude of critical listening" in the individual. This involves being attentive to the subtle differences among sounds and can involve a considerable amount of drill work on the discrimination of phonemes which are difficult for the adult to perceive. Lists of matched syllables/words which contain the troublesome phonemes, such as she-fee, so-tho, met-let, or mash-math, are read to the individual who repeats them back. Such training should also include phrases and sentences, with the goal of developing as rapid and precise a recognition of the phonetic elements as is possible within the limitations imposed by the person's hearing loss. Speechreading combined with a person's hearing was also encouraged by Carhart during auditory-training sessions.

Because we often communicate under less than ideal listening circumstances, Carhart advocated including training of auditory discrimination in three commonly encountered situations: (a) relatively intense background noise, (b) the presence of a competing speech signal, and (c) listening on the telephone. This emphasis on practice in speech perception under listening conditions with decreasing amounts of redundancy has been emphasized more recently by Sanders (1982).

According to Carhart hearing aids were vital in auditory training and he recommended they be utilized as early as possible in the auditory-training program, particularly with adults. These recommendations were consistent with Carhart's belief that systematic exposure to sound during auditory training was an ideal means of allowing a person to adequately adjust to amplification.

Persons interested in more specific information concerning Carhart's auditory-training strategies should review his chapter in the second edition of Davis and Silverman's *Hearing and Deafness* (1960).

more recent approaches to auditory training

Although the basic intent of auditory training is to maximize communication potential by developing the auditory channel to its fullest, several unique approaches to this form of aural rehabilitation have emerged in recent years, representing a departure from traditional methods. In this section we will identify and briefly describe the underlying features of a selected number of the more recent developments.

Verbotonal Method. Perhaps the most innovative auditory-training approach to appear in some time is the Verbotonal Method, developed in 1954 at the University of Zagreb, Yugoslavia, by Guberina (1964, 1987).

Although designed originally to teach foreign language, the method was modified for use with hearing-impaired children and adults. Specifically, the approach aims at developing auditory and speech skills simultaneously, with speech stimuli being employed at all times during training exercises. Early emphasis is placed on determining "the optimal field" of hearing for each individual. This is done in conjunction with an extensive array of auditory training equipment known as SUVAG I and II, as well as special test material designed to determine each person's optimum frequency response for speech perception. According to Asp (1973), the "optimum field" usually corresponds to the individual's most sensitive frequency range of hearing. Once the student has achieved acceptable levels of auditory perception in the optimal field of hearing, the frequency response is gradually broadened to resemble that of a conventional hearing aid, with some additional low-frequency amplification. Hearing aids are individually fit at a later stage in training. The use of visual cues during therapy is encouraged, but no speechreading instruction is provided.

For prelingual deaf children development of normal intonation and rhythm patterns is essential for acquisition of intelligible speech, according to the Verbotonal Method. To facilitate acquisition of these speech parameters, a series of kinesthetic or rhythmic body movements are used. The filtered auditory signal is further enhanced by simultaneous tactile stimulation using a vibrotactile device. Syllables and single words are presented in early training sessions, and the child attempts to repeat each accurately. Later, phrases and sentences are incorporated as the child's perceptual and speech skills progress. A child's progress is measured by how well he/she can imitate the speech presented.

The Verbotonal Method of auditory and speech training has received a considerable amount of attention in recent years in this country, and has achieved an admirable degree of success (Asp, 1984, 1985). Although the approach has been most frequently utilized with children, Guberina has recommended its use with adults as well. Santose (1978) reported on the successful use of the Verbotonal Method with a large number of adults with varying degrees of hearing impairment.

Erber. A generalized approach to auditory training with children has been described by Erber (1982). This adaptive method is based on a careful analysis of a child's auditory perceptual abilities through the use of the *Glendonald Auditory Screening Procedure* (GASP). Evaluation of the child's perception skills takes into account two major factors: (a) the complexity of the stimuli to be perceived (speech elements to connected discourse), and (b) the form of the response required (detection, discrimination, identification, comprehension). Several levels of stimuli and

TABLE 3.3
Three General Auditory Training Methods

Natural conversational approach:

1) The teacher eliminates visible cues and speaks to the child in as natural a way as possible, while considering the general situational context and ongoing classroom activity. 2) The auditory speech-perception tasks may be chosen from any cell in the stimulus-response matrix, for example, sentence comprehension. 3) The teacher adapts to the child's responses by presenting remedial auditory tasks in a systematic manner (modifies stimulus and/or response), derived from any cell in the matrix.

Moderately structured approach:

1) The teacher applies a closed-set auditory identification task, but follows this activity with some basic speech development procedures and a related comprehension task. Thus, the method retains a degree of flexibility. 2) The teacher selects the nature and content of words and sentences on the basis of recent class activities. 3) A few neighboring cells in the stimulus-response matrix are involved (for example, word and sentence identification and sentence comprehension).

Practice on specific tasks:

1) The teacher selects the set of acoustic speech stimuli and also the child's range of responses, prepares relevant materials, and plans the development of the task—all according to the child's specific needs for auditory practice. 2) Attention is directed to a particular listening skill, usually represented by a single cell in the stimulus-response matrix (for example, phrase discrimination).

From *Auditory Training* by N. Erber, 1982, Washington, DC: Alexander Graham Bell Association for the Deaf. Reprinted by permission.

responses are involved as shown in Figure 3.6. However, the GASP evaluates only the three stimulus-response combinations indicated in the figure.

Once the child's auditory capabilities are determined, an auditory-training program is outlined—taking into consideration the same model when establishing goals and beginning points for therapy. Erber proposed three styles of auditory training which differ in specificity, rigidity, and direction. These are described in Table 3.3. Adaptive procedures, where the child's responses to speech stimuli are used to determine the next activity, can be employed with any of these styles.

In implementing this approach to auditory training, Erber (1982) stated:

Auditory training need not follow a developmental plan where, for instance, you practice phoneme detection first and attempt comprehension of connected discourse last. Instead, you might use the "conversational approach" during all daily conversation, and apply the "moderately structured approach" as a follow-up to each class activity. During each activity, you will note consistent errors. Later, you might provide brief periods of specific practice with difficult material. In this way, you can incorporate auditory training into conversation and instruction, rather than treat listening as a skill to be developed independent of communication. (p. 105)

The emphasis on integrating development of auditory skills in all activities with hearing-impaired children is shared by Ling and Ling (1978), who recommended that auditory training "be viewed as a supplement to auditory experience and as an integral part of language and speech training" (p. 113).

Programmed Self-Instruction. Innovative approaches to auditory training have not been confined exclusively to use with children. Staff at the National Technical Institute for the Deaf (NTID) at the Rochester Institute of Technology in Rochester, NY, have developed a comprehensive program in auditory training for use with deaf students attending

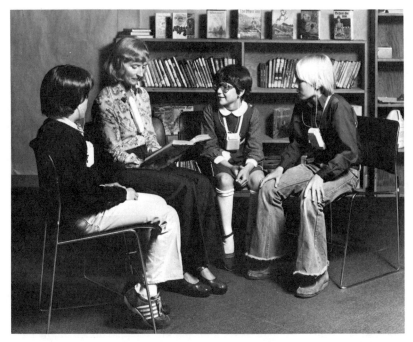

Figure 3.8. Group auditory training session. (Courtesy of H. C. Electronics.)

the Institute (Durity, 1982; Sims, 1985) who utilize hearing aids. A unique aspect of this program is the incorporation of self-instructional listening exercises recorded on audio cassettes.

Prospective students are placed in one of three courses based primarily on their auditory discrimination of the *CID Everyday Sentence Test* (Davis & Silverman, 1978), which is a subtest of NTID's Communication Profile (Johnson, 1976). Students unable to perceive any of the test material generally are placed in the basic auditory training course (Level I). Students with scores up to 49% are enrolled in the intermediate course (Level II), while those scoring from 50-100% are placed in the advanced auditory training course (Level III). A portion of the curriculum for each course is similar, and includes lecture and discussion of topics pertaining to hearing loss and speech perception, communication strategies, as well as sensory aids and/or assistive listening devices. Because of the degree of the students' impairment, the emphasis in the basic course is on detection, discrimination, and identification of: (a) syllabification, (b) word/sentence stress, (c) time-based cues, (c) intonation, and (d) environmental sounds. Substantial improvement has been noted in speechreading performance in the presence of auditory input among many of the students in the basic course, and an increase in the amount of daily hearing aid use has also occurred.

The intermediate and advanced courses contain a greater degree of work with perception of words and sentences in quiet and against a background of noise, as well as vocabulary development. The intermediate course emphasizes consonant recognition through drills concentrating on phonetic feature recognition, as well as attention to visual distinctive feature recognition. The advanced course emphasizes speech recognition within connected discourse in the individual and group activities in which each student participates. Tracking techniques are used routinely. The successful use of communication strategies is also emphasized at each level. To facilitate communication with hearing people, students learn to use "coping" techniques, such as rephrasing, repetition, and gesturing.

An important and unique aspect of NTID's auditory training courses is the use of programmed self-instruction with audio cassettes. Students individually are assigned a certain number of cassettes to complete during the semester. Each cassette or unit consists of a series of exercises which emphasize specific aspects of listening. Vocabulary and expressions from the units used by students in the intermediate and advanced courses have been specifically selected as being commonly encountered in the students' academic programs as well as in social situations. Students utilize the audio cassettes in NTID's Auditory Learning Center, which contains individualized auditory training carrels equipped with instrumentation as described in detail by Durity (1982).

Programmed self-instruction has proven to be an effective means of providing auditory training for severely hearing-impaired young adults at NTID (Sims, 1985). Boothroyd (1986) also reported on a computer-assisted program of speech perception training which utilizes interactive audio and video systems. The success of these computerized programs undoubtedly will foster attempts in the near future to apply similar self-instructional techniques with hard-of-hearing adults in the traditional clinical setting. Caution should be exercised, however, if self-instruction is used without guidelines and active participation on the part of a clinician. As Durity (1982) pointed out, the clinician's direct involvement is integral to the success of the self-instruction process.

Communication Training. All forms of aural rehabilitation, including auditory training, have received careful scrutiny and evaluation in the past decade. This questioning of traditional approaches to rehabilitation of the hearing disabled has led to a number of alternative philosophies and methodologies regarding the form of the services to be provided and the manner in which they are to be delivered. Specifically, a number of professionals dealing with those with hearing loss share the belief that while auditory training, speechreading, and other forms of aural rehabilitation are helpful, each has definite limitations. Associated with this is the conviction that long-term, intensive auditory training or speechreading therapy does not result in enough improvement in communication ability for most hearing-handicapped individuals to justify devoting long periods of time and energy by client and clinician on a routine basis.

Recognizing the potential of aural rehabilitation for improving communication skills in many persons, several professionals have initiated aural rehabilitation programs which are short term and comprehensive in scope. Recent reports of similar programs include Hardick (1977), Schow, Christensen, Hutchinson, and Nerbonne (1978), and Giolas (1982). Rather than concentrating on one aspect of aural rehabilitation, such as auditory training, over a prolonged period of time, these alternative approaches cover a number of key elements associated with successful communication. Topics typically include how we hear, characteristics of hearing loss in general and those associated with the particular person in therapy, hearing aid adjustment, basic principles of speechreading, the acoustical properties of speech, good listening habits, psychosocial adjustment to hearing loss, and other related areas. In a majority of cases, these topics are covered in informal group sessions, accompanied by individual exercises. Most programs vary in length from 6 to 10 weeks, with 1 to 2 hours devoted to sessions each week. This type of program seems to provide many of the same gains in communication skills which were previously achieved in prolonged, unisensory or bisensory therapy with adults having mild to severe hearing losses. For the most part, the programs have been well received and appear to meet the needs of many hard-of-hearing adults routinely seen in clinical settings.

However, developers of these short-term, comprehensive aural rehabilitation programs do not maintain that their approach is appropriate for everybody. To the contrary, it is generally felt that certain clients, particularly those with severe to profound hearing losses, may best profit from auditory training provided on a one-to-one basis over an extended period of time. Of importance in determining the length of an auditory training program is the hearing-impaired person's attitude toward his/her disability and the entire rehabilitation process (Goldstein & Stephens, 1981).

Consonant Recognition Training. Investigating the effects of consonant recognition training on the perception of speech, Walden, Erdman, Montgomery, Schwartz, and Prosek (1981) described an intensive, short-term approach for adults developed at the Walter Reed Army Medical Center which shows promise as an effective procedure. The training materials, developed originally by Walden, Prosek, Montgomery, Scherr, and Jones (1977) for speechreading training, consist of 38 exercises, each concentrating on a select number of consonants presented in a syllable context. The listener's task is to make same-different judgments between syllable pairs and to identify the nonsense syllables presented individually. The position of the consonants within the syllable is varied between exercises. Listeners receive immediate feedback regarding the correctness of their response. This procedure allows for hundreds of syllables to be presented during a 30-minute training session.

This approach to auditory training has proven effective with 10 hearing-impaired adults who produced significant improvement in speech perception. Thus, Walden et al. noted an 11.6% average improvement in consonant recognition. More impressively, a 28.2% average improvement was found in subjects' perception of sentences presented in a combined audiovisual mode. A recent study by Montgomery, Walden, Schwartz, and Prosek (1984) utilized a similar protocol in investigating the effectiveness of speech-recognition training involving a combined auditory-visual approach. Using sentence material to assess performance, researchers noted a substantial improvement in speech recognition for the hearing-impaired group receiving concentrated auditory-visual integration training. Though further research is needed before this approach can be recommended for widespread use, the authors consider it to be of great promise. Their work emphasizes increasing interest on the part of some professionals in providing auditory training within a bisensory context, where visual as well as auditory skills are worked on simultaneously to facilitate integration of information taken in by these two sensory channels.

Tracking. DeFilippo and Scott (1978) developed a method to provide perception practice with sentence-length material, referred to as *tracking*, which has been applied recently to aural rehabilitation (Danz & Binnie, 1983; Erber, 1982; Owens & Telleen, 1981). As it is utilized with auditory training, the method involves having the clinician read short segments of a story in an auditory-only communication mode. The hearing-impaired listener then attempts to repeat verbatim what was read. When the listener fails to provide a verbatim response, the clinician selects one or more of a series of strategies to help the listener achieve 100% recognition. Strategies include repeating the word(s) missed, repeating the words heard correctly, and using a synonym for the word missed. Strategies are selected at the clinician's discretion. Visual cues can be added for bisensory training. Performance in the tracking procedure is monitored by calculating the number of words correctly repeated by the listener per minute during a therapy session. An example of how the tracking method is applied in a therapy session is provided below. (The topic of the passage is fishing.)

Clinician: Dry flies float on the surface.

Listener: .....flies float.....

Clinician: Dry flies float on the surface.

Listener: .....flies float on the water.

Clinician: The opposite of wet is dry.

Listener: Dry?

Clinician: Yes. Dry flies float on the surface.

Listener: Dry flies float on the water.

Clinician: No. On the surface of the water.

Listener: Surface. Dry flies float on the surface.

Clinician: Yes.

Results of work with tracking by Owens and Telleen (1981), Danz and Binnie (1983), and others suggest that it is an effective tool for the clinician engaged in auditory training and other forms of aural rehabilitation. Its application is expected to increase.

current trends in auditory training

Traditional approaches to auditory training continue to be employed in aural rehabilitation. The emergence of several alternative approaches, however, signifies a trend to explore new forms of training. The difficulties experienced in demonstrating significant improvement in the perception of speech following lengthy periods of traditional auditory training have led to skepticism regarding several of the common features of these older approaches. Rodel (1985) presented an excellent review of some of the areas of concern which have been identified in the literature, including the questionable use of extensive environmental sounds rather than linguistic stimuli during auditory training (Ling, 1978). Rodel summarized this concern by stating:

> The value of using nonlinguistic stimuli in auditory training procedures for young hearing-impaired children appears limited. While responding to bells, whistles, drums and animal sounds might be an enjoyable therapy activity for the young child, his parents and the clinician, gross nonverbal, environmental sound discrimination evidently does little to facilitate the development of speech perception skill, or, ultimately, to build a solid foundation for adequate aural-oral communication ability.....In general, gross discrimination tasks using nonspeech sounds should constitute only a minor portion of a young child's auditory training program. (p. 1010)

Rodel also cited the need to carefully evaluate the linguistic structures presented in auditory training. Rather than bombarding the child with auditory stimulation of all types and levels of linguistic sophistication, the clinician should attempt to use linguistic forms which are consistent with the normative information available concerning the emergence of language in children. Also needed is a more careful selection of speech material for auditory training whose phonetic composition is conducive to perception by hearing-impaired individuals (Asp, 1973). This requires close examination of the audiometric results for each case as well as the intensity and frequency properties of individual speech sounds.

As pointed out, another trend in present-day aural rehabilitation consists of conducting an increasing proportion of the training activities within a combined bisensory process which facilitates integration of auditory and visual cues. The importance of emphasizing auditory-visual integration was discussed by Montgomery and Sylvester (1984), whose thought-provoking comments are recommended for those interested in exploring this aspect of aural rehabilitation. These, and other issues involving auditory training, are currently receiving the attention of professionals involved in management of the hearing impaired. Careful evaluation of current procedures will lead to improvement in the effectiveness of auditory training, which ultimately will be reflected in improved communication skills on the part of the hearing disabled.

summary

This chapter has presented an overview of the role of audition in the communication process and the part auditory training plays in aural rehabilitation of the hearing disabled. Specifically, the complexity of speech perception was emphasized along with the ways in which auditory training techniques can be utilized to maximize the contribution of the impaired auditory channel to overall communication. Its potential for improving the communication skills of the hearing impaired is substantial. Application of auditory training and its importance in the total aural rehabilitation process will be further discussed in later chapters.

recommended readings

Danz, A., & Binnie, C. (1983). Quantification of the effects of training the auditory-visual reception of connected speech. *Ear and Hearing, 4,* 146-151.

Durity, R. (1982). Auditory training for severely hearing-impaired adults. In D. Sims, G. Walter, & R. Whitehead (Eds.), *Deafness and communication: Assessment and training* (pp. 296-311). Baltimore: Williams and Wilkins.

Erber, N. (1988). *Communication therapy for hearing-impaired adults.* Abbotsford, Vic. 3067/Australia: Clavis Publishing.

Erber, N. (1982). *Auditory training.* Washington, DC: Alexander Graham Bell Assoc. for the Deaf.

Ling, D., & Ling, A. (1978). *Aural habilitation.* Washington, DC: Alexander Graham Bell Assoc. for the Deaf.

Sims, D. (1985). Adults with hearing impairment. In J. Katz (Ed.), *Handbook of clinical audiology* (3rd ed., pp. 1017-1045). Baltimore: Williams and Wilkins.

references

Alpiner, J., & McCarthy, P. (Eds.). (1987). *Rehabilitative audiology: Children and adults.* Baltimore: Williams and Wilkins.

Asp, C. (1973). The verbo-tonal method as an alternative to present auditory training techniques. In J. Wingo & G. Holloway (Eds.), *An appraisal of speech pathology and audiology: A symposium* (pp. 134-145). Springfield, IL: Charles C. Thomas.

Asp, C. (1984). The verbo-tonal method for establishing spoken language and listening skills. In W. Perkins (Ed.), *Current therapy of communication disorders* (pp. 95-100). New York: Thieme-Stratton.

Asp, C. (1985). The verbational method for management of young, hearing-impaired children. *Ear and Hearing, 6,* 39-42.

Bench, R. (1968). Sound transmission to the human fetus through the maternal abdominal wall. *Journal of Genetic Psychology, 113,* 85-87.

Bilger, R., Rzcezkowski, C., Nuetzel, J., & Rabinowitz, W. (1979). *Evaluation of a test of speech perception in noise (SPIN).* Paper presented at the convention of the American Speech-Language-Hearing Association, Atlanta.

Bilger, R., & Wang, M. (1976). Consonant confusions in patients with sensorineural hearing loss. *Journal of Speech and Hearing Research, 19,* 718-748.

Boothroyd, A. (1978). Speech perception and sensorineural hearing loss. In M. Ross & T. Giolas (Eds.), *Auditory management of hearing-impaired children* (pp. 117-144). Baltimore: University Park Press.

Boothroyd, A. (1982). *Hearing impairments in young children.* Englewood Cliffs, NJ: Prentice-Hall.

Boothroyd, A. (1986). *Computer-assisted speech perception training and testing.* Presentation at the Annual Convention of the American Speech-Language-Hearing Association, Detroit.

Byers, V. (1973). Initial consonant intelligibility by hearing impaired children. *Journal of Speech and Hearing Research, 16,* 48-55.

Carhart, R. (1960). Auditory training. In H. Davis & R. Silverman (Eds.), *Hearing and deafness* (2nd ed., pp. 368-386). New York: Holt, Rinehart & Winston.

Crandall, I. (1925, October). Sounds of speech. *Bell System Technical Journal,* 586-626.

Danhauer, J., Lewis, A., & Edgerton, B. (1985). Normally hearing children's responses to a nonsense syllable test. *Journal of Speech and Hearing Disorders, 50,* 100-103.

Danz, A., & Binnie, C. (1983). Quantification of the effects of training the auditory-visual reception of connected speech. *Ear and Hearing, 4,* 146-151.

Davis, J., & Hardick, E. (1981). *Rehabilitative audiology for children and adults.* New York: Wiley and Sons.

Davis, H., & Silverman, R. (1960). *Hearing and deafness* (2nd ed.). New York: Holt, Rinehart & Winston.

Davis, H., & Silverman, R. (1978). *Hearing and deafness* (4th ed.). New York: Holt, Rinehart & Winston.

DeFillippo, C., & Scott, B. (1978). A method for training and evaluating the reception of ongoing speech. *Journal of the Acoustical Society of America, 63,* 1186-1192.

Denes, P. (1967). On the motor theory of speech perception. In W. Wathen-Dunn (Ed.), *Models for the perception of speech and visual form* (pp. 309-314). Cambridge: The MIT Press.

Denes, P., & Pinson, E. (1973). *The speech chain.* Garden City, NJ: Anchor Press.

Durity, R. (1982). Auditory training for severely hearing-impaired adults. In D. Sims, G. Walter, & R. Whitehead (Eds.), *Deafness and communication: assessment and training* (pp. 296-311). Baltimore: Williams & Wilkins.

Edgerton, B., & Danhauer, J. (1979). *Clinical implications of speech discrimination testing using nonsense stimuli.* Baltimore: University Park Press.

Eimas, P. (1975). Developmental studies in speech perception. In L.B. Cohen & P. Salapatek (Eds.), *Infant perception* (Vol. 2, pp. 193-231). New York: Academic Press.

Eisenberg, R. (1965a). Auditory behavior in the human neonate. I. Methodologic problems and the logical design of research procedures. *Journal of Auditory Research, 5,* 159-177.

Eisenberg, R. (1965b). Auditory behavior in the human neonate. *Journal of International Audiology, 4,* 65-68.

Eisenberg, R. (1970). The develoment of hearing in man: An assessment of current status. *Asha, 12,* 110-123.

Eisenberg, R. (1976). *Auditory competence in early life.* Baltimore: University Park Press.

Eisenberg, R., Griffin, D., Coursin, D., & Hunter, M. (1964). Auditory behavior in the human neonate: A preliminary report. *Journal of Speech and Hearing Research, 7,* 245-269.

Erber, N. (1979). Speech perception by profoundly hearing-impaired children. *Journal of Speech and Hearing Disorders, 122,* 255-270.

Erber, N. (1982). *Auditory training.* Washington, DC: Alexander Graham Bell Association for the Deaf.

Fletcher, H. (1953). *Speech and hearing in communication.* Princeton: D. VanNostrand Co.

Fletcher, S. (1970). Acoustic phonetics. In F.S. Berg & S.G. Fletcher (Eds.), *The hard of hearing child* (pp. 57-84). New York: Grune & Stratton.

Garstecki, D. (1980). Alternative approaches to measuring speech discrimination efficiency. In R. Rupp & C. Stockdell (Eds.), *Speech protocols in audiology* (pp. 119-144). New York: Grune & Stratton.

Giolas, T. (1982). *Hearing-handicapped adults.* Englewood Cliffs, NJ: Prentice-Hall.

Goldstein, D., & Stephens, S. (1981). Audiological rehabilitation: Management model I. *Audiology, 20,* 432-452.

Goldstein, M. (1939). *The acoustic method of the training of the deaf and hard of hearing child.* St. Louis: Laryngoscope Press.

Guberina, P. (1964). *Studies in the verbo-tonal system.* Columbus: The Ohio State University Press.

Hardick, E. (1977). Aural rehabilitational programs for the aged can be successful. *Journal of the Academy for Rehabilitative Audiology, 10,* 51-68.

Hirsh, I., Davis, H., Silverman, S.R., Reynolds, E., Eldert, E., & Bensen, R. (1952). Development of materials for speech audiometry. *Journal of Speech and Hearing Disorders, 17,* 321-337.

House, A., Williams, C., Hacker, M., & Kryter, K. (1965). Articulation-testing methods: Consonantal differentiation with a loud-set response. *Journal of the Acoustical Society of America, 37,* 158-166.

Jerger, S., Jerger, J., & Abrams, S. (1983). Speech audiometry in the young child. *Ear and Hearing, 4,* 56-66.

Jerger, S., Lewis, S., Hawkins, J., & Jerger, J. (1980). Pediatric speech intelligibility test I. Generation of test materials. *International Journal of Pediatric Otorhinolaryngology, 2,* 217-230.

Johansson, B., Wedenberg, E., & Westin, B. (1964). Measurement of tone response by the human fetus. *Acta Otolaryngologica, 57,* 188-192.

Johnson, D. (1976). Communication characteristics of a young deaf adult population: Techniques of evaluating their communication skills. *American Annals of the Deaf, 121,* 409-424.

Kalikow, D., Stevens, K., & Elliott, L. (1977). Development of a test of speech intelligibility in noise using sentence materials with controlled word predictability. *Journal of the Acoustical Society of America, 61,* 1337-1351.

Katz, D., & Eliott, L. (1978, November). *Development of a new children's speech discrimination test.* Paper presented at the convention of the American Speech-Language-Hearing Association, Chicago.

Lehiste, I. (1970). *Suprasegmentals.* Cambridge: The MIT Press.

Lehiste, I. (1976). Suprasegmental features of speech. In N.J. Lass (Ed.), *Contemporary issues in experimental phonetics* (pp. 225-242). New York: Academic Press, Inc.

Levitt, H., & Resnick, S. (1978). Speech reception by the hearing impaired. Methods of testing and the development of new tests. *Scandinavian Audiology, 6* (Suppl. 1), 107-130.

Ling, D. (1976). *Speech and the hearing-impaired child: Theory and practice.* Washington, DC: Alexander Graham Bell Association for the Deaf.

Ling, D. (1978). Auditory coding and recoding: An analysis of auditory training procedures for hearing-impaired children. In M. Ross & T. Giolas (Eds.), *Auditory management of hearing-impaired children* (pp. 181-218). Baltimore: University Park Press.

Ling, D., & Ling, A. (1978). *Aural rehabilitation.* Washington, DC: Alexander Graham Bell Association for the Deaf.

Lisker, L. (1957). Closure duration and the intervocalic voiced-voiceless distinction in English. *Language, 33,* 42-49.

McGlone, R. (1966). Vocal pitch characteristics of children aged one and two years. *Speech Monographs, 33,* 178-181.

McKay, D. (1956). The epistemological problems for automata. In C.E. Shannon & J. McCarthy (Eds.), *Automata studies* (pp. 235-251). Princeton: Princeton University Press.

Miller, G., & Nicely, P. (1955). Analysis of perceptual confusions among some English consonants. *Journal of the Acoustical Society of America, 27,* 338-352.

Minifie, F. (1973). Speech acoustics. In F. Minifie, T. Hixon, & F. Williams (Eds.), *Normal aspects of speech, hearing and language* (pp. 235-284). Englewood Cliffs, NJ: Prentice-Hall.

Moffitt, A. (1971). Consonant cue perception by twenty- to twenty-four week-old infants. *Child Development, 42,* 717-732.

Montgomery, A., & Sylvester, S. (1984). Streamlining the aural rehabilitation process. *Hearing Instruments, 35,* 46-50.

Montgomery, A., Walden, B., Schwartz, D., & Prosek, R. (1984). Training auditory-visual speech recognition in adults with moderate sensorineural hearing loss. *Ear and Hearing, 5,* 30-36.

Moore, E. (1975). Programmed self-instruction in auditory training. *Journal of the Academy of Rehabilitative Audiology, 8,* 90-94.

Myatt, B., & Landes, B. (1963). Assessing discrimination loss in children. *Archives of Otolaryngology, 77,* 359-362.

Newby, H. (1958). *Audiology.* New York: Appleton-Century-Crofts.

Northern, J., & Downs, M. (1984). *Hearing in children* (3rd ed.). Baltimore: Williams & Wilkins.

Orr, D., Friedman, H., & Williams, J. (1965). Trainability of listening comprehension of speeded discourse. *Journal of Educational Psychology, 56,* 148-156.

Owens, E. (1978). Consonant errors and remediation in sensorineural hearing loss. *Journal of Speech and Hearing Disorders, 43,* 331-347.

Owens, E., Benedict, M., & Schubert, E. (1972). Consonant phoneme errors associated with pure tone configurations and certain types of hearing impairment. *Journal of Speech and Hearing Research, 15,* 308-322.

Owens, E., Benedict, M., & Schubert, E. (1971). Further investigation of vowel items in multiple-choice discrimination testing. *Journal of Speech and Hearing Research, 14,* 814-847.

Owens, E., Kessler, D., Roggio, M., & Schubert, E. (1985). Analysis and revision of the *minimal auditory capabilities (MAC) battery. Ear and Hearing, 6,* 280-287.

Owens, E., Kessler, D., Telleen, C., & Schubert, E. (1981). The minimal auditory capabilities (MAC) battery. *Hearing Journal, 34*(9), 32-34.

Owens, E., & Schubert, E. (1977). Development of the California Consonant Test. *Journal of Speech and Hearing Research, 20,* 463-474.

Owens, E., & Telleen, C. (1981). Tracking as an aural rehabilitative process. *Journal of the Academy of Rehabilitative Audiology, 14,* 259-273.

Oyer, H. (1966). *Auditory communication for the hard of hearing.* Englewood Cliffs, NJ: Prentice-Hall.

Palmer, L., & Wallber, J. (1984, November). *Auditory trainer for the new hearing aid user.* Paper presented at the convention of the American Speech-Language-Hearing Association, San Francisco.

Perkins, W. (1971). *Speech pathology: An applied behavioral science.* St. Louis: C.V. Mosby.

Peterson, G.E., & Barney, H.L. (1952). Control methods used in the study of the vowels. *Journal of the Acoustical Society of America, 32,* 693-703.

Resnick, S., Dubno, D., Howie, G., Hoffnung, S., Freeman, L., & Slosberg, R. (1976). *Phoneme identification on a closed-response nonsense syllable test.* Paper presented at the convention of the American Speech-Language-Hearing Association, Houston.

Rodel, M. (1985). Children with hearing impairment. In J. Katz (Ed.), *Handbook of clinical audiology* (3rd ed., pp. 1004-1016). Baltimore: Williams & Wilkins.

Ross, M., & Lerman, J. (1970). A picture identification test for hearing impaired children. *Journal of Speech and Hearing Research, 13,* 44-53.

Sanders, D. (1977). *Auditory perception of speech.* Englewood Cliffs, NJ: Prentice-Hall.

Sanders, D. (1982). *Aural rehabilitation* (2nd ed.). Englewood Cliffs, NJ: Prentice-Hall.

Santore, F. (1978). The verbotonal aural rehabilitation program. *Journal of the Academy of Rehabilitative Audiology, 11,* 33-44.

Scher, A., & Wens, E. (1974). Consonant confusions associated with hearing loss above 2,000 Hz. *Journal of Speech and Hearing Research, 17,* 669-681.

Schow, R., Christensen, J., Hutchinson, J., & Nerbonne, M. (1978). *Communication disorders of the aged.* Baltimore: University Park Press.

Schulman, C. (1970). Heart rate response habituation in high-risk premature infants. *Psychophysiology, 6,* 690-694.

Schultz, M., & Schubert, E. (1969). A multiple choice discrimination test (MCDT). *Laryngoscope, 79,* 382-399.

Schwartz, D., & Surr, R. (1979). Three experiments on the California Consonant Test. *Journal of Speech and Hearing Disorders, 44,* 61-72.

Sims, D. (1985). Adults with hearing impairment. In J. Katz (Ed.), *Handbook of clinical audiology* (3rd ed., pp. 1017-1045). Baltimore: Williams & Wilkins.

Stevens, S., & Davis, H. (1938). *Hearing: Its psychology and physiology.* New York: John Wiley & Sons.

Tillman, T., & Carhart, R. (1966). *An expanded test for speech discrimination utilizing CNC monosyllabic words.* Northwestern University Auditory Test No. 6 (Technical Report No. SAM-TR-66-55). Brooks Air Force Base, TX: USAF School of Aerospace Medicine.

Tramwell, J., & Owens, S. (1977). *The test of auditory comprehension (TAC).* Paper presented at the annual convention of the American Speech-Language-Hearing Association, Chicago.

Walden, B., Erdman, J., Montgomery, A., Schwartz, D., & Prosek, R. (1981). Some effects of training on speech recognition by hearing-impaired adults. *Journal of Speech and Hearing Research, 24,* 207-216.

Walden, B., & Montgomery, A. (1975). Dimensions of consonant perception in normal and hearing-impaired listeners. *Journal of Speech and Hearing Research, 18,* 444-455.

Walden, B., Prosek, R., Montgomery, A., Scherr, C., & Jones C. (1977). Effects of training on the visual recognition of consonants. *Journal of Speech and Hearing Research, 20,* 130-145.

Watson, T. (1961). *The use of residual hearing in the education of deaf children.* Washington, DC: The Volta Bureau.

Wedenberg, E. (1951). Auditory training of deaf and hard of hearing children. *Acta Otolaryngologica* (Suppl. #110).

Wedenberg, E., & Wedenberg, M. (1970). The advantage of auditory training. In F. Berg & S. Fletcher (Eds.), *The hard of hearing child* (pp. 319-330). New York: Grune & Stratton.

Whitehurst, M. (1966). *Auditory training for children.* Washington, DC: Alexander Graham Bell Association for the Deaf.

Zemlin, W. (1981). *Speech and hearing science* (2nd ed.). Englewood Cliffs, NJ: Prentice-Hall.

chapterfour

VISUAL STIMULI IN COMMUNICATION

NICHOLAS M. HIPSKIND

contents

introduction

When engaged in conversation, we tend to rely on our hearing to receive and subsequently comprehend the message being conveyed. In addition, given the opportunity, we *look at the speaker* in order to obtain further information related to the topic of conversation. The speaker's mouth movements, facial expressions and hand gestures as well as various aspects of the physical environment in which the communication takes place are potential sources of useful information. Humans learn to utilize vision for communication to some extent, even though most of us enjoy the benefits of normal hearing and find it unnecessary to depend on vision to communicate.

The hearing-impaired person, on the other hand, is much more dependent on visual cues for communication. The degree to which the hearing impaired need visual information when conversing with someone is proportional to the amount of information that is lost due to hearing impairment. In other words, a person with a severe hearing loss is likely to be more dependent on visual information to communicate than an individual with a mild auditory impairment (see Chapter 1 for a classification of *auditory impairment*).

Visual information may be transmitted by means of a manual or an oral system. In oral communication, the listener utilizes visual cues by observing the speaker's mouth, facial expressions, and hand movements to help perceive what is being said. This process is referred to by such terms as *lipreading, visual hearing, visual communication, visual listening,* or *speechreading*. Among lay personnel the most popular of these terms is *lipreading*. The term seems to imply only the use of visual cues for purposes of identifying various articulatory gestures. However, since the use of vision for communication involves more than watching the speaker's mouth, most professionals prefer the term *speechreading*. Thus, *speechreading* is used in the remainder of this chapter to refer to visual perception of oral communication. An exception to this is a speechreading method termed *TADOMA*, in which vibratile cues are used for speech perception by placing the fingers and hand on the speaker's lips, face, and neck. This method has proven successful with some deaf-blind individuals.

Manual communication, or "sign language," also relies on a visual system. *Manual communication* is transmitted via special signs and symbols made with the hands and is received and interpreted visually. This complex form of communication allows for transfer of information via the visual channel when both the sender and the receiver are familiar with the same system of symbols.

The intent of this chapter is to discuss the advantages and limitations of vision as part of the aural rehabilitation process. Emphasis will be given to the factors that affect speechreading as well as a discussion of manual communication methods. The reader is reminded that the hearing impaired comprise two populations: the hard of hearing and the deaf. Although frequently classified under the generic term *hearing impaired*, these groups have different communication needs and limitations (Davis, 1978). Therefore, it is unrealistic to expect that a single rehabilitation method can satisfy all their communication needs. Ultimately, it is the clinician's responsibility to select strategies that will enable the hard of hearing and the deaf to use vision to effectively enhance their communicative skills, to achieve educational and vocational success, and to mature emotionally and socially.

factors related to speechreading

The variables that affect the speechreading process usually fall in four general areas: the speaker, the signal/code, the environment, and the speechreader. While research has contributed to a better understanding of how speech is processed visually, some of the findings are equivocal and have been found to be difficult to duplicate in the clinical setting (Alpiner & McCarthy, 1987; Best, 1978; Hardick, 1977). This is not to imply that aural rehabilitationists should ignore available laboratory findings; rather, they must realize the significance of these findings in order to provide individualized patient programming. The following section presents selected experimental evidence regarding factors that have been reported to influence the efficacy of speechreading. Figure 4.1 provides a summary of these factors.

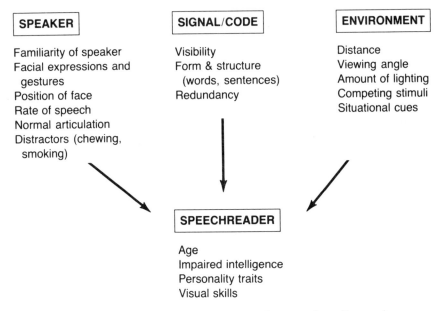

Figure 4.1. Summary of various factors related to speechreading performance. *Note.* Arrows have been drawn from the Speaker, Signal/Code, and Environmental lists to Speechreader to signify that all these factors impact on the speechreader's performance in addition to those variables that are directly related to the speechreader.

speaker

Differences among speakers have a greater effect on speechreading than on listening. Over 50 years ago a positive correlation was shown to exist between speaker-listener familiarity and the information received from speechreading (Day, Fusfeld, & Pintner, 1928). That is, speechreading performance improved when the speaker was familiar to the receiver (speechreader). Speakers who used appropriate facial expressions and common gestures and who positioned themselves face to face or within a 45° angle of the listener also facilitated communication for the speechreader (Berger, 1972a; Stone, 1957; Woodward & Lowell, 1964).

The rate of normal speech results in as many as 15 phonemes/sec (Orr, Friedman, & Williams, 1965). Evidence suggests that the eye is capable of recording only 8 to 10 discrete movements/sec (Nitchie, 1951). Thus, a speaker's normal speaking rate may exceed the listener's visual reception capabilities. The normal rate of speech may be too fast for optimum visual processing; on the other hand, slowed and exaggerated speech production does not assure improved comprehension. Rather, investigators have reported that speakers who use a normal speech rate accompanied by precise, not exaggerated, articulation are the easiest for the speechreader to understand (O'Neill, 1951; Rios-Escerla & Davis, 1977). The speaker should avoid simultaneous oral activities such as chewing, smoking, and yawning when conversing with a hearing-impaired person. While the "masking effects" of these coincidental activities have not been documented, they seem likely to complicate an already trying task.

The speaker may enhance conversational efficiency by complementing speechreading with appropriate facial expressions and gestures (Sanders, 1982). From infancy, we learn that the spoken word "no" is accompanied by a stern facial expression and shaking of the head and/or index finger from side to side. Salutations are made in conjunction with a smile and the extension or wave of the hand, opening of the arms and/or puckering of the lips. Similarly, shrugging of the shoulders has become a universal gesture that augments the verbal phrases, "I don't know" or "I don't care." Thus, *appropriate* nonverbal communication is closely associated with the verbal message and is used simultaneously with speech to provide emphasis and redundancy. Nitchie (1912) was one of the earliest to stress that the hearing impaired must learn to be cognizant of nonverbal cues when attempting to understand speech that to them is acoustically and visually distorted.

signal/code

Speech consists of acoustic information that is efficiently received and effectively interpreted by the normal auditory mechanism. It possesses physical characteristics that are compatible with the receptive capabilities of the normal ear. The basic units of speech are consonants and vowels, classified as *phonemes*. A phoneme has distinctive acoustic features that enable the listener to distinguish it from all other speech sounds.

Vowels embody the major concentration of acoustic energy found in speech, and are termed *resonanted* phonemes. Vowel production is accomplished by directing vocalizations through the oral cavity, which is altered in shape and size by different tongue and lip positions. These subtle alterations are responsible for providing each vowel with specific acoustic features.

Consonants, which are primarily responsible for the intelligibility of speech, are termed *articulated* phonemes, *articulate* meaning "to join or put together." As pointed out in Chapter 3, these phonemes possess articulatory features that permit a listener to recognize them. Miller and Nicely (1955) classified these features as *voicing, nasality, affrication, duration,* and *place of articulation.* Except for place of articulation, the identifying characteristics of consonants are perceived well on the basis of acoustic information. Although difficult to distinguish acoustically, the place of articulation may be processed to some extent visually due to the visibility of the articulators.

Since many of the approximately 41 phonemes used in English demonstrate ambiguous or very limited visible features, an individual who relies solely on vision to understand speech faces much uncertainty. Knowledge of the visual components of speech depends, for the most part, on research using small speech units, that is, consonant-vowel combinations or monosyllabic words (e.g., Binnie, Jackson, & Montgomery, 1976; Brannon & Kodman, 1959; Fisher, 1968; Franks & Kimble, 1972; Greenberg & Bode, 1968; Montgomery & Binnie, 1976; O'Neill, 1954; Woodward, 1957; Woodward & Lowell, 1964).

Visemes. The number of distinctive visual features of vowels and consonants is reduced to the shape of the mouth for vowels and the place of articulation for consonants. Since the perception of phonemes is primarily an auditory function based on acoustic features, Fisher (1968) coined the term *viseme* to indicate the distinguishable visual characteristics of speech sounds. A viseme, therefore, is a speech sound (phoneme) that has been classified by its place of articulation or by the shape of the mouth. This creates a major limitation for the observer of speech compared to the listener. Whereas combinations of auditory distinctive features are unique to each phoneme, several phonemes yield the same viseme, thus limiting the speechreader to the conclusion that one of a group of sounds was uttered.

Woodward (1957) and Woodward and Barber (1960) concluded that, since groups of consonants are produced at the same points of articulation, the phonemes within these groups cannot be differentiated visually without grammatical, phonetic, or lexical information. These visually confusable units of speech are labeled *homophemes* —speech sounds that look the same. Similarly, words that look alike are referred to as *homophenous* words. Look in the mirror and say aloud or have a friend utter the syllables /pʌ/ /bʌ/ and /mʌ/. As you watch and listen simultaneously, the syllables sound so different that you may not notice their visual similarities. However, when these same syllables are formed without voice, you will note that their visual characteristics are indistinguishable. This same type of confusion occurs among the word groups: pet, bed and men; tip, limb and dip; and cough and golf. Nearly 50% of the English phonemes are homophenous in conversation (Berger, 1972b).

Consonant visemes. Several studies have been conducted to determine the number of visemes in spoken English. Woodward and Barber (1960) classified consonants into four visually contrastive groups based on their place of articulation: bilabials, rounded labials, labiodentals, and nonlabials. Fisher (1968) later tested for confusion among these same consonants when they occurred in the initial and final positions of words. In general, his results were in agreement with Woodward and Barber's (1960) classification of homophenous groupings; however, his viseme classes resulted in five clusters, rather than four, for both the initial and final positions. Franks and Kimble (1972) found that their viewers were able to recognize seven distinct groups of consonants. Data on this issue also were collected by Binnie and his associates (1976) who concluded that individuals are capable of correctly identifying nine homophenous clusters. Table 4.1 lists the homophenous classifications proposed by several authors.

Table 4.1 also illustrates the chance for error a listener has when required to interpret phonemes visually. Except for the cases of /r/ and /w/ reported by Binnie et al. (1976), all viseme clusters contain at least two phonemes. On the average, the speechreader has at best a 50% chance of correctly identifying a specific isolated phoneme within any group when relying solely on vision.

Vowel visemes. Although vowels are not considered articulated phonemes, Jeffers and Barley (1971) suggested that vowels can be visually recognized by their movements, that is, by "a recognizable visual motor pattern, usually common to two or more speech sounds" (p. 42). These authors observed seven visible movements when the vowels were produced at a slow rate accompanied with pronounced movement and normal rhythm. When the same phonemes were produced in conversational speech the number of different movements was reduced to four.

TABLE 4.1
Visemes for English Consonants Determined by Various Researchers

Woodward & Barber (1960)	Viseme Groups Fisher (1968)		Binnie et al. (1976)
	Initial*	Final**	
1. /f, v/—labiodentals	1. /f, v/	/f, v/	1. /f, v/
2. /p, b, m/—bilabials	2. /p, b, m, d/	/p, b/	2. /p, b, m/
3. /w, r/—rounded labials	3. /ʍ, w, r/	/ʃ, ʒ, dʒ, tʃ/	3. /w/
4. /t, d, n, θ, ð, ʃ, dʒ, h, s, z, k, g, ŋ, ʒ/— nonlabials	4. /ʃ, t, n, l, s, z, dʒ, j, h/	/t, d, n, θ, ð, s, z, r, l/	4. /l, n/
			5. /ʃ, ʒ/
			6. /r/
			7. /θ, ð/
			8. /t, d, s, z/
			9. /k, g/

* Observed in the initial position.
** Observed in the final position.
The order of the visemes is based on Binnie et al.'s (1976) rank-ordering of the visual clustering of these phonemes.

These findings prompted Jackson et al. (1976) to study the visemic characteristics of vowels. The following five traits appeared to enable their viewers to group vowels:

1. Lip extension versus lip rounding (e.g., *tea* vs. *to*)

2. Vertical lip separation (e.g., *key* vs. *car*)

3. General size opening (e.g., *bird* vs. *sad*)

4. Vertical movements from 1st to 2nd nucleus (e.g., *tie* vs. *lay*)

5. Size of opening of the 2nd nucleus (e.g., *out* vs. *ate*)

According to these authors the last two traits only provide information for diphthong recognition. The distinctive visible characteristics of vowels as determined by Jeffers and Barley (1971) and Jackson et al. (1976) are shown in Table 4.2.

In general, it has been demonstrated that there are consistent visual confusions among vowels, frequently with vowels that have similar lip positions and movement (Bruhn, 1929; Kinzie & Kinzie, 1931; Nitchie, 1950; Woodward & Lowell, 1964). Further, there are vowels that are seldom recognized visually and, as might be expected, the vowels that are perceived correctly in isolation are not necessarily comprehended visually in conversational speech.

TABLE 4.2
Visemes for English Vowels, as Determined by Two Separate Studies

Viseme Groups

Jeffers & Barley (1971)	Jackson, Montgomery, & Binnie (1976)
Ideal Viewing Conditions	Dimension 1. Lip Shape — from Lips
1. Lips Puckered-Narrow Opening — /u, U, O, OU, ɝ/	Extended to Lips Rounded — /aI, æ, a, eI, ɛ, ʌ/ vs. /u, ʊ, ɝ,
2. Lips Back-Narrow Opening — /i, I, eI, e, ʌ/	aʊ, oʊ, ɔI/
3. Lips Rounded-Moderate Opening — /ɔ/	Dimension 2. Vertical Dimension of the Lips — /i, I, E/
4. Lips Relaxed-Moderate Opening to Lips Puckered-Narrow Opening — /aU/	vs./aI, æ, a/
5. Lips Relaxed-Moderate Opening — /ɛ, æ, a/	Dimension 3. General Size of Mouth Opening — Small vs. Large — /u, ʊ, ɝ, i/
6. Lips Rounded-Moderate Opening to Lips Back-Narrow Opening — /ɔI/	vs./æ, a, ɛ/
7. Lips Relaxed-Moderate Opening to Lips Back-Narrow Opening — /aI/	Dimension 4. Size of Movement from Nucleus 1 to Nucleus 2 in Diphthong Production — /aI/vs./eI/
Usual Viewing Conditions	Dimension 5. Size of Lip Opening for Nucleus 2 in
1. Lips Puckered-Narrow Opening — /u, ʊ, o, oʊ, ɝ/	Diphthong Production — /aʊ/vs./aI/
2. Lips Relaxed-Moderate Opening to Lips Puckered-Narrow Opening — /aʊ/	
3. Lips Rounded-Narrow Opening — /ɔ, ɔI/	
4. Lips Relaxed-Narrow Opening — /i, I eI, ʌ, E, æ, a, aI/	

Visual Intelligibility of Connected Discourse. Researchers have enumerated the visemes that viewers can identify at the syllable and word levels, but they are less certain about what is visibly discernible when these units are portions of lengthier utterances. The visual properties of isolated speech units change when placed in sentence form, as does the acoustic waveform itself. Unless there is a visible pause between words, a speechreader presumably perceives an uninterrupted series of lip movements of varying degrees of inherent visibility. This sequence is broken only when the speaker pauses, either deliberately or for a breath. As a result, the written message, "There is a blue car in our driveway," is spoken, /ðɛrɪzəblukarɪnauɚdraivwel/. Connected speech contains numerous articulatory positions and movements that occur in a relatively short period of time. The majority of phonemes in conversational speech occur in the medial position. The example just given contains an initial consonant /ð/ and a final vowel /e/ and numerous sounds (positions and movements) between these phonemes. Ironically, researchers have not determined the number of visemes which are identifiable when phonemes occur in the medial position.

The nature of grammatical sentence structure imposes constraints on word sequences that are not present when the words exist as isolated units. These word-arrangement rules change the probabilities of word occurrence. Thus, the receiver's task is altered (theoretically in a positive direction) because of the linguistic information and redundancy provided by connected discourse. Language is structured in a way that provides more information than is absolutely necessary to convey a given meaning or thought. Even if certain fragments of the spoken code are missed, cues or information inherent in the message may assist the receiver in making an accurate prediction of the missing parts. That is, oral language is an orderly process that is governed by the rules of structure, context, and situation and is characterized by a great amount of redundancy.

Briefly, the constraints of linguistic structure dictate how sentences are constructed. That is, if a plural noun is used, an agreeing verb can be predicted with a high degree of certainty. Similarly, contextual rule limits conversation to a specific topic, which, in turn, governs the vocabulary that is appropriate to describe the topic. We use this rule consistently, even though we frequently introduce it in a negative manner. For example, how many times have you said, "Not to change the subject," and then promptly deviated from the original topic of conversation? You are engaging the rule of contextual information, and regardless of how it is initiated it provides your receiver with a preparatory set that allows him to expect a specific vocabulary concerned with a specific event. The situational constraint refers to how the environment determines the manner in which the speaker will describe a certain event. Comedians are masters at using this rule; they alter the language of their "stories" based on the makeup of their audience. Contextual and situational constraints are closely allied and are used interchangeably by some authors. For example, during a televised sporting event when a coach disputes a decision by a referee have you noticed how well you perceive what the coach says even though you only have limited auditory and visual cues available? Contextually you perceive an argument while the situation causes the coach to express himself by using a rather limited and "heated" vocabulary that enables you to predict the words being used. As illustrated in this instance, the situation in which the conversation occurs provides information that otherwise you may not have been able to obtain by relying solely on the articulatory features of the message.

Redundancy, the result of these constraints, contributes significantly to the information afforded by language. Thus, redundancy allows the receiver to predict missed information from the information that has been perceived. To illustrate, "Dogs going" means the same as "The dogs are going away." The latter is grammatically correct and contains redundant information. Plurality is indicated twice (dogs, are), present tense twice (are, going), and the direction twice (going, away). Consequently, it would be possible to miss the words "are" and "away" while yet comprehending the message ("dogs are going"). If we miss part of a message, linguistic redundancy can enable us to synthesize correctly what we missed. However, as will be mentioned in the discussion of perceptual closure, a minimum amount of information must be perceived before accurate predictions can be made. In the preceding example, the words *dogs* and *away* would have to be processed visually in order for the speechreader to conceptualize the message, "The dogs are going away."

While the constraints of language do not enhance the physical visibility of oral sentences, they assist the receiver in visually understanding what has been said. Albright, Hipskind, and Schuckers (1973) demonstrated that speechreaders obtain more total information from the redundancy and linguistic rules of spoken language than from phoneme and word visibility. This finding has been supported by Hipskind (1977). Clouser (1976) concluded that the ratio between the number of consonants and vowels did not determine the visual intelligibility of sentences; rather, he found that short sentences were easier to speechread than longer sentences. In another study related to visual perception of speech, Berger (1972b) determined that frequently used words were identified visually more often than were words used infrequently.

environment

The environments in which the speechreader must communicate tend to be the most inflexible factors in the speechreading process. Although the environment and situation may provide the listener with valuable cues, the speechreader can do little to alter many of the physical surroundings among which communication occurs. For example, investigators have demonstrated that such factors as distance and viewing angles between speaker and receiver influence speechreading performance (Berger, 1972a; Erber, 1971, 1974; Woodward & Lowell, 1964). Erber's (1971c) study regarding the influence of distance on the visual perception of speech revealed that speechreading performance was optimal when the speaker was about 5 feet from the speechreader. Although performance decreased beyond 5 feet, it did not drop significantly until the distance exceeded 20 feet. Similarly, there is evidence that simultaneous acoustic and visual competition can have an adverse effect on speechreading under certain conditions (Leonard, 1968; O'Neill & Oyer, 1981). Although the amount of lighting is not an important factor in speechreading, provided a reasonable amount of light is present (Thomas, 1969), Erber (1974) suggested that, for optimal visual reception of speech, illumination should provide a contrast between the background and the speaker's face.

Based on independent studies, Pelson and Prather (1974) and Garstecki (1977) concluded that speechreading performance improved when the spoken message was accompanied by relevant pictorial and auditory cues. This finding was given further support by Garstecki and O'Neill (1980), whose subjects had better speechreading scores when the CID Everyday Sentences were presented with appropriate situational cues. In essence, environmental cues afford listeners with contextual and situational information, thereby increasing their ability to predict what is being conveyed verbally.

speechreader

Reduction of a person's ability to *hear* (auditory sensitivity) acoustic events is only one of several parameters that contribute to the handicapping effects of hearing impairments. The factors of auditory perception (recognizing, identifying, and understanding), age at onset of the impairment, progressivity, site(s) of lesions, and educational/therapeutic management result in making the hearing-impaired population extremely heterogeneous (Hipskind, 1978). This heterogeneity appears to extend to speechreading, since hearing-impaired individuals demonstrate considerable variability in their ability to use vision to speechread. Since beginning to use speechreading as an educational and clinical approach to aural rehabilitation, clinicians and researchers have attempted to determine what personal characteristics account for success/failure in speechreading, including age, intelligence, personality traits, and visual acuity (Berger, 1972a; O'Neill & Oyer, 1981). In general, it is impossible to identify what characteristics lead to success in speechreading. The following is a sampling of the research that has been conducted in this area.

Age. There appears to be some interactions between a speechreader's age and other attributes that contribute to speechreading ability. Specifically, evidence suggests that speechreading proficiency tends to develop and improve throughout childhood and early adulthood (Berger, 1972a; Craig, 1964; Evans, 1960, 1965; Heider, 1947; Jeffers & Barley, 1971; Wynn, 1964). Even though their speechreading abilities are not fully developed, younger children, even infants, may use speechreading to some extent (Pollack, 1970).

Some older people demonstrate *phonemic regression,* that is, an inability to understand speech which is not consistent with their audiometric profiles (Gaeth, 1948). This same type of phenomenon may account, in part, for the finding that older individuals do less well in speechreading than their counterparts who are between the ages of 21 and 30 years old (Farrimond, 1959; Garstecki, 1983; Goetzinger, 1964; Pelsen & Prather, 1974). Shoop and Binnie (1979) suggested several reasons why the elderly perform more poorly on experimental speechreading tasks, including (a) inability to process abstract stimuli as one becomes older, (b) unfamiliarity with the stimuli used to assess speechreading ability, and (c) the questionable reliability between scores obtained on a speechreading test and a person's ability to speechread messages that occur in daily life. Finally, decreased visual acuity may also contribute to reduced speechreading skill among the elderly.

Intelligence. An abundance of research describes the relationship between speechreading and mental abilities. Generally, no demonstrable positive correlation has been found between understanding speech visually and intelligence, assuming intelligence levels in or above the "low normal" range (Cavender, 1949; Lewis, 1972; O'Neill, 1951; O'Neill & Davidson, 1956; Reid, 1946; Simmons, 1959). Nevertheless, a study conducted by Smith and his colleagues (1964) with a population of mentally impaired individuals revealed that reduced intelligence levels did affect speechreading scores in a predictable manner.

Personality Traits. As may be expected from the preceding discussion, investigators have not been able to ferret out specific personality traits that differentiate among levels of speechreading proficiency. While motivation is tenuous to assess, most clinicians intuitively concur that highly motivated (competitive) clients tend to speechread more effectively than do unmotivated clients. Nitchie (1912, 1950) and Kinzie (1931) discussed the necessity of motivation in their methods of teaching speechreading. However, various persons have concluded that good and poor speechreaders cannot be stereotyped based on personality patterns (Giolas, Butterfield, & Weaver, 1974; O'Neill, 1951).

Visual Skills. Since speechreading is a visual activity, the acuity of vision is critical in the decoding process. As discussed in the Visual Assessment section of this chapter, vision has received meager attention from researchers in aural rehabilitation.

Visual Acuity. In the early 1960s Goetzinger (1964) reported that there was no demonstrable relationship between visual acuity and the ability to decode speech visually. In 1969, however, results of Lovering's research in the area of visual acuity and speechreading performance contradicted previous findings. Thus, he demonstrated that visual acuity of 20/40 and less had an appreciable, negative affect on speechreading scores. A year later, Hardick, Oyer, and Irion (1970) found that they could rank order successful and unsuccessful speechreaders on the basis of visual acuity. Furthermore, these authors observed a significant relationship between eye blink rate and speechreading ability, with poorer speechreaders demonstrating higher eye blink rates.

In support of the argument that good visual acuity is important for successful speechreading performance, Romano and Barlow (1974) concluded that visual acuity must be at least 20/80 before speech can be decoded visually. Recently, a line of research has compared visually evoked responses and speechreading ability. According to the results of this research, a viewer's ability to process speech visually is, in part, a function of the rapidity (latency) with which physical visual stimuli are transduced to neural energy for interpretation at the cortical level (Samar & Sims, 1983, 1984; Shepard, 1982; Shepard et al., 1977). While the clinical applicability of this research has not yet been fully realized, visually evoked responses can assist the clinician in understanding a client's ability to process visually oriented information. Potentially, visually evoked responses may provide aural rehabilitationists with information regarding a viewer's ability to speechread various types of oral stimuli.

Visual Perception. Dependent on and relevant to visual acuity is visual perception. Based on Gibson's (1969) definition of perception, our eyes receive visual stimuli that are interpreted at a cortical level and provide us with visual information. This information, in turn, enables us to make a selective response to the original stimuli. Thus, when interpreting speech visually, the speechreader first "sees" the movement of the lips, which the cortex classifies as speech. The accuracy of the speechreader's response to these stimuli is a function of how well the peripheral-to-central visual process enables him to discriminate among the speaker's articulatory movements.

At present, explanations of the way in which the perceptual process develops are theoretical. However, two strategies appear predominant in connection with obtaining information from the environment. The first, *figure-ground patterning* is achieved by identifying a target (meaningful) signal that is embedded in similar, but ambient, stimuli. Observe the following letters:

W	A	B	R	I	O	D	R	A	Z
O	P	A	I	B	L	O	H	Y	E
L	I	P	R	E	A	D	I	N	G
I	L	R	A	C	R	A	X	O	L
M	U	A	L	Y	O	C	E	P	L

The letters within this rectangle are of the same case (capitals) and are placed in an order that meets the criterion of structural ordering. That is, all the letter combinations are possible and probable in written English. As noted, however, there is only one string of letters that creates a meaningful word—LIPREADING (see line 3). Thus, this sequence of printed symbols is the *figure* while all the other letters are merely spurious background stimuli. The development of *figure-ground patterning* permits the hearing impaired to separate meaningful visual and auditory events from ambient stimuli.

As early as 1912 Nitchie claimed that successful speechreaders are intuitive and able to synthesize limited visual input into meaningful wholes. More recently, Sanders and Conscarelli (1970), Sharp (1972), and Hipskind (1977) concurred that effective speechreaders possess the ability to visually piece together fragmented pictorial and spoken stimuli into meaningful messages. This ability, *closure*, is yet another strategy used to obtain information from environmental events. Before this strategy can be used effectively, we must receive at least minimal stimulation, and, more importantly, must have had prior experience (familiarity) with the whole. Both of the following sentences require that the reader use closure to obtain accurate information.

1. Humpty _____/_____/_____/_____/wall.

2. When you _____ time, you murder _____.

In all probability you had little difficulty supplying the four words, Dumpty sat on a, to the first sentence. The second sentence may have been more difficult unless you are familiar with the adage, "When you kill time, you murder opportunity." The first sentence provides considerably fewer physical cues than does the second; but experience with and exposure to nursery rhymes permitted you to perceive the whole figure. Effective visual closure skills are essential for the hearing impaired, because, due to their disorder and the limited visual cues afforded by speech, they receive fragmented/distorted auditory and visual stimuli. In trying to understand the role of prediction or predictability it is probably very important to realize that we do not merely get some information by perception (processing the stimuli) and some from the context (prediction), and then add the two. If we did, the total information received would be equal to, or *less* than (because of redundancy, or correlation), the sum of what we can get from either channel alone. The fact that the total is greater than the sum of both channels (as measured above) implies a facilitating or "feedback" effect from one to the other ... the aural information facilitates visual processing, and the visual information enhances auditory processing.

It is apparent that numerous factors have an impact on speechreading success. The successful clinician will be familiar with these and take each into account when assisting the hearing impaired in effectively utilizing visual information for communication.

speechreading and the hearing impaired

Assessing speechreading ability and providing effective speechreading instruction to the hearing impaired are two primary responsibilities of the aural rehabilitationist. The next section outlines some of the ways in which a person's visual communication ability can be evaluated. It also describes several traditional and current approaches to speechreading instruction.

measurement of speechreading ability

Because of the complexities associated with the process, accurate evaluation of speechreading performance is difficult. Professionals have attempted for several decades to develop a means of reliable and valid measurement, yet no universally acceptable test or battery of tests has emerged for this purpose to date. Nevertheless, clinicians recognize the importance of assessing speechreading ability to determine if visual communication training is warranted for a particular individual as well as to evaluate the effectiveness of speechreading training. Consequently, a number of formal and informal approaches of measuring speechreading are currently in use.

Formal Speechreading Tests. Since the mid 1940s, speechreading tests have been developed, published, and used. These tests, designed either specifically for adults or to measure children's speechreading abilities, may consist of syllables, words, sentences, stories, or a combination of these stimuli. Tests are usually presented without acoustic cues on film, videotape, or in a "live", face-to-face manner. While test contents remain constant, the manner of presentation may vary considerably among clinicians. Some of these tests are listed in Table 4.3

Informal Speechreading Tests. Informal tests are presented live by the clinician who selects and employs stimulus materials. Contents vary as a function of the client's age and the information sought by the rehabilitationist. This type of test may include such items as "What is your name?", "Where do you work?", "Do you like candy?", and "Show me (a particular object or picture; for example, pig, dog, chicken, car, airplane)." This type of assessment allows the tester to select stimuli that are more pertinent for a particular client than items on *formal* speechreading tests. As a result of the format and intent of these tests, the obtained results do not lend themselves well to comparative analysis. Sanders (1971) presented a thorough discussion of informal speechreading assessment. The reader is encouraged to consult this source for further information.

limitations of speechreading tests

Formal speechreading tests have met with some criticism. These criticisms include:

1. Absence of accompanying auditory cues

2. Unnatural and limited gestures

3. Unnatural and inappropriate facial expression

4. Nonfunctional sentences

5. Use of a single speaker

6. Scored as an identification task rather than as a person's ability to perceive thoughts visually

7. No differentiation between skilled and unskilled speechreaders

8. Poor predictors of speechreading success

TABLE 4.3
Chronological Listing of Speechreading Tests for Adults and Children

Date Developed	Title of Test	Author(s)	Content Format
	ADULTS		
1946	How Well Can You Read Lips?*	Utley	Words Sentences Stories
1957	A Film Test of Lipreading	Taaffe	Sentences
1967	Multiple-Choice Test of Lipreading	Donnelly & Marshall	Sentences
1971	Barley-CID Sentences	Barley	Sentences
1976	Lipreading Screening Test	Binnie, Jackson, & Montgomery	CV-Syllables
1978	Denver Quick Test of Lipreading Ability*	Alpiner	Sentences
	CHILDREN		
1949	Cavender Test of Lipreading Ability	Cavender	Sentences
1957	Costello Test of Speech-Reading	Costello	Words Sentences
1959	Semi-Diagnostic Test	Hutton, Curry, & Armstrong	Words
1964	Craig Lipreading Inventory*	Craig	Words Sentences
1968	Butt Children's Speechreading Test	Butt & Chreist	Questions/ Commands
1970	Diagnostic Test of Speechreading	Myklebust & Neyhaus	Words, Phrases & Sentences

* See Appendix for more information.

Whether using formal or informal speechreading tests, it is important that the stimuli not be so difficult that they discourage the client, nor so easy that test scores reflect a ceiling effect (100% correct for each viewer). Materials should be selected so that they approximate various types of stimuli encountered by the individual in everyday situations. For children and certain adults (such as those with severe speech or writing problems) the response mode should involve pointing with a multiple-choice format; most adults are capable of responding to (writing or repeating) open-set tests. Because of the various shortcomings of existing speechreading tests, these instruments cannot be expected to provide completely valid measures of speechreading ability, but may yield data of some clinical usefulness.

The use of live, face-to-face presentation, while widespread, should be conducted carefully with optimal consideration for distance (5-10 feet), lighting (no shadows), and viewing angle (0°-45°). Even following these precautions, speaker variability will introduce uncertainty into the test situation. Not only will two speakers produce the same speech stimuli differently, but a single talker, producing the same stimuli twice, will not do so in precisely the same manner each time. Therefore, it is difficult to compare a person's skills from one testing to another (pre- and post-therapy) or to directly compare the performance of two individuals. Scores obtained through face-to-face test administration, while useful, need to be interpreted carefully.

Assessment of speechreading most often involves the presentation of visual stimuli without any associated acoustic cues. While this yields meaningful information regarding the basic skill of speechreading, additional testing of speechreading ability in a combined auditory/visual fashion is also advocated (Binnie, 1973), since it more closely resembles ordinary person-to-person communication. Such testing provides a measure of how well a person integrates visual and auditory information (Garstecki, 1983; see also Chapter 9). Auditory/visual presentation is meaningful only when the hearing loss is great enough to preclude 100% performance on the basis of hearing alone. For research purposes, however, auditory processing can be artificially limited by earplugs or masking noise.

visual assessment and speechreading measurement

As discussed, there is clear evidence that even mild visual acuity problems can have adverse effects on speechreading performance. It is amazing, therefore, that aural rehabilitationists have given only limited attention to measuring visual abilities in connection with assessment/instruction of speechreading with hearing-impaired persons. Concern for this is further reinforced by research on visual disorders among those with hearing loss. Thus, evidence indicates that the incidence of occular anomalies among hearing-impaired students is greater than for normally hearing children of the same age (Johnson & Caccamise, 1982). Campbell and her associates (1981) surveyed the literature and found that 38-58% of the hearing impaired reportedly have accompanying visual deficiencies. Even more alarming are data from the National Technical Institute for the Deaf showing that of the total number of students entering in 1978 and 1979, 65% demonstrated defective vision (Johnson, Caccamise, Rothblum, Hamilton, & Howard, 1981). Additional information by Karp (1983) concerning visual defects among individuals with hearing loss is provided in Chapter 13 of this text.

It is obvious that assessment of speechreading skills must be preceded by a measure of visual acuity. Berger (1972a) argued that visual acuity is a poor and inaccurate predictor of speechreading ability since visual acuity is determined by having the viewer observe a static target whereas the ability to speechread requires detection of dynamic stimuli (rapid movements). This opinion is difficult to refute; however, if a person is not capable of differentiating among static visual stimuli, it seems logical that he or she would have considerable difficulty discriminating visually the rapid movements of speech.

Riggs (1965) suggested that visual tasks of *detection, recognition, resolution,* and *localization* are fundamental when assessing a person's visual acuity. (These tasks are described in Figures 4.2, 4.3, 4.4, and 4.5.)

1. *Detection.* The viewer states whether or not the object is present in the field of vision (Figure 4.2).

2. *Recognition.* The viewer names the test object or specifies the location of some critical aspect of it (Figure 4.3).

3. *Resolution.* The viewer responds to the separation between elements of particular patterns (Figure 4.4).

4. *Localization.* The viewer discriminates among displacements of one part of the test object with respect to other parts (Figure 4.5).

Another visual measurement, *dynamic visual acuity* (DVA), is made when the target, the viewer, or both, are moving. This test is not designed to determine the eye's ability to differentiate among similar and rapid movements, but evaluates the viewer's visual acuity for a moving target. The only area of visual acuity that is reported routinely in the aural

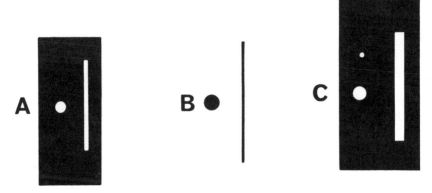

Figure 4.2. The task of detection. *A*: Bright test objects against a dark field. *B*: Dark test objects against a bright field. *C*: Low contrast objects. The subject states whether the object is present. He or she is not required to name, discriminate parts, or indicate a position. (From "Visual Acuity" by L. A. Riggs in *Vision and visual perception* (p. 322) by C. Graham (Ed.), 1965, New York: John Wiley & Sons. Reprinted by permission.)

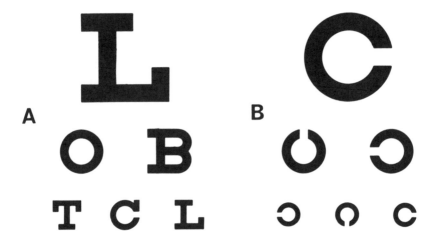

Figure 4.3. The task of recognition. *A*: Snellen letters of the alphabet. *B*: Landolt ring test object. The subject is required to name specific aspects of the object; for example, what the letters are, where the gaps are located. (From "Visual Acuity" by L. A. Riggs in *Vision and visual perception* (p. 324) by C. Graham (Ed.), 1965, New York: John Wiley & Sons. Reprinted by permission.)

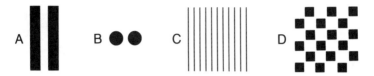

Figure 4.4. The task of resolution. *A*: Double line target. *B*: Double line target. *C*: Acuity grating. *D*: Checkerboard. The basic measurement is to determine the minimal distance between objects for the discrimination of separateness. (From "Visual Acuity" by L. A. Riggs in *Vision and visual perception* (p. 325) by C. Graham (Ed.), 1965, New York: John Wiley & Sons. Reprinted by permission.)

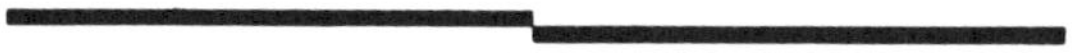

Figure 4.5. The task of localization. The task is to appreciate small lateral displacements of one segment of a line. (From "Visual Acuity" by L. A. Riggs in *Vision and visual perception* (p. 326) by C. Graham (Ed.), 1965, New York: John Wiley & Sons. Reprinted by permission.)

rehabilitation literature is that of *recognition*. Thus, most clinicians are not well prepared to discuss the potential significance of the other visual acuity tests for speechreading.

hearing impairment and dependence on vision

The degree to which the hearing impaired depend on vision for information is related to the extent of their hearing loss. To paraphrase Ross (1982), there is a world of difference between the deaf, who must communicate through a visual mode (speechreading or manual communication), and the hard of hearing, who communicate "primarily" through an auditory mode (albeit imperfectly).

Deaf. The deaf, who receive little or no meaningful auditory cues, must rely on their vision to keep in contact with their environment. Myklebust (1954) and others have determined that the deaf use their vision projectively and are visually oriented. However, as stated throughout this chapter, vision is inferior to audition when used to decode spoken language. The deaf are further handicapped in that, before they can gain meaning from speechreading stimuli, they must have developed language, which, in turn, is most naturally acquired through auditory stimulation. Speechreading refers to the ability to perceive verbal language visually. Using this definition, it is evident that language development is a prerequisite for obtaining meaning from speechreading. Thus, deaf persons face the monumental challenge of having to speechread words that they may never have conceptualized.

Hard of Hearing. Hard-of-hearing individuals, by definition, possess functional residual hearing, which permits them to receive auditory cues within their environment. This ability would suggest that they are less dependent on their vision than are the deaf when having to recognize speech. Even so, the hard of hearing, who employ their vision to supplement distorted and reduced acoustic stimuli, receive considerably more information from the spoken code than is provided solely by their auditory channel.

Various investigators have assessed the advantages that audition, vision, and a combination of these sensory modalities afford the receiver when decoding spoken stimuli (Binnie et al., 1976; Erber, 1971a, 1971b, 1972, 1979; Hutton, 1959; Neely, 1956; O'Neill, 1954; Sanders & Goodrich, 1971; Sumby & Pollack, 1954). Few would disagree that using these senses simultaneously produces better speech reception and speech discrimination than using either alone. Likewise, it is clear that vision provides information to the receiver when decoding speech in the absence of auditory cues. More importantly, however, even limited auditory input allows the listener to establish a referent from which additional information can be gained visually. Thus, the contributions made by these sensory mechanisms as receptors of speech fall into a hierarchy. That is, when both residual hearing and speechreading are available, the impaired listener tends to do better on a communicative task. For example, if a person gets a speech discrimination score of 50% and a speechreading score of 20% with similar test material, that individual may achieve a combined auditory/visual score which could approach 90%. In other words, there is more than a simple additive effect from the combination of auditory and visual information. Consequently, speechreading used as a unisensory approach (visual only) to rehabilitate the hard of hearing is normally not encouraged. A point forgotten by many clinicians is that the ultimate goal is to provide their clients with experiences that will alleviate limitations rather than stressing a procedure that exaggerates the existing impairment. The utility of vision in decoding speech should be exploited in audiological communication training. However, this particular decoding process should not be emphasized at the expense of denying auditory input, except under special circumstances.

traditional speechreading methods

During the early 1900s, four methods of teaching speechreading were popularized in the United States (O'Neill & Oyer, 1981). Three of these methods were nurtured by individuals who had normal hearing until adulthood, at which time they acquired significant hearing losses. Initially, they sought assistance to overcome the limitations placed on them by their sensory deprivation. Subsequently, they became interested in assisting other hearing-impaired persons in developing speechreading skills, eventually establishing methods that bear their names: the Bruhn method (1929), the Kinzie method (1931), and the Nitchie method (1912). Later Bunger (1944) wrote a book describing a speechreading method developed by Brauckman in Jena, Germany, the Jena method.

Analytic and Synthetic Approaches. Each of these methods primarily reflects one of two approaches (analytic or synthetic) to teach speechreading. The *analytic* approach, advocated by Bruhn and Brauckman, is based on the concept that before the whole can be identified, it is necessary to perceive each of its basic parts. That is, since a word is constructed by placing phonemes in a given sequential order and since sentences (thoughts) are constructed by correctly ordering words, it is essential that the viewer initially identify phonemes visually in isolation before attempting to perceive words. Likewise, we must be able to identify individual words before attempting to recognize strings of words (sentences/phrases). Said differently, this approach considers the syllable to be the basic unit of speech; therefore, these units must be recognized in isolation before comprehension of the whole is probable.

Conversely, the *synthetic* approaches of Nitchie and Kinzie emphasize that the perception of the whole is paramount regardless of which of its parts is perceived visually. Consequently, the speechreader is encouraged to comprehend the general meaning of oral utterances rather than concentrating on accurately identifying each component within the oral message. As noted earlier, a considerable number of English phonemes are not visible or distinguishable on the speaker's lips; thus, the receiver must predict and synthesize information from fragmented visual input. The synthetic approach considers the sentence to be the basic unit and backbone of visual speech perception.

When reviewing these four methods, it becomes evident that each reveals the author's philosophy of how speechreading skills are most efficiently and effectively developed; however, they also share several characteristics. First, each method stresses the importance of explaining to the speechreader the difference between articulatory position and articulatory movement. Position refers to the placement of the articulators during the production of isolated phonemes; movement is the action of the articulators progressing from one position to another. Second, the authors emphasize that voice should accompany all speechreading stimuli. This practice assures that the stimuli are produced in a natural and realistic manner. Third, the primary goal is to develop skills that will enable the speechreader to recognize connected discourse. Synopses of these methods follow.

Bruhn method (1929). Martha Bruhn, who acquired a hearing loss during early adulthood, studied speechreading with Julius Mueller-Walle in Hamburg, Germany and later returned to the United States where she opened her own school in Boston for the hearing impaired. Bruhn's method emphasizes the need to quickly recognize the position and movement of speech sounds produced in rapid rhythmic succession. This is accomplished by having the receiver initially view syllables rather than words so that he concentrates on seeing specific movements and positions rather than concerning himself with identifying a particular word. The method proceeds to words and sentences, at which time the speechreader is encouraged to develop the ability to obtain the general meaning of the sentences rather than concentrating on correctly identifying each word.

Jena method (1944). This method is considered the most analytic of all speechreading training. It was developed by Karl Brauckman in Jena, Germany, and promoted in Michigan by Anna Bunger, who later wrote a book based on Brauckman's format. The method emphasizes syllable drills, rhythm practice, and kinesthetic awareness. Syllables are presented in a rhythmic pattern and the student is required to imitate them simultaneously with the teacher. This activity permits the student to experience how the various phonemes feel during production. The advantage of presenting the stimuli in a rhythmic manner is to reinforce the fact that speech is a rhythmical event; consequently, the development of rhythm may produce greater speechreading success.

Nitchie method (1912, 1950). Edward Nitchie became deaf during his adolescence and immediately enrolled in speechreading therapy. He eventually established his own school for the deaf in New York, stressing the analytic approach. Later, Nitchie altered his philosophy and has been given credit for developing the synthetic approach to speechreading. The speechreader studies articulatory movements by viewing meaningful monosyllabic words. Nitchie used this exercise to develop eye training. Since communication involves processing words strung together to form thoughts and ideas, the speechreader must develop the ability to transfer the observed movements into language. To achieve this, Nitchie advocated the use of sentences and stories whereby the mind is trained to comprehend the general meaning of connected discourse, rather than accurately identifying each of the words within the sentences and stories.

Kinzie method (1931). Cora Kinzie acquired a hearing loss while a medical student in Pennsylvania. She studied speechreading with Bruhn and subsequently opened her own school in Philadelphia. Shortly thereafter she studied with Nitchie and at his urging she and her sister developed their own method of speechreading training by combining the best features of the Bruhn and Nitchie methods. A uniqueness of Kinzie's method was the construction of graded lessons for both adults and children. These lessons were designed to provide materials for speechreaders of varying abilities. The Kinzies considered the sentence the basis of speechreading therapy and that, consequently, teachers should be masters of sentence construction. They recommended that all sentences used in speechreading instruction be "definite, natural, interesting, pleasing, rhythmical, and dignified" (p. 7).

recent trends in speechreading instruction

In recent years few new approaches to speechreading instruction have emerged. Berger (1972a) traced the history of speechreading methods following the Mueller-Walle, Nitchie, Kinzie, and Jena eras, and referred to the more recent work of McNutt (1952), Ewing (1959), Wyatt (1960), and Haspiel (1964). As he indicated, most of the newer instructional methods are modifications or combinations of the earlier well-known approaches. This finding is reinforced by Rodel (1978), who observed:

> Few visual training programs ... today adhere exclusively to techniques described in the traditional approaches to lipreading. Most often an eclectic approach, which includes principles and practice material from several different methods, is emphasized. (p. 586)

The improvements in personal amplification devices which have occurred in the past two decades have made it possible for the hearing impaired, especially those with moderate to severe losses, to more effectively utilize speechreading in an integrated manner with their hearing. In a sense, this increased potential to greatly improve the communication abilities of those with hearing loss through hearing aids has led to less emphasis on speechreading in rehabilitation programs for many individuals. The next two sections briefly discuss some of the more recent ways in which speechreading has been incorporated into rehabilitation strategies for both children and adults.

Children. Therapeutic approaches used with hearing-impaired children by Wedenberg (1951), Huizing (1952), Griffiths (1964), and Pollack (1964, 1985) focused almost exclusively on the auditory channel. Despite the unisensory orientation of these approaches, children trained by them often emerged with effective speechreading skills. Neither Wedenberg nor Pollack generally prevented their students from watching the lips, although the teaching clearly focuses on auditory input. Apparently this skill develops synergistically with the acquisition of auditory and language skills. Pollack (1964) also noted the excellent visual-perception abilities exhibited by those trained using the acoupedic approach, which maximizes the auditory potential of hard-of-hearing infants.

Methods that incorporate both auditory and visual input are frequently favored currently (Rodel, 1985; Whitehurst, 1964), even though the auditory input often receives the initial emphasis (Pollack, 1985). In short, the use of visual stimuli in remediation of children with hearing loss continues to be an important component in early training. However, there is a tendency to allow this aspect of rehabilitation to develop naturally in conjunction with the acquisition of auditory, speech, and linguistic skills (see Chapter 8). Thus, more emphasis is placed on integration of auditory and visual cues, rather than exclusive work in isolation on either speechreading or auditory skills. Recent research (Boothroyd & Hnath, 1986) has also demonstrated that speechreading skills can be enhanced through the simultaneous use of vibrotactile cues.

As with adults, aural rehabilitation for children should be client oriented. That is, activities must be interesting and give the child the opportunity to experience success in correctly recognizing what is being said. Figure 4.6 is an example of such an activity. The child is given a worksheet with a picture on it and asked to speechread the *key* words presented by the clinician or other children, if in a group session. Beyond providing contextual and situational information, the picture also has the potential to stimulate client motivation and interest. As a reward the clinician may ask the child to color the picture. Numerous exercises and materials for speechreading training with children are described in Berg (1976), Sanders (1982), and Whitehurst (1964).

Adults. In the past, speechreading instruction was often provided to hearing-impaired adults in an intensive manner over a sometimes lengthy period of time. This approach is still utilized in some instances, such as the program at the National Technical Institute for the Deaf (NTID)

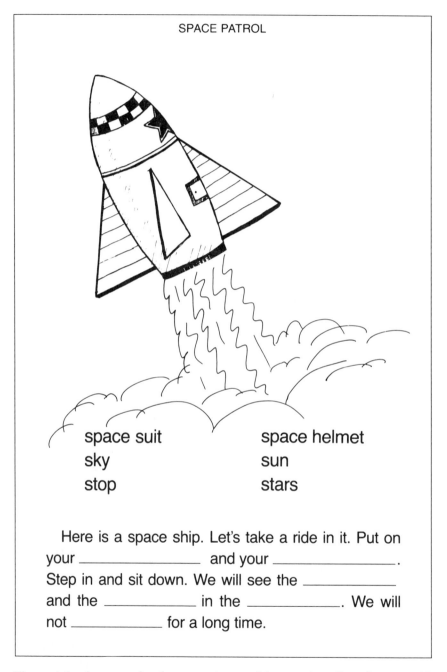

Figure 4.6. An example of an exercise used in speechreading therapy with children.

(Jacobs, 1982; Sims, 1985), and speechreading therapy conducted with some individuals at Walter Reed Army Hospital (Walden et al., 1977, 1981). There has been a growing interest, however, in including speechreading instruction as part of a general orientation to effective communication skills. This type of program is comparatively short-term and emphasizes the general listening and visual attentiveness aspects of auditory training and speechreading. Giolas outlines such an approach in Chapter 13. Fleming (1972) and Hardick (1977) also described similar methodologies.

Whether or not speechreading therapy is conducted over a short- or long-term basis, or is carried out in an analytic or synthetic manner, a growing awareness has been expressed in recent times (Garstecki, 1983; Montgomery & Sylvester, 1984) of the wisdom of working with adults on auditory and visual skills simultaneously.

In emphasizing the need for integration of visual and auditory training, Sanders (1982) stated:

> Except for the person with little or no residual hearing, visual communication training is inseparable from auditory training. To consider it as a separate aspect of communication requiring separate training sessions is to ignore the indisputable finding that audiovisual speech processing is superior to auditory or visual processing alone under degraded listening conditions. (p. 436)

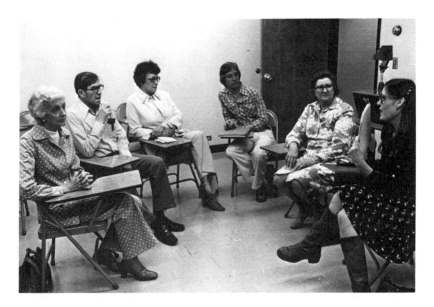

Figure 4.7. Speechreading instruction with adults.

A number of activities may be utilized during speechreading therapy to emphasize the synergistic effects between vision and audition. For example, the therapist may present selected sentences live or videotaped—auditorily and visually. For the first several sentences the last word is presented solely as a visual stimulus; for example, The girl wore a pretty pink (*dress*). All the words except *dress* are verbalized—*dress* is merely "mouthed." Another group of sentences are given with the last two words presented solely as visual stimuli. This procedure is continued until the reduction in auditory information no longer causes a corresponding reduction in the listener's ability to understand the meaning of the utterance. The same type of activity can be used to eliminate the auditory cues from any of the words within the sentences.

Since a frequent complaint by the hard of hearing is that they have difficulty understanding speech in noise or during group conversations, conducting therapy in the presence of controlled competitions is another useful and practical technique. This may be accomplished by developing a tape (auditory only) of meaningful sentences and another tape of multi-talker speech babble. Next, a sample of meaningful sentences (targets) is presented to the client (auditorily and visually). These may be delivered live or on videotape. The target sentences and the competition (speech babble or similar signal) are introduced simultaneously at various signal/competition ratios. The competition is more effective and creates a more realistic environment when sentences of the same topic as the target sentences are used. That is, Competition—"We saw a horse at the farm;" Target—"The brown horse didn't run very far." Or Competition—"Successful students develop good study habits;" Target—"The student was successful in achieving good grades." Rehabilitationists must select appropriate signal-to-competition ratios for each client based on the client's hearing and visual abilities (see Chapter 9 for further discussion regarding adults).

Binnie's (1976) pseudo-dialogue format is an effective strategy for developing listener/viewer confidence. This procedure involves selecting a specific topic such as carpentry, cooking, economics, hobbies, natural resources, and so forth, from which a number of questions and answers are developed. The client reads (out loud to himself) a question prepared by the clinician such as: "What type of leisure-time activities do you enjoy?" He then observes the clinician who replies, without voice, "My favorite summer activity is golfing." The client then writes down what he thinks the clinician has said and reads the next question which may be, "How often do you get to play?" to which the clinician may answer, "I usually play on Saturday morning." The client's next printed question would be, "Is that all you get to play?", to which the clinician's "mouthed" response would be, "Every now and then I sneak out during the week.'' This give-and-take provides the listener with a preparatory set while attempting to interpret speech visually.

In describing the general strategies used with the hearing-impaired adult in the remediation process, Alpiner and McCarthy (1987) stressed the "progressive" approach. Basically, this is a client-centered, individualized approach to rehabilitation which emphasizes the use of counseling techniques to deal with specific communication problems. The use of the progressive approach in conjunction with traditional forms of aural rehabilitation such as speechreading is described thoroughly by Alpiner and McCarthy.

As discussed with regard to auditory training, the tracking method (DeFilippo & Scott, 1978) is now being utilized in speechreading therapy. This method requires the individual to speechread verbatim passages presented live, with performance measured by the number of words correctly identified per unit of time. Owens and Telleen (1981), Robbins, Osberger, Miyamoto, Kienle, and Myers (1985), and Levitt, Waltzman, Shapiro, and Cohen (1986) confirmed that their subjects demonstrated significant learning effects when using the tracking procedure. Continued research is needed concerning tracking to determine the amount of carryover from therapy to everyday situations.

Other innovative approaches which incorporate speechreading training have utilized computer-based instruction. For example, Cronin (1979) and his colleagues at NTID devised such a system for self-instruction in speechreading and auditory training for students of the school. The student makes use of videotaped exercises which provide structured speechreading drill in a variety of material at beginning, intermediate, and advanced levels of instruction. The student uses a microcomputer interface to access the videotapes and to type in responses to drill work. The computer also provides a means of monitoring student performance. This system, referred to as DAVID (Dynamic Audio Video Interactive Device), appears to have potential for a variety of applications within communication rehabilitation (Sims, 1985).

Another computerized program, the Lip-Reader Trainer (Universe Electric Research Co., 1987) has been introduced recently for use with a microcomputer. It incorporates 19 high-resolution, three-color, graphic mouth shapes to simulate speech production. The program has an unlimited vocabulary and is capable of animating words or sentences up to 115 characters in length. There is little doubt that more computer-generated speechreading programs will be developed in the future for use by the hearing impaired.

Other Considerations. It is not unusual for clinicians to lament the lack of carryover between therapy sessions or between therapy and everyday activities. One reason for this is that little may be occurring in therapy that is appropriate for the client to "carryover" or apply to the real world. Materials presented during speechreading therapy should be meaningful and useful, and applicable to the client's daily needs. If they are, the odds of successful carryover are greatly increased.

To further increase the chances of carryover, clinicians are encouraged to conduct a portion of the therapy sessions on visual training or other aspects of aural rehabilitation outside the confines of the therapy cubicle. Frequently, therapy becomes unduly artificial because of *where* as well as *how* it is conducted. Most hearing-impaired clients communicate adequately, if not normally, during individual therapy sessions. Conversely, many of these same clients experience considerable difficulty conversing in everyday situations. Clinicians may learn a great deal by taking their clients to auditoriums, playgrounds, coffeeshops, shopping malls, and other community locations. Finally, the clinician's creativity should be devoted to providing experiences that are client oriented.

manual communication

Physical gestures and facial expressions have always been used by humans to express emotions and to share information. The transmission of thoughts in this manner undoubtedly preceded the verbal form of communication. As stated earlier in this chapter, manual communication is comprised of specific gestural codes. That is, a message is transmitted by the fingers, hands, arms, and bodily postures using specific signs or fingerspelling.

In general, *manualism* is used by a high percentage of the deaf and profoundly hard of hearing to communicate with other individuals having manual communication skills. The various forms of manual communication are used in isolation or in combination with speech.

types of manual communication

Numerous forms of manual communication have evolved. The major types, along with spoken English, are briefly described and compared in Table 4.4 (Smith, 1984). Smith pointed out that the only two pure languages represented in this group are English and American Sign Language.

TABLE 4.4
Forms of Manual and Spoken Communication

American Sign Language (ASL)	Pidgin Sign English (PSE)	Signed English	Linguistics of Visual English (LOVE)	Signing Exact English (SEE 2)	Seeing Essential English (SEE 1)	Finger Spelling	Cued Speech	English
Independent language; visual manual mode; own grammar; own syntax; signs are meaning based; has dialects, regionalisms, slang, puns; can be written; wide range of vocabulary covering minute differences in meaning; may borrow from other languages; is verbal, but also makes use of nonverbal elements.	A combination of elements from ASL and the sign systems, ranging from the more ASL-like (occasionally called Ameslish) to the more English-like (sometimes called CASE—Conceptually Accurate Signed English). Usually contains few if any sign markers (see Signed English), yet makes frequent use of finger-spelled English words. Used in conjunction with speech in interpreting and college teaching. Signs are meaning based.	Signed in accordance with English grammar, but signs are meaning based; specially invented sign markers for important affixes in English; invented by Bornstein; used widely in education.	Essentially the same as SEE 2, but has a method of writing each sign; used in education; invented by Wampler; usage is diminishing.	Signs are word based; special signs for all affixes in English; signed in strict accordance with English; invented by Zawolkow, Pfetzing and Gustason; widely used in education; very influential.	Signs are based on word roots (morphemes) (trans/port/a/tion); an extreme form of word-based signs; invented by Anthony; not popular in U.S., but still common in Iowa and Colorado schools for the deaf; signs for all affixes.	Manual representation of the written language; one hand shape for each letter of alphabet; used to borrow English words into ASL; when used with speech and speechreading, it is called the Rochester Method.	Employs 8 hand shapes in 4 positions on the face, and used in conjunction with lip movements to enable a deaf person to lipread more easily; based on sound with the syllable as the basic unit; devised by Orin Cornett at Gallaudet College.	Independent language; aural-oral mode; own grammar; own syntax; words are meaning based; contains dialects, regionalisms, slang, puns; can be written; wide range of vocabulary covering minute differences in meaning; may borrow from other languages; is verbal, but also makes use of nonverbal elements.

Artificial pedagogical systems, invented for educational purposes

Nonverbal communication: natural gestures, facial expression, body movements, body language, pantomime

From W. H. Smith, personal communication, 1984.

American Sign Language (ASL).   The first form of manual communication was established, independent of existing oral languages, by the deaf. Consequently, the original sign language was indeed a unique "natural" language. The genesis and evolution of American Sign Language (ASL) is not without controversy. Today approximately one-half million deaf and hearing individuals use this language (O'Rourke, Medina, Thames, & Sullivan, 1975). The signs associated with ASL have been shown to possess identifying physical characteristics analogous to the distinctive features of speech (Stokoe, 1960; Stokoe, Casterline, & Croneberg, 1965). The physical features of ASL signs, *cheremes*, are described by Stokoe and his associates as:

1. DEZ—which *designates* the handshape of the sign.

2. SIG—which is the *movement/signation* of the hand during the production of a sign.

3. TAB—which signifies where (*tabulation*) on the body the sign is produced.

Approximately 10 years after Stokoe's classification of signs, researchers agreed that the palmar direction of the hands was a viable and independent parameter during signing. Consequently, the fourth classification, known as *orientation*, should be included (Battison, Markowicz, & Woodward, 1975).

An example of these features can be seen in the signs illustrated in Figure 4.8.

Since ASL is a language, it consists of words. However, there is no corresponding sign to represent each English word, just as there is no unique relationship between the words used in English, French, Portuguese, Chinese, or Japanese.

All languages developed using a common code for exchange of information. Also, the structure of each language is as unique as is its vocabulary (code). Thus, "Ni qui guo zhong-guo mei-you?" probably looks and sounds "funny" to those of us native to the United States, but the sentence is logical and meaningful to someone in Taiwan. Similarly, ASL is not a form of English but rather a language produced manually that requires just as unique a translation of English as does any foreign language.

Some of the over 6,000 signs that have been identified can be decoded intuitively. These signs are classified as *iconic*, meaning that they are imageries of English words. The signs in Figure 4.9 will be familiar to most readers, even those who have never been exposed to manual communication—specifically ASL.

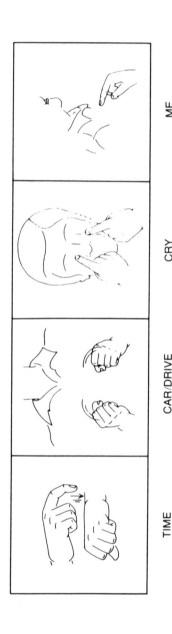

TIME   CAR/DRIVE   CRY   ME

Figure 4.8. Four signs used in ASL representing the features of designation of handshape (DEZ); tabulation where sign is produced (TAB); and movement/signation (SIG); and palmar direction of the hands. (From *The Joy of Signing* by L. Riekehof, 1978, Springfield, MO: Gospel Publishing House.)

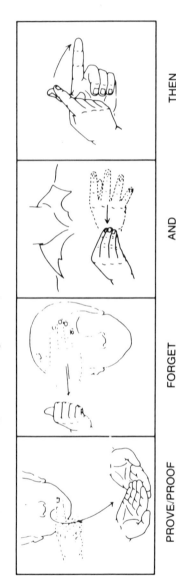

PROVE/PROOF   FORGET   AND   THEN

Figure 4.9. Four iconic signs. The signs are an imagery of the English words they represent. From *The Joy of Signing* by L. Riekehof, 1978, Springfield, MO: Gospel Publishing House.)

Signed English Systems.   A counterpart to sign language is a *sign system*. Sign systems are an effort to duplicate manually spoken English. Four sign systems have been developed and accepted with varying degrees of enthusiasm in this country. These systems, Seeing Essential English, Signing Exact English, Linguistics of Visual English and Signed English, are briefly described in the following paragraphs.

Seeing Essential English (SEE 1).   In 1969 a group of educators/ researchers headed by David Anthony created a manual communication system designed to incorporate American Sign Language and English (Anthony, 1971). The philosophy underlying SEE 1 is that the sender of a message uses a sign for each word in the message. Also, the word order of the message parrallels the word order used in English. However, the number of signs used is predicated on how a word is spelled, how it is pronounced, and what it means. When words are spelled the same and pronounced the same way, a single sign (ASL) is to represent the word regardless of the context in which it is used. However, if two words are spelled the same but are pronounced differently or have a different meaning, a separate sign is used for each. Thus, when two words meet two of the criteria (identical spelling, pronunciation, or meaning), one sign is used to express them. For example; The word "hit" can mean "to smack/strike," "to find" (they hit oil) or "a success" (he was a hit with the teenagers); since it is spelled the same and pronounced the same it is indicated manually with a single sign even though it has a variety of meanings. In contrast, the words "lead" (a soft heavy metal) and "led" (she led the band) are pronounced identically, are spelled differently, and have different meanings. Therefore, they are expressed using different signs. Specific signs are also used to denote the word markers: *-ed, -ing, -ist, -ity, -ly, -ment, -ous,* and *-s.* SEE 1 creates new signs by placing the hands in a particular fingerspelling position while making an ASL sign; therefore, the words "people" and "person" are made with the handshape in the "p" position but using a different hand movement for each word. Syntactically, SEE 1 has signs for articles and pronouns; these are used structurally in the same order as they are used in English.

Signing Exact English (SEE 2).   Because most of the rules of SEE 1 were arbitrarily determined, Gustason, Pfetzing, and Zawolkow (1972) developed SEE 2, *Signing Exact English*. The intent of these authors was to maintain the syntactic structure of SEE 1 without making the system unintelligible for those using ASL. SEE 2 uses the same criteria as SEE 1 for signing words that have either the same pronunciation, spelling, or meaning. The signed word used when English meets two out of the three criteria may be selected from ASL or a new sign may be created.

Linguistics of Visual English (LOVE). At approximately the same time SEE 2 was being developed, Wampler (1971, 1972) was refining another sign system aimed at approximating English. The vocabulary suggested by Wampler is more limited than that of SEE 1 and SEE 2. It attempts to mirror spoken English by making signed movements that correspond to the number of syllables uttered in a spoken word. Yet, LOVE is primarily a manual system identical to the ones created by Anthony and Gustason and their colleagues.

Signed English. This system is also known as *Gallaudet Signed English* as it was designed by Bornstein and his associates at Gallaudet (Bornstein, 1974). The system, created for young deaf children (preschoolers through elementary school-age students), adheres basically to ASL; however, special syntactic markers that are familiar to a young age group, as well as articles, auxiliary verbs, and pronouns are also signed.

Fingerspelling. Another method of duplicating speech manually is to have senders spell the words with their fingers. That is, instead of using pencil and paper, speakers write their message in the air by using various handshapes to represent the letters in the English alphabet. This mode of communication, *fingerspelling*, represents the 26 letters of the English alphabet by 25 handshapes and two hand movements (see Figure 4.10). Collectively these are also referred to as the *manual alphabet* . The letters *i* and *j* are produced by the same handshape with the *j* being produced by moving the hand in a hook of *j*-like motion. The letter *z* is made by moving a unique handshape in the form of a *z*. Although fingerspelling is an exact and effective means of communication, it is the least efficient form of manual communication as each letter of each word must be produced. Since no additional characters are included in the alphabet nor digits in the numeric system, a person can learn to transmit a message via fingerspelling in a relatively short time. However, because of the rapidity in which one learns to "spell" a message and because of the similarity in the production of *e, o, m* and *n,* and between the letters *a* and *s* , the reception of fingerspelling requires considerable practice and concentration. As mentioned in the discussion of speechreading, the similarity among letters and sounds becomes more confounding during discourse than in isolation. But, as in every other form of communication, predictability mitigates this problem. Today, fingerspelling is used to supplement all forms of manual communication by expressing proper names, technical terms, and events that cannot be conveyed by signs. A popular application of fingerspelling is the *Rochester Method,* in which the teachers and students simultaneously "spell" what they are expressing orally.

Cued speech. Some professionals have been promoting the use of *cued speech* as an ancillary tool in speechreading instruction (Cornett,

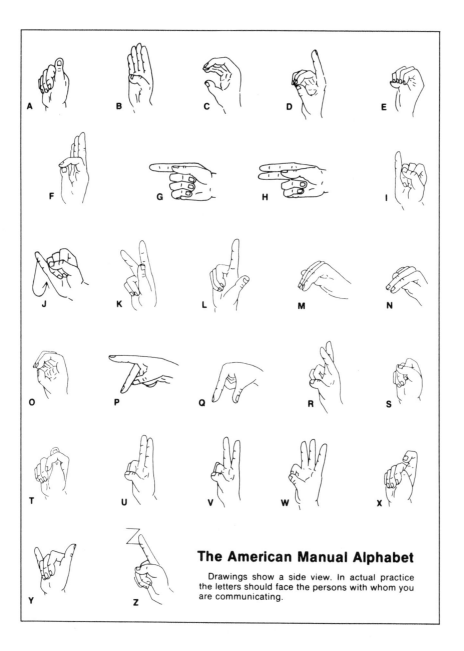

The American Manual Alphabet

Drawings show a side view. In actual practice the letters should face the persons with whom you are communicating.

Figure 4.10. American manual alphabet. The hand positions are shown as they appear to the person reading them. (Courtesy of Gallaudet College, Washington, DC.)

1967, 1972; Ling & Ling, 1978). The intent of Cornett's (1967) cued speech system (some would prefer to classify it as a *manual system*) is to use hand cues to reduce the confusion produced by homophenous words. Cornett selected four hand positions to accompany the spoken vowels and eight handshapes to be used by the speaker near the mouth when producing the consonants (see Figure 4.11). These are used in combination and presented simultaneously with speech as a supplement to the visual information already present for the speechreader.

Although the Lings recommended cued speech as a means of clarifying speechreading reception (Ling & Ling, 1978), the method has received some criticism (Moores, 1969). Specifically, Wilbur (1976) summarized the pros and cons of the technique by adding that it may be used for speech instruction but discouraged its use for initial language learning.

summary

This chapter has reviewed information related to the various ways in which vision can be utilized effectively by the hearing impaired. Philosophies differ considerably concerning the role of vision and the way it is utilized in aural rehabilitation. Yet, most would urge maximizing the use of the visual channel to facilitate communication in the overall management of the hearing impaired.

recommended readings

Alpiner, J., & McCarthy, P. (Eds.). (1987). *Rehabilitative audiology: Children and adults* (3rd ed.). Baltimore: Williams and Wilkins.

Berger, K. (1972). *Speechreading*. Baltimore: National Educational Press.

Binnie, C. (1976). Relevant aural rehabilitation. In J. Northern (Ed.), *Hearing disorders*. Boston: Little, Brown & Co.

DeFilippo, C., & Sims, D. (1988). New reflections on speech reading. *Volter Review, 90*(5), 3–313.

Hipskind, N. (1978). Aural rehabilitation for adults. *Otolaryngologic Clinics of North America, 11*, 823–834.

Jeffers, J., & Barley, M. (1971). *Speechreading*. Springfield, IL: Charles C. Thomas.

O'Neill, J., & Oyer, H. (1981). *Visual communication for the hard of hearing* (2nd ed.). Englewood Cliffs, NJ: Prentice-Hall.

CHART I
Cues for English Vowels

	Group I (base position)	Group II (larynx)	Group III (chin)	Group IV (mouth)
open	[a:] (fäther) (gŏt)	[a] (thăt)	[o:] (fôr) (ought)	
flattened-relaxed	[ʌ] (but) [ə] (the)	[i] (ĭs)	[e] (gĕt)	[i:] (fe͞et) (meat)
rounded	[ou] (nōte) (boat)	[u] (go͝od) (put)	[u:] (blue) (fo͞od)	[ə] (ûrn) (hẽr)

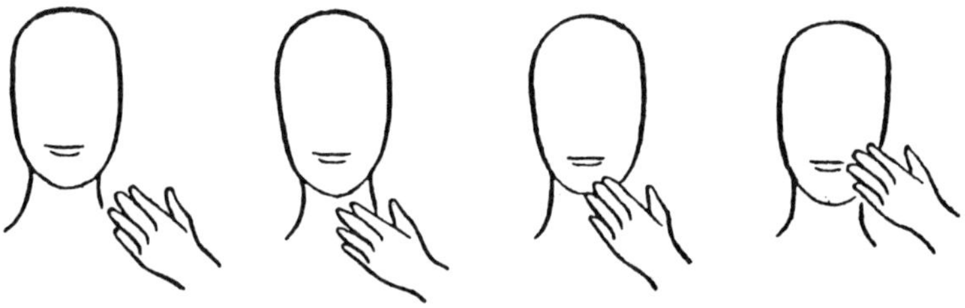

CHART III
Cues for English Consonants

T Group*	H Group	D Group	ng Group	L Group	K Group	N Group	G Group
t	h	d	(ng)	l	k	n	g
m	s	p	y (you)	sh	v	b	j
f	r	zh	ch	w	th (the)	hw**	th (thin)
					z		

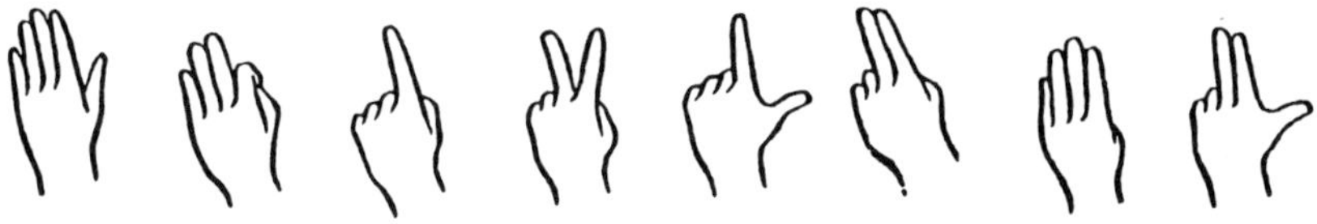

*Note: The T group cue is also used with an isolated vowel—that is, an initial vowel not run with a final consonant from the preceding syllable.

Figure 4.11. An illustration of the hand positions and handshapes used in cued speech. (From "Cued Speech" by R. Cornett, 1967, *American Annals of the Deaf, 112,* 3–13.)

Sims, D., Walter, G., & Whitehead, R. (Eds.). (1982). *Deafness and communication: Assessment and training.* Baltimore: Williams and Wilkins.

Vernon, M. (1987). Controversy within sign language. *The Deaf American, 28*(1), 22-25.

references

Albright, P., Hipskind, N., & Schuckers, G. (1973). A comparison of visibility and speechreading performance on English and Slurvian. *Journal of Communication Disorders, 6,* 44-52.

Alpiner, J., & McCarthy, P. (Eds.). (1987). *Rehabilitative audiology: Children and adults* (3rd ed.). Baltimore: Williams & Wilkins.

Anthony, D. (1971). *Seeing essential English* (Vols. 1 and 2). Anaheim, CA: Anaheim Union School District, Educational Service Division.

Battison, R., Markowicz, H., & Woodward, J. (1976). A good rule of thumb; variable phonology in American Sign Language. In R. Shuy & R. Fasold (Eds.), *New ways of analyzing variation in English. Volume II* (pp. 250-280). Baltimore: Williams & Wilkins.

Berg, F. (1976). *Educational audiology: Hearing and speech management.* New York: Grune and Stratton.

Berger, K. (1972a). *Speechreading: Principles and methods.* Baltimore: National Educational Press.

Berger, K. (1972b). Visemes and homophenous words. *Teacher of the Deaf, 70,* 396-399.

Best, L.G. (1978). Research aspects of rehabilitative audiology. In J.G. Alpiner (Ed.), *Handbook of adult rehabilitative audiology* (pp. 250-260). Baltimore: Williams & Wilkins.

Binnie, C.A. (1973). Bi-sensory articulation functions for normal hearing and sensorineural hearing loss patients. *Journal of the Academy of Rehabilitative Audiology, 3,* 43.

Binnie, C.A. (1976). Relevant aural rehabilitation. In J.L. Northern (Ed.), *Hearing disorders* (pp. 213-227). Boston: Little, Brown & Co.

Binnie, C.A., Jackson, P., & Montgomery, A. (1976). Visual intelligibility of consonants: A lipreading screening test with implications for aural rehabilitation. *Journal of Speech and Hearing Disorders, 41,* 530-539.

Bode, D., Nerbonne, G.P., & Salstrom, L. (1970). Speechreading and the synthesis of distorted printed sentences. *Journal of Speech and Hearing Research, 13,* 115-121.

Bornstein, H. (1974). Signed English: A manual approach to English language development. *Journal of Speech and Hearing Disorders, 39,* 330-343.

Boothroyd, A., & Hnath, R. (1986). Lipreading with tactile supplements. *Journal of Rehabilitation Research and Development, 23*(1), 139-146.

Brannon, J.B., Jr., & Kodman, Jr., F. (1959). The perceptual process in speechreading. *AMA Archives of Otolaryngology, 98,* 114-119.

Bruhn, M.E. (1929). *The Mueller-Walle method of lip reading for the deaf.* Lynn, MS: Nicholas Press.

Bunger, A.M. (1944). *Speech reading - Jena method.* Danville, IL: The Interstate Co.

Campbell, C., Polomeno, R., Elder, J.M., Murray, J., & Altosaar, A. (1981). Importance of an eye examination in identifying the cause of congenital hearing impairments. *Journal of Speech and Hearing Disorders, 46,* 258-261.

Cavender, B. (1949). *The construction and investigation of a test of lip reading ability and a study of factors assumed to affect the results.* Unpublished master's thesis, Indiana University.

Clouser, R.A. (1976). The effects of vowel consonant ratio and sentence length on lipreading ability. *American Annals of the Deaf, 121,* 513-518.

Cornett, R. (1967). Cued speech. *American Annals of the Deaf, 112,* 3-13.

Cornett, R.O. (1972). Cued speech parent training and follow-up program. Washington, DC: Bureau of Education for the Handicapped, DHEW.

Craig, W. (1964). Effects of preschool training on the development of reading and lipreading skills of deaf children. *American Annals of the Deaf, 109,* 280-296.

Cronin, B. (1979). The DAVID system: The development of an interactive video system at the National Institute for the Deaf. *American Annals of the Deaf, 124,* 615-618.

Davis, H. (1978). Abnormal hearing and deafness. In H. Davis & S.R. Silverman (Eds.), *Hearing and deafness* (4th ed., pp. 87-146). New York: Holt, Rinehart & Winston.

Day, H., Fusfeld, I., & Pintner, R. (1928). *A survey of American schools for the deaf 1924-25.* Washington, DC: National Research Council.

DeFilippo, C., & Scott, B. (1978). A method for training and evaluating the reception of ongoing speech. *Journal of the Acoustical Society of America, 63*(4), 1186-1192.

Erber, N.P. (1971a). Auditory and audiovisual reception of words in low-frequency noise by children with normal hearing and by children with impaired hearing. *Journal of Speech and Hearing Research, 14,* 496-512.

Erber, N.P. (1971b). Auditory detection of spondaic words in wide-band noise by adults with normal hearing and by children with profound hearing losses. *Journal of Speech and Hearing Research, 14,* 372-382.

Erber, N.P. (1971c). Effects of distance on the visual reception of speech. *Journal of Speech and Hearing Research, 14,* 848-857.

Erber, N.P. (1972). Auditory, visual and auditory-visual recognition of consonants by children with normal and impaired hearing. *Journal of Speech and Hearing Research, 15,* 413-422.

Erber, N.P. (1974). Effects of angle, distance and illumination on visual reception of speech by profoundly deaf children. *Journal of Speech and Hearing Research, 17,* 99-112.

Erber, N.P. (1979). Auditory-visual perception of speech with reduced optical clarity. *Journal of Speech and Hearing Research, 22,* 212-223.

Evans, L. (1960). Factors relating to listening and lipreading. *Teacher of the Deaf,* *58,* 417-423.

Evans, L. (1965). Psychological factors related to lipreading. *Teacher of the Deaf,* *63,* 131-136.

Ewing, I. (1959). *Lipreading and hearing aids.* Manchester, England: Manchester University Press.

Farrimond, T. (1959). Age differences in the ability to use visual cues in auditory communication. *Language and Speech, 2,* 174-192.

Fisher, C.G. (1968). Confusions among visually perceived consonants. *Journal of Speech and Hearing Research, 11,* 796-800.

Fleming, M. (1972). A total approach to communication therapy. *Journal of the Academy of Rehabilitative Audiology, 5,* 28-31.

Franks, J.R., & Kimble, J. (1972). The confusion of English consonant clusters in lipreading. *Journal of Speech and Hearing Research, 15,* 474-482.

Gaeth, J.H. (1943). *A study of phonemic regression in relation to hearing loss.* Unpublished doctoral dissertation, Northwestern University.

Garstecki, D. (1977). Identification of communication competence in the geriatric population. *Journal of the Academy of Rehabilitative Audiology, 10,* 36-45.

Garstecki, D. (1983). Auditory, visual and combined auditory-visual speech perception in young and elderly adults. *Journal of the Academy of Rehabilitative Audiology, 16,* 221-233.

Garstecki, D., & O'Neill, J.J. (1980). Situational cues and strategy influence on speechreading. *Scandinavian Audiology, 9,* 1-5.

Gibson, E.J. (1969). *Principles of perceptual learning and development.* New York: Appleton-Century-Crofts.

Giolas, T., Butterfield, E.C., & Weaver, S.J. (1974). Some motivational correlates of lipreading. *Journal of Speech and Hearing Research, 17,* 18-24.

Goetzinger, C. (1964). A study of monocular versus binocular vision in lipreading. *Proceeding—International Congress on Education of the Deaf, and the 41st Meeting of the Convention of American Instructors of the Deaf.* Washington, DC: Document No. 106. U.S. Gov't Printing Office.

Greenberg, H.L., & Bode, D.L. (1968). Visual discrimination of consonants. *Journal of Speech and Hearing Research, 11,* 869-874.

Griffiths, C. (1964). The auditory approach for pre-school deaf children. *Volta Review, 66,* 387.

Gustason, G., Pfetzing, D., & Zawolkow, E. (1972). *Signing exact English.* Silver Spring, MD: Modern Signs Press.

Hardick, E.J. (1977). Aural rehabilitational programs for the aged can be successful. *Journal of the Academy of Rehabilitative Audiology, 10,* 51-66.

Hardick, E.J., Oyer, H.J., & Irion, P.E. (1970). Lipreading performance is related to measurements of vision. *Journal of Speech and Hearing Research, 13,* 92.

Haspiel, G. (1964). *A synthetic approach to lip reading.* Magnolia, MA: The Expression Co.

Heider, G. (1947). The Utley lipreading test. *Volta Review, 49,* 457-458.

Hipskind, N.M. (1977). *The relationship of linguistic redundancy to speechreading.* Paper presented at the Speech-Language-Hearing Association National Convention, Chicago.

Hipskind, N.M. (1978). Aural rehabilitation for adults. *Otolaryngologic Clinic of North America, 11,* 823-834.

Hipskind, N.M., Nerbonne, G.P., & Gravel, J.S. (1973). The intelligibility of C.I.D. Auditory Test W-1 words as speechreading stimuli. *Journal of Communication Disorders, 6,* 1-10.

Huizing, H. (1952). Auditory training. *Acta Otolaryngologica* (Suppl. 110), 158-163.

Hutton, C. (1959). Combining auditory and visual stimuli in aural rehabilitation. *Volta Review, 61,* 316-319.

Jackson, P.L., Montgomery, A.A., & Binnie, C.A. (1976). Perceptual dimensions underlying vowel lipreading performance. *Journal of Speech and Hearing Research, 19,* 796-812.

Jacobs, M. (1982). Visual communication for the severely and profoundly hearing-impaired young adult. In D. Sims, G. Walter, & R. Whitehead (Eds.), *Deafness and communication: Assessment and training.* Baltimore: Williams & Wilkins.

Jeffers, J., & Barley, M. (1971). *Speechreading.* Springfield, IL: Charles C. Thomas Publisher.

Johnson, D., & Caccamise, F. (1982). *Visual assessment of hearing-impaired persons: Options and implications for the future.* Chicago: John C. Winston.

Johnson, D., Caccamise, F., Rothblum, A., Hamilton, L., & Howard, M. (1981). Identification and follow-up of visual impairments in hearing-impaired populations. *American Annals of the Deaf, 126,* 321-360.

Karp, A. (1983). Aural rehabilitation strategies for the visually and hearing impaired patient. *Journal of the Academy of Rehabilitative Audiology, 16,* 23-32.

Kinzie, C.E., & Kinzie, R. (1931). *Lipreading for the deafened adult.* Chicago: John C. Winston.

Leonard, R. (1968). *The effects of continuous auditory distractions on lipreading performance.* Unpublished master's thesis, Michigan State University.

Levitt, H., Waltzman, S.B., Shapiro, W., & Cohen, N.L. (1986). Evaluation of a cochlear prosthesis using connected discourse tracking. *Journal of Rehabilitation Research, 23*(1), 147-154.

Lewis, D.N. (1972). Lipreading skills of hearing impaired children in regular schools. *Volta Review, 74,* 303-311.

Ling, D., & Clarke, B.R. (1975). Cued speech: An evaluative study. *American Annals of the Deaf, 120,* 480-488.

Ling, D., & Clarke, B.R. (1976). The effects of using cued speech: A follow-up study. *Volta Review, 78,* 23-34.

Ling, D., & Ling, A. (1978). *Aural rehabilitation: The foundations of verbal learning in hearing-impaired children.* Washington, DC: Alexander Graham Bell Association for the Deaf.

Lovering, L. (1969). *Lipreading performance as a function of visual acuity.* Unpublished doctoral dissertation, Michigan State University.

McNutt, E. (1952). *Hearing with our eyes.* Washington, DC: The Volta Bureau.

Miller, G.A. (1960). Speech and language. In S. Stevens (Ed.), *Handbook of experimental psychology* (pp. 789-810). New York: John Wiley & Sons, Inc.

Miller, G.A., & Nicely, P.E. (1955). An analysis of the perceptual confusions among some English consonants. *Journal of the Acoustical Society of America, 27,* 338-352.

Montgomery, A., & Sylvester, S. (1984). Streamlining the aural rehabilitation process. *Hearing Instruments, 35,* 46-50.

Moores, D. (1969). Cued speech: Some practical and theoretical considerations. *American Annals of the Deaf, 114,* 23-27.

Myklebust, H. (1954). *Auditory disorders in children.* New York: Grune & Stratton.

Neely, K. (1956). Effects of visual factors on intelligibility of speech. *Journal of the Acoustical Society of America, 28,* 1276-1277.

Nitchie, E.B. (1912). *Lip reading: Principles and practice.* New York: Frederick A. Stokes Co.

Nitchie, E.B. (1950). *New lessons in lip reading.* Philadelphia: J.B. Lippincott.

O'Neill, J.J. (1951). An exploratory investigation of lipreading ability among normal-hearing students. *Speech Monographs, 18,* 309-311.

O'Neill, J.J. (1954). Contributions of the visual components of oral symbols to speech comprehension. *Journal of Speech and Hearing Disorders, 19,* 429-439.

O'Neill, J.J., & Davidson, J.A. (1956). Relationship between lipreading ability and five psychological factors. *Journal of Speech and Hearing Disorders, 21,* 478-481.

O'Neill, J.J., & Oyer, H.J. (1961). *Visual communication for the hard of hearing.* Englewood Cliffs, NJ: Prentice Hall.

O'Neill, J.J., & Oyer, H.J. (1981). *Visual communication for the hard of hearing* (2nd ed.). Englewood Cliffs, NJ: Prentice Hall.

O'Rourke, T., Medina, T., Thames, A., & Sullivan, D. (1975, April). *National Association Skills Program. Programs Hand,* 27-30.

Orr, D., Friedman, H., & Williams, J. (1965). Trainability of listening comprehension of speeded discourse. *Journal of Educational Psychology, 56,* 148-156.

Owens, E., & Telleen, C. (1981). Tracking as an aural rehabilitation process. *Journal of the Academy of Rehabilitative Audiology, 34*(11), 9.

Pelsen, R.O., & Prather, W. (1974). Effects of visual mess, age-related cues, age and hearing impairment on speechreading performance. *Journal of Speech and Hearing Research, 17,* 518-525.

Pollack, D. (1964). Acoupedics. *Volta Review, 66,* 400.

Pollack, D. (1985). *Educational audiology for the limited hearing infant and preschooler.* Silver Spring, MD: Fellendorf Assoc.

Reid, G.A. (1946). A preliminary investigation in the testing of lipreading achievement. *American Annals of the Deaf, 91,* 403-413.

Riekehof, L. (1978). *The joy of signing.* Springfield, MO: Gospel Publishing House.

Riggs, L. (1965). Visual acuity. In C. Graham (Ed.), *Vision and visual perception* (pp. 321-349). New York: John Wiley & Sons.

Rios-Escalera, A., & Davis, J. (1977). An investigation of lipreading performance as a function of speaking rate. In K. Berger (Ed.), *Research studies in speechreading* (pp. 60-70). Kent, OH: Herald Publishing House.

Robbins, A., Osberger, J.J., Miyamoto, R., Kienle, M., & Myers, W. (1985). Speech-tracking performance in single-channel cochlear implant subjects. *Journal of Speech and Hearing Research, 28*(4), 565-578.

Rodel, M. (1985). Children with hearing impairment. In J. Katz (Ed.), *Handbook of clinical audiology* (3rd ed., pp. 1004-1016). Baltimore: Williams & Wilkins.

Romano, P., & Barlow, W. (1974). Vision requirements for lipreading. *American Annals of the Deaf, 119*, 393-386.

Ross, M. (1982). *Hard of hearing children in regular schools*. Englewood Cliffs, NJ: Prentice-Hall.

Samar, V.J., & Sims, D.G. (1983). Visual evoked response correlates of speechreading performance in normal-hearing adults: A replication and factor analytic extension. *Journal of Speech and Hearing Research, 26*, 2-9.

Samar, V.J., & Sims, D.G. (1984). Visual evoked response components related to speechreading and spatial skills in hearing and hearing impaired adults. *Journal of Speech and Hearing Research, 27*, 23-26.

Sanders, D.A. (1971). *Aural rehabilitation*. Englewood Cliffs, NJ: Prentice-Hall.

Sanders, D.A. (1982). *Aural rehabilitation* (2nd ed.). Englewood Cliffs, NJ: Prentice-Hall.

Sanders, D.A., & Conscarelli, J.E. (1970). The relationship of visual synthesis skill to lipreading. *American Annals of the Deaf, 115*, 23-26.

Sanders, D.A., & Goodrich, S.J. (1971). The contribution of vision to speech intelligibility under the conditions of frequency distortion. *Journal of Speech and Hearing Research, 14*, 154-159.

Sharp, E.Y. (1972). The relationship of visual closure to speechreading. *Exceptional Children, 38*, 729-734.

Shepherd, D.C. (1982). Visual-neural correlate of speechreading ability in normal-hearing adults: Reliability. *Journal of Speech and Hearing Research, 25*, 521-527.

Shepherd, D.C., DeLavergne, R.W., Fruek, F.X., & Clobridge, C. (1977). Visual-neural correlate of speechreading ability in normal-hearing adults. *Journal of Speech and Hearing Research, 20*, 752-765.

Shoop, C., & Binnie, C.A. (1979). The effects of age upon the visual perception of speech. *Scandinavian Audiology, 8*, 3-8.

Simmons, A. (1959). Factors related to lipreading. *Journal of Speech and Hearing Research, 2*, 340-352.

Sims, D. (1985). Adults with hearing impairment. In J. Katz (Ed.), *Handbook of clinical audiology* (3rd ed., pp. 1017-1045). Baltimore: The Williams & Wilkins Co.

Smith, R. (1964). *An investigation of the relationships between lipreading ability and the intelligence of the mentally retarded*. Unpublished master's thesis, Michigan State University.

Smith, W.H. (1984). Personal communication.

Stokoe, W. (1960). Sign language structure: An outline of the visual communication system of the American deaf. *Studies in Linguistic Science*, Occasional Papers No. 8.

Stokoe, W., Casterline, D., & Croneberg, C. (1965). *A dictionary of American sign language on linguistic principles*. Washington, DC: Gallaudet College Press.

Stone, L. (1957). *Facial clues of context in lipreading*. Los Angeles, CA: John Tracy Clinic Research Papers, V.

Sumby, W.H., & Pollack, I. (1954). Visual contribution to speech intelligibility in noise. *Journal of the Acoustical Society of America, 26*, 212-215.

Thomas, S.L. (1969). *Lipreading performance as a function of light levels*. Unpublished master's thesis, Michigan State University.

Universe Electric Research Co. (1987). *The lip-reader trainer*. Unpublished brochure. Webster-Groves, MO 63119.

Utley, J. (1946). A test of lipreading ability. *Journal of Speech and Hearing Disorders, 11*, 109-116.

Walden, B., Erdman, S., Montgomery, A., Schwartz, D., & Prosek, R. (1981). Some effects of training on speech perception by hearing-impaired adults. *Journal of Speech and Hearing Research, 24*, 207-216.

Walden, B., Prosek, R., Montgomery, A., Scharr, C., & Jones, C. (1977). Effects of training on the visual recognition of consonants. *Journal of Speech and Hearing Research, 20*, 130-145.

Wampler, D. (1971). *Linguistics of visual English*. Santa Rosa, CA: Early Childhood Education Department, Aurally Handicapped Program, Santa Rosa City Schools.

Wampler, D. (1972). *Linguistics of visual English*. Santa Rosa, CA: Early Childhood Education Department, Aurally Handicapped Program, Santa Rosa Schools.

Wedenberg, E. (1951). Auditory training of deaf and hard of hearing children. *Acta Otolaryngology* (Suppl. 94), *39*, 1-139.

Whitehurst, M. (1964). *Integrated lessons in lipreading and auditory training*. North Merrick, NY: Hearing Rehabilitation.

Wilbur, R. (1976). The linguistics of manual languages and manual systems. In L. Lloyd (Ed.), *Communication assessment and intervention strategies* (pp. 423-500). Baltimore: University Park Press.

Wong, W., & Taaffe, G. (1958). *Relationships between selected aptitude and personality tests of lipreading ability*. Los Angeles, CA: John Tracy Clinic Research Papers, VII.

Woodward, M.F. (1957). *Linguistic methodology in lip reading research*. Los Angeles, CA: John Tracy Clinic Research Papers, IV.

Woodward, M.F., & Barber, C.G. (1960). Phoneme perception in lipreading. *Journal of Speech and Hearing Research, 3*, 212-222.

Woodward, M., & Lowell, E. (1964). *A linguistic approach to the education of aurally-handicapped children*. Washington, DC: DHEW (Project # 907).

Wyatt, O. (1960). *Lipreading*. London: The English Universities Press.

Wynn, M. (1964). *Norms for a film presentation of the semi-diagnostic tests in aural rehabilitation*. Unpublished master's thesis, Michigan State University.

APPENDIX FOUR A

utley—how well can you read lips?

This test, commonly referred to as the "Utley Test," consists of three subtests: Sentences (Forms A and B), Words (Forms A and B) and Stories accompanied by questions that relate to each of the stories. Utley (1946) demonstrated that the Word and Story subtests are positively correlated with the Sentence portion of the test. Therefore, these are the stimuli most often used and associated with the *Utley Test*.

Utley evaluated her viewers' responses by giving one point for each word correctly identified in each sentence. A total of 125 words are contained in the 31 sentences on each form (Forms A and B). Consequently, a respondent's score may range from 0 to 125 points. Utley suggested that homophenous words not be accepted when scoring the sentence subtest.

Utley administered the sentence subtest to 761 hearing-impaired children and adults, and the following descriptive statistics summarize her findings:

	Form A	Form B
Range	0-84	0-89
Mean	33.63	33.80
SD	16.36	17.53

Practice Sentence
 1. Good morning.
 2. Thank you.
 3. Hello.
 4. How are you?
 5. Goodbye.

Utley Sentence Test, Form A
 1. All right.
 2. Where have you been?
 3. I have forgotten.
 4. I have nothing.
 5. That is right.
 6. Look out.
 7. How have you been?
 8. I don't know if I can.
 9. How tall are you?
10. It is awfully cold.
11. My folks are home.
12. How much was it?
13. Good night.
14. Where are you going?
15. Excuse me.
16. Did you have a good time?
17. What did you want?
18. How much do you weigh?
19. I cannot stand him.
20. She was home last week.

From "A Test of Lipreading Ability" by J. Utley, 1946, *Journal of Speech and Hearing Disorders, 11*, pp. 109–116. Reprinted with permission.

21. Keep your eye on the ball.
22. I cannot remember.
23. Of course.
24. I flew to Washington.
25. You look well.
26. The train runs every hour.
27. You had better go slow.
28. It says that in the book.
29. We got home at six o'clock.
30. We drove to the country.
31. How much rain fell?

APPENDIX FOUR B

the denver quick test of lipreading ability

The *Denver Quick Test* is designed to measure adult ability to speechread 20 common everyday sentences. Sentences are presented "live" or taped by the tester and are scored on the basis of meaning recognition. No normative data are available to which individual scores may be compared; however, when the Quick Test was given without acoustic cues to 40 hearing-impaired adults, their scores were highly correlated (0.90) with their results on the *Utley Sentence Test* (Alpiner, 1982).

The Denver Quick Test of Lipreading Ability

1. Good morning.
2. How old are you?
3. I live in (state of residence).
4. I only have one dollar.
5. There is somebody at the door.
6. Is that all?
7. Where are you going?
8. Let's have a coffee break.
9. Park your car in the lot.
10. What is your address?
11. May I help you?
12. I feel fine.
13. It is time for dinner.
14. Turn right at the corner.
15. Are you ready to order?
16. Is this charge or cash?
17. What time is it?
18. I have a headache.
19. How about going out tonight?
20. Please lend me 50 cents.

From "Evaluation of Communication Function" by J. Alpiner. In *Handbook of Adult Rehabilitative Audiology* (pp. 18–79) by J. Alpiner (Ed.), 1982, Baltimore: Williams & Wilkins. Reprinted by permission.

APPENDIX FOUR C

craig lipreading inventory

The *Craig Lipreading Inventory* consists of two forms of 33 isolated words and 24 sentences. The vocabulary for these stimuli was selected from words used by children enrolled in kindergarten and first grade. A filmed version of the test is available. The test is usually presented "live" or may be videotaped by a clinician.

The viewer should be positioned 8 feet from the speaker. Each of the isolated words is preceded by a contextually meaningless carrier phrase, "show me". The respondent is provided with answer sheets that contain four choices for each stimulus. A single point is awarded for each of the words and sentences identified correctly. Consequently, maximum scores are 33 and 24 for the word test and sentence test, respectively.

Individual performances may be compared to the following mean scores obtained by Craig with deaf children:

	Preschool	*Nonpreschool*
Words	62.5%-68%	68%-69%
Sentences	52.5%-62%	61.5%-63%

Craig Lipreading Inventory
Word Recognition — Form A

1. white	12. woman	23. ear
2. corn	13. fly	24. ice
3. zoo	14. frog	25. goat
4. thumb	15. grapes	26. dog
5. chair	16. goose	27. cat
6. jello	17. sled	28. nut
7. doll	18. star	29. milk
8. pig	19. sing	30. cake
9. toy	20. three	31. eight
10. finger	21. duck	32. pencil
11. six	22. spoon	33. desk

From "Effects of Preschool Training on the Development of Reading and Lipreading Skills of Deaf Children" by W. Craig, 1964, *American Annals of the Deaf, 109*, pp. 280-296. Reprinted by permission.

VISUAL STIMULI

Sentence Recognition — Form A

1. A coat is on a chair.
2. A sock and shoe are on the floor.
3. A boy is flying a kite.
4. A girl is jumping.
5. A boy stuck his thumb in the pie.
6. A cow and a pig are near the gate.
7. A man is throwing a ball to the dog.
8. A bird has white wings.
9. A light is over the door.
10. A horse is standing by a new car.
11. A boy is putting a nail in the sled.
12. A big fan is on a desk.
13. An owl is looking at the moon.
14. Three stars are in the sky.
15. A whistle and a spoon are on the table.
16. A frog is hopping away from a boat.
17. Bread, meat and grapes are in the dish.
18. The woman has long hair and a short dress.
19. The boys are swinging behind the school.
20. A cat is playing with a nut.
21. A man has his foot on a truck.
22. A woman is carrying a chair.
23. A woman is eating an apple.
24. A girl is cutting a feather.

CRAIG LIPREADING INVENTORY

Word Recognition

NAME: _____

AGE: _____ DATE: _____ SCHOOL: _____

EX.	fish	table	baby	ball
1.	kite	fire	white	light
2.	corn	fork	horse	purse
3.	two	zoo	spoon	shoe
4.	cup	jump	thumb	drum
5.	hair	bear	pear	chair

	WORD RECOGNITION		PAGE 2.
6.	yoyo	hello	Jello	window
7.	doll	ten	nail	suit
8.	pig	pie	book	pear
9.	two	toe	tie	toy
10.	Flower	finger	fire	feather
11.	six	sing	sit	kiss

WORD RECOGNITION				**PAGE 3.**
12.	table	apple	woman	rabbit
13.	fire	tie	fly	five
14.	four	frog	fork	flag
15.	grapes	airplane	tables	cups
16.	goose	tooth	shoe	school
17.	desk	sled	leg	nest

WORD RECOGNITION

18.	dog	sock	star	car
19.	wing	sing	ring	swing
20.	three	teeth	key	knee
21.	duck	rug	truck	gun
22.	moon	school	spoon	boot
23.	ear	hair	eye	egg

WORD RECOGNITION   PAGE 5.

24.	horse	house	ice	orange
25.	goat	gate	kite	girl
26	dish	duck	desk	dog
27.	cat	cake	gun	coat
28.	nail	nut	nest	ten
29.	man	bat	milk	bird

WORD RECOGNITION   PAGE 6.

30.	egg	cake	key	car
31.	eight	egg	cake	gate
32.	pencil	picture	mitten	pitcher
33.	wet	dress	nest	desk

chapterfive

LANGUAGE AND SPEECH OF THE HEARING IMPAIRED

DEBORAH NOALL SEYFRIED
JOHN M. HUTCHINSON
LINDA LOU SMITH

contents

introduction

Aural habilitation focuses on establishing competence in standard English for the hearing-impaired child. The following chapter will provide an overview of the standard English abilities of hearing-impaired children. Speech skills, although representing the phonologic component of the language system, will also be discussed. In addition, a brief treatment will focus on the speech problems encountered by those who are adventitiously deafened as adults. Both the language and the speech sections will include descriptive research, assessment, and management concerns. The term *language* will be used in reference to standard English unless otherwise indicated. Consideration of language in hearing-impaired children presupposes a knowledge of information related to normal language development. Because no brief summary could adequately describe normal language acquisition, readers are referred to Brown (1973), deVilliers and deVilliers (1978), Bloom and Lahey (1978), and Leonard (1986).

language

"critical period" for language intervention

Until recently, it has been fairly common for professionals to wait until the hearing-impaired child was 3 to 4 years of age before providing language intervention (see Chapter 8). Arguments for early language intervention are based upon the concepts of "critical period for language acquisition" and "natural language acquisition within parent-child communication." These concepts will be briefly discussed in relation to the hearing-impaired child inasmuch as they are important precursors to any complete discussion of speech and language habilitation in this population.

Lenneberg (1967) posited a "critical period" for language learning related to the maturation of the nervous system (predominantly from birth to five years, with an endpoint at puberty). During this period, the child's brain is believed to mature from a state of bilateral representation of language (involvement of both hemispheres of the brain) to a state of lateralized language representation (dominance of one hemisphere). Theoretically, the earlier period of bilateral language representation results in a heightened facility for language learning (deVilliers & deVilliers, 1978). As children reach puberty, language learning is considered to progress more slowly, and, according to Lenneberg, language acquired after puberty is not acquired in the same manner as in normal language development.

The concept of more bilateral language representation during infancy has been disputed (Entus, 1975; Goldberg & Costa, 1981). As a result, the original notion of a "critical period" has also been called into question. Northern and Downs (1984) offered an alternative viewpoint that nonetheless salvages the idea of a critical period by suggesting that the critical period may be viewed as the period during which auditory language perceptions are formed. To support their contention, these authors cited animal studies in which early auditory deprivation was associated with permanent alterations in the auditory nervous system. Accordingly, early auditory impairment may hinder or preclude the formation of auditory language perceptions and result in a language disorder. However, to date, this alternate interpretation of "critical period" has not received broad, data-based support.

Natural Language Acquisition within Parent-Child Communication.
Parent-child communication is essential to normal language development. For the normal-hearing child, language is not only used directly for communication; language is observed. The child watches others and learns when, why, and where different language forms are used. Thus, the normal-hearing child learns how language forms are used and the settings in which they are appropriate (Kolzak, 1983). When speaking to young children, parents use utterances which are short, syntactically and semantically simple, grammatical, fluent, repetitive, and relevant to the child's immediate environment (Bloom & Lahey, 1978; deVilliers & deVilliers, 1978). Such parent-child communication allows the child to discover the phonologic, syntactic, semantic, and pragmatic principles of English.

However, the young hearing-impaired child may not receive the same richly embedded parent-child communication. English is primarily coded by the acoustic speech waveform. Thus, whether with or without amplification, hearing-impaired children may receive reduced and/or distorted acoustic cues. Further, early parent-child communication is mostly available in the home environment. Without early home intervention, hearing-impaired children may learn early language skills in the classroom rather than during the more abundant, early parent-child communication. The majority of deaf children (90%; Altshuler, 1974) have hearing parents who may attempt to use simultaneous communication (i.e., sign language and oral English). Incorporation of sign language into daily communication is not a simple task. Bornstein, Saulnier, and Hamilton (1980) reported that hearing parents of deaf children often do not achieve beyond a beginner's level of sign proficiency. Deaf children who have little useful hearing, therefore, may receive only a limited set of signs in the home environment. The teacher of the deaf may then become a dominant language model and communication partner (Newton, 1985).

Parental communication style may differ with hearing-impaired as opposed to normal-hearing children. Parental interactions with hearing-impaired children appear to be more directive than interactive with parents using more direct imperatives, fewer questions, and shorter utterances (Goss, 1970; Kretschmer & Kretschmer, 1978; Matey & Kretschmer, 1985). Matey and Kretschmer (1985) suggested a possible explanation for the differences in parental communication to hearing-impaired children. They compared maternal language forms directed to young Down's syndrome, hearing-impaired, and normal-hearing children. Significant differences were found between the maternal language directed to normal-hearing vs. Down's children, and between the maternal language directed to normal-hearing and hearing-impaired children. According to Matey and Kretschmer, the use of comparable language with Down's and hearing-impaired children suggests that mothers adjust their language to their child's language level rather than to the child's cognitive level. If maternal language were adjusted to cognitive level, differences would be expected between Down's children (delayed cognition and language) and the hearing-impaired children (normal cognition and delayed language).

Early home intervention and formal training are established for the purpose of broadening the hearing-impaired child's language experience. Recently, such intervention has focused on providing child-centered and functional language experiences according to the normal developmental sequence of language (Kolzak, 1983). In contrast to previous intervention strategies which emphasized language drillwork and passive instruction, current attempts aim at presenting language within a communication context.

Establishing functional communication is critical, not only to the child's academic career but to the learning of social customs and interpersonal roles and relationships. According to Schum (1987), hearing-impaired children may be delayed in social growth because they ''have two experiential deficits: no common communication method to receive information from other people in their life, particularly family in the early stages of development, and no fully developed language system to enable them to process, code, and manipulate experiential information'' (p. 6).

Early Intervention and Communication Mode. Ideally, early amplification and speech/language stimulation should facilitate normal or near-normal communicative development in most hearing-impaired children. Clinicians have reported that early intervention often permits even severely hearing-impaired children to progress through normal developmental sequences (Ling, 1976). The benefits of early intervention may not be evident in the literature in that, until recently, hearing-impaired children were not receiving special services until after the ages of 3 or 4 years (Davis et al., 1986). In regard to the severely hearing impaired,

Monsen (1982) noted that "all contemporary approaches advocate the development of oral communication skills to whatever extent possible" (p. 845). While English may represent a second language for some deaf children (Charrow, 1977; Kretschmer & Kretschmer, 1978), English competency remains essential to academic success and communication in our society. According to Kretschmer and Kretschmer, most deaf children have the potential for attaining "fluency in interpersonal communication, ability to read a range of printed materials, and ability to write a coherent sentence" (pp. 87-88).

It has been speculated that manual communication may provide a language base that facilitates the development of English language skills—a contention that has been used as a major support for the total communication approach (Nix, 1975). However, Kretschmer and Kretschmer (1978) noted that early sign acquisition may interfere with early spoken language because,

> Normally hearing children of deaf parents seem to develop manual and spoken language systems that are relatively independent of one another; with regard to some structural issues (e.g., word order) there may be direct but temporary confounding influences of manual language acquisition. (p. 104)

Further study is needed to establish whether manual language acquisition interferes with English acquisition in hearing-impaired children. Deaf children may use the word order rules of American Sign Language when speaking or writing English (Osberger et al., 1986a). This apparent confounding of rules may not, however, be due to the availability of sign language but to a lack of acoustic data and exposure to English forms.

Parasnis (1983) presented a study addressing the issue of manual language as a facilitator for development of standard English. In this study, two groups of congenitally deaf college students were compared on English reading and writing skills. One group consisted of deaf native speakers of American Sign Language (ASL), the other of individuals who were not taught sign until 6 to 12 years of age. If early manual acquisition were to facilitate English language development, native ASL users would be expected to perform better on English skills tests. Yet, no difference was found in English reading and writing test scores between the groups. Results of two other measures used by Parasnis, speechreading and speech intelligibility, were significantly better in the "delayed" sign group. This finding was related to the group's earlier and more consistent exposure to speech.

Another form of manual communication, Signed English (signs used with English inflections and word order), may facilitate English acquisition. Ideally parents and teachers would speak and use signed English simultaneously with the deaf child. However, very few individuals are able to do so (Marmor & Pettito, 1979). Even if exact mirroring of spoken English may not be possible, consistent use of Signed English may facilitate young hearing-impaired children's acquisition of English morphemes (Gilman, Davis, & Raffin, 1980). For communication ease, deaf children may revert to the use of ASL in less formal communication situations (e.g., on the playground). In view of this, Bornstein et al. (1980) suggested that Signed English be considered a model of standard English rather than the only acceptable communication mode for deaf children.

Incorporation of sign language is essential for providing some deaf children with a means of communication. Early exposure to spoken English appears beneficial for speechreading and speech production skills. Osberger et al. (1986) observed that students in auditory-oral schools appear "to achieve significant gains in speech intelligibility, whereas students in total communication programs do not" (p. 31). Those investigators cautioned, however, that these differences may be related to the more intense and systematic speech training provided to students in the auditory-oral programs rather than to the use of total communication per se. Their greatest concern was that "regardless of communication approach, hearing-impaired children score significantly below their normal-hearing peers on English language measures" (Kretschmer & Kretschmer, 1978, p. 86). Because of the proven need to give these children every communicative advantage as early as possible, a constant theme of this chapter will be the imperative to achieve early intervention at all costs.

relationship between language deficit and hearing loss

Language function in the hearing-impaired child cannot be solely predicted on the basis of severity of hearing loss. Thus, Norlin and Van Tasell (1980) commented that the range of language skills for children with similar audiograms is not surprising considering other important factors such as speech-discrimination abilities, ability to use amplification, the individual child's ability to learn language, and the child's ability to tolerate and use incomplete data. That is to say, for a variety of yet undetermined reasons some children may be able to arrive at a Gestalt from a limited set of data far more easily than others. Hence, when presented with a limited or restricted auditory signal, they may be able to extrapolate better and thereby more readily understand the message and its context. While emphasizing the potential range of language abilities, these authors noted that "in general, an increase in the severity of hearing-impairment is associated with progressively greater difficulty in the capacity to extract and learn the rules of an oral language system'' (p. 24).

More recently, Davis et al. (1986) reported that this assumption did not hold true for the 40 mild and moderately hearing-impaired children in their study. They emphasized the heterogeneous language performance within hearing-loss categories, concluding that ''the motivation and efforts of parents, educational programming and other factors may be much more important....''(p. 61). Although variable language abilities may be expected, the following characteristics generally apply to the language of hearing-impaired children:

1. Language delay

2. Plateau of language skills which may be partly attributed to teaching methods

3. Deviant language forms usually restricted to children with profound hearing losses (>90 dB HL).

Most hearing-impaired children will exhibit language deficits/delays related to the aforementioned factors. It appears that the deteriorated speech acoustic signal robs the hearing-impaired child of information regarding the form (phonology, syntax, morphology), content (semantics), and use (pragmatics) of language. Language delay may be a primary consequence of this information loss. For the profoundly hearing-impaired child, the lack of sufficient speech information may preclude normal language acquisition through audition. Thus, in this population deviant language forms may accompany severe language delay. As mentioned previously, profoundly hearing-impaired children's standard English may be considered and treated as a second language. A cautious distinction between the majority of hearing-impaired (i.e., hard-of-hearing children, <80-90 dB HL) and the profoundly hearing-impaired (i.e., deaf children, >80-90 dB HL) may be appropriate.

Phonology. A few studies (Oller, Jensen, & Lafayette, 1978; Oller & Kelly, 1974) indicate that the hard-of-hearing child's phonologic system resembles that of younger, normal-hearing children. Normal phonological processes (i.e., simplification of sounds and sound combinations) and delay in articulation skills indicate a normal but delayed acquisition of speech sounds. Jensema, Karchmer, and Trybus (1978) noted that this speech delay may not be resolved and these children's speech skills may plateau at seven years of age. It is unknown whether this reflects inadequate cues for speech production and/or inadequate speech training.

Primarily due to the limited availability of temporal cues (e.g., syllabic stress and number), profoundly hearing-impaired children may have insufficient information to allow them to learn appropriate speech movements (Fletcher & Hasegawa, 1983; Tye-Murray, 1987). Thus, their speech is commonly characterized by deviant respiratory, laryngeal, and articulatory movements. Such inappropriate physiological movements in the speech systems result in errors in the production of consonants and vowels as well as disturbances in voice patterns and suprasegmental integrity. As in the hard-of-hearing population, severely hearing-impaired children appear to evidence little speech improvement beyond seven years of age (Jensema et al., 1978). The reader is referred to the Speech section of this chapter for a more thorough discussion of the phonological deviations.

Syntax. A large number of descriptive studies of language have focused on the syntactic abilities of hearing-impaired children as measured by reading comprehension and writing production tasks. Although these measures tap secondary language skills, results of these and more recent measures paint the following picture of hearing-impaired children's syntactic skills:

1. Restricted knowledge of word classes as evidenced by overuse of nouns and verbs and omission of function words

2. Restricted knowledge of syntax as evidenced by overuse of the subject-verb-object sentence structure

3. Syntactic delay with subsequent plateau in regard to syntactic abilities

4. Deviant syntax in profoundly hearing-impaired children.

Investigators have implied that these language characteristics are by-products of hearing loss. More recently, Hasenstab and Horner (1982) noted that hearing-impaired and language-disordered children generally exhibit language delay rather than language deviance. In other words, the language deficits resemble immature language development. These authors indicated further that these populations have the potential for acquiring language through the normal developmental sequence. Other investigators (Simmons-Martin, 1977) have suggested that such language deficits may reflect rigid training methods rather than the linguistic potential of the hearing-impaired child since rigidity in training can reduce the expressive linguistic structure to the point that a limited subset of linguistic forms is displayed.

Restricted knowledge of word classes. Hearing-impaired children tend to use a greater proportion of nouns and verbs than their normal-hearing peers. Analyses of written language samples (Brannon, 1968; MacGuintie, 1964; Tervoort, 1967) concur with this observation, noting hearing-impaired children's sparse use of adverbs, auxiliaries, pronouns, prepositions, and Wh-questions. The same preferential use of nouns, verbs, and articles is observed in young normal-hearing children. However, normal-hearing children gradually decrease their use of these forms while increasing the use of pronouns, prepositions, adjectives, adverbs, and conjunctions with age (Myklebust, 1964). A similar pattern is evidenced in oral language analyses (Brannon & Murry, 1966; Griswold & Cummings, 1974). Specifically, Brannon and Murry reported that the tendency to omit function words increased with severity of hearing loss.

Restricted knowledge and use of syntactic forms. The length of written sentences has been used to distinguish between the communication skills of hearing-impaired and normal-hearing children of the same chronologic age. Thus, the average sentence length is shorter for the hearing-impaired child, partly as a function of a larger proportion of simple sentences vs. compound and complex sentences used by this population. Further, hearing-impaired children often use a stereotypic phrase in sentences where a noun phrase (e.g., "the boy _____") introduces a series of related sentences on a given topic (Heider & Heider, 1940; Kretschmer, 1975; Simmons, 1962). In addition, the hearing-impaired child commonly adheres to a subject-verb-object sentence structure format rather than more complex sentence structures which may not be comprehended (Davis & Blasdell, 1975). In this regard, Davis and Blasdell observed that young normal-hearing children and older children faced with unfamiliar structures tend to adhere to subject-verb-object structures. Using this strategy, the child with limited syntactic flexibility may attempt to reduce communications to the more familiar subject-verb-object pattern. The inability to comprehend more complex forms poses serious problems for reading (Osberger et al., 1986).

Lack of syntactic flexibility has also been revealed in word recall tasks. Odom and Blanton (1967) studied severely to profoundly hearing-impaired children's recall of four-word strings in a paired-associates task. Well-formed partial sentences, fragments of partial sentences, and scrambled nonsyntactic strings were developed. Syntactic order was found to facilitate recall for normal-hearing subjects but not for the hearing impaired. Tomblin (1977) assessed recall for four-, six-, and eight-word strings of syntactically well-formed and randomly ordered "phrases." As in the Odom and Blanton study, Tomblin's hearing-impaired subjects did not benefit from four-word strings by syntax. Syntax did facilitate their recall of six- and eight-word strings, however. It was speculated that the training approach might explain the differential use of syntactic information in regard to shorter vs. longer strings. That is, children taught via a grammatical "slot filler" approach (in which longer declarative sentences predominate) may fail to recognize short phrases as having syntactic structure, instead interpreting them as "nonsentences."

Syntactic delay and plateau.   Geffner and Freeman (1980) assessed the language comprehension of 65 six-year-old profoundly hearing-impaired children using the *Assessment of Children's Language Comprehension* (Foster, Giddan, & Stark, 1972) and the *Syntax Screening Test* (Gaffney, 1977). The following basic structures proved most effective (a) nouns and verbs, (b) noun + verb and noun + noun, and (c) negation and rejection. The performance of these hearing-impaired children was reportedly comparable to that of normal-hearing children in the three- to four-year age range. Based on these findings, Geffner and Freeman tentatively concluded that hearing-impaired children acquire syntax in the normal developmental sequence but at a slower rate. Wilcox and Tobin (1974) also reported that their hard-of-hearing subjects' performance was comparable to that of younger normal-hearing children. They too postulated that the hard of hearing acquire language in a normal but delayed sequence.

Quigley, Steinkamp, and Jones (1978) developed the *Test of Syntactic Ability* to assess the syntactic skills of adolescent hearing-impaired children. They found that the order of difficulty for syntactic structures was similar for hearing-impaired children and normal-hearing children. However, older hearing-impaired subjects evidenced mastery of only the simplest forms (e.g., negation and conjunction). Certain grammatical skills such as verb formation and use of pronouns and the passive voice were rarely seen in correct form in these children. The investigators concluded that deaf children follow the normal developmental sequence of syntactic acquisition, but differ in the rate of development and apparent plateau of syntactic skills.

Studies equating hearing-impaired and normal-hearing children on the basis of mean length of utterance (MLU) further support language delay as opposed to language deviance as a characteristic of children with hearing impairments. For example, Hess (1972) equated a hearing-impaired boy and a normal-hearing boy on their mean lengths of utterance and found the two children's ability to perform linguistic operations over a 5-month period to be essentially the same. Hess concluded that the hearing-impaired child evidenced essentially the same sequence of acquisition as the normal-hearing child.

Using a somewhat different strategy, Smith (1972) evaluated nine oral hearing-impaired children on the basis of MLU. The MLUs were used to place children into one of three stages of language development. Oral language comprehension tasks employed in the study involved picture pointing in response to subject-verb, verb-object, subject-verb-object, and fully developed grammatical strings. The hearing-impaired children performed at the same level as the normal children within each stage of language development. Furthermore, all children at a particular stage, regardless of hearing status, dealt with stimuli differently than did children in other stages. When equated on the basis of MLU, the hearing-impaired and normal-hearing appeared to use similar comprehension strategies. In addition, a change in strategies occurred as a result of changes in language development.

Although limited in number, studies of oral language also support the theory of syntactic delay and plateau of skills in hearing-impaired children. Pressnell (1973) assessed oral language of 47 hard-of-hearing and deaf children using the *Northwestern Syntax Screening Test* (Lee, 1969) and *Developmental Sentence Scoring* (Lee & Canter, 1971). Both measures indicated language delay and little apparent improvement in syntax with age for hearing-impaired children. Using a sentence-generation task to identify syntactic skills in deaf children, Stoutenburgh (1971) reported a similar plateau of syntactic skills. The grammatical complexity of normal-hearing children's productions increased by 20% between the ages of 9 and 14. In contrast, the oldest deaf children were still using predominantly simple sentences.

Deviant syntax in profoundly hearing-impaired children. Despite remarkable similarity in syntactic development between normal and hearing-handicapped children, the latter, particularly in severely involved cases, manifest certain unique syntactic structures (Quigley et al., 1976). For example, Tervoort (1967) assessed the videotaped language samples of 48 deaf children between 7 and 12 years of age. Structures were categorized as "grammatical," "acceptable" (i.e., comprehensive), or "agrammatical." It was discovered that 35% of these children's productions were categorized as "agrammatical" (free order and absence of morphologic markers). Such agrammaticality has also been observed among deaf adults. In a sentence-recall task, Sarachan-Deily and Love (1974) observed non-sentence forms which involved omission of major sentence constituents, use of incorrect endings and asequential word orders. These non-English forms were judged to reflect unstable or limited syntactic competence in English.

Morphology and vocabulary. Studies of hearing-impaired children's morphology and vocabulary use suggest two principal disturbances: (a) delay and plateau in morphologic skills and (b) reduced vocabulary and difficulty with function words. When compared to normal-hearing peers, hearing-impaired children evidence delay in their use of common morphologic inflections (Cooper, 1967; Gilman et al., 1980). In studies of morphologic inflections, deaf children were observed to be markedly delayed, yet their performance appeared related to exposure or lack of exposure to a morpheme-based sign system on a consistent basis. Thus, deaf children with consistent exposure to Seeing Essential English (a morpheme-based system) used morphologic inflections with much greater accuracy.

Reduced vocabulary is common among hearing-impaired populations. This restricted vocabulary has been discussed, in part, in relation to restricted use of word classes (i.e., predominance of nouns and verbs). Thus, Brannon (1968) and Simmons (1962) noted less diverse vocabulary in hearing-impaired children's written compositions. Restricted vocabulary was also reported by Young and McConnell (1957). Similarly, students with hearing losses scored substantially lower on the *Ammons Full Range Picture Vocabulary Test* (Ammons & Ammons, 1948) than did their normal peers.

Restricted word knowledge has also been reported by Moeller et al. (1986) for a sample of hearing-impaired students from a state residential school for the deaf. These investigators administered the *Peabody Picture Vocabulary Test* (PPVT) and the Picture Vocabulary subtest (TO-PV) of the *Test of Language Development* to hearing-impaired children between the ages of 4 and 20. The students' age-equivalent scores evidenced severe delays relative to the normative data for normal-hearing children. Age-equivalent scores on the PPVT, for example, indicated that, on the average, these children's performance was comparable to that of normal-hearing children 6-8 years of age. In addition, the PPVT scores for the hearing-impaired children showed little growth beyond 12 years of age. In a sample of 40 mild-to-moderately hearing-impaired children, PPVT scores were also found to indicate delays in vocabulary development (Davis et al., 1986). According to Davis et al., "age deviation scores on the PPVT-R indicated vocabulary development ranging from a delay of about 1 year for the older, moderately hearing-impaired children to more than 3 years for the older severely hearing-impaired children" (p. 57).

While not a true vocabulary measure, the *Boehm Test of Basic Concepts* (Boehm, 1971) has been used to assess concepts related to early school curricula. Davis (1974) reported that 75% of her population of hard-of-hearing children scored below the 10th percentile on the *Boehm*. In addition, no difference in performance was noted between younger and older hearing-impaired children.

Moeller et al. (1986) reported on the administration of the *Boehm Test of Basic Concepts* to a population of hearing-impaired students from a state residential school for the deaf. They concluded that even by 16-18 years of age, many students were not comprehending basic linguistic concepts (space, quantity, time) mastered by 6- to 8-year-old children with normal hearing.

Semantics. Oral language analyses (Curtiss, Prutting, & Lowell, 1979; Skarakis & Prutting, 1977) of severe and profoundly hearing-impaired preschool children provide evidence of a delay in acquisition of semantic functions; that is, the number and variety of semantic operations were restricted in comparison to those of normal-hearing peers. Most of the hearing-impaired youngsters used several different semantic functions, although few used words to express these semantic functions (i.e., they relied on nonverbal forms of communication). However, the sequence of acquisition of various semantic competencies was comparable to that of normal children.

McKnight and Davis (1983) assessed semantic knowledge using a unique judgment task. Profoundly hearing-impaired children of primary-school age were required to judge and provide necessary corrections for the following types of imperative sentences: (a) semantically and syntactically correct, (b) syntactically reversed, and (c) semantically anomalous. The investigators discovered that linguistically unsophisticated language users are better able to use semantic information in making metalinguistic judgments. This tendency was evidenced in the hearing-impaired children's superior performance in judging semantic correctness. Interestingly, the MLU did not equate hearing-impaired and normal-hearing children as the former performed much more poorly than did normal subjects at a given MLU. For all subjects, however, higher MLUs were associated with better task performance. As with other language measures, it was concluded that the hearing impaired develop semantic and syntactic metalinguistic awareness in a sequence similar to that of their normal counterparts but at a slower rate.

The study of semantic knowledge in older hearing-impaired children has typically involved pencil-and-paper inventories using essentially two approaches to measurement: (a) the semantic differential and (b) word-association tests. The *semantic differential* (rating stimulus words with respect to a series of bipolar adjectives) has been used to uncover similarities between normal and hearing-impaired subjects on some factors, such as evaluation (e.g., good-bad) and potency (e.g., little-big), but not others, including activity (e.g., fast-slow) and warmth (e.g., hot-cold) (Green & Shepherd, 1973). Further insight concerning semantic structure was offered by Holmes and Green (1974) who evaluated two groups of hearing-impaired children, one averaging 8, the other 12 years of age. These researchers reported that the younger group did not demonstrate a definite semantic structure as measured by the semantic differential approach. However, the older group's judgments were similar to those of normal-hearing children.

The results of word-association tests indicate that hearing-impaired individuals' responses are comparable to those of younger hearing subjects of the same reading achievement level. That is, hearing-impaired subjects tend to give more *syntagmatic* responses (different form class, as in the example where the stimulus is "table" and the response is "eat") than *paradigmatic* response (same form class, as in the example where the stimulus is "table" and the response is "chair") (Koplin, Odom, Blanton, & Nunnaly, 1967). There is also some evidence that the hearing impaired use a more concrete (as opposed to abstract) form of language (Blanton & Nunnaly, 1964).

Impact of training has been a constant theme of this discussion concerning language deficiencies and delays among the hearing impaired. This theme has also been reflected in word-association tasks. For example, Restaino (1968) evaluated word-association responses from hearing-impaired children in two schools for the hearing impaired as well as for normal-hearing children in elementary school. A difference in responses obtained from children in the two schools for the hearing impaired emerged. Restaino interpreted this finding by pointing out that the schools differed in method of language instruction. One used an analytic/grammatical approach, the other a normal language development approach. The hearing-impaired children from the latter gave responses more similar to those of normal children. Restaino emphasized that, even though the two groups of hearing-impaired children were instructed under the auspices of an oral method, the differences in actual "instruction" of language probably affected their word-association capabilities.

In a second related study, McGettigan and Rosenstein (1969) evaluated the ability to identify synonyms and associations by normal-hearing children and by hearing-impaired children from two different schools for the hearing impaired. The hearing-impaired children were less able to correctly identify associations and synonyms compared to normal-hearing children. However, the subjects from one school for the hearing impaired made significantly more errors than the students from the other school. McGettigan and Rosenstein concluded that differences in training between the two schools accounted for the group differences. Osberger et al. (1986a) also suggested that synonyms are more difficult than antonyms for hearing-impaired children, perhaps due to training strategies. These investigators analyzed the error patterns of hearing-impaired children from a state residential school for the deaf on the Antonyms/Synonyms subtest of the *Woodcock-Johnson Psychoeducational Test Battery*. They attributed the greater number of synonym errors to the fact that deaf children are often taught concepts using polar opposite (e.g., hot-cold). In addition, due to restricted vocabulary these children may have only one label for any given referent.

Pragmatics. While pragmatics is a major topic in connection with language-delayed children, generally to date, little experimental work has been published regarding the pragmatic skills of children with hearing impairments. Skarakis and Prutting (1977) and Curtiss et al. (1979) analyzed the pragmatic function of hearing-impaired children between 2 and 4 years of age. Finding that these children evidenced a wide range of pragmatic functions both verbally and nonverbally, Kolzak (1983) emphasized the need to consider hearing-impaired children's pragmatic function in that children with severe hearing losses often do not initiate communication, exchange social forms such as "please" and "thank you", and have difficulty sustaining or repairing conversations.

language assessment in the hearing impaired

Two broad groups need to be considered in evaluating language function of hearing-impaired children. For the majority of these children, appropriate language assessments are the same as for language-delayed children. A second group involves severely hearing-impaired children who evidence notable language delays and deviant forms.

Regardless of the assessment strategy chosen, several factors must be kept in mind when evaluating the language of a child with hearing impairment (for additional detail on this issue, refer to Chapter 6). First, by their very nature, nearly all language tests are verbal tests—a fact which obviously puts the hearing impaired at a disadvantage. Therefore, effort must be made to maximize the use of visual cues to insure that the task is clearly understood. Though by no means an ideal compensation, it may be necessary to supplement verbal cues with sign language and fingerspelling. Second, the examiner should speak distinctly and economically, avoiding unnecessary comments during the examination. Third, as with all language testing, environmental distractions— particularly background noise—should be avoided. Fourth, hearing aids should be checked for proper functioning prior to evaluation.

Formal Language Assessment. Formal assessment methods developed for normal-hearing children include tests of expressive and receptive language and tests of phonologic, morphologic, syntactic, and semantic development. When dealing with the hearing impaired, the clinician must determine what modifications should be made in the test, in the presentation of items, in the instructions, or in the evaluation of responses. A first step would be to optimize the test environment and test instructions. Perhaps the clinician should then provide decreasing redundancy in the presentation of items. If formal tests are administered, not for the purpose of assessing normative development, but to gain information regarding baseline behavior and directions for intervention, their use with the hearing impaired seems both logical and appropriate.

The major communication assessment technique recommended for use with the hearing impaired, however, is "informal," namely, a spontaneous language sample (Ling, 1976). Rules for sampling techniques, transcription, calculation of MLU, determination of stage of development, and analysis of form and function of utterances within the sample have been discussed by Larson (1976) and Tyack and Gottsleben (1974). This technique yields information relative to baseline language information and intervention approaches.

Language Assessment Designed for the Hearing Impaired. Language assessment measures for the hearing-impaired child can be categorized as follows: (a) communication checklists, (b) formal tests of syntax, and (c) language sample analyses. The assessment formats within these categories will be described in the following sections.

Communication checklists. Although communication checklists fail to provide indepth information regarding language function, they may be used as a cross-check on data derived from formal tests (Kretschmer & Kretschmer, 1978). Moog and Geers (1975) developed the CID *Scales of Early Communication Skills for Hearing-Impaired Children* to assess children between the ages of 2 and 8 years. The scales consist of a teacher checklist on which the child is rated on receptive language skills, expressive language skills, nonverbal receptive language skills, and nonverbal expressive skills. Ling (1976) and Chalfant (1977) also introduced developmental checklists for the hearing impaired. Ling's checklist assesses audition, speech, language, and general communication skills whereas Chalfant's instrument includes items related to motor performance, speech imitation skills, gestural language, receptive language, and expressive language.

Tests of syntax. Of the several tests designed to assess the syntax of hearing-impaired children, most evaluate expressive syntactic skills rather than receptive syntactic ability. The following discussion will describe briefly four such tests: (a) *Grammatical Analysis of Elicited Language (GAEL)*, (b) *Test of Expressive Language Ability (TEXLA)*, (c) *Test of Syntactic Ability (TSA)*, and (d) *Test of Receptive Language Ability (TERLA)*.

The GAEL provides an indepth analysis of prompted and imitated sentence structures at the simple and the complex sentence level. Comparison scores are provided for severely and profoundly hearing-impaired children between 2½ and 11 years and for normal-hearing children between 3 and 6 years.

The TEXLA assesses basic grammatical structures in a written response format, thereby limiting its use to children with at least basic writing skills. The authors provide normative data for 7- to 12-year-old hearing-impaired children and first-grade normal-hearing youngsters.

The companion test to the TEXLA, the TERLA, also is designed to assess basic grammatical structures in young hearing-impaired children. The child reads a single word or verb phrase and is required to point to the "best" picture. Norms are provided for hearing-impaired children between 6 and 12 years of age as well as normal-hearing first graders.

Quigley et al. (1976) devised the TSA, a series of reading and writing tasks, to assess the syntax of older hearing-impaired children. A variety of syntactic structures is probed on 20 subtests of 70 items each. Sentence completion and grammatical judgments or corrections are used to indicate the child's syntactic function. The accompanying 120-item screening test may be more practical at times inasmuch as each subtest requires approximately one hour to administer (Thompson et al., 1987).

Language sample analyses. A language sample analysis for the hearing impaired was proposed by Lehman (1970), who developed the structural complexity response index to measure syntactic complexity of oral productions from a spontaneous language sample. Although this test only focuses on language form (i.e., syntax), it was an initial step toward more complete assessment of younger hearing-impaired youngsters.

Kretschmer and Kretschmer (1978) provided a very comprehensive and elegant spontaneous language analysis procedure. They also thoroughly outlined and depicted the means by which they analyzed the pragmatic, semantic, and syntactic functions of hearing-impaired children. Assessment categories include preverbal behaviors, single-word and two-word productions, semantic classes, single-proposition productions, complex sentence productions, communication competence, and restricted form types. Although this analysis requires both clinician sophistication and time, its apparent excellence justifies its clinical use or use of similar strategies. Samples of both expressive and receptive language should be obtained and analyzed. In the expressive area several strategies may be used, including (a) having the mother keep a diary, and (b) recording the words the child uses while noting the context in which they are used. Receptively, samples should be taken which detail (a) the words to which the child responds consistently (e.g., action verbs that he/she will act out), and (b) how the child responds to direction words in connection with a specific task.

For a more comprehensive discussion of language-assessment issues, the reader is referred to Thompson et al.'s (1987) text, *Language Assess-*

ment of Hearing-Impaired School Age Children. This work also includes a listing and discussion of 36 tests which may be useful for assessing hearing-impaired children.

habilitation procedures for the hard-of-hearing child

Materials and procedures for the language-delayed, normal-hearing child may be used with hearing-impaired children, particularly since most hearing-impaired children exhibit language delay rather than language deviance. For further reference, Hasenstab and Horner (1982) present an excellent listing of goals for hearing-impaired and language-delayed children in general. The prevention approach to language intervention would also be appropriate with hard-of-hearing children. This approach is further discussed in the following section on intervention methods used with the most severely hearing-impaired children.

habilitation procedures for the severely hearing-impaired child

The purpose of this section on language is to identify strategies that historically have been used for language improvement among the severely hearing impaired. Comprehensive treatment programs cannot be presented because of space limitations. Consequently, the reader is invited to consult the references cited for more information.

General Considerations. Issues surrounding approaches to teaching hearing-impaired children include such questions as whether a "multisensory" (visual/aural/oral) or a "unisensory" (aural/oral, acoupedic) method should be used. The multisensory approach historically has focused on speechreading as one of the major input channels of a language development program. The unisensory approach, on the other hand, does not focus on speechreading per se, but on the "impaired" sense modality—hearing—for language learning. This does not mean that children are forced not to look or not allowed visual information. Rather, using a unisensory approach, the child is generally allowed to speechread in a different way. That is, he may observe ongoing nonlinguistic stimuli in the environment and connect the nonlinguistic information to the linguistic information that is being received auditorily. However, the child has the option of looking at the speaker's face and, in essence, the child determines what visual information is necessary for understanding.

Hasenstab and Horner (1982) provided an excellent outline of language intervention techniques for young hearing-impaired children. A few of their general language goals are as follows:

1. Development of concepts pertinent to the child's environment and functioning.

2. Association of words with a referent: Understanding of familiar objects and names through the use of speechreading and audition.

3. Development of visual attention combined with listening activity.

4. Recognition of similarities in shapes and familiar objects through matching.

5. Awareness of size differences and color concepts.

6. Control of tongue, lips, and facial muscles.

7. Control of breathstream and blowing.

8. Imitation of meaningful gestures and actions.

9. Vocalization through imitation and spontaneity.

10. Vocalization of meaningful words.

The reader is referred to Hasenstab and Horner's text (1982) for subskills and suggested activities for attaining these goals.

Historical Methods. Various systems have traditionally been used to teach language to hearing-impaired children, including grammatical systems, such as the Barry Five Slate System (Barry, 1899) and the Fitzgerald Key (Fitzgerald, 1929). These systems focus on the form of the child's utterance to the exclusion of understanding; words are categorized with respect to parts of speech; and written language is generally used as a first mode of communication. "Slot filler" techniques such as these as well as sentence-patterning techniques are associated with a grammatical system and there is a focus on drills and formal exercises. The Fitzgerald Key emphasizes analysis of relations among discrete units of language through the visual aid of written language for the purpose of helping the child understand syntactic rules. The Key is placed on the chalkboard with vertical lines drawn to reflect potential divisions within sentences. Columns are then labeled to indicate the most common word order in English sentences that can be placed within a column.

Techniques like the Key tend to lend themselves best to simple, active, affirmative, declarative sentences (recall the review of language development in the hearing impaired). In addition, they do not account for idiomatic or incomplete utterances. The who/what distinction is initially advocated in the Key. A review of systematic development of question behavior will indicate that initial learning of the who/what distinction is not within guidelines of developmental order of question behavior (Brown, 1969; Ervin-Tripp, 1970). Specific grammatical approaches such as the Key are slowly being replaced by all-purpose sentence patterns.

Several more recent patterning techniques have been introduced for use with the hearing impaired. For example, Caniglia, Cole, Howard, Krohn, and Rice (1972) introduced a sequential, patterned language program for teaching written language structure and vocabulary. This program includes strategies for teaching negation and question transformation. McCarr (1973) presented a structured transformational approach to teaching written language through a series of lessons and also developed an approach to transferring reading skills to writing skills using language patterning and a cloze procedure. Although these programs tend to be sequential and use some psycholinguistic information, they rely on the written form. Yet, written language as the major mode of teaching oral language has been questioned (Doehring, 1976; Ling, 1974). Furthermore, these strategies focus on syntax/structure/form rather than the function of language. The authors point out that the programs were not intended as an exclusive language-development plan. Since techniques like these can be used to initiate a particular language skill or to review and/or stabilize a structure, they should be considered supplemental.

The major problem with the aforementioned traditional approaches to language remediation is that they have been used as entire language programs and have not been sensitive to normal language development. While they have utility as individual implementors for facilitating specific objectives, they should not constitute the overall language-development program.

Natural Language Intervention. The experiential or natural approach to rehabilitation was first advocated by Groht (1958) and Harris (1963). The basis for this approach is that language should involve expressing thoughts and ideas that are interesting to the child using meaningful repetition of language rather than drills. Further, language should be learned through meaningful experiences (Kolzak, 1983). This approach to language teaching is activity oriented and directs the setting for therapeutic intervention as well as the nonlinguistic information and activities that might be provided. The content/unit approach (Croker, Jones, & Pratt, 1928; Streng, 1968) is based upon the notion that subject matter can contribute to increased vocabulary as well as clarification and practice of spoken or written language. A content-based curriculum would provide units on such items as transportation as a framework for learning language.

As an example of the natural approach to language intervention, consider the case of a child who is having difficulty with relative adjectives. Rather than develop a lesson plan that involves drill work on "little, littler, littlest" or "big, bigger, biggest," a session could be constructed around familiar household items, the child's toys, or family members of different sizes. The child would have the opportunity to master these concepts in a meaningful context.

The prevention approach to language intervention for hearing-impaired children uses data on the developmental sequence of language forms and functions as they appear to be acquired by normal-hearing children. (The reader is referred to the excellent treatment by Kretschmer and Kretschmer [1978].) This method assumes that, although certain areas of language behavior may be emphasized at a particular time, there are no subsidiary skill areas. For example, function is not taught without form and form is not taught without function. Auditory training becomes "listening to language" rather than bells or drums. Similarly, speech becomes "spoken language" rather than individual phoneme and syllable drills (Ling, 1981; Ling & Milne, 1980). The linguistic approach has been described under a variety of labels including the *acoupedic method* (Pollack, 1970) and the *auditory-global system* (Calvert & Silverman, 1975; Simmons-Martin, 1977). This general concept emphasizes strengthening of language processing through the auditory sense modality with reference to normal language development.

Emerging Techniques: Tactile Aids and Cochlear Implants. Researchers have sought to develop the "perfect sensory aid—some type of replacement ear, so to speak, that would be useful for a broad spectrum of speech training and reception applications" (Rothenberg, 1979, p. 232). Attempts to achieve this goal have led to the development of (a) tactile aids which code speech as vibratory patterns on the skin, and (b) cochlear implants which code speech as electrical pulses directly to the eighth nerve. Although these devices do not generally permit complete perception of speech, they do provide considerable information (duration, timing, intensity, and low-frequency speech components) that allows for some speech perception. Equally important, tactile aids and cochlear implants supply supplemental information which facilitates speechreading and allows some monitoring of speech production. These alternative sensory aids are generally considered for use when traditional amplification is unsuccessful. In the case of tactile aids they sometimes are used to supplement conventional amplification. Chapter 2 contains additional information concerning these devices.

Use of alternative sensory aids with prelingually deafened children has been questioned because these youngsters have no English language base for speechreading. Yet, proponents of such use report that children with these aids demonstrate simple speech discrimination abilities (e.g., long vs. short sounds, syllable number) and increased and more modulated vocalizations (Chouard, Fugain, Meyer, & Lacomb, 1983; Eisenberg, Berliner, House, & Edgerton, 1983; Geers, Miller, & Gustus, 1983). In a recent report, Geers et al. (1983) also noted an increase in spoken language vocabulary with use of a vibrotactile aid. The benefits of these sensory aids for speech and language development in the prelingually deaf may be substantial in the future.

speech

As mentioned, speech may be viewed as the oral component of language expression. In a recent article, Monsen (1982) noted that "all of the contemporary approaches in the education of the hearing impaired encourage and advocate the development of oral communication skills to whatever extent possible" (p. 845). The focus of the present chapter on oral communication skills reflects this attitude. However, this perspective is not meant to deny that other means of communication are beneficial and essential. Given this stance, the following section will provide a general information base for rehabilitation as well as data that may help the reader begin to question certain fallacies and misconceptions previously reported in the literature regarding the speech of hearing-impaired persons. Two general sections, one on early vocalizations of the hearing impaired and one on speech intelligibility, will be followed by a review of speech production in the mild-to-moderately hearing-impaired child as well as a review of speech production in the severe-to-profoundly impaired child. In the latter two sections, speech behaviors, assessment strategies, and management concerns for both populations of hearing-impaired youngsters will be discussed.

early vocalization of the hearing impaired

Historically, it has been argued that at the early stages of speech/language development the hearing-impaired and the normal-hearing child

cannot be differentiated. Thus, the babbling stage is presumably characterized by vocalizations that are quantitatively and qualitatively similar
for hearing and hearing-impaired infants. This contention was supported
by Smith (1982) in a study comparing the vocalizations of hearing, hearing-
impaired, and Down syndrome children from 3 to 15 months of age.
Smith found that velar/back consonants dominated in the 12- to 15-month
range for all three groups. Likewise vocalic productions for all three groups
were similar with a predominance of front, mid-central, and low vowels
being the most frequent. In contrast, some investigators have reported
quantitative and/or qualitative differences between the babbling of normal-
hearing and hearing-impaired children (Lenneberg, 1967; Stark, 1983;
Stoel-Gammon & Otomo, 1986).

Stark (1983) found that hearing-impaired children's babbling differed
primarily with respect to the range of speech-like sounds that occurred.
More recently, Stoel-Gammon and Otomo (1986) analyzed and compared
babbling samples from 11 normal-hearing children from 4-18 months
of age and 11 hearing-impaired subjects between 4 and 28 months. When
compared to normal-hearing infants of similar age, the hearing-impaired
babies evidenced a smaller variety of consonant sounds. The difference
in consonantal repertoire was particularly noticeable at ages beyond 8
months. Hearing-impaired infants also tended to produce fewer multi-
syllabic utterances containing "true consonants" (i.e., consonants other
than the glides [w, j, h] and glottal stop).

Some evidence suggests that there may be a decline in vocalizations
of hearing-impaired children after the age of 15 months. Thus, Mavilya
(1972) recorded the vocalizations of three hearing-impaired children once
a week for 12 consecutive weeks beginning at the age of 16 months.
These vocalizations were compared with those of a normal-hearing baby.
Unlike the normal-hearing child, the children with hearing losses evidenced a peak in quantity of vocalizations followed by a noticeable decrement. In addition, a relatively low proportion of consonant production
was found among the three hearing-impaired infants when compared
to the normal-hearing infant. Degree of hearing loss was considered to
be a factor in that differences in babbling were greatest when comparing
the children with moderately severe to profound hearing losses with
the normal-hearing children. Kent, Osberger, Netsell, and Hustedde
(1987) recently described a unique "natural experiment" which allowed
for the investigation of the effects of hearing loss on babbling. They studied a pair of identical twins one of whom had normal hearing, the other
a severe-to-profound hearing loss. Audio and video recorded samples
were taken at 8, 12, and 15 months. The hearing-impaired twin was
found to have a more limited repertoire of consonants, a more restricted

range of first and second formants in vowels, and a highly variable fundamental frequency. Differences in babbling were noted even though the hearing-impaired twin had used binaural amplification since age 3 months. Menyuk (1977) contended that "prelinguistic" babbling behaviors signal

> a period during which the normally hearing infant makes both perceptual and productive categorization of the speech signal which may be crucially important for later language development. In contrast, the severely hearing-impaired infant ceases to spontaneously vocalize to a marked degree and is obviously losing acoustic information of vital importance. (p. 625)

Systematic studies of the development of early vocalizations beyond the babbling state are scanty. Occasionally, however, one may find a study enumerating the phonetic profile of deaf children at various age levels (e.g., Carr, 1953; Lach, Ling, Ling, & Ship, 1970).

speech intelligibility

Although speech intelligibility may not be predicted solely on the basis of hearing levels, research supports a cautious distinction between the speech of mild-to-moderately hearing-impaired children (25-70 dB HL) and that of severe-to-profoundly hearing-impaired children (> 70 dB HL). Nober (1967), for example, reported substantially poorer performance on the *Templin-Darley Test of Articulation* (Templin & Darley, 1969) for children with hearing levels greater than 80 dB HL versus children with lesser degrees of hearing impairment. Similarly, as seen in Table 5.1, a nationwide survey of Jensema et al. (1978) indicated considerably poorer intelligibility ratings for children with hearing levels exceeding 70 dB HL. Further inspection of Table 5.1 reveals that a majority of children with hearing levels of 70 dB HL or better demonstrated "intelligible" or "very intelligible" speech. Intelligibility ratings are more variable in the population of children with hearing levels exceeding 70 dB HL. Degree of hearing loss appears to have a great impact on speech intelligibility. Markides (1983) recommended that correlations between speech intelligibility and hearing levels in the better ear be interpreted with caution. He plotted the intelligibility scores and hearing levels from an investigation (Markides, 1967) in which a correlation of − .71 had been obtained between these variables. A 90% confidence interval was plotted around the best fitting curve, illustrating that children with similar hearing losses have widely different speech intelligibility scores, especially in cases with hearing losses of 50 dB HL or greater. Monsen (1983) also observed that

TABLE 5.1
Speech Intelligibility Ratings as a Function of Hearing Loss

Degree of Hearing Loss[a]	Very Intelligible		Intelligible		Barely Intelligible		Not Intelligible		Would Not Speak		Total	
	N	%	N	%	N	%	N	%	N	%	N	%
<27dB ISO	6	60.0	3	30.0	1	10.0	0	0	0	0	10	100.0
27-40dB ISO	10	43.5	10	43.5	2	8.7	1	4.3	0	0	23	100.0
41-55dB ISO	31	52.5	22	37.3	6	10.2	0	0	0	0	59	100.0
56-70dB ISO	40	38.8	46	44.7	9	8.7	5	4.9	3	2.9	103	100.0
71-90dB ISO	41	15.6	103	39.3	53	20.2	35	13.4	30	11.5	262	100.0
≥91dB ISO	15	3.1	96	20.0	135	28.2	149	31.1	84	17.5	479	100.0
All Categories	143	15.3	280	29.9	206	22.0	190	20.3	117	12.5	936	100.0

χ^2 = 310.7, df = 20, p < .001.

[a]Estimates of hearing loss were not available for 42 students.

From *The Rated Speech Intelligibility of Hearing-Impaired Children: Basic Relationships* by C. J. Jensema, M. A. Karchmer, and R. J. Trybus, 1978, Washington, DC: Gallaudet College of Demographic Studies.

children with more severe hearing losses may span the whole range from *very intelligible* to *very unintelligible*.

The production of intelligible speech may be of greater concern with children whose hearing levels exceed 70 dB HL. Children with milder hearing impairments may require a focus on speech precision and refinement. Whereas the Jensema et al. survey pointed to the child's "better" ear pure-tone average as the single most important predictor of speech intelligibility, other factors such as onset of hearing loss, age at intervention, and family attitudes should also be considered.

By referring to Table 5.2 the reader will note that hearing-impaired children in both populations (i.e., mild-to-moderately and severe-to-profoundly hearing impaired) showed no improvement in speech intelligibility beyond age 7. This finding suggests the need to reassess our orientation to speech therapy in these populations and the techniques used, especially with older children.

the mild-to-moderately hearing-impaired child

Characteristic Errors. Reports in the literature, although primarily anecdotal, indicate that most children with mild-to-moderate hearing losses produce intelligible speech. The Jensema et al. (1978) data provide empirical support for this contention, noting that vowel articulation, voice quality, and suprasegmental features for this group are generally comparable to those of normal-hearing peers. Weiss et al. (1985) assessed use of contrastive stress in a sample of 20 severely hearing-impaired children. All subjects were prejudged to be "intelligible with the exception of a few words" or "intelligible." When compared to normal-hearing children matched on mean length of utterance, the hearing-impaired children's use of contrastive stress was found to be comparable. Cozad (1974) and others have reported that the primary speech errors of mild-to-moderate hearing-impaired children are related to the articulation of single consonants and consonant blends. Knowledge of speech acoustics and the typical, sloping audiometric configuration would suggest that sounds characterized by low intensity, high frequency, and/or short duration might be more commonly in error. Complexity of formation, visibility, and developmental order of acquisition are also considerations in the speech errors of this population. Thus, the reported occurrence of final consonant omissions and the omission/distortion of blends and affricates is consistent with the above-mentioned factors. In this context, Markides (1970) provided the following data for his population of partially hearing children:

TABLE 5.2

Speech Intelligibility Ratings as a Function of Age

Age in Years[a]	Very Intelligible		Intelligible		Barely Intelligible		Not Intelligible		Would Not Speak		Total	
	N	%	N	%	N	%	N	%	N	%	N	%
≤7	18	9.7	66	35.5	34	18.3	36	19.4	32	17.2	186	100.0
8-11	67	17.8	100	26.6	83	22.1	88	23.4	38	10.1	376	100.0
12-15	37	15.1	69	28.2	58	23.7	49	20.0	32	13.1	245	100.0
≥16	28	16.6	52	30.8	39	23.1	27	16.0	23	13.6	169	100.0
All Categories	150	15.4	287	29.4	214	21.9	200	20.5	125	12.8	976	100.0

$\chi^2 = 19.146$, $df = 12$, $p > .05$ (nonsignificant).

[a]The age of two students was not available.

From *The Rated Speech Intelligibility of Hearing-Impaired Children: Basic Relationships* by C. J. Jensema, M. A. Karchmer, and R. J. Trybus, 1978, Washington, DC: Gallaudet College of Demographic Studies.

1. An average intelligibility rating between 76% (when rated by experienced listeners) and 83% (when rated by teachers of the hearing impaired).

2. A vowel error rate of 9%, with the greatest number of errors related to diphthong production.

3. A consonant error rate of 26%, with the greatest number of errors related to final consonant omissions and the distortion of fricatives and affricates.

Markides' findings support anecdotal reports of generally intelligible speech: (a) adequate vowel production; and (b) omission/distortion of fricatives, affricates, and final consonants.

Two phonologic analyses (Oller & Kelly, 1974; West & Weber, 1974) have indicated that children with mild-to-moderate hearing losses produce speech errors comparable to younger normal-hearing peers. These investigators sought to describe the phonology of a single hearing-impaired child and a normal-hearing child. Both children reportedly produced accurate vowels. Their consonant errors could be related to phonological processes used by younger, normal-hearing children (e.g., voicing avoidance, fronting of consonants). Oller and Kelly tentatively proposed that hard-of-hearing children develop and use speech sounds in the same order as normal-hearing children. The findings of these investigations provide a basis for assessment and remediation of speech errors in the mild-to-moderately hearing-impaired child.

Speech Assessment. The mild-to-moderately hearing-impaired child and the normal-hearing, articulation-delayed child apparently share articulation errors. Therefore, the practice of using standard articulation tests with hearing-impaired children appears justified. Use of phonologic analyses, voice assessment, and/or suprasegmental assessment tools would depend upon the individual child and time restrictions.

Speech Management. As suggested previously, with early and appropriate amplification, many children with mild-to-moderate losses can be expected to have essentially normal language and highly intelligible speech. Individuals with earlier onsets and/or later detection, on the other hand, may be expected to experience more serious articulation problems. Nevertheless, it is conceivable that the clinician's only efforts will be directed toward articulation therapy. Standard articulation therapy techniques are appropriate with this population.

Several factors, however, should be kept in mind while undertaking such therapy. First, while articulatory-impaired children with normal hearing generally present a full complement of intact sensory systems, those with hearing loss do not. Therefore, it may be necessary to heighten the use of visual, tactile, and kinesthetic cues to compensate for any auditory deficiencies. Second, the speech clinician must be familiar with the child's audiometric profile to ascertain those sound productions that are beyond the range of audibility. There must be nearly total reliance upon alternate sensory modalities to facilitate and habituate correct sound production. Third, the clinician should be familiar with the impact of context on articulatory configuration and its acoustic consequence. Rather than spending inordinate amounts of time on isolated speech-sound production, therapists should concentrate on sounds in context. Fourth, those investing time in speech rehabilitation must become familiar with the wide variety of treatment approaches (e.g., traditional, distinctive feature, coarticulatory/contextual, phonological processes) available for speech remediation.

For example, once a child has mastered or nearly mastered isolated sound production of the phoneme /t/, the clinician should consider moving quickly into syllabic drills. Rapid patterning such as the following would be appropriate:

/titi tite tita tito titu/
/teti tete teta teto tetu/
etc.

These patterned drills could be accompanied by a clapping or tapping activity that both heightens the rhythmic character of the exercise and adds to the enjoyment of the exercise. When the child has become skilled in producing accurately these permuted patterns, work on meaningful words and short phrases would be warranted.

the severe-to-profoundly hearing-impaired child

Characteristic Errors. For convenience, the characteristic speech errors of children with severe-to-profound hearing impairment will be subsumed under the conventional categories of respiration, phonation, and articulation. However, such division is at times hazardous because there is always an interaction among processes. In this context, Smith (1980) cautioned that the speech of deaf children represents ''stacks of errors which are complex and interrelated'' (p. 27). In addition to the three categories mentioned, some attention will also be directed to suprasegmental errors and recent work on speech-voice profiling in the severe-to-profoundly impaired.

Respiration. Although clinicians and researchers have repeatedly acknowledged the presence of respiratory disturbances in the speech of the deaf, few experiments have been conducted to confirm these impressions and fewer still have employed adequate physiologic assessment methods. For this review, a major paper by Forner and Hixon (1977) serves as a basis for discussion. These researchers employed a well-developed technique for assessing abdomen and rib cage movement with 10 young adult males with severe-to-profound bilateral hearing losses. With respect to continuous discourse, Forner and Hixon found deviancies in three areas underlying respiratory function for speech: (a) linguistic programming, (b) mechanical adjustments of respiratory origin, and (c) mechanical adjustments of the larynx and upper airway. More recently, Whitehead (1983) used similar measurements on a sample of 15 young deaf males and found results similar to those reported by Forner and Hixon.

Disturbances in linguistic programming were evidenced by respiratory intake at unusual linguistic junctures. Specifically, the subjects often uttered a few syllables at a time, segmented by inappropriately long silences. Several findings led to the conclusion that deaf subjects experienced difficulty with the mechanical adjustments of the respiratory system. Rather than initiating speech at roughly twice the volume for tidal exchange, as observed in normal individuals, the deaf subjects often started the utterance within the tidal range or lower. Such an adjustment would require substantially greater expiratory muscular effort for longer periods of time to preserve acceptable pulmonary pressure levels for speech. In addition, Forner and Hixon described a "wastage" phenomenon wherein the deaf expelled considerable amounts of air during pauses, thereby encroaching further on the expiratory reserve volume. The "wastage" of air was also observed during speech production, leading to the conclusion that the larynx and upper airway were not efficiently valving the stream of pulmonary air.

Additional support for the suggestion of inefficiency in the valving provided by the upper airway was introduced by Hutchinson and Smith (1976), who studied intraoral air pressure and airflow patterns in the speech of seven young deaf adults. Figure 5.1 displays two commonly observed disturbances in these patterns. In the first, the airflow was substantially greater than would be expected, suggesting a low mechanical resistance to the airstream. The second pattern, which reflects an abnormally low flow, could have been the result of high resistive loads, low pulmonary volume, or diminished expiratory muscle effort. Similar findings were discovered in a later study involving hard-of-hearing children (Hutchinson, Smith, Kornhauser, Beasley, & Beasley, 1978).

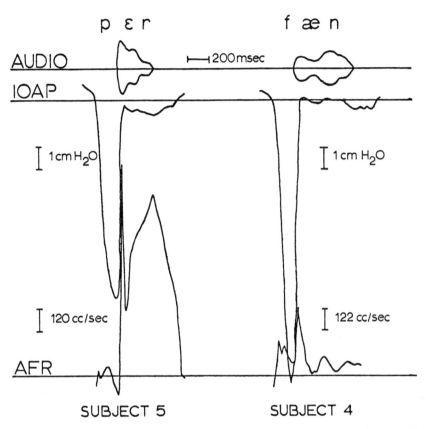

Figure 5.1. Disturbances in airstream valving. Subject #5 exhibited unusually high airflow rate for the vocalic portion of the word "pair." Subject #6 produced a very low airflow rate for the fricative /f/ in the word "fan." (From Aerodynamic Functioning during Consonant Production by Hearing-Impaired Adults" by J. M. Hutchinson and L. L. Smith, 1976, *Audiology and Hearing Education, 2,* p. 23.)

Phonation. With respect to phonation, the reduction in acoustic cues available to the deaf and hard of hearing might be expected to affect voice characteristics. Indeed, this is the case. Several studies have documented aberrations in fundamental frequency (f_0) of the voice, and usually deaf talkers are observed to have higher f_0s than their normal-hearing counterparts. For example, Angelocci, Kopp, and Holbrook (1964) measured f_0 in two groups of 18 male subjects (hearing impaired and normal) ranging in age from 11 to 14 years. Their results confirmed that the group of deaf boys had f_0s that were noticeably higher than those of normal boys.

Some evidence suggests that the disparity in f_0 between normal and deaf persons may be a function of age. Thus, Boone (1966) reported data on f_0 from 44 deaf subjects and 44 matched controls; in each group 22 subjects were 7 to 8 years old, the remaining 22 were 17 to 18 years of age. No appreciable differences in f_0 were found between groups at the younger age level, but the older group exhibited f_0s qualitatively similar to those reported by Angelocci et al. (1964). In addition, Monsen (1979) reported f_0 scores for 24 young hearing-impaired children to be within normal limits.

The range of fundamental frequency is also often reduced in the contextual speech for the deaf. Hood and Dixon (1969) provided strong support for this observation. Figure 5.2 presents a summary of some of their observations. During utterance of the phrase, "There's a big piece of cake left over from dinner," the deaf generally exhibited f_0 patterns that were qualitatively similar to those of normal subjects. However, the variability was reduced.

Control of fundamental frequency is primarily a function of laryngeal events (Shipp, 1975; Shipp & McGlone, 1971). However, these laryngeal events are not independent of respiratory and upper airway influences. Consequently, disturbances in the operation of these compo-

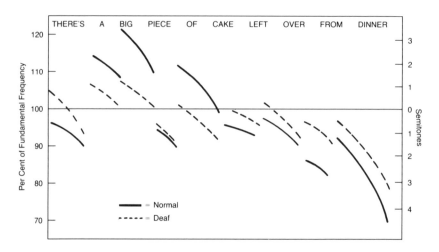

Figure 5.2. Mean intonation patterns of 6 normal and 12 hearing-impaired subjects during production of the sentence, "There's a big piece of cake left over from dinner." (From "Physical Characteristics of Speech Rhythm of Deaf and Normal-Hearing Speakers" by R. B. Hood and R. F. Dixon, 1969, *Journal of Communication Disorders, 2,* p. 224.)

nents of the speech mechanism can result in phonatory problems. Certainly, the voice-quality deviations present in the speech of the hearing impaired result from such interactive deviations.

With respect to voice-quality deviations, historically, clinicians and teachers of the deaf have reported voice-quality disturbances suggestive of breathiness and tension among typical deaf clients (Subtelny, 1977). Some of these deviations reflect primary valving problems at the level of the larynx. This is particularly true for breathiness. However, in the case of tension, it is possible for respiratory problems to provoke laryngeal hypervalving. As mentioned previously, the deaf often speak with lung volumes well below the functional residual capacity, thereby necessitating excessive activity in the muscles of forced exhalation to preserve acceptable levels of alveolar pressure. It is conceivable that this physiologic effort could "overflow" to the laryngeal muscles, resulting in increased adductor and tensor activity, thereby yielding the perception of tension. Furthermore, one could argue that phonatory tension results from abnormally high resistive loads supplied by the upper airway. This increased impedence could prompt greater effort lower in the vocal tract leading to increased laryngeal muscle activity and the perception of tension.

Yet another aspect of phonation—intensity, although primarily a function of laryngeal activity—involves the interactive control of all components of the speech production system. Isshiki (1964) and Hirano, Ohala, and Vennard (1969) provided evidence that laryngeal control accounts for most variations in vocal intensity, at least in the modal register. The data on intensity are limited for the hearing impaired. Essentially, three problems have been mentioned in the literature. First, Calvert and Silverman (1975) suggested that overall intensity is generally reduced in the deaf. Indeed, the presence of a pervasive breathiness and low pulmonary volume during speech would tend to support such a conclusion. In the study reported by Angelocci et al. (1964), it was discovered that the average intensity of vowels was reduced in the hearing impaired.

A second problem occasionally encountered in the deaf and hard of hearing is an abnormally loud voice. Penn (1955), for example, reported that of 1,086 subjects with marked sensorineural hearing losses, excessive volume was a common vocal characteristic. Excessive vocal intensity could result from an abnormally high respiratory driving force, excessive glottal resistance, or both. It may seem inconsistent to report both excessive and reduced vocal intensity in this group, but both problems have been observed. The reason for this heterogeneity is currently not understood.

Finally, Hood and Dixon (1969) reported reduced intensity variability in contextual speech. Reduced auditory feedback is undoubtedly the principal reason for decrements in intensity variability. However, speaking at the lower extremes of lung volume increases the mechanical stiffness of the respiratory system, thereby rendering the "pulsatile" variations in respiratory adjustment necessary for intensity (stress) increments less probable (see Hixon, 1973).

Articulation. As suggested earlier, variability seems to be one of the hallmarks of speech production among the hearing impaired. This is certainly true of articulation. However, despite the variability a clinician encounters, some disturbances may be expected in most hearing-impaired persons. Two general conclusions are possible: (a) Patterns of consonant and vowel error can be identified in this population. (b) Consonant misarticulation is much more common than vowel or diphthong misarticulation.

With respect to the latter, the following categorizations of error patterns, offered originally by Hudgins and Numbers (1942), have been substantiated in more recent research:

1. Vowel substitution and neutralization (i.e., the tendency for all vowels to resemble the neutral schwa /ə/);

2. Diphthongalization (e.g., /ai/ for /a/);

3. Diphthong distortion (e.g., /a/ for /ai/ or /ə/ for /ai/);

4. Nasalization of vowels (Markides, 1970, 1983; Smith, 1975).

Greater experimental insight into errors in vowels and diphthongs was offered by Monsen (1978), who observed that hearing-impaired persons failed to produce significant formant variations in short time periods. In particular, these rapid and dramatic formant variations characterize the acoustic spectra of diphthong production. Monsen reported minimal second-formant transitions for these sounds, which would be suggestive of limited lingual movement. Further, he did not find disturbances in transitions for the first formants in the same diphthongs. He suggested two explanations for this discrepancy. First, the frequency range of the first formant is considerably lower than that of the second and hence more audible for those with high-frequency hearing losses. Consequently, deaf persons may be able to produce changes in the first formant more easily because they hear them more clearly. Second, and perhaps more persuasive, variations in the first formant can be accomplished by alterations in oral opening. Such alterations are much more visible than lingual adjustments, which are apt to underlie the variations in second formant position. Oral openings are more easily imitated.

Another experimentally documented disturbance in vowel production concerns vowel duration. Contrary to popular opinion, available evidence does not support the suggestion that vowel durations are longer in the hearing impaired. Specifically, Monsen (1974) discovered that a tense vowel (e.g., /i/) and a lax vowel (e.g., /I/) occupy mutually exclusive duration ranges in the deaf regardless of phonetic context. That is, the tense vowel is unconditionally longer. Normal subjects, in contrast, do not exhibit such mutual exclusivity. In normal talkers, the tense vowel is longer than its lax counterpart only in the same phonetic context. Monsen observed that the tense/lax contrast depends upon two acoustic cues, frequency of the second formant and duration. Perceptually, for hearing-impaired persons duration may be a much more prominent cue than the frequency of the second formant. Consequently, their tense/lax distinction, from a productive standpoint, is based more directly on the duration parameter. Such a finding implies fundamental differences in phonologic organization among the deaf. The therapeutic implications of such differences, although unknown, are apt to be profound.

Whereas vowel errors are not uncommon in the speech of deaf talkers, the less intense, less visible consonants are more commonly found to be misarticulated. Hudgins and Numbers (1942) categorized the most common consonant errors of deaf children as follows:

1. Voicing errors (e.g., substitution of /b/ for /p/);

2. Omission and distortion of consonants;

3. Omission of consonants in blends;

4. Nasalization of consonants.

Although the majority of investigators report a greater proportion of voiced/voiceless errors (Gold, 1980), the voiceless/voiced error may also be observed in the speech of deaf children. Voicing errors noted include voiced/voiceless confusions, devoicing of final consonants, and omission of final voiced consonants (Hutchinson et al., 1978; Hutchinson & Smith, 1976; Stark, 1979; Oller, Jensen, & Lafayette, 1978; McGarr & Osberger, 1978; Nober, 1967).

Omission of both initial and final consonants appears to be common among the hearing impaired. Geffner and Freeman (1980) suggested that the greater preponderance of initial versus final omissions reported in the literature is related to the age of subjects studied and/or differences in stimuli employed. Specifically, consonants which required greater articulatory precision and/or were less visible were most likely to be produced incorrectly. Finally, whereas hypernasality has been used to characterize the speech of the deaf child, some investigators (Miller, 1980) have reported a high incidence of hyponasality as well.

In addition to individual phoneme errors, investigators have suggested that deaf speakers do not move their articulators correctly when proceeding from one sound to the next. Thus, Calvert's (1961) study of the perceptual categorization of "deaf speech" indicates that faulty transition between sounds provides the best clue to "deaf speech." In addition, deaf speech is sometimes characterized by reduced coarticulatory effects (Whitehead & Jones, 1978; Tye-Murray, 1987). For example, Tye-Murray found that her two least intelligible subjects rarely, if ever, demonstrated context effects in either jaw or tongue dorsum positioning for CVC words with differing vowels. She offered this finding in support of the contention that deaf speakers often produce speech sounds as a series of separate events. Also, deaf speakers appear to use extremely slow tongue movements. This phenomenon has been partly attributed to the training of static articulatory positions.

Suprasegmental aspects. Suprasegmental errors (i.e., errors in the relative variation of duration, intensity, and fundamental frequency across the utterance) may contribute substantially to the poor intelligibility of the deaf child (Gold, 1980; Hudgins & Numbers, 1942; Smith, 1975). Suprasegmentals may communicate an individual's emotional intent or the urgency of the message (Lehiste, 1976). More essential to speech intelligibility, suprasegmentals encode linguistic stress. According to Allen (1975), linguistic stress allows a listener to "organize the incoming acoustic elements into coherent packages which allow for the perceptual separation of words and phrases" (p. 84). Consequently, the deaf child's suprasegmental errors may be expected to reduce speech intelligibility.

Overall slow speaking rate and abnormal pause behaviors represent two major duration errors produced by deaf talkers. The former (Markides, 1983; Voelker, 1935) has been related to the prolongation of individual phonemes and the presence of lengthy pauses within utterances. Forner and Hixon's (1977) observation of improved rate for numerical strings versus sentences led them to conclude that deaf speakers do not adjust their rate in accordance with linguistic structure. It is interesting to note that some investigators have reported improved intelligibility for slower speaking rates (Osberger & Levitt, 1979). Thus, overall slow speaking rate may, in part, be an appropriate compensatory adjustment. On the other hand, excessively slow rates may interrupt the perceived successiveness of speech thereby reducing intelligibility. Markides (1983) noted that "a considerable number of hearing-impaired children's oral reading was so slow that the listeners had difficulty in organizing the speech of the children into meaningful wholes" (p. 188).

The research on abnormal pause behaviors (John & Howarth, 1965; Miller, 1980) indicates that deaf speakers use more and longer pauses in addition to within-phrase pauses. Normal-hearing speakers, in contrast, tend to avoid the use of within-phrase pauses (Osberger & Levitt, 1979). Although deaf speakers often exhibit abnormal pause behaviors, Osberger and Levitt reported little effect of such abnormal pause behaviors on intelligibility.

Whereas linguistic stress is communicated by a combination of differences in duration, intensity, and fundamental frequency, faulty intonation has been most consistently associated with reduced speech intelligibility (Formby & Monsen, 1982; Monsen, Engbretson, & Vemulla, 1979; Wingfield, Buttett, & Sandoval, 1979). Both excessive pitch variation and less-than-normal pitch variation have been reported (Boone, 1966; Formby & Monsen, 1982; Green, 1956; Miller, 1980; Monsen, 1979; Voelker, 1935). Monsen's (1979) differentiation between a "flat fundamental frequency contour" (variation less than 10 Hz/100 msec) and a "short-falling contour" (uncontrolled direction of frequency change over relatively large time segments) supports reports of both reduced and excessive pitch variations in deaf speakers. For example, Formby and Monsen (1982) noted that hearing-impaired speakers with excessive and less-than-normal pitch variation received lower intelligibility scores. Inappropriate pitch variation may result in faulty stress and the "stacatto speech" associated with some deaf talkers.

In summary, deaf speakers may inappropriately adjust durational, intensity, and intonational cues within an utterance. These suprasegmental errors may result in faulty linguistic stress and hence reduce speech intelligibility. Faulty intonation appears to contribute most substantially to reduced speech intelligibility.

Speech/voice profiling. Following the lead offered by Darley, Aronson, and Brown (1969) in profiling deviations in speech and voice patterns among dysarthrics, Miller (1980) and Miller and Hutchinson (1982) developed a profiling system for the hearing impaired. Speech samples, obtained from 72 hearing-impaired and deaf adolescents, were rated by five experienced listeners on 34 dimensions of speech and voice. The deviant patterns were related to the general parameters of loudness, resonance, pitch, voice quality, and rate. Statistical analysis revealed that the noted deviances clustered into five general voice patterns: (a) disfluent vocal pattern, (b) reduced vocal variability, (c) stereotyped prosodic pattern, (d) laryngeal hyperfunction, and (e) laryngeal hypofunction.

From a clinical perspective, it was noted that different subjects among the 72 presented rather unique profiles wherein different combinations of the five factors appeared. For example, a subject might exhibit factors (c) and (e). If this were the case, a clinician could focus on reducing the stereotype present in the speech pattern as well as work to increase phonatory tension to overcome laryngeal hypofunction.

From the foregoing review, it should be clear that severe-to-profound hearing impairment may do enormous violence to speech production. Virtually all aspects of speech generation may be disrupted from articulatory placement to long-term prosodic patterning. To complicate matters further, the hearing impaired demonstrate considerable heterogeneity with respect to the sorts of deviations clinicians may encounter. Therefore, as the clinician approaches a hearing-impaired child with an eye toward remediation, assessment assumes great urgency. In the section that follows, we will conceptualize the process of speech assessment so critical to appropriate, efficient, and durable therapy.

Speech Assessment. In this section four general areas of evaluation will be considered. First, attention will be directed toward conventional procedures for evaluating the physiological and acoustic dimensions of speech production. Second, measures of intelligibility will be considered. Third, strategies for assessing articulation are reviewed. Fourth, several methods of perceptual assessment of the voice will be offered. It is advisable in most circumstances for clinicians to derive a comprehensive picture of the speech characteristics of hearing-impaired clients. Accordingly, it is suggested that physiologic/acoustic data, estimates of intelligibility, articulation profiles, and perceptual features be obtained whenever possible before making any decisions regarding remediation of speech.

Physiologic and acoustic measures. It is beyond the scope of this chapter to discuss, in depth, instrumentation and procedures used to measure the physiologic and acoustic aspects of speech. Further, budgetary limitations may prevent some clinicians from acquiring sophisticated equipment for making these assessments. Nevertheless, an overview of this area is warranted.

With respect to respiratory assessment, a skilled clinician *may* be able to infer respiratory deviations by simply listening to and observing the client during contextual speech utterances. However, physiologic assessment in the form of respirometry is far more sensitive and accurate. For example, respirometric techniques can provide data regarding speech initiatory volumes and other patterns of respiratory adjustment used by a given hearing-impaired speaker. In addition to instrumental measures of respiratory function, attention should be directed to assessment of voice of fundamental frequency and range of fundamental frequency. Several instruments and software have been developed for voice analysis, including the Tunemaster III (Berkshire Instruments, Inc.); the f_o - Indicator (S.I. America, Inc.); Visi-Pitch (Kay Elemetrics, Inc.); and MacSpeech Lab II (G.W. Instruments, Inc.).

Measures of intelligibility. "Percent intelligible word" measures and intelligibility rating scales are most widely used for speech intelligibility assessment. The former requires an individual or a panel of judges to identify words spoken by a person reading a standard reading passage, describing a picture, or producing conversational speech. The percent intelligibility score represents the percentage of words correctly identified by the judge or the average of several judges. Although the use of several judges is preferable, many clinicians may be limited to a one-judge panel. Although reading passages allow for standardized results, Geffner and Freeman (1980) noted that the variable intelligibility associated with various speech sampling (e.g., common words versus spontaneous speech) necessitates a measure of intelligibility in spontaneous speech. Ling (1976) incorporated the percent intelligible word measure in his phonologic evaluation, which requires clinicians to determine the number of intelligible words and complete utterances produced in conversation.

The oral speech intelligibility of hearing-impaired talkers has been found to differ significantly depending upon whether (a) simple sentences, sentences with consonant clusters, polysyllabic words, or complex syntax are used; (b) listeners are experienced or inexperienced with regard to hearing-impaired speech; (c) sentences are in or out of context; and (d) sentences are heard or seen (Monsen, 1983). According to Monsen, these factors become less influential as speakers' productions come closer to normal speech. Sitler et al. (1983) postulated that contextual effects are related to the hearing-impaired speaker's single-word intelligibility. These investigators found that sentence intelligibility (CID Everyday Sentences) was superior to single-word intelligibility for only the better speakers. Poorer speakers (scores below 30%) had roughly equivalent single-word and sentence-intelligibility scores. Sitler et al. suggested that the sentence-intelligibility score was preferable in assessment by being a measure of the speaker's maximal performance and more generalizable to the real world. Markides (1978) suggested that a picture elicitation task rather than a reading task be used to obtain a speech-intelligibility sample. He argued that the reading task does not allow for normal speech rhythm, and that it suppresses the intelligibility scores of hearing-impaired children, many of whom have reading difficulties.

The second most commonly used assessment tool, the rating scale, has been presented by the National Technical Institute for the Deaf (NTID) as a rapid and efficient means of intelligibility assessment for the deaf (Johnson, 1975). NTID provides training tapes which allow clinicians to associate the five points on the NTID rating scale with various levels of speech intelligibility. It is suggested that five judges assess each speaker. These judges are familiarized with the tapes and the following scale.

Rate   Description

1   Speech cannot be understood.

2   Speech is very difficult to understand—only isolated words and phrases are intelligible.

3   Speech is difficult to understand; however, the gist of the content can be understood.

4   Speech is intelligible with the exception of a few words and phrases.

5   Speech is completely intelligible.

The judges listen to a recording of a standard reading passage and assign values between 1 and 5. A major benefit of the rating scale is that it provides a rapid means of assessing speech intelligibility. Different judges, however, may disagree substantially on assigning these ratings. Due to interjudge differences in ratings, Osberger et al. (1986b) recommended the use of multiple judges and an average intelligibility rating. A major criticism of the rating scale approach—the subjectivity of individual judges—may be reduced by use of the NTID training tapes.

Monsen (1982) proposed the use of the *Speech Intelligibility Evaluation* (SPINE) as a rapid and easy speech-intelligibility measure. Ten sets of words are used to assess two major speech errors: (a) indistinct vowels and (b) voicing errors. The word sets are printed on 10 ''decks'' of cards and the child is dealt the cards in such a way that the examiner cannot see the word printed on a given card. It is the examiner's task to decide which word was spoken and record it. Scores range from below chance (25%) to ''excellent speech intelligibility'' (100%). Monsen reported that test scores for 10- to 16-year-old children were highly correlated with percent intelligible word measures. Obviously, this speech intelligibility measure cannot be used with very young hearing-impaired children who cannot read.

Measures of articulation.   With respect to articulation, perceptual evaluation using any of the conventional phonemic inventories would be valuable. However, the limitations of such tests must be appreciated (Noll, 1970) and assessment of articulation in context is crucial for determining an accurate phonologic profile. For example, recently, experts in disorders of articulation have focused increasing attention on what is broadly termed ''phonological process analysis.'' In such analyses (e.g., Shriberg & Kwiatkowski, 1980), the clinician examines speech samples for the presence of certain processes such as final consonant deletion, cluster reduction, stopping, and so forth. These processes are thought to be natural in the speech of young children and, presumably, analysis of them can guide therapy decisions.

To date, adaptation of conventional methods of articulation assessment for the hearing-impaired population has been rather limited. Geffner and Freeman (1980) recommended restricting test stimuli to words known to be in the vocabulary of young deaf children. Consequently, they have modified the *Goldman-Fristoe Test of Articulation* (Goldman & Fristoe, 1969) such that "difficult" vocabulary items were replaced with items more likely to fall within a deaf child's vocabulary. Markides (1983) presented an articulation test he had specifically devised for hearing-impaired children. The list consists of 24 monosyllabic words "within the vocabulary of the children to test a representative number of vowels, diphthongs and consonants in the English language" (p. 44). Another procedure developed rather exclusively for the deaf is that of Ling (1976), whose phonetic evaluation requires the child to imitate sounds in syllables. This test has been noted for its systematicity and the ease with which test findings may be related to Ling's speech training program. However, the procedure may be fatiguing for the younger child.

Perceptual assessment of speech and voice. Over the past decade, several procedures have been developed for perceptual assessment of speech and voice patterns. Typically, such procedures permit clinicians to focus on a number of perceptual dimensions and rate each using a scaling procedure. In view of the wide variety of speech and voice deviations that can be observed among the deaf, such strategies for perceptual analysis are of value.

Currently, perhaps the most widely used system is that of Wilson (1977). This evaluative technique allows the clinician to make judgments on three "major" and two "minor" dimensions of voice. Major factors are laryngeal valving (scale points range from *laryngeal air wastage* to *extreme tension*), pitch, and nasality. The minor factors include intensity and pitch variability. In addition, Wilson urges the clinician to check for the presence of such voice deviations as diplophonia, audible inhalation, pitch breaks, phrasing irregularities, and so forth.

A system has also been developed to help clinicians assess disturbed suprasegmental features among the hearing impaired. Thus, the *Prosodic Feature Production* (Stark & Levitt, 1974) evaluates the child's ability to produce simple prosodic contrasts. Four short sentences are marked in relation to the presence of the following: (a) statement, (b) question with a final rising pitch, (c) specified pauses, and (d) different stress patterns. The authors emphasize the experimental nature of this test which is not yet in widespread use. While investigators search for more objective measures, the clinician's subjective judgment of suprasegmentals appears to be the most widely used assessment format.

Speech Management. The purpose of this last section is to outline available procedures for improving speech production in the severely hearing impaired. While it is beyond the scope of this discussion to provide comprehensive lesson plans for various goals, general habilitation principles are offered and the reader is referred to Calvert and Silverman (1975), Ling (1976), Osberger et al. (1978), Hochberg, Levitt, and Osberger (1983), and Vorce (1974) for more information on speech therapy techniques for the hearing impaired.

General considerations. Nearly all investigators who have studied speech production in the deaf are struck by the extreme variability in error patterns both between and within subjects. Such variability highlights the importance of diagnostic evaluation of speech production skills. Speech habilitation procedures should be developed for individual cases, and techniques found to be effective for one subject may be useless for another. Despite this variability and the premium on individual programming, some general principles of speech teaching are applicable to all cases.

First, speech sounds are rarely produced in isolation, hence extensive therapeutic effort on sounds out of phonetic context is unwarranted. This is not to say that initial phonemic training cannot involve some work at the individual sound level (e.g., Ling, 1976). However, as soon as possible, the clinician should move from isolated sound production to contextual speech. A variety of meaningful contexts can be employed, and it must be recognized that coarticulatory influences will alter the target characteristics of the phonemes involved.

A second general consideration concerns the programming strategies employed by the therapist. Careful attention to the principles of reinforcement and programmed instruction is very important. Furthermore, once the client has mastered sounds in the clinical situation, every effort should be made to highlight their significance and use in the child's everyday communication milieu.

The final consideration relates to the techniques employed to teach correct sound production. Even if the deaf and the hard of hearing are at least partially deprived of perhaps the most important channel for monitoring correct sound production, techniques for speech habilitation used with normal-hearing children are applicable. Although perhaps requiring greater ingenuity and instrumental assistance, conventional speech remediation procedures can readily be modified for hearing-impaired children. Four major approaches are recommended for developing better sound production in the hearing impaired: (a) use of residual hearing, (b) anatomic and pictorial monitoring, (c) visual stimulation, and (d) complex feedback aids. These strategies are not mutually exclusive and their combined use is probably warranted in most cases.

Use of residual hearing.   Auditory discrimination and auditory monitoring through use of residual hearing represents one approach to developing better sound production. Fortunately, most hearing-impaired individuals possess some residual hearing and its use should be maximized. Conventional wisdom emphasizes the need for early amplification. Amplification at an appropriately early age will facilitate codification of auditory cues associated with speech communication. It is well established that speech production skills of children with early amplification are superior to those of children who receive aids later in life (Hirsh, 1966; Markides, 1983). Chase (1968) echoed this finding when he stated:

> It is noteworthy that the provision of hearing aids during the first two years of life greatly facilitates the speech acquisition process in the child with profound hearing loss . . . The importance of providing amplification at an early age reminds us about the probable existence of a critical period for speech learning. (p. 249)

The tremendous acoustic redundancy in the speech signal permits even the profoundly deaf child a limited subset of cues upon which to base an internal phonologic organization (Fry, 1966). This organization is undoubtedly different from that of persons with normal hearing, for whom a much richer set of cues is available. Insights into the importance of this phonologic organization process for the hearing impaired can be found in several experiments. For example, DiCarlo (1960) observed that delayed auditory feedback was particularly disruptive to the fluency of speech in deaf children who relied heavily upon auditory feedback to monitor speech accuracy. The experiments reported earlier by Monsen (1974, 1978) reveal that acoustic differences in speech production by deaf talkers may be explained on the basis of perceptual cues available.

Anatomic and pictorial monitoring.   The second approach to developing improved sound production is *anatomic* or *pictorial modeling.* Such aids as anatomic charts, sagittal sections of the head with a mobile tongue, and pictures of labial geometry for certain sounds are useful in some cases. Some of these models are available commercially, otherwise they can be made without undue expense. The central problem with such aids is that they give only a snapshot of the proper articulatory position. Usually, they represent the ideal articulatory target while being grossly insensitive to the impact of coarticulatory movements upon vocal tract shape. Accordingly, it may be wise to use anatomic and pictorial models only in the initial stages of sound production, and only as a last resort.

Visual stimulation.   The third general approach to improving speech production is visual stimulation by the clinician and visual monitoring in the mirror. A tremendous amount of information is available from just the visible aspect of speech. However, excessive attention to visual feedback may be hazardous for two related reasons. First, the visual characteristics of sounds change dramatically as a function of context. For example, the visual parameters of /w/ are considerably different in the words "wound" and "weed". Second, extensive demands by the clinician to focus on visual cues may distract attention from available auditory cues. This assumption requires further experimental validation, but it is logical that an undue load on visual processing could have a deleterious effect on auditory monitoring. Some support for this position was provided by Gaeth (1963).

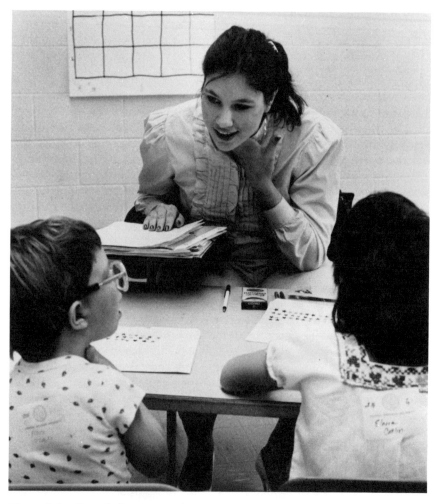

Figure 5.3. Speech therapy emphasizing voicing with a hearing-impaired child.

Complex feedback aids. The final approach to assisting hearing-impaired talkers in acquiring more natural speech is the use of complex feedback aids, generally in the form of mechanical and electronic instrumentation. Such devices may be subsumed under the generic label of *vocoding devices* or *biofeedback systems*. Collectively, they are designed to provide conscious awareness of events not easily monitored through extant feedback channels. For the deaf, this generally means providing visual and touch-pressure representations and acoustic and physiologic events associated with speech production. The accelerated growth of electronic instrumentation has greatly enhanced the use of such aids with the hearing impaired. Although these devices hold great promise for the improvement of speech, *carte blanche* acceptance and use of vocoding devices is unwise. Clinicians are cautioned to preview devices of this sort and to examine any outcome research that might confirm their utility.

The clinician should be aware of two important facts. First, few of the commercially available biofeedback aids for the deaf have been subjected to rigorous experimental scrutiny. In spite of frequent appeals to authority for testimony as to their effectiveness, outcome data are typically sparse. Second, many of the devices cannot perform what they purport to. Thus, there may be no feature detectors in the visual or touch-pressure systems that are sensitive to the critical acoustic dimensions (e.g., second formant transitions) important for speech perception. Further, the process of transducing an auditory signal to a visual or touch-pressure signal may obliterate important perceptual cues or introduce additional unimportant cues that act as "noise" in the visual system. As further support for the notion that visual, and auditory perceptual systems, in particular, function differently, Jakobson (1967) pointed out that, with visual signs, the spatial aspect is not important. Instead, auditory perception is based primarily on the temporal aspect. Accordingly, it seems reasonable to conclude that the eye simply cannot do what the ear is designed to accomplish. Consequently, biofeedback aids based on the assumption of such intersensory equivalence are apt to be of little value in speech training. As a general principle, devices designed to provide feedback regarding manner of production (e.g., nasality, voicing, continuance), temporal features, physiologic gestures, or suprasegmental parameters like f_0 and intensity hold greater promise than aids engineered to help the subject recognize individual phonemes (Bargstadt, Hutchinson, & Nerbonne, 1978).

Fletcher and Hasegawa (1983) pointed out that acoustic signals are already abstractions from the basic articulatory events and that visual and touch-pressure transformation displays are abstractions of abstractions. They suggested that devices which provide more direct information on speech movements may be more beneficial to the young hearing-impaired child. Fletcher and Hasegawa discussed the training of a 3-½-year-old deaf child with dynamic orometric modeling. The child was presented with a side-by-side video display of the trainer's linguapalatal contact pattern and her own linguapalatal contact pattern. Coarticulatory gestures (/i/, /a/, /t/) were learned rapidly with respect to position and timing features. These investigators did not mention whether the child was able to produce the target sounds when no linguapalatal contact feedback was available.

speech in the adventitiously hearing impaired

Descriptions of speech abilities in individuals with acquired hearing loss have not been well documented in the literature, but generally consist of anecdotal reports. Adventitious deafness appears to produce a gradual rather than immediate deterioration of speech. Zimmerman and Rettaliata (1981) posited that "...while auditory information may not be necessary on a gesture-to-gesture basis, it plays a critical role in the long-term monitoring and maintenance of speech coordinative structures" (p. 177). The apparently wide variation in speech production may be attributed to the degree of hearing loss, age at onset of hearing loss, hearing aid history, and other factors (Cowie, Douglas-Cowie, & Kerr, 1982; Jackson, 1982). According to Calvert and Silverman (1975), typical speech errors in this population affect production of siblants, final consonants, voice quality, loudness control, and speech rhythm. However, in a recent report, Goehl and Kaufman (1984) evaluated the speech of five adventitiously deafened adults with hearing losses of at least 10 years' duration and concluded that "...there is no clinically significant deterioration of speech sound production" (p. 63).

Cowie and Douglas-Cowie (1983) reported data from their assessment of the speech of 13 adults with severe or profound adventitious hearing losses. Speech intelligibility was assessed by first having the hearing-impaired speakers read a series of short passages. Normal-hearing judges then listened to a passage and immediately repeated what they heard (i.e., tracking). The percent of words correctly identified in the tracking procedure on a given passage was averaged for 10 listeners. Intelligibility scores ranged from below 10% to above 90%. Cowie and Douglas-Cowie claimed that the tracking procedure is more sensitive to speech aberrations than the speech intelligibility measures used with prelingually deafened speakers because the latter typically involve presentation of a single sentence at a time thereby eliminating time pressure. Age at onset of hearing loss was related to the rank ordering of speakers by intelligibility with those deafened before 18 years of age generally being less intelligible than those deafened later. Cowie and Douglas-Cowie also reported that normal-hearing listeners had negative reactions (i.e., adverse comments on education and intelligence) to these deaf speakers' productions. One of their subjects reportedly carried a letter explaining that his speech was slurred because he was deaf—not because he was drunk. Cowie and Douglas-Cowie concluded that both reduced speech intelligibility and negative reactions to voice quality/slurring were possible effects of adventitious hearing loss.

It may be argued that appropriate amplification should provide acoustic cues to improve this type of speech errors in most individuals with acquired hearing loss. Cochlear implant users reportedly also show improvement in loudness control and voice quality (Chouard et al., 1983; Eisenberg et al., 1983; Engelmann, Waterfall, & Hough, 1981; Fourcin et al., 1983; Hochmair-Desoyer, Hochmair, Burian, & Fischer, 1981). In addition, kinesthetic cues may provide information for speech cues which are not audible with amplification/prostheses. In cases where intervention is deemed necessary, the reader is referred to Jackson (1982) for a comprehensive discussion of speech conservation issues and techniques.

summary comments: training of clinicians and teachers

Who should be responsible for the habilitation of speech and language in the hearing impaired? The answer to this question depends on education and training. If the clinician or teacher has sufficient background and practical training in speech and language remediation for the deaf and hard of hearing, there should be no barrier to proceeding with their clinical endeavors. However, most audiologists and educators of the deaf do not have a proper understanding of the physiologic and acoustic parameters of speech in the hearing impaired. Unfortunately, many speech pathologists are also poorly trained in the nature and impact of hearing impairment on speech production.

The obvious and imperative solution to this problem is expanded emphasis upon the speech and language problems of the hearing-impaired in professional courses offered by university training programs. In a rather extensive study of personnel preparation for teaching speech to the hearing-impaired child, Subtelny, Webster, and Murphy (1980) uncovered areas of educational deficiency among educators of the deaf and speech/language pathologists. Specifically, deaf educators were found to be lacking in diagnostic skills for detection of speech and voice problems. In addition, they expressed a need for more information on speech science and therapeutic strategies. Professionals in the field of speech and language pathology were reported to demonstrate somewhat different deficiencies. Specifically, they appeared to need more information in language diagnosis and intervention for the hearing impaired, speech rehabilitation of the hearing impaired, and issues related to counseling individuals with hearing problems and their families. It is hoped that training programs will expand their curricula to obviate these deficiencies.

recommended readings

Bloom, L., & Lahey, K. (1978). *Language development and language disorders*. New York: John Wiley & Sons.

Boone, D.R. (1966). Modification of the voices of deaf children. *Volta Review, 68*, 686-692.

Bunch, G.O. (1987). *The curriculum and the hearing-impaired student: Theoretical and practical considerations*. San Diego: College Hill-Little, Brown & Company.

Easterbrooks, S.R. (1987). Speech/lanugage assessment and intervention with school-age hearing impaired children. In J. Alpiner & P. McCarthy (Eds.), *Rehabilitative audiology: Children and adults* (pp. 188-240). Baltimore, MD: Williams and Wilkins.

Frisina, R. (Ed.). (1976). A bicentennial monograph of hearing impairment: Trends in the USA. *Volta Review, 78*(4). Washington, DC: Alexander Graham Bell Association for the Deaf.

Hochberg, I., Levitt, H., & Osberger, M. (Eds.). (1983). *Speech of the hearing impaired*. Austin, TX: Pro-Ed.

King, C.M., & Quigley, S.P. (1985). *Reading and deafness*. San Diego: College-Hill Press.

Kretschmer, R., & Kretschmer, L. (1978). *Language development and intervention with the hearing impaired*. Baltimore, MD: University Park Press.

Ling,D. (1976). *Speech and the hearing impaired child: Theory and practice*. Washington, DC: Alexander Graham Bell Association for the Deaf.

McAnally, P.L., Rose, S., & Quigley, S.P. (1987). *Language learning practices with deaf children*. San Diego: College Hill-Little, Brown and Company.

Osberger, M.J., Moeller, M.P., Eccarius, M., Robbins, A.M., & Johnson, D. (1986). Expressive language skills. In M.J. Osberger (Ed.), *Language and learning skills of hearing-impaired students* (pp. 54-65). ASHA Monographs #23.

Quigley, S.P., & Paul, P.V. (1984). *Language and deafness.* San Diego: College-Hill Press.

Subtelny, J.D. (1980). *Speech assessment and speech improvement for the hearing impaired.* Washington, DC: Alexander Graham Bell Association for the Deaf.

Thompson, M., Biro, P., Vethivelu, S., Pious, C., & Hatfield, N. (1987). *Language assessment of hearing impaired school age children.* Seattle: University of Washington Press.

references

Allen, G.D. (1975). Speech rhythm: Its relation to performance universals and articulatory timing. *Journal of Phonetics, 3,* 75-86.

Altshuler, K. (1974). The social and psychological development of the deaf child: Problems, their treatment, and prevention. *American Annals of the Deaf, 119,* 365-376.

Ammons, R.B., & Ammons, H.S. (1948). *Full-Range Picture Vocabulary Test.* Missoula, MT: Psychological Test Specialists.

Angelocci, A.A., Kopp, G.A., & Holbrook, A. (1964). The vowel formants of deaf and normal-hearing eleven-to-fourteen year old boys. *Journal of Speech and Hearing Disorders, 29,* 156-170.

Bargstadt, G.H., Hutchinson, J.J., & Nerbonne, M.A. (1978). Learning visual correlates of fricative production by normal-hearing subjects: A preliminary evaluation of the video articulator. *Journal of Speech and Hearing Disorders, 43,* 200-207.

Barry, K.E. (1899). *The five slate system: A system of objective language teaching.* Philadelphia: Sherman & Co.

Blanton, R.L., & Nunnaly, J.C. (1964). Evaluational language processes in the deaf. *Psychological Reports, 15,* 891-894.

Bloom, L., & Lahey, M. (1978). *Language development and language disorders.* New York: John Wiley and Sons.

Boehm, A.E. (1971). *Boehm Test of Basic Concepts.* New York: The Psychological Corporation.

Boone, D.R. (1966). Modification of the voices of deaf children. *Volta Review, 68,* 686-692.

Bornstein, H., Saulnier, K., & Hamilton, L. (1980). Signed English: A first evaluation. *American Annals of the Deaf, 125,* 467-481.

Brannon, J. (1968). Linguistic word classes in spoken language of normal, hard-of-hearing and deaf children. *Journal of Speech and Hearing Research, 11,* 279-287.

Brannon, J.B., & Murray, T. (1966). The spoken syntax of normal, hard of hearing and deaf children. *Journal of Speech and Hearing Research, 9,* 604-610.

Brown, R. (1969). The development of questions in child speech. *Journal of Verbal Learning and Verbal Behavior, 7,* 279-290.

Brown, R. (1973). *A first language: The early stages.* Cambridge, MA: Harvard University Press.

Calvert, D.R. (1961). *Some acoustic characteristics of the speech of profoundly deaf individuals.* Unpublished doctoral dissertation, Stanford University.

Calvert, D.R., & Silverman, S.R. (1975). *Speech and deafness.* Washington, DC: Alexander Graham Bell Association for the Deaf.

Caniglia, J., Cole, N.J., Howard, W., Krohn, E., & Rice, M. (1972). *Apple tree: A patterned program of linguistic expansion through reinforced experiences and evaluations.* Beaverton, OR: Dormac, Inc.

Carr, J. (1953). An investigation of spontaneous speech sounds of five-year-old deaf children. *Journal of Speech and Hearing Disorders, 18,* 22-29.

Chalfant, J.S. (1977). *A communication checklist for hearing impaired pre-schoolers.* Paper presented at the Annual Convention of the American Speech and Hearing Association, Chicago.

Charrow, V.R. (1977). A psycholinguistic analysis of "deaf English". *Sign Language Studies, 7,* 139-150.

Chase, R.A. (1968). Motor organization of speech. In S.J. Freeman (Ed.), *The neuropsychology of spatially oriented behavior* (pp. 261-264). Homewood, IL: Dorsey Press.

Chouard, C.H., Fugain, C., Meyer, B., & Lacomb, H. (1983). Long-term results of the multi-channel cochlear implant. In C.W. Parkings & S. W. Anderson (Eds.), *Cochlear prostheses: An international symposium.* New York: The New York Academy of Sciences.

Cooper, R. (1967). The ability of deaf and hearing children to apply morphological rules. *Journal of Speech and Hearing Research, 10,* 77-86.

Cooper, W.E., & Sorensen, J.M. (1977). Fundamental frequency contours at syntactic boundaries. *Journal of the Acoustical Society of America, 62,* 783-792.

Cowie, R.I.D., & Douglas-Cowie, E. (1983). Speech production in profound postlingual deafness. In M.E. Lutman & M.P. Haggard (Eds.), *Hearing science and hearing disorders.* New York: Academic Press.

Cowie, R., Douglas-Cowie, E., & Kerr, A.G. (1982). A study of speech deterioration in post-lingually deafened adults. *Journal of Laryngology and Otology, 96,* 101-112.

Cozad, R.L. (1974). *The speech clinician and the hearing-impaired child.* Springfield, IL: Charles C. Thomas.

Croker, G.W., Jones, M.K., & Pratt, M.E. (1928). *Language stories and drills.* Brattleboro, VT: Vermont Printing.

Curtiss, S., Prutting, C.A., & Lowell, E.L. (1979). Pragmatic and semantic development in young children with impaired hearing. *Journal of Speech and Hearing Research, 22,* 534-552.

Darley, F.L., Aronson, A.E., & Brown, J. (1969). Clusters of deviant speech dimensions in the dysarthrias. *Journal of Speech and Hearing Research, 12,* 246-269.

Davis, J. (1974). Performance of young hearing-impaired children on a test of basic concepts. *Journal of Speech and Hearing Research, 17*, 342-352.

Davis, J., & Blasdell, R. (1975). Perceptual strategies employed by normal-hearing and hearing-impaired children in the comprehension of sentences containing relative clauses. *Journal of Speech and Hearing Research, 17*, 342-352.

Davis, J.M., Elfenbein, J., Schum, R., & Bentler, R.A. (1986). Effects of mild and moderate hearing impairments on language, educational and psychosocial behavior of children. *Journal of Speech and Hearing Disorders, 51*(1), 53-62.

deVilliers, J.G., & deVilliers, P.A. (1978). *Language acquisition.* Cambridge, MA: Harvard University Press.

DiCarlo, L.M. (1960). The effect of hearing one's own voice among children with impaired hearing. In A. Ewing (Ed.), *The modern educational treatment of deafness.* Manchester, England: Manchester University Press.

Doehring, D.G. (1976). Reading theories and hearing impairment. In S.K. Hirsh, D.H. Eldredge, I.J. Hirsch, & S.R. Silverman (Eds.), *Hearing and Davis: Essays honoring H. Davis* (pp. 313-319). St. Louis: Washington University Press.

Eisenberg, L.S., Berliner, K.I., House, W.F., & Edgerton, B.J. (1983). Status of the adults' and children's cochlear implant programs at the House Ear Institute. In C.W. Parkins & S.W. Anderson (Eds.), *Cochlear prostheses: An international symposium.* New York: The New York Academy of Science.

Engelmann, L.R., Waterfall, M.K., & Hough, J.V.D. (1981). Results following cochlear implantation and rehabilitation. *Laryngoscope, 91*, 1821-1833.

Entus, A.K. (1975). *Hemispheric asymmetry in processing of dichotically presented speech and nonspeech stimuli by infants.* Paper presented at the Biennial Meeting of the Society for Research in Child Development, Denver.

Ervin-Tripp, S. (1970). Discourse agreement: How children answer questions. In W. Hayes (Ed.), *Cognition and the development of language* (pp. 79-107). New York: John Wiley and Sons.

Fitzgerald, E. (1929). *Straight language for the deaf.* Staunton, VA: The McClure Co.

Fletcher, S.G., & Hasegawa, A. (1983). Speech modification by a deaf child through dynamic orometric modeling and feedback. *Journal of Speech and Hearing Disorders, 48*, 178-185.

Formby, C., & Monsen, R.B. (1982). Long-term average speech spectra for normal and hearing-impaired adolescents. *Journal of the Acoustical Society of America, 71*, 196-202.

Forner, L.L., & Hixon, T.J. (1977). Respiratory kinematics in profoundly hearing-impaired speakers. *Journal of Speech and Hearing Research, 20*, 373-407.

Foster, R., Giddan, J., & Stark, J. (1972). *Assessment of children's language comprehension.* Palo Alto, CA: Consulting Psychologists Press.

Fourcin, A.J., Douek, E.E., Moorel, B.C.J., Rosen, S., Walliker, J.R., Howard, D.M., Abberton, E., & Frampton, S. (1983). Speech perception with promontory stimulation. In C.W. Parkins & S.W. Anderson (Eds.), *Cochlear prostheses: An international symposium.* New York: The New York Academy of Science.

Fry, D.B. (1966). The development of the phonological system in the normal and the deaf child. In F. Smith & G. A. Miller (Eds.), *The genesis of language* (pp. 187-206). Cambridge, MA: The MIT Press.

Gaeth, J. (1963). *Verbal and nonverbal learning in children including those with hearing losses.* Washington, DC: U.S. Office of Education, Project #1001.

Gaffney, R., Sr. (1977). *Comprehension of syntax by six year old deaf children.* Unpublished doctoral dissertation, City University of New York Graduate Center.

Geers, A.E., Miller, J.D., & Gustus, C. (1983). *Vibrotactile stimulation - Case study with a profoundly deaf child.* Paper presented at the American Speech-Language-Hearing Association, Cincinnati.

Geffner, D.S., & Freeman, L.R. (1980). Assessment of language comprehension of six-year-old deaf children. *Journal of Communication Disorders, 13,* 455-470.

Gilman, M., Davis, J., & Raffin, M. (1980). Use of common morphemes by hearing-impaired children exposed to a system of manual English. *Journal of Auditory Research, 20,* 57-69.

Goehl, H., & Kaufman, D.K. (1984). Do the effects of adventitious deafness include disordered speech? *Journal of Speech and Hearing Disorders, 49,* 58-64.

Gold, T. (1980). Speech production in hearing-impaired children. *Journal of Communication Disorders, 13,* 397-418.

Goldberg, E., & Costa, L.D. (1981). Hemisphere differences in the acquisition and use of descriptive systems. *Brain and Language, 14,* 144-173.

Goldman, R., & Fristoe, M. (1969). *The Goldman-Fristoe Test of Articulation.* Circle Pines, MN: American Guidance Service.

Goss, R. (1970). Language used by mothers of deaf children and mothers of hearing children. *American Annals of the Deaf, 115,* 93-96.

Green, D.S. (1956). *Fundamental frequency characteristics of the speech of profoundly deaf individuals.* Unpublished doctoral dissertation, Purdue University.

Green, W.B., & Shepherd, D.C. (1973). *The semantic structure in deaf children.* Paper presented at the Annual Convention of the American Speech and Hearing Association, Detroit.

Griswold, E., & Cummings, J. (1984). The expressive vocabulary of preschool deaf children. *American Annals of the Deaf, 119,* 16-28.

Groht, M.A. (1958). *Natural language for deaf children.* Washington, DC: Alexander Graham Bell Association for the Deaf.

Harris, G. (1963). *Language for the preschool deaf child.* New York: Grune and Stratton.

Hasenstab, M.S., & Horner, J.S. (1982). *Comprehensive intervention with hearing-impaired infants and pre-school children.* Rockville, MD: Aspen Systems, Inc.

Heider, F.K., & Heider, G.M. (1940). Comparisons of sentence structure of deaf and hearing children. *Psychological Monographs, 52,* 42-103.

Hess, L. (1972). *A longitudinal transformational generative comparison of the emerging syntactic structure in a deaf child and a normal hearing child.* Unpublished master's thesis, University of Cincinnati.

Hirano, M., Ohala, J., & Vennard, W. (1969). The function of laryngeal muscles in regulating fundamental frequency and intensity of phonation. *Journal of Speech and Hearing Research, 12,* 616-628.

Hirsh, I.J. (1966). Teaching the deaf child to speak. In F. Smith & G.A. Miller (Eds.), *The genesis of language* (pp. 207-216). Cambridge, MA: MIT Press.

Hixon, T.J. (1973). Respiratory function in speech. In F.D. Minifie, T.J. Hixon, & F. Williams (Eds.), *Normal aspects of speech, hearing and language* (pp. 73-126). Englewood Cliffs, NJ: Prentice-Hall.

Hochberg, I., Levitt, H., & Osberger, M.J. (Eds.). (1983). *Speech of the hearing impaired: Research, training, and personal preparation.* Baltimore, MD: University Park Press.

Hochmair-Desoyer, I.J., Hochmair, E.S., Burian, K., & Fischer, R.E. (1981). Four years of experience with cochlear prostheses. *Medical Progress in Technology, 8,* 107-119.

Holmes, D.W., & Green, W.B. (1974). *A developmental study of deaf children's semantic system.* Paper presented at the annual convention of the American Speech-Language-Hearing Association, Las Vegas.

Hood, R.B., & Dixon, R.F. (1969). Physical characteristics of speech rhythm of deaf and normal-hearing speakers. *Journal of Communication Disorders, 2,* 20-28.

Hudgins, C.V., & Numbers, F.C. (1942). An investigation of the intelligibility of speech of the deaf. *Genetic Psychology Monographs, 25,* 289-392.

Hutchinson, J.M., & Smith, L.L. (1976). Aerodynamic functioning during consonant production by hearing-impaired adults. *Audiology and Hearing Education, 2,* 16-24.

Hutchinson, J.M., Smith, L.L., Kornhauser, R.L., Beasley, D.S., & Beasley, D.C. (1978). Aerodynamic functioning in consonant production in hearing-impaired children. *Audiology and Hearing Education, 4,* 23-31.

Isshiki, N. (1964). Regulatory mechanism of voice intensity variation. *Journal of Speech and Hearing Research, 7,* 17-29.

Jackson, P.L. (1982). Techniques for speech conservation. In R. Hull (Ed.), *Rehabilitative audiology* (pp. 129-152). New York: Grune and Stratton.

Jakobson, R. (1967). About the relation between visual and auditory signs. In W. Wathen-Dunn (Ed.), *Models for the perception of speech and visual form* (pp. 1-10). Cambridge, MA: The MIT Press.

Jensema, C.J., Karchmer, M.A., & Trybus, R.J. (1978). *The rated speech intelligibility of hearing-impaired children: Basic relationships.* Washington, DC: Gallaudet College Office of Demographic Studies.

John, J.E., & Howarth, J.N. (1965). The effect of time distortion on the intelligibility of deaf children's speech. *Language and Speech, 8,* 127-134.

Johnson, D.D. (1985). Communication characteristics of NTID students. *Journal of the Academy of Rehabilitative Audiology, 8*(1), 17-32.

Kent, R.D., Osberger, M.J., Netsell, R., & Hustedde, C.G. (1987). Phonetic development in identical twins differing in auditory function. *Journal of Speech and Hearing Disorders, 52*(1), 64-75.

Kolzak, J. (1983). The impact of child language studies on mainstreaming decisions. *Volta Review, 85*(5), 129-137.

Koplin, J.H., Odom, P.B., Blanton, R.L., & Nunnally, J.C. (1967). Word association test performance of deaf subjects. *Journal of Speech and Hearing Research, 10,* 126-132.

Kretschmer, R. (1975). *The written language of hearing-impaired children: Delayed, deviant, or dialect?* Paper presented at the annual convention of the American Speech and Hearing Association, Washington.

Kretschmer, R., & Kretschmer, L. (1978). *Language development and intervention with the hearing impaired.* Baltimore: University Park Press.

Lach, R., Ling, D., Ling, A., & Ship, N. (1970). Early speech development in deaf infants. *American Annals of the Deaf, 115,* 522-526.

Larson, V. (1976). *Informal language assessment, influence of situational factors on sampling and analysis of the spontaneous language sample.* Unpublished manuscript, University of Wisconsin at Eau Claire.

Lee, L.L. (1969). *Northwestern Syntax Screening Test.* Evanston, IL: Northwestern University Press.

Lee, L.L., & Canter, S. (1971). Developmental sentence scoring: A clinical procedure for estimating syntax development in children's spontaneous speech. *Journal of Speech and Hearing Disorders, 36,* 315-340.

Lehiste, I. (1976). Suprasegmental features in speech. In N.J. Lass (Ed.), *Contemporary issues in experimental phonetics* (pp. 225-239). New York: Academic Press.

Lehman, J. (1970). A suggested approach to the evaluation of expressive oral syntactic competence of the hearing-impaired child. *The Hearing Impaired.* (ERIC Reproduction Service No. ED039 #381)

Lenneberg, E.H. (1967). *Biological foundations of language.* New York: Wiley Press.

Leonard, L. (1986). Normal language acquisition: Some recent findings and clinical implications. In J. Costello & A. Holland (Eds.), *Handbook of speech and language disorders* (pp. 543-578). San Diego: College-Hill Press.

Ling, D. (1974). Discussant comment. In R.E. Stark (Ed.), *Sensory capabilities of hearing-impaired children* (pp. 185-217). Baltimore, MD: University Park Press.

Ling, D. (1976). *Speech and the hearing-impaired child: Theory and practice.* Washington, DC: Alexander Graham Bell Association for the Deaf.

Ling, D. (1981). Early speech development. In G.T. Mencher & S.E. Gerber (Eds.), *Early management of hearing loss.* New York: Grune and Stratton.

Ling, D., & Milne, M.M. (1980). The development of speech in hearing-impaired children. In F. Bess (Ed.), *Amplification in education.* Washington, DC: Alexander Graham Bell Association for the Deaf.

MacGuintie, W. (1964). Ability of deaf children to use different word classes. *Journal of Speech and Hearing Research,* 141-150.

Markides, A. (1967). *The speech of deaf and partially-hearing children with special reference to factors affecting intelligibility.* Unpublished master's thesis, University of Manchester.

Markides, A. (1970). The speech of deaf and partially hearing children with special reference to factors affecting intelligibility. *British Journal of Disorders of Communication, 5,* 126-140.

Markides. A. (1978). Assessing the speech intelligibility of hearing-impaired children. Oral reading vs. picture description. *Journal of the British Association of Teachers of the Deaf, 2,* 185-189.

Markides, A. (1983). *The speech of hearing-impaired children.* Oxford: Manchester University Press.

Marmor, G., & Pettito, L. (1979). Simultaneous communication in the classroom: How well is English grammar represented? *Sign Language Studies, 23*, 99-136.

Matey, C., & Kretschmer, R. (1985). A comparison of mother speech to Down's syndrome, hearing impaired, and normal hearing children. *Volta Review, 87*(4), 205-214.

Mavilya, M. (1972). Spontaneous vocalization and babbling in hearing-impaired infants. In G. Fant (Ed.), *International symposium on speech communication ability and profound deafness* (pp. 163-171). Washington, DC: Alexander Graham Bell Association for the Deaf.

McCarr, D. (1973). *I can write.* Beaverton, OR: Dormac, Inc.

McGarr, N.S., & Osberger, M.J. (1978). Pitch deviancy and intelligibility of deaf speech. *Journal of Communication Disorders, 11*, 237-248.

McGettigan, J.F., & Rosenstein, J. (1969). The influence of associative strength on identification of word meanings. In J. Rosenstein & W. MacGuintie (Eds.), *Verbal behavior: Studies of word meanings and associations* (pp. 39-44). New York: Teacher's College, Columbia University.

McKnight, P., & Davis, K.A. (1983). *Metalinguistic awareness in profoundly hearing-impaired children.* Unpublished manuscript, University of Iowa.

Menyuk, P. (1977). Effects of hearing loss on language acquisition in the babbling stage. In B. Jaffe (Ed.), *Hearing loss in children* (pp. 621-629). Baltimore, MD: University Park Press.

Miller, M.L. (1980). *Deviant vocal parameters in the speech of hearing-impaired children and adolescents.* Unpublished master's thesis, Idaho State University.

Moeller, M.P., Osberger, M.J., & Eccarius, M. (1986). Receptive language skills. In M.J. Osberger (Ed.), *Language and learning skills of hearing impaired students* (pp. 41-53). ASHA Monograph #23. Washington, DC: ASHA.

Monsen, R.B. (1974). Durational aspects of vowel production in the speech of deaf children. *Journal of Speech and Hearing Research, 17*, 386-398.

Monsen, R.B. (1978). Toward measuring how well deaf children speak. *Journal of Speech and Hearing Research, 21*, 197-219.

Monsen, R.B. (1979). Acoustic qualities of phonation in young hearing-impaired children. *Journal of Speech and Hearing Research, 22*, 270-288.

Monsen, R.B. (1982). A usable test for the speech intelligibility of deaf talkers. *American Annals of the Deaf, 71*, 845-852.

Monsen, R.B. (1983). The oral speech intelligibility of hearing-impaired talkers. *Journal of Speech and Hearing Research, 48*, 286-296.

Monsen, R.B., Engbretson, A.M., & Vemulla, N.R. (1979). The effects of deafness on the generation of voice. *Journal of the Acoustical Society of America, 66*, 1680-1690.

Moog, J.S., & Geers, A.E. (1975). *Scales of early communication skills for hearing impaired children.* St. Louis: CID.

Myklebust, H. (1964). *The psychology of deafness.* New York: Grune and Stratton.

Newton, L. (1985). Linguistic environment of the deaf child: A focus on teacher's use of nonliteral language. *Journal of Speech and Hearing Research, 28*(3), 336-344.

Nix, G.W. (1975). Total communication: A review of the studies offered in its support. *The Volta Review, 11*, 470-474.

Nober, E.H. (1967). Articulation of the deaf. *Exceptional Child, 33,* 611-621.

Noll, J.D. (1970). Articulatory assessment. *Speech and the dentofacial complex: State of the art* (ASHA Report #5), 283-298. Washington, DC: ASHA.

Northern, J.L., & Downs, M.P. (1984). *Hearing in children* (3rd ed.). Baltimore, MD: Williams and Wilkins.

Norlin, P.F., & Van Tasell, D.J. (1980). Linguistic skills of hearing-impaired children. *Monographs in Contemporary Audiology, 1,* 1-32.

Odom, P.B., & Blanton, R.L. (1967). Phrase learning in deaf and hearing subjects. *Journal of Speech and Hearing Research, 10,* 816-827.

Oller, D., Jensen, H., & Lafayette, R. (1978). The relatedness of phonological processes of a hearing impaired child. *Journal of Communication Disorders, 11,* 97-105.

Oller, D., & Kelly, C.A. (1974). Phonological substitution processes of a hard-of-hearing child. *Journal of Speech and Hearing Disorders, 39,* 65-74.

Osberger, M.J., Johnstone, A., Swarts, E., & Levitt, H. (1978). The evaluation of a model speech training program for deaf children. *Journal of Communication Disorders, 11,* 293-313.

Osberger, M.J., & Levitt, H. (1979). The effect of timing errors on the intelligibility of deaf children's speech. *Journal of the Acoustical Society of America, 66,* 1316-1324.

Osberger, M.J., Moeller, M.P., Eccarius, M., Robbins, A.M., & Johnson, D. (1986). Expressive language skills. In M.J. Osberger (Ed.), *Language and learning skills of hearing-impaired students* (pp. 54-65). ASHA Monographs #23. Washington, DC: ASHA.

Osberger, M.J., Robbins, A.M., Lybolt, J., Kent, R.D., & Peters, J. (1986). Speech evaluation. In M.J. Osberger (Ed.), *Language and learning skills of hearing-impaired students* (pp. 24-31). ASHA Monograph #23. Washington, DC: ASHA.

Parasnis, I. (1983). Effects of parental deafness and early exposure to manual communication on the cognitive skills, English language skill and field independence of young deaf adults. *Journal of Speech and Hearing Research, 26,* 588-594.

Penn, J.P. (1955). Voice and speech patterns of the hard-of-hearing. *Acta Otolaryngologica* (Supple. 124).

Pollack, D. (1970). *Educational audiology for the limited hearing infant.* Springfield, IL: Charles C. Thomas.

Pressnell, L.M. (1973). Hearing-impaired children's comprehension and production of syntax in oral language. *Journal of Speech and Hearing Research, 16,* 12-21.

Quigley, S.P., Monranelli, D.S., & Wilbur, R.B. (1976). Some aspects of the verb system in the language of deaf students. *Journal of Speech and Hearing Research, 19,* 536-550.

Quigley, S.P., Steinkamp, M.W., & Jones, B.W. (1978). The assessment and development of language in hearing-impaired individuals. *Journal of the Academy of Rehabilitative Audiology, 11,* 24-41.

Restaino, L. (1968). Word association of deaf and hearing children. In J. Rosenstein & W. MacGuintie (Eds.), *Verbal behavior of the deaf child: Studies of word meanings and associations* (pp. 1-12). New York: Teacher's College Press, Columbia University.

Rothenberg, M. (1979). Optimizing sensory substitution. In D. L. McPherson & M.S. Davis (Eds.), *Advances in prosthetic devices for the deaf: A technical workshop.* Rochester, NY: National Technical Institute for the Deaf.

Sarachan-Deily, A.B., & Love, R.J. (1974). Underlying grammatical rule structure in the deaf. *Journal of Speech and Hearing Research, 17,* 689-698.

Schum, R.L. (1987). *Communication and social growth: A development model of deaf social behavior.* Paper presented at the Mayo Clinic Audiology Symposium, Rochester, MN.

Shipp, T. (1975). Vertical laryngeal position during continuous and discrete vocal frequency change. *Journal of Speech and Hearing Research, 18,* 707-718.

Shipp, T., & McGlone, R. (1971). Laryngeal dynamics associated with voice frequency change. *Journal of Speech and Hearing Research, 14,* 761-768.

Shriberg, L.D., & Kwiatkowski, J. (1980). *Natural process analysis.* New York: John Wiley and Sons.

Simmons, A.A. (1962). A comparison of the type-token ratio of spoken and written language of deaf and hearing children. *Volta Review, 64,* 417-421.

Simmons-Martin, A.A. (1977). Natural language and auditory input. In F. Bess (Ed.), *Childhood deafness, causation, assessment and management* (pp. 305-312). New York: Grune and Stratton.

Sitler, R.W., & Schiavetti, N., & Metz, D.E. (1983). Contextual effects in the measurement of hearing-impaired speakers' intelligibility. *Journal of Speech and Hearing Research, 26,* 30-34.

Skarakis, E.A., & Prutting, C.A. (1977). Early communication: Semantic functions and communication intentions in the communication of the preschool child with impaired hearing. *American Annals of the Deaf, 122,* 392-394.

Smith, B.L. (1982). Some observations concerning pre-meaningful vocalization of hearing-impaired infants. *Journal of Speech and Hearing Disorders, 47,* 439-441.

Smith, C.R. (1975). Residual hearing and speech production in deaf children. *Journal of Speech and Hearing Research, 18,* 795-811.

Smith, C.R. (1980). Speech assessment at the elementary level: Interpretation relative to speech training. In J.D. Subtelny (Ed.), *Speech assessment and speech improvement for the hearing impaired* (pp. 18-29). Washington, DC: The Alexander Graham Bell Association for the Deaf.

Smith, L.L. (1972). *Comprehension performance of oral deaf and normal hearing children at three stages of language development.* Unpublished doctoral dissertation, University of Wisconsin, Madison.

Stark, R.E. (1979). Speech of the hearing-impaired child. In L.J. Bradford & W.G. Hardy (Eds.), *Hearing and hearing impairment* (pp. 209-233). New York: Grune and Stratton.

Stark, R.E. (1983). Phonatory development in young normally hearing and hearing-impaired children. In I. Hochberg, H. Levitt, & M.J. Osberger (Eds.), *Speech of the hearing impaired: Research, training, and personnel preparation* (pp. 251-266). Baltimore, MD: University Park Press.

Stark, R.E., & Levitt, H. (1974). Prosodic feature reception and production in deaf children. *Journal of the Acoustical Society of America, 55,* 563.

Stoel-Gammon, C., & Otomo, K. (1986). Babbling development of hearing-impaired and normally hearing subjects. *Journal of Speech and Hearing Disorders, 51*, 33-41.

Stoutenburgh, G. (1971). *A psycholinguistic approach to the study of language deficits in the language performance of deaf children.* Unpublished doctoral dissertation, Syracuse University.

Streng, A. (1968). The language arts in the curriculum for deaf children. In H. Kopp (Ed.), Curriculum, cognition, and content. *Volta Review, 70*, 487-492.

Subtelny, J.D. (1977). Assessment of speech with implications for training. In F. Bess (Ed.), *Childhood deafness: Causation, assessment, and management* (pp. 183-194). New York: Grune & Stratton.

Subtelny, J.D., Webster, P.E., & Murphy, L.E. (1980). Personal preparation for teaching speech to the hearing impaired: Current status and recommendations. In J.D. Subtelny (Ed.), *Speech assessment and speech improvement for the hearing impaired* (pp. 366-388). Washington, DC: The Alexander Graham Bell Association for the Deaf.

Templin, M.O., & Darley, F.L. (1969). *The Templin-Darley Tests of Articulation.* University of Iowa, Iowa City: Bureau of Education, Research and Service.

Tervoort, B. (1967). Language development of deaf children. In *International conference on oral education of the deaf* (Vol. II, pp. 1289-1295). Washington, DC: Alexander Graham Bell Association for the Deaf.

Thompson, M., Biro, P., Vethivelu, S., Pious, C., & Hatfield, N. (1987). *Language assessment of hearing impaired school age children.* Seattle: University of Washington Press.

Tomblin, J.B. (1977). Effects of syntactic order on serial-recall performance of hearing-impaired and normal-hearing subjects. *Journal of Speech and Hearing Research, 20*, 421-429.

Tyack, D. & Gottsleben, R. (1974). *Language sampling and training.* Palo Alto, CA: Consulting Psychologists Press.

Tye-Murray, N. (1987). Effects of vowel context on the articulatory closure postures of deaf speakers. *Journal of Speech and Hearing Research, 30*, 99-104.

Voelker, C.H. (1935). A preliminary phostroboscopic study of the speech of the deaf. *American Annals of the Deaf, 80*, 243-259.

Vorce, E. (1974). *Teaching speech to deaf children.* Washington, DC: Alexander Graham Bell Association for the Deaf.

Weiss, A.L., Carrey, A.E., & Leonard, L.B. (1985). Perceived contrastive stress production in hearing-impaired and normal-hearing children. *Journal of Speech and Hearing Research, 28*(1), 26-35.

West, J.J., & Weber, J.L. (1974). A phonological analysis of the spontaneous language of a four-year-old hard-of-hearing child. *Journal of Speech and Hearing Disorders, 38*, 25-35.

Whitehead, R.L. (1983). Some respiratory and aerodynamic patterns in the speech of the hearing impaired. In I. Hochberg, H. Levitt, & M. J. Osberger (Eds.), *Speech of the hearing impaired* (pp. 97-116). Baltimore, MD: University Park Press.

Whitehead, R. L., & Jones, K.O. (1978). The effect of vowel environment on duration of consonants produced by normal-hearing, hearing-impaired and deaf adult speakers. *Journal of Phonetics, 6,* 77-81.

Wilcox, J., & Tobin, H. (1974). Linguistic performance of hard-of-hearing and normal-hearing children. *Journal of Speech and Hearing Research, 17,* 286-293.

Wilson, F.B. (1977). *Voice disorders.* Austin, TX: Learning Concepts.

Wingfield, A. (1975). Acoustic redundancy and the perception of time-compressed speech. *Journal of Speech and Hearing Research, 18,* 96-104.

Wingfield, A., Buttett, J., & Sandoval, A.W. (1979). Intonation and intelligibility of time-compressed speech: Supplementary report. *Journal of Speech and Hearing Research, 22,* 708-716.

Young, C., & McConnell, F. (1957). Retardation of vocabulary development in hard of hearing children. *Exceptional Child, 23,* 368-370.

Zimmerman, G., & Rettaliata, P. (1981). Articulatory patterns of an adventitiously deaf speaker: Implications for the role of auditory information in speech production. *Journal of Speech and Hearing Research, 24,* 169-178.

chaptersix

PSYCHOSOCIAL ASPECTS OF HEARING IMPAIRMENT

McCAY VERNON

PAULA J. OTTINGER

contents

introduction

No professional groups have been more instrumental in establishing the attitudes that determine the psychologic and sociologic adjustments of persons with hearing loss than those representing audiology, speech-language pathology, and education of the hearing impaired. These persons are often central in the key decision-making points of a hearing-impaired individual's life. Therefore, it is vital that those who have professional powers that influence the eventual psychologic and sociologic fate of deaf and hard-of-hearing persons possess a thorough understanding of deafness and the hearing-impaired population, as well as the evaluation processes that guide them at these decision points. The information presented in this chapter addresses a number of relevant psychologic and sociologic aspects of deafness, including the dynamics surrounding diagnosis and a brief review of evaluation procedures and instruments.

the hearing-impaired population

Hearing impairment is the single most prevalent chronic physical disability in the United States. Current estimates indicate that at least 22 million people in this country have hearing impairment (Goldstein, 1984).

This population represents a wide variety of hearing losses, with the two key factors affecting an individual's abilities and disabilities being age at onset of the loss (pre- or postlingual) and degree of impairment, ranging from persons for whom the loss is a mild inconvenience to those who are unable to understand conversational speech in most situations. Of this latter group, those who incurred their deafness prelingually are defined as *educationally* and *socially deaf* for the purposes of this chapter.

the deaf

Intelligence and Education. Extensive research has been conducted on the intelligence of deaf persons; results indicate that the deaf and hearing populations have essentially the same distribution of intelligence (Vernon, 1968b). Thus, no causal relationship exists between hearing loss and IQ, nor do the difficulties with speech and with written language experienced by hearing-impaired persons reflect an absence of cognitive potential.

A common fallacy related to hearing-impaired persons is that they demonstrate lower capacities for abstract thought. However, research on the relationship of language and thought, as manifested in deaf and hard-of-hearing persons, demonstrates that the potential for abstract thought is as prevalent among deaf as among hearing people (Furth, 1966; Lenneberg, 1967; Vernon, 1967, 1985).

In some cases the disease or condition causing a hearing loss may leave residual brain damage which affects intelligence and thought patterns; for example, meningitis, complications of Rh factor, premature birth, maternal rubella, and certain genetic syndromes (Mindel & Vernon, 1987). Also, a lower overall IQ may be expected in the minority of deaf children affected by chronic brain syndromes.

In sharp contrast to these facts regarding their intelligence, the educational achievement level of deaf persons and many who are hard of hearing has been, on the average, shockingly low. Although some have attained advanced academic degrees, most are grossly undereducated. While this is an acknowledgment, to an extent, of the tremendous challenge hearing loss and its effects on language development present to academic learning, in larger measure it is an indictment of the educational system for failing to develop the intellectual capacity of deaf students.

Many surveys of the educational achievement of the deaf provide data indicating that deaf children are being failed educationally (Trybus & Karchmer, 1977). Large numbers never achieve beyond the elementary grade levels; until recently, an appallingly small percentage attended college.

Thus, despite having potential, too many hearing-impaired youth still do not receive adequate and appropriate opportunities to learn. The crippling psychologic and sociologic implications of this educational deprivation are self-evident; the equally dismal vocational ramifications are discussed below.

Family Patterns. The majority (roughly 90%) of deaf children are born to hearing parents (Schein & Delk, 1974). As adults, about 95% of deaf persons marry deaf spouses, the most frequent exceptions being those who are hard of hearing or adventitiously deafened. Marriage between deaf individuals is a realistic adjustment to deafness. In turn, the majority of offspring of deaf couples (roughly 88%) have normal hearing (Schein & Delk, 1974). These figures have important ramifications for the communication patterns that develop within families, and, as a corollary, the psychologic health of the family unit, as discussed later.

Vocational Trends. Despite having the same intelligence as hearing people, deaf persons usually engage in unskilled or semi-skilled labor because of the prevailing lack of opportunity for higher level employment. Thus, a disproportionately high percentage of deaf persons are engaged in some form of manual labor, paralleled by a disproportionately small number holding white-collar jobs. Underemployment—working at jobs below one's educational level and other levels of capabilities—is a serious and chronic problem for deaf workers (Schein & Delk, 1974).

In planning for the vocational future of deaf clients, the following employment trends must be kept in mind (Vernon, 1987):

1. There is a general shift to increasing numbers of white-collar jobs and decreasing numbers of manual, unskilled, and semi-skilled jobs. Thus, the area where the majority of deaf people find employment is one of decreasing opportunity, whereas the areas of increasing opportunity are those where deaf persons experience the greatest difficulty finding and maintaining employment.

2. The urban shift imposes hardships on some deaf persons. However, in general it has resulted in making a higher level of professional services more accessible.

3. The rapid advances in technology within the world of work have important implications for deaf persons.. The increasing need for retraining is a potential problem for deaf workers because of their communication problems (this may be overcome with some flexibility on the part of the employer).

4. A growing increase in the educational requirements for employment is evident throughout the job market. This presents difficulties for deaf persons in view of their generally lower levels of educational achievement.

5. Finally, employment opportunities in the service sector (education, health and medical care, hotels) are rapidly increasing. The majority of jobs in these areas are white-collar jobs, a classification where deaf people are not well represented. In addition, many require civil service examinations, the language levels of which are difficult for many deaf persons.

The resolution of this vocational crisis lies in using the potential of deaf persons, that is currently largely untapped. Specifically, improvement of educational techniques, of communication opportunities through manual communication and other methods, and of counseling services can do much to alleviate what otherwise seems to be a dim vocational future for many deaf persons.

Communication. Any analysis of the psychologic and sociologic functioning of severely hearing-impaired persons must carefully examine the issue of communication and its implications for persons with a hearing loss. Among the basic aspects of communication, in addition to hearing, which must be considered are speech, speechreading, written English, fingerspelling and sign language.

Speech. Learning speech when one is significantly hearing impaired is extremely difficult. A rough parallel can be drawn by imagining the problems normal-hearing persons would encounter trying to learn to speak a foreign language without being able to hear it and without being able to monitor their own voice, or with only partial and imperfect input and feedback. Because of such difficulties, many prelingually deaf persons are unable to develop speech that can be understood in most social situations. This is not to imply that speech training should be ignored, but the reality of the extreme difficulty of this task must not be forgotten by professionals or parents.

Speechreading. Although helpful, skill in speechreading has been demonstrated to be only of limited value for most hearing-impaired persons (Erber, 1979). Since 40% to 60% of English speech sounds are homophenous (i.e., they look the same on the lips), persons without a sound language base, for example, a deaf child, are unable to fill in the gaps, therefore understanding very little (Mindel & Vernon, 1987). This places heavy demands on hearing-impaired individuals and on those with whom they try to communicate. Again, we are not implying that the ability to speechread has no value or that opportunities to develop it should not be provided. Rather, this communication tool must be approached realistically and with a sense of balance regarding its role in the communication functioning of persons with hearing impairments.

Written English. Communication by reading and writing is a severely limited outlet for many deaf persons, as discussed in the section on education.

Fingerspelling and sign language. These communication methods are preferred by most deaf people; those knowing the language of signs and fingerspelling do not encounter the problems of ambiguity and frustration inherent in speech and speechreading. In addition to the social and psychologic benefits of a fluent and viable communication system, there is mounting evidence of educational benefits, as discussed previously.

The psychologic significance of the available data on communication is crucial. Specifically, many families do not communicate fluently and comfortably with their severely hearing-impaired members. Very few learn sign language or other effective communication methods. Such a lack of communication is devastating educationally, psychologically, and sociologically. In addition, many school programs turn out a high percentage of students who do not possess adequate means of communication and social interaction—skills which would have been possible to acquire given a combined manual/oral education. As a result, many deaf adults function as isolates, ignorant about much of the world in which they live. (See Chapter 7 on Oral, Manual and Total Communication for recent trends in educational programming.)

Mental Health Concerns. Since a major consequence of hearing impairment often is social isolation, studies have been conducted to determine the influences of deafness on mental health. Research findings on major mental illnesses among the deaf population have not always been consistent. For example, Rainer, Altschuler, Kallmann, and Deming (1963), in an extensive study of psychotic illness among deaf persons, found that schizophrenia was not more common among hospitalized deaf patients than among hearing patients. Studies by this group of researchers and others have disagreed on the relationship between deafness and other conditions, such as depressive illness and paranoid patterns (Mindel & Vernon, 1971).

Among less severe mental health problems, some of the more frequent difficulties relate to social isolation due to communication problems, pervasive underachievement (among school-age patients), and "primitive personality"—a term for deaf persons who possess normal intellectual potential but almost totally lack verbal or manual language (Mindel & Vernon, 1987). As illustrated, inadequate communication has serious implications for the mental health of many hearing-impaired individuals.

the hard of hearing

The term "hard of hearing" covers a broad degree of impairments, but is generally used to refer to persons who are able, with or without amplification, to use residual hearing for purposes of communication. In addition, speechreading techniques may be needed to supplement aural methods. The extent to which this definition is applicable depends on a variety of factors, including the degree and type of loss and the efficiency of amplification. Generally, hard-of-hearing persons are classified in terms of the severity of their loss, ranging from slight to mild (25 to 40 dB HL), mild to moderate (41 to 70 dB HL), and severe (71 to 90 dB HL). Persons with hearing losses above 90 dB demonstrate profound losses and are generally considered audiologically deaf. Regardless of degree of loss, persons may psychologically identify or consider themselves either deaf or hard of hearing; this perception, in turn, will impact preferred modes of communication and functioning.

Children who are hard of hearing face tremendous educational challenges. Unlike deaf children, who are more likely to receive appropriate educational placement in a school for the deaf or in a mainstreamed environment, hard-of-hearing children, depending on their individual abilities and needs, are given few educational or communication options. They are expected to perform as hearing children do, in a mainstreamed classroom using aural and oral communication. These settings are sufficient for learning and participation only in the ideal. Often amplification appropriate to the room size and ambient noise is not provided. In addition, close positioning of the child to and visibility of the teacher and other members of the class may be random, and the child may miss critical educational and social learning. Boredom and pressure from teacher and parents to perform better often result, leading many hard-of-hearing youngsters to counter their feelings of inadequacy with asocial behavior. Since behavior problems are common in hard-of-hearing children, audiologists should advise parents, teachers and school counselors of available means for remediation, including exploring classroom amplification, pursuing logistical support, and obtaining possible tutelage for these children. Socialization is another important part of the educational process; the child's relationship with peers and adults may also benefit from use of appropriate intervention strategies.

Adults with mild-to-moderate hearing losses experience persistent communication difficulties which vary in degree depending upon a number of variables. Such communication deficiencies can, in turn, lead to problems related to psychosocial adjustment. For example, the hard-of-hearing adult may experience strong feelings of frustration and inadequacy stemming from the inability to hear as effectively as before. Withdrawal from situations in which hearing difficulties often occur, such as meetings, church, and social events, therefore, is commonplace. Because the hearing-impaired person may restrict his/her activity, a sense of isolation and loneliness can result which may eventually lead to depression. Professionals must be alert to the potential for hard-of-hearing adults to experience a variety of difficulties in adjusting to their impairment. While most will adjust reasonably well, some individuals will require counseling to resolve psychosocial problems resulting from their hearing loss.

Patterns of reaction and adjustment in adults trying to cope with hearing loss will vary. However, some patterns are commonly (though not universally) seen in initial reactions, including denial of the disability, procrastination in seeking diagnosis and treatment, and feelings of anxiety regarding the medical and personal implications of the hearing loss. Such feelings are not surprising; in fact, the same patterns may also be seen in persons experiencing other disabilities and illnesses.

Especially if significant, hearing impairment imposes on clients the need to adjust various aspects of their lives. As clients learn to deal with the day-to-day reality of impaired hearing, their adjustment patterns and coping strategies remain individual. This is to be expected since they bring to the experience of hearing loss the same gamut of individual variation one would encounter in the general population. A few of the myriad of factors involved in adjustment to hearing loss include such auditory factors as the degree, type, etiology, permanence, and rate of onset of the loss; personal factors such as age, sex, education, general health, and socioeconomic status, and the personal and professional support systems available to the client (Wylde, 1987).

The diversity within the hearing-impaired population should serve as a reminder that we cannot develop and impose on clients a set of stereotyped expectations regarding what hearing-impaired people are like, how they behave, and what they need. Sometimes it is easy to judge and label clients according to their behaviors, especially if they are not in keeping with our expectations. For example, the client who experiences a sudden significant hearing loss may drop certain social activities which have become stressful and unrewarding due to the hearing impairment, and adopt others which are enjoyable. Such changes may be labeled by one professional as "pathological withdrawal" or "giving in to the disability", yet another may consider the same reaction a healthy and realistic adjustment to a significant change in the client's life circumstance.

A hearing-impaired client may attempt to compensate for loss of background environmental sounds and increased difficulty in understanding speech by increasing attentiveness to visual stimuli and cues, and by frequently asking what other people are saying. Such coping mechanisms have been labeled *suspiciousness* or *paranoia* by some clinicians. Such judgmental attitudes should be resisted, however; they may ultimately cause clients to feel defensive and become less able to seek and accept necessary support services.

In spite of resistance from some clients to accepting suggestions, clinicians should strive to consistently maintain client involvement in decisions regarding the direction and pace of the rehabilitation program. If such resistance exists, whatever its source, those feelings are real and cannot be overcome by "railroading" the client. It is beneficial in such situations to attend to the information only clients themselves can offer regarding the demands of their life styles and what resources are available to them (both intrapersonal and those in the environment). As they continually adjust to new ways of managing the tasks of daily living, hearing-impaired persons' ability to turn to others for both informational and emotional support can be a key variable.

A special consideration in working with certain moderate to severely hard-of-hearing clients is that they may find themselves unable to find a "niche" in which they are comfortable. Thus, many hard-of-hearing persons feel that they are "neither fish nor fowl"; they are not truly deaf and find it psychologically threatening or otherwise difficult to identify with and be accepted by the deaf community. (In fact, many members of this population have no exposure to and awareness of the deaf community.) At the same time, they discover that, because of the limitation imposed by their hearing loss, interaction with hearing persons means (a) constant struggle to comprehend, (b) frequent misunderstandings, and (c) much emotional stress. Often they are encouraged by well-meaning family and professionals to push themselves to be as nearly "hearing" as possible—not to allow themselves to "be deaf."

Yet, it is not uncommon for hard-of-hearing persons (more so those with a significant loss) to identify with deaf persons. Although they may make maximal use of their residual hearing and speech skills in situations where this is appropriate, some hard-of-hearing individuals find, once they have had the opportunity to experience sign language, a sense of relief or respite in the ease and confidence of communication that is available to them only through use of manual communication systems. This need for comfortable and viable communication should not be overlooked. Although it is essential to aid each client in achieving the best possible aural/oral functioning, the difficulty and emotional demands that may be imposed by a hearing loss must be acknowledged and the client's feelings and wishes be considered.

counseling with the hearing-impaired client

Until recently, almost no counseling or therapeutic services were available specifically for deaf persons. For example, hearing-impaired patients admitted to mental hospitals often faced a prolonged stay, which was more custodial than therapeutic. There still exists an acute shortage of persons who are trained in both mental health and deafness and who possess the necessary communication skills. However, the picture is improving as a result of new training programs, additional research on deafness, and increasing attention to deafness from psychologists as well as professionals in other disciplines.

Since the client perspective has already been examined, the counseling process with deaf clients will be examined here from three other perspectives: the counselor, interprofessional coordination, and the counseling process.

the counselor

Under the rubric of *counselor* may fall such diverse specialties as mental health, vocational, and aural rehabilitation. In general, however, counselors share certain skills and focal areas.

First, the qualifications of counselors are rising. Thus, increasing numbers have developed familiarity with the implications of hearing impairment and sensitivity to the communication needs of their hearing-impaired clients—including personally learning sign language. This is vital, because there can be no true counseling relationship without true communication. In addition to being willing to learn to sign (Sullivan & Vernon, 1979), counselors of the deaf also need to learn to understand and deal with the practical, everyday realities of hearing impairment, as well as to master the theoretical concepts. Overall, it is important that counselors not stereotype deaf clients, their abilities, or disabilities.

One of the best ways to accomplish these goals is to maintain frequent and direct contact with persons having a hearing loss.

interprofessional coordination in counseling

The best provision of services often results from the combined efforts of a variety of professionals. This is true also in the provision of mental health services for hearing-impaired clients.

Professionals with a background in audiology, speech-language pathology, and aural rehabilitation have valuable services to offer persons confronted with hearing impairment. Because of their involvement at crucial points in these individuals' lives, professionals from such disciplines must acquire basic grounding in the psychodynamics surrounding hearing loss and its diagnosis. At the same time, it is helpful to have as a resource a psychologist experienced in the various facets of hearing impairment. Unfortunately, such backup is rare.

One of the most frequent needs of hearing-impaired clients is psychologic evaluation and follow-up counseling. Another relates to parent/family therapy, either individual or group. For children such services often fall within the realm of the school psychologist. For adults, a psychologist may be consulted in mental health centers, through vocational rehabilitation, or other state agencies. Throughout, however, clients and their families are provided a disservice if these functions are carried out by mental health professionals unfamiliar with hearing impairments. The same holds true when such services are performed by professionals experienced in hearing impairment but not in psychology. Often state schools for the deaf are important resources, and most of them will have staff who possess the appropriate background or can provide referral information. Also, psychologists in public school programs that serve hearing-impaired children may be experienced with the population. In the absence of individuals with qualifications in both mental health and hearing impairment, clinicians may be well served to invest time and effort on orienting relevant professionals about deafness (in return, they may gain valuable skills in the field of mental health). Such an approach offers the possible advantage of developing a pool of personnel that share professional growth and are able to work together as a team.

the counseling process

Assuming that the counselor possesses the basic skills necessary to be effective, what are the special considerations in counseling a hearing-impaired client?

Communication Modality. As noted, hearing-impaired clients present a broad range of skills, preferences, and comfort levels in communication strategies. Therefore, the counselor must initially determine the client's preferred mode of communication, assess its adequacy, and be prepared to use it. Among clients who sign, the level and type of signing used will vary greatly, and the counselor may need considerable skill to meet this challenge. If needed, an interpreter may be called in. It is rare to find a client with significant hearing impairment with whom written communication can be used effectively in the counseling relationship. Finally, the counselor must also be prepared to deal with clients who have been limited to "oral-only" communication, but have experienced limited success. In such situations, clients (and counselor) are left with severely restricted communication.

Concrete vs. Abstract. Some hearing-impaired clients may have difficulty dealing with concepts that have no immediate or specific referent. This may result from language or educational deficiencies, isolation, lack of general information, or other factors. For such clients counseling must be related directly to their concrete environment.

General Information. For some hearing-impaired persons hearing loss may result in the loss of a great deal of "incidental" knowledge. Therefore, professionals should be prepared for what may seem to be extreme naiveté on the part of some clients, and not mistake it for a lack of intelligence.

Familiarity with Specialized Services. It is helpful for persons working with hearing-handicapped clients, in whatever capacity, to become familiar with area agencies and facilities that serve, or may be adapted to serve, hearing-impaired clients, as well as with regional and national resources.

psychological aspects of diagnosing hearing loss in the child

An understanding of the psychodynamics surrounding the diagnosis of a child's hearing loss is essential for all professionals who work with the hearing impaired. However, this is particularly true for those professionals who make the actual diagnosis and inform the parents of their findings.

The way in which the diagnosis of deafness, and the trauma that surrounds it, is handled has long-term consequences for both child and family. Thus, conveying such sensitive and psychologically threatening information is often very stressful for both parents and professionals. Use of a constructive approach, based on knowledge of all relevant psychodynamics and the way they develop, may help avoid irreversible psychological damage and counterproductive reactions. The discussion that follows traces the factors relevant to these parental dynamics, beginning with pregnancy.

pregnancy

Many pregnancies are not planned, and may not be wanted. Even couples who plan and desire pregnancy often feel ambivalent about it. High hopes, excitement, and feelings of bonding and closeness may be dampened by fearfulness and hostility toward the added responsibilities, demands, and discomfort of parenthood. Often unplanned pregnancies result in one partner blaming the other for the carelessness that led to the conception.

Such mixed feelings usually find some form of expression, ranging from simple disgruntlement over the physical discomforts of pregnancy or necessary changes in established routines to wishful fantasies that the pregnancy will somehow end prematurely. Indeed, there may be deliberate violations of obvious canons of prenatal care, and, in some cases, more direct attempts to abort.

The point to be made here is that variations of these feelings are normal. However, they can have tremendous implications in terms of guilt and denial for parents if their child is later diagnosed as hearing-impaired.

factors influencing acceptance of deafness

Diagnosis of deafness is usually made 1 to 3 years after birth. Usually actual diagnosis is preceded by a period of gradually unfolding knowledge about the child and building suspicions that something is wrong. This process is influenced by a number of factors relevant to parental personalities and backgrounds. (For a more complete treatment of this topic, see Mindel and Feldman, 1987.)

The first relevant factor in parents' personalities is their adaptive capacities. How able are they to cope with unusual or unanticipated events, specifically, having a hearing-impaired child? The coping mechanisms of the mother and father in rearing young children may differ significantly. This results, at least partially, from the psychologic processes experienced by the mother during gestation (when strong emotions, positive or negative, may be projected onto the fetus) and following the child's birth (when the newborn and parents, especially the mother, enter into a relationship that is both demanding and rewarding). The manner in which the parent deals with events in this period provides significant clues about his or her ability to cope with unanticipated events, such as those that will be encountered in having a disabled child.

Although parents' individual personalities are significant, so too are their collective personality factors, as they are influenced by the marriage relationship. The relationship of both spouses to their own mothers and fathers will also have considerable bearing on the nature of the marriage and how they handle the discovery of deafness and their disabled child.

Finally, the hearing-impaired child's ordinal position in the family and the family's cultural background are significant. New parents may not know how a child should react to sound, and therefore not suspect the hearing loss as early as experienced parents. Additionally, in families where the child's language development is highly valued (generally among parents with higher levels of education), detection of deafness is more apt to occur earlier because of increased attention to articulation and grammatical correctness.

the early years

As stated previously, actual diagnosis of hearing loss is usually preceded by a period during which parents begin to suspect a problem. They may not consider the possibility of hearing impairment, partly because many infants having significant losses demonstrate enough residual hearing to respond to gross sounds, thereby masking their inability to understand speech sounds, which will have a profound impact on development. During this period, parents' anxiety will mount along with their suspicions. It is not uncommon for both parents to suspect, separately, that something is wrong, but not discuss this with one another.

When these concerns are presented to the physician, they may be interpreted as common manifestations of the anxieties experienced by many parents of normal babies. Thus, the doctor may minimize parental concerns with such comments as, "It's just a phase - he'll outgrow it"; or "Everything is fine - you're just a worrier." Although such remarks may be well intended, they only serve to increase frustration, anxiety, and confusion in the family. In addition, they also have the serious consequence of delaying diagnosis and habilitation during what is believed by many to be a crucial point in the child's psychologic, linguistic, and educational development.

The high rate of misdiagnosis of deafness further complicates the diagnosis crisis (Mindel & Vernon, 1987). Some of these misdiagnoses arise out of the complex problems surrounding the differential diagnosis between brain damage, aphasia, delayed speech, autism, childhood schizophrenia, mental retardation, and deafness (Sullivan & Vernon, 1979). This is especially true for the hearing-impaired child with additional handicaps. However, some misdiagnoses also must be attributed to errors on the part of physicians and psychologists employing inappropriate evaluation techniques (Vernon, 1973). Finally, the delay in obtaining an accurate diagnosis may result from the unconscious denial of deafness on the part of some parents who do not acknowledge the child's symptoms or associate them with hearing loss.

the diagnosis

As stated previously, the child may be 2 or 3 years old before deafness is conclusively diagnosed. For some parents, the diagnosis results in a sense of relief initially, especially if the child's problem was previously believed to be retardation, autism, or some other condition perceived as being worse than deafness. For most parents, however, being confronted with the child's deafness is a traumatic disappointment, the full depth of which is rarely sensed by the professional who delivers the diagnosis.

When confronted with the realization that their child is hearing impaired, parents experience what they often describe as "shock." Parents commonly will relate, "I don't remember a thing the doctor said after I was told my child was deaf." This reaction is a mixture of disbelief, grief, and helplessness, followed by feelings of anger and guilt. In this condition parents feel suddenly alone, set apart from the rest of society.

The noted disbelief is an extension of the earlier period of doubts felt about the child and his condition. Thus, parents may ask themselves, "Why did this happen to me?" Consciously or unconsciously they may regard the child's hearing impairment as punishment for some supposed transgression. Specifically, the ambivalent feelings toward the child during pregnancy and early infancy may be recalled by the parent and interpreted as somehow being the cause of the child's disability, resulting in intense feelings of guilt. Parents may torture themselves with feelings of guilt for having produced a disabled child, and seek out some reason, some cause—real or imagined.

Feelings of disappointment and frustration are common to parents having to deal with the reality of their child's disability. They experience helplessness, confusion, and either real or potential loss of some of the gratifications of parenthood. Anger is the natural consequence of this frustration, and, like all emotions, their anger seeks an object. While they consciously recognize that their child is not responsible for the disability, parents will nevertheless find themselves inexplicably harboring negative feelings toward the child, which stimulates further guilt. Clearly, families in the midst of the crisis surrounding diagnosis associated with a child who is seriously and irreversibly disabled have a great deal to cope with. Excellent research by Siller (1969), Luterman (1979), and Moses (1985) provides some crucial general principles for helping parents and families cope better with their realization of hearing impairment.

According to the first of these principles, the patient and family can begin to cope effectively only after they are fully aware of the reality of the condition, its implications, and its irreversibility. If false hopes for a cure, or indications that the ramifications of the disability can be overcome are extended, patients and families do not begin to develop the kind of constructive adaptations that are based on the reality of the disability. Thus, the potential for successful rehabilitation may rest, in large part, with the person who informs parents of their child's hearing impairment, and how he or she handles this delicate situation.

A second principle derived from research on reaction to disability is that certain coping mechanisms or defenses are almost universal. The most important of these is the denial of the defect or its implications. Denial is a normal coping mechanism through which we initially protect ourselves at a time of trauma. It is when denial becomes chronic that it takes on a pathologic and counterproductive nature.

Parents often go through a long period of denying indications that their child has a problem, and when the deafness is finally diagnosed, it is typically initially denied. This denial syndrome is often compounded by the professional community. Frequently, in the diagnostic conference with parents, the full implications of the hearing disability are not explained (Mindel & Vernon, 1987). Perhaps almost nothing is said about what the disability will mean in the lives of the family and child. Sometimes the presentation of life with a "handicapped" child is so bleak that it becomes even more difficult for parents to confront this reality. More commonly, however, in an effort to help parents through this difficult time, the professional creates false impressions and hopes, glossing over the real ramifications of significant hearing impairment. Consequently, parents may be led to believe that amplification and oral skills training will enable their child to function as if there were no hearing loss. Although subtle and usually unintentional, this leading of parents into what frequently are unrealistic beliefs about the potential benefits of amplification, speech, and speechreading fosters denial and may lead to feelings of anger and frustration as parent and child eventually confront the inevitable communication difficulties.

Another aspect related to diagnosis is an inevitable sense of mourning over loss of hearing. This feeling is rarely experienced as an intense grief, which is worked through psychologically (Vernon, 1973, 1979). Thus, misdirected kindness of professionals often encourages parents to deny the loss, and it is uncommon for parents informed about deafness to be allowed time to talk through the very intense feelings that occur at the diagnosis and for some time thereafter. Thus, the mourning that should be experienced is repressed, and chronic denial is substituted for constructive coping.

constructive coping

The difficulties and limitations posed by speechreading and speech for persons with severe hearing losses are discussed elsewhere in this chapter. Unfortunately, it is unusual for professionals to share with parents the difficulties they and their child will face in attempting to establish viable oral communication, often, at least in part, because the professionals themselves are unaware of these facts. To present these facts is painful; yet is a reality. Until this reality is known, denial is prolonged and constructive coping cannot begin. The consequences are a communication breakdown and a great discrepancy between parents' expectations and their child's actual achievement. This circumstance may have many sequelae: frustration, avoidance of parent-child interaction, lowered levels of academic achievement, and emotional isolation of the deaf individual from the family.

A reasonable resolution of the communication problems faced by many severely-to-profoundly impaired individuals is offered by total communication (TC), that is, the use of fingerspelling, the language of signs, speech, speechreading, and amplification. The major advantage of total communication is that it does not entail the ambiguity inherent in speech and speechreading alone. Although not a panacea, it represents a step forward, and has been endorsed as such by the National Association of the Deaf—the world's largest organization for the deaf.

Communication methodology, however, is only one of the many issues parents will confront. For the vast majority, the process of revising their concept of their infant's future to one that includes realistic acknowledgment of the deafness is long and at times difficult.

The professional community can do a great deal to foster a true understanding and acceptance of the hearing loss. Primary among them is presenting a realistic picture of the limitations imposed by hearing impairment, balanced by the possibility of a happy and rewarding relationship with the child if appropriate measures are taken. Counseling services that provide an accepting atmosphere and help parents understand their own emotional turmoil are of great value, as, too, is information about numerous facets of hearing disabilities, contact with hearing-impaired adults and other parents of children with hearing loss. Centers offering a comprehensive, multidisciplinary approach can be of great help. Such programs, however, presuppose that professionals first become knowledgeable about and comfortable with deaf persons and deafness in all its aspects.

psychological aspects of diagnosing hearing loss in adults

A majority of persons with significant hearing loss become impaired post-educationally, that is, after the age of 17. For those who were normally hearing during their formative educational and social years, a sudden loss of hearing in adult life can be a psychologically traumatic event. Unlike adults who had hearing impairments as children and for whom the disability has become part of their identity, those who face onset of hearing loss as adults identify as hearing persons, even though they can no longer function as such. In addition to impacting on personal image and identity, hearing loss in adulthood may impact significantly on social and family relationships, career, and living styles—all of which are patterned and established in the formative years of those becoming hearing impaired as youths.

For adults who lose their hearing, the term "hearing loss" has true significance, because the longer they have had normal hearing, the more they perceive its absence as a true "loss." The major loss for both deafened and hard-of-hearing adults is in communication, where easy conversation and the appreciation of music, religious liturgies, the sounds of nature, and so forth is affected. New modes of communication can be learned but, especially for those with severe hearing losses, the joy of music and the sounds of nature may be permanently lost. For those who are totally deafened, the signals that once kept them in touch with their environments—the sounds of airplanes, of sirens, of doorbells, and telephones—will be missed, as will the sounds of their own bodies, like breathing, that once, although perhaps not noticed, reassured them or alerted them to ill health.

Common reactions to hearing loss among adults may include denial, anger, guilt, and depression. They may deny their hearing impairments, insisting that communication difficulties are caused by others who do not speak clearly or loudly enough. They may be angry at physicians who cannot restore their hearing or at audiologists for not providing complete rehabilitative relief. They may turn their anger inward, feeling guilty that perhaps if they had done something differently they could have saved their hearing. After experiencing a spectrum of emotions, and realizing that nothing can be done to restore their hearing, depression may ensue; if prolonged, such depression can lead to feelings of isolation.

Hearing-impaired adults face problems related to adjustment, change, and relearning. Their success in making this adjustment depends on a combination of factors—the degree and type of hearing loss, general physical and mental health, interest in life and motivation to adapt, and support of family, friends, employers, and co-workers. These factors interact to affect the success of most rehabilitative efforts, including the fitting of hearing aids and use of other amplification devices, aural rehabilitation, speechreading training, fingerspelling, and/or sign language instruction.

Generally, the younger one is at the onset of hearing impairment, the easier it is to adapt. But age is a state of mind—one can be old at 45 and young at 80—and no prognosis should be assumed based solely on the client's age. The elderly, however, may face special problems adapting to hearing loss. For example, they may be more isolated by their families or by care providers in institutions. The tendency to treat elderly persons like children, using conversation only to give commands or to inquire about their basic needs, makes acceptance of a hearing loss that further isolates them even more difficult. Family members may also deny the existence of a hearing loss, even after differential diagnosis has been made by physicians and audiologists, instead attributing the elderly's behavior to senility, brain damage, or stubbornness. In addition to the mental health and environmental support factors affecting the elderly hearing impaired, general physical health also affects acceptance and motivation to adapt. Thus, hearing impairment may be only one of the disabilities faced by the elderly person, and it may not be the most debilitating.

Efforts to fit elderly clients with hearing aids may be welcomed with a sense of relief—or with rebellion. Clients may complain about the earmolds or the noises the aid emits. The audiologist must take into consideration the difficulty of finding an appropriate aid for presbycusic clients, and also pay attention to the psychological components of rejecting the aid. The success of aural rehabilitation efforts for those who have residual hearing will depend on motivation as well as the effectiveness of amplification. Elderly clients who have not yet accepted their hearing loss are not likely to be motivated to learn compensatory methods. Similarly, speechreading efforts for both deaf and hard-of-hearing clients may be thwarted by lack of client motivation and, especially with elderly clients, success may be affected by reduced visual acuity and attention span.

For some clients, fingerspelling and sign language may be used to indicate sounds missed in speechreading or to spell proper names. Manual signs for concepts used on a daily basis may also be learned. Realistically, however, for many elderly hearing-impaired persons these methods have limited applicability as alternatives to speechreading and aural methods because they must be learned not only by the hearing-impaired person, but by others in the environment as well. Such manual methods may be most successful when used only to supplement aural and speechreading methods, and when everyone's motivation is high.

Regardless of age, many means of support are available whereby deaf and hard-of-hearing adults can improve the quality of their daily lives. For example, although the family can provide emotional and practical support, counseling is required to explain the difficulties experienced by the client as well as the family's role in providing emotional and communication support. The family or care provider should be involved in rehabilitative approaches to foster communication effectiveness outside the therapy environment. The hearing-impaired person is only one member of the communication event; to be successful, it requires willing and knowledgeable participation of hearing members. Often the necessary participation of hearing persons in the relearning process increases the hearing-impaired person's guilt feelings upon realizing his or her dependency.

Self-help groups of hearing-impaired adults are springing up across the country, providing another means of emotional support through problem sharing. (Some groups are limited to elderly hearing-impaired persons.) These groups are most effective when they are led by a professional—a social worker or psychologist—specializing in the psychosocial aspects of hearing impairment.

Although human support is most critical to the adaptive process, many practical devices can enhance the daily lives of hearing-impaired persons. Specifically, in addition to hearing aids, hard-of-hearing persons may benefit from a variety of amplification devices in various settings. The auditory loop, for example, once used only for amplification in theatres and lecture halls, has now been adapted for use on a smaller scale in meetings or even in one-to-one communication. Some of these devices eliminate distracting environmental sounds which a standard hearing aid may not. Deaf and hard-of-hearing persons may find that certain light- or vibration-dependent warning devices are helpful, such as telephone or doorbell lights, flashing or vibrating alarm clocks, and vibrating beeper systems. Television decoders provide closed captioning of news programs, serials, movies, and sports. Captioned films, available through public libraries and film clubs, make first- and second-run movies accessible to hearing-impaired persons. Finally, telephone communication can be facilitated through built-in phone amplifiers or telecommunication devices for the deaf (TDDs), which enable complete telephone accessibility for the deaf by carrying typed messages over the telephone lines. Presently a TDD is required by both parties in a phone conversation; increasing numbers of agencies and businesses are installing TDDs, and some communities have message services which provide a relay link between those using a TDD and a party using a regular voice phone. Most of the devices mentioned are relatively low cost and convenient. In addition, new technological developments are constantly increasing their capabilities and effectiveness leading toward fuller, richer, more normal lives for hearing-impaired persons.

psychological evaluation of deaf and hard-of-hearing persons

As schools, speech and hearing clinics, rehabilitation agencies, and mental health centers strive to offer coordinated, comprehensive services to hearing-impaired persons, it is vital that the professionals involved become familiar with the basic components of psychologic and educational evaluation: available instruments, how they should be administered with the deaf and hard of hearing, what to request and expect in a psychologic evaluation report, and how to interpret such reports. It is the purpose of this section to provide a practical guide in these areas.

general considerations in evaluation of hearing-impaired persons

A number of elements are fundamental to all types of evaluation with deaf clients, regardless of age (Sullivan & Vernon, 1979; Vernon, 1976). Many of these testing principles also apply (although sometimes to lesser degrees) to deafened persons or the hard of hearing, who will demonstrate varying degrees of hearing loss and language and communication competencies. The principles include:

1. Psychologic tests involving use of verbal language are not generally valid with hearing-impaired clients. Use of such tests will produce a score that measures the language deficiencies imposed by the client's hearing loss; therefore, it does not validly measure intelligence, emotional stability, or other aptitudes.

2. Tests administered by professionals who are not experienced with hearing-impaired clients are subject to appreciably greater error than are those administered by somebody familiar with this population.

3. Group testing with deaf and hard-of-hearing individuals is not recommended, but should be regarded as a screening technique at best.

4. Congenitally hard-of-hearing clients are often more like congenitally deaf individuals in terms of psychodiagnosis than their speech and response to sound seem to suggest. Therefore, these clients should be administered tests that are appropriate for both the profoundly

hearing impaired and the normally hearing. If discrepancy in the results indicates that a client performed better on the nonlanguage measure, results of this instrument should be judged as the more valid.

types of testing and their use with hearing-impaired clients

Various types of information may be sought in a psychologic evaluation. The major types of testing and general assessment guidelines are reviewed below, with recommended testing batteries listed at the end of this section. A helpful reference in this area is Ziezula (1982).

Intelligence Testing. Three primary guidelines apply to intelligence testing with hearing-impaired adults and children:

1. The importance of avoiding verbal, language-based tests in evaluating the IQ of hearing-impaired persons must be reemphasized. To be valid as measures of intelligence (rather than of language impairment), nonverbal performance-type tests must be used (Sullivan & Vernon, 1979). With the use of such performance scales, and provided they are administered correctly, it is possible to obtain valid intelligence test scores for the hearing impaired. However, "nonverbal" tests still require verbal directions (Sullivan & Vernon, 1979). Results obtained from testing a client who may be unable to understand the task are questionable, and use of such inappropriate instruments and methods has resulted in tragic misdiagnoses (Vernon, 1976).

2. Evaluation with hard-of-hearing clients should begin with a performance measure, followed by verbal instruments if desired. Such procedures often result in an appreciably higher score on the former; in all probability, these instruments are more valid than the language-dependent test.

3. The use of only the nonverbal portion of an IQ test reduces by roughly half (or more) the items used; therefore, at least two performance scales should be given to improve validity.

Special considerations in intelligence testing with children. Testing and test results obtained with children present several considerations beyond those listed previously:

1. Test scores of preschool and early elementary-age hearing-impaired children tend to be unreliable (Sullivan & Vernon, 1979). Therefore,

these scores should be viewed as questionable, especially if low, and if no other data support them. Many factors may affect a child's performance in the testing situation in a negative way, leading to artificially low scores (Sullivan & Vernon, 1979).

2. Tests that have time limits or in other ways emphasize the time factor are not as valid as those that do not. Children may respond to being timed by working very hastily or by ignoring the time factor. Untimed tests are, therefore, preferable.

3. The questionable validity of tests administered by those unfamiliar with deafness is even more true when working with children. These children's atypical attentive set to testing, which has been frequently cited in the literature, is felt to be one of the reasons for this (Sullivan & Vernon, 1979; Zierzula, 1982).

Personality Evaluation. Personality evaluation, even with normal-hearing clients, is much more demanding and complex than evaluation of intelligence. Therefore, additional information from case history data and personal experience with the client should be taken into considera-

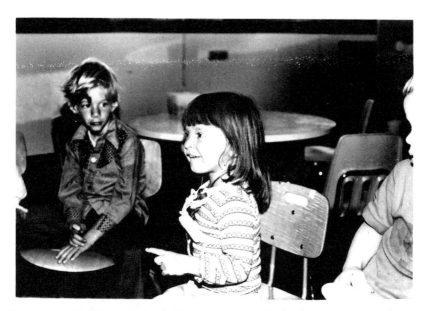

Figure 6.1. Valid psychological assessment with the hearing impaired must take into account communication skills. (From *Introduction to Aural Rehabilitation* (p. 200) by R. L. Schow and M. A. Nerbonne (Eds.), 1980, Austin, TX: PRO-ED. Reprinted with permission.)

tion when interpreting test results in this area—especially results obtained by an examiner who is unfamiliar with deafness.

One of the complicating factors is that the hearing-disabled person's communication problems make personality tests more difficult to administer (Sullivan & Vernon, 1979). In addition, many of these tests require a relatively high level of reading skills or extensive verbal exchange in addition to assuming a level of confidence and rapport that is often difficult to achieve if the subject is unable to fully understand what is being said or written. If projective tests (such as the *Rorschach*) are used, it is often necessary for the examiner to be fluent in manual communication.

In an attempt to deal with the communication problems posed by hearing-impaired clients, psychologists unfamiliar with deafness sometimes use an interpreter to translate their conversations into fingerspelling and sign language. However, use of an interpreter in psychologic evaluations may result in conclusions of questionable validity.

Whether or not the norms established for personality structure in the general population may be appropriately applied to deaf and hard-of-hearing persons must be considered when interpreting the personality evaluations of those with a hearing loss (Vernon, 1976). Although this issue remains unresolved, it is conceivable that deafness alters the environment in ways that result in a different personality organization. Consequently, with hearing-impaired clients "normality" would differ from that of persons with normal hearing (Vernon, 1976).

Clinicians not familiar with the language difficulties of hearing-impaired persons may draw inappropriate conclusions based on writing samples from deaf clients, especially those having low levels of verbal skills. Although such samples often seem to reflect confusion and disassociation, this effect is usually the result of language difficulties, not an indication of disordered or deranged thought processes.

As a result of these factors, few personality tests have gained wide acceptance for use with hearing-impaired persons.

Screening for Brain Injury. Many of the major etiologies of deafness may cause other types of damage to the central nervous system (Vernon, 1987). Psychologic evaluations should, therefore, include testing for brain damage, supplemented with information from such sources as neurologic and audiologic diagnostic techniques (Rose, 1978).

Case History Data. Because past history is the best predictor of the future, complete background information on the client is of great import. With hearing-impaired children, and sometimes with adults, contact with their school(s) is often a source of complete and perceptive information.

In addition to the usual information, a child's case history should include information relevant to the disability, such as the parents' description of the nature of the problem; its etiology and onset; history of diagnosis, including past and present professional services; and communication at home. Parental interviews often offer an insight into the parents' and child's attitudes and coping behaviors toward the hearing loss.

In addition to routine information, adult case histories should not overlook such factors as job history, family circumstances, and educational and vocational skills.

Communication Skills.   Since hearing loss manifests itself most clearly in communication skills, the evaluation process should include an assessment in this area. Although the primary responsibility for this assessment may lie with the speech pathologist and audiologist, input from the psychologist, parents, and the school's language specialist (as appropriate for young clients) may also be valuable.

Specifically, both receptive and expressive skills should be appraised in the following areas (in addition to an audiologic workup):

1. Ability with written language may be evaluated through use of school records, educational and language tests, or sentence completion. The verbal subtests of the *Wechsler* may be used by the psychologist to yield some information.

2. Speech and speechreading have considerable relevance for both the child in school and the adult at work. Thus, psychologists, counselors, and others may be involved in practical "lay" assessment in this area. Their conclusions may be questionable, however, if they are not aware of the extreme difficulty of attaining these skills. It is crucial that difficulty in communication (oral and written) not be confused with lack of intelligence. Professionals trained in these areas, especially those experienced with individuals having hearing loss, are better prepared to assess these skills and interpret the results.

3. Finally, an evaluation of the client's manual communication skills is helpful. Manual communication is the means most often employed by deaf adults to communicate among themselves, and it is gaining increasingly wide use in school settings as part of the total communication approach. Such an evaluation requires that the evaluator possess sufficient expertise to draw legitimate conclusions.

Educational Achievement.   A complete evaluation should also include an assessment of educational level. School records should be consulted for younger clients. In addition, numerous tests cover a wide range of content and skill areas. Two of the most appropriate are the *Metropolitan Achievement Tests* and the *Stanford Achievement Test*. The former has norms for both hearing and deaf subjects. The latter has recently been revised for use with deaf students by the Office of Demographic Studies at Gallaudet College (Washington, DC), and is one of the most widely used achievement tests in schools for the deaf. Both tests are easy to administer. Care must be taken that the subject understands and successfully completes the sample items in each subtest. It is also crucial that the battery chosen is at the appropriate level for the person being tested to avoid invalid results. Scores on these achievement tests, taken by hearing-impaired subjects, should be interpreted in light of the data on educational achievement presented previously in this chapter.

Aptitude and Interest Testing. Aptitude and interest are basic areas of evaluation for older teens and adults, that is, they assess any particular abilities the client may have. Hundreds of relevant tests are available. For a more complete discussion, consult Myklebust (1962) and Ziezula (1982). In general, evaluation for hearing-impaired individuals should not be based on aptitude tests that depend on language; instead, they should measure such general areas as manual dexterity, mechanical aptitudes, and spatial relations, because these types of aptitudes are directly related to the kind of work and activity carried out by most hearing-handicapped people.

Interest tests present a special challenge, since they are almost without exception highly verbal. One of these, the *General Aptitude Test Battery* (GATB), yields much misinformation when administered to hearing-impaired persons in its language-dependent form. A recent adaptation specifically for the deaf is available through the Rehabilitation Services Administration, Washington, DC.

Additional Areas of Evaluation. Although not treated in depth here, the information contributed by the audiologist, speech-language pathologist, and physician (based on physical examination and medical history) also constitutes an important part of a meaningful and complete psychologic evaluation.

recommended tests and testing batteries

The following test batteries are recommended for the age groups specified.

Preschool. Measurement of intelligence should be based on at least two of the following IQ tests: the *Leiter International Performance Scale,* the *Merrill-Palmer Scale of Mental Tests,* or the *Randalls Island Performance Tests.*

No suitable personality tests or tests for brain injury are available for deaf preschool children. Hence, clinical judgment and medical, audiologic, and case history data must be depended on exclusively for evaluation in these areas.

Beginning School Age through Age 9. IQ tests should include at least two of the following: the *Leiter International Performance Scale, Wechsler Intelligence Scale for Children-Revised* (WISC-R), *Hickey-Nebraska Test of Learning Aptitude, Goodenough-Harris Drawing Test,* or *Raven's Progressive Matrices.* Human figure drawing interpretation and *Bender-Gestalt* responses should be used to screen for personality deviations and organic brain damage.

Ages 9 through 15. The most appropriate measure of intelligence for this age range is the WISC-R. It can best be supplemented with *Raven's Progressive Matrices* or the *Leiter International Performance Scale.* Human figure drawings and the *Bender-Gestalt* become increasingly valid measures in this age range and are the best screening techniques for personality disturbance and brain damage.

Ages 16 through High School Graduation. The *Wechsler Adult Intelligence Scale - Revised* (WAIS-R) stands out as the superior measure of intelligence for this age range. The second most valid measure for intelligence is *Raven's Progressive Matrices.* In addition, the *Memory-for-Designs Test* can be added to or substituted for the *Bender-Gestalt* and *Draw-A-Person Test* and can be used as a screening measure for organic brain damage. Vocational tests should also be included at this time. Their selection is a highly individual matter that depends on the subject as well as available vocational educational facilities.

Adults. The WAIS-R, *Raven's Progressive Matrices,* or *Revised Beta* may be used as IQ tests. The *Bender-Gestalt* is useful for detection of brain damage and may be an effective projective test for personality, along with the *Draw-A-Person* and *House-Tree-Person Test.* The latter two require skilled interpretation. Finally, the *Thematic Apperception Test* may be used for personality evaluation if the psychologist and the subject can communicate fluently with each other.

recommended readings

Jacobs, L. (1980). *A deaf adult speaks out* (2nd ed.). Washington, DC: Gallaudet College Press.

Luterman, D. (1979). *Counseling parents of hearing-impaired children*. Boston: Little, Brown and Co.

Mindel, E., & Vernon, M. (1987). *They grow in silence: Understanding deaf children and adults* (2nd ed.). San Diego: College-Hill Press.

Moores, D.F. (1987). *Educating the deaf: Psychology, principles and practices* (3rd ed.). Boston: Houghton Mifflin.

Orlans, H. (Ed.). (1985). *Adjustment to adult hearing loss*. San Diego: College-Hill Press.

Quigley, S.P., & Kretschmer, R.E. (1982). *The education of deaf children: Issues, theory and practice*. Baltimore, MD: University Park Press.

Vernon, M., & Inskip, R. (1988). *Success for hard of hearing people*. Silver Spring, MD: National Association of the Deaf.

Wylie, M.A. (1987). Psychological counseling aspects of the adult remediation process. In J. Alpiner & P. McCarthy (Eds.), *Rehabilitative audiology: Children and adults* (3rd ed.). Baltimore, MD: Williams & Wilkins.

references

Erber, N. (1979). Auditory-visual perception of speech with reduced optical clarity. *Journal of Speech and Hearing Research, 22*, 212-223.

Furth, H.G. (1966). *Thinking without language*. New York: The Free Press.

Goldstein, D. (1984). Hearing impairment, hearing aids, and audiology. *Asha, 26*, 24-35.

Lenneberg, E.H. (1967). *Biological foundations of knowledge*. New York: John Wiley & Sons.

Luterman, D. (1979). *Counseling parents of hearing-impaired children*. Boston: Little, Brown and Co.

Maurer, J.F. (1982). The psychosocial aspects of presbycusis. In R.H. Hull (Ed.), *Rehabilitative audiology* (pp. 221-232). New York: Grune and Stratton.

Mindel, E., & Feldman, V. (1987). The impact of deaf children on their families. In E. Mindel & M. Vernon (Eds.), *They grow in silence* (pp. 1-30). San Diego: College-Hill Press.

Mindel, E., & Vernon, M. (1987). *They grow in silence: Understanding deaf children and adults* (2nd ed.). San Diego: College-Hill Press.

Moses, K. (1985). Dynamic intervention with families. In *Hearing-impaired children and youth with developmental disabilities* (pp. 82-98). Washington, DC: Gallaudet College Press.

Rainer, J.D., Altschuler, K.Z., Kallmann, F.J., & Deming, W.E. (Eds.). (1963). *Family and mental health problems in a deaf population.* New York: New York State Psychology Institute.

Rose, D. (1978). *Audiological assessment.* Englewood Cliffs, NJ: Prentice-Hall.

Schein, J., & Delk, M. (1974). *The deaf population of the United States.* Silver Spring, MD: National Association of the Deaf.

Siller, J. (1969). Psychological situation of the disabled with spinal cord injuries. *Rehabilitation Literature, 30,* 290-296.

Sullivan, P., & Vernon, M. (1979). Psychological assessment of hearing impaired children. *School Psych Digest, 8,* 271-290.

Trybus, R.J., & Karchmer, M.A. (1977). School achievement scores of hearing impaired children: National data on achievement status and growth patterns. *American Annals of the Deaf, 122,* 62-69.

Vernon, M. (1967). Prematurity and deafness: The magnitude and nature of the problem among deaf children. *Exceptional Children, 38,* 5-12.

Vernon, M. (1968). Fifty years of research on the intelligence of the deaf and hard-of-hearing. A survey of literature and discussion of implications. *Journal of Rehabilitation of the Deaf, 1,* 1-11.

Vernon, M. (1973, February). Psychological aspects of the diagnosis of deafness in a child. *Eye, Ear, Nose, Throat Monthly, 52,* 60-66.

Vernon, M. (1976). Psychologic evaluation of hearing-impaired children. In L. Lloyd (Ed.), *Communication assessment and intervention strategies* (pp. 195-224). Baltimore, MD: University Park Press.

Vernon, M. (1979). Parental reactions to birth defective children. *Postgraduate Medicine, 65,* 183-189.

Vernon, M. (1985). The relationship of language and thought, bilingualism, and critical stage theory to reading. In M. Douglass (Ed.), *Proceedings of Claremont reading conference, 1985* (pp. 21-30). Claremont, CA: Claremont Graduate School.

Vernon, M. (1987). Outcomes: deaf people at work. In E. Mindel & M. Vernon (Eds.), *They grow in silence* (pp. 187-196). San Diego: College-Hill Press.

Wylde, M. (1987). Psychological and counseling aspects of the adult remediation process. In J. Alpiner & P. McCarthy (Eds.), *Rehabilitative audiology: Children and adults* (3rd ed.). Baltimore, MD: Williams and Wilkins.

Ziezula, F.R. (Ed.). (1982). *Assessment of hearing-impaired people.* Washington, DC: Gallaudet College Press.

chapterseven

EDUCATIONAL ALTERNATIVES FOR THE HEARING IMPAIRED

JULIA MAESTAS Y MOORES

DONALD F. MOORES

contents

introduction

The education of the hearing impaired has a long and fascinating history, longer than any other area of special education. The first documented systematic instruction of exceptional children took place in a Spanish monastery in the 1500s where a number of recessively deaf children of the Spanish aristocracy resided (Chaves & Solar, 1974). Techniques and methods related to the facilitation of speech, speechreading, language, and cognitive development were perfected in the following two centuries and were then introduced to France by the Spanish/Portuguese educator of the deaf, Pereira (Seguin, 1866). The contributions of the Spanish pioneers provided the basis for the work of the original French educators of the deaf and of the retarded (Rosen, Clark, & Kivitz, 1976), which in turn provided the major guidelines for the first programs for the handicapped in the United States. Specifically, the deaf French educator Laurent Clerc was the major influence on the development of educational programs in America in the early 1800s (Moores, 1982), while Edward Seguin performed a similar function in educational programs for the retarded in the middle part of the 1800s (Rosen et al., 1976). Today much of the instruction of severely hearing-impaired children in the United States utilizing analytical speech and language exercises and sense training has a history of 400 years of application. Even the ''American'' Manual Alphabet is an almost exact copy of the Spanish Manual Alphabet. In addition, sense training as exemplified by Seguin's physiological method and many of the techniques developed by Montessori may be traced back to the same roots (Maestas y Moores, in press).

It should be pointed out, however, that most of the work with the hearing impaired has concentrated on individuals with severe hearing losses, those who would traditionally be characterized as *deaf*. It is relatively easy to document trends in research, educational practices, and school placement for this population due to the enormous bodies of literature in each of these areas. Although mild and moderate hearing losses are far more frequent, much less information is available on the population traditionally classified as *hard of hearing* in regard to difficulties in the development of phonologic, grammatic, semantic, academic, and linguistic skills (see chapters 5, 8, & 11). At present, a large majority of children with severe and profound hearing losses receive special services, whereas a majority of those with mild and moderate losses are not being served.

hearing impairment and hearing handicap defined

Part of the difficulty of securing proper services lies in the process of identification. Many children, especially those with mild losses, are misdiagnosed as mildly retarded or learning disabled. Even when correctly diagnosed, these children have not received top priority for services because they are not perceived as suffering from as great a handicap as a child with deafness, blindness, or highly restricted mobility. Additional difficulties arise over the confusion between the terms *impairment* and *handicap*. A hearing impairment is measured by reception of speech and other sounds calibrated for frequency and intensity. A handicap, on the other hand, cannot be stated in such easily quantifiable terms. Rather, it refers to the extent to which impairment limits an individual's functioning.

One example of the different ideas about the relationship between handicap and impairment can be observed in connection with a statement from the Conference of Executives of American Schools for the Deaf (CEASD—now known as the Conference of Educational Administrators Serving the Deaf). This group established a four-level system based on impairment for classification of hearing loss (Frisina, 1974). Based on the impairment level, different amounts of handicap were predicted and rehabilitation services recommended. It has been several years since the system was devised, and it is no longer considered to be an acceptable general guideline in view of advances in our knowledge about hearing impairment and its complications. For one thing, the classification system assumes that unless a child has at least a 35 dB loss he/she will not need special speech, hearing, language, and educational services. However, considerable evidence suggests that this is a very questionable level for initiating services. As noted in Chapter 1, the lower fence should probably be about 20 dB. Even though the authors clearly stated that the resulting handicap may vary, it is clear that there are not only individual differences but also needed revisions in this outdated interpretation of impairment findings.

The complexity of the situation was noted in Chapter 1. As suggested, two individuals may have identical audiograms while differing greatly in development of speech, use of residual hearing, academic achievement, or language. Contributing factors include age at onset of hearing loss, age at identification of loss and provision of services, appropriateness and adequacy of services, and presence of other potentially handicapping conditions. Approximately 30% of children in programs for the hearing impaired in the United States suffer from additional handicapping conditions (Gentile & McCarthy, 1973). A hearing-impaired child with additional difficulties, such as visual perception dysfunction, mental retardation, cerebral palsy, or neurologic impairment, is unlikely to respond as effectively to aural management as a child suffering from hearing impairment alone.

estimates of incidence

Hearing loss is relatively common in the general population and most individuals experience a lessening of hearing acuity with age. In the most extensive study of hearing loss in the United States, Schein and Delk (1974) determined that of the nearly 2 million who are described as deaf, approximately 200,000 became deaf prelingually, another 200,000 became deaf between 3 and 19 years of age.

Only a portion of these persons are presently in the educational system. Since the majority of hearing losses are acquired in adulthood, they are not of concern in the present chapter. Prevalence figures for the hearing-impaired school-age population are discussed in detail in Chapters 1 and 8. The shocking statistics, however, have to do with the level of services provided. Over 90% of the children classified as deaf are being served educationally. On the other hand, less than 25% of the hard-of-hearing children have been identified as receiving adequate services (Sontag, Smith, & Certo, 1977). Thus, using even conservative estimates, less than one-third of the total number of hearing-impaired school-age children are receiving special services. Those provided intensive educational treatment tend to be classified as deaf. Individuals in the hard-of-hearing category fortunate enough to be provided any special assistance receive training primarily in speech and hearing and, to a lesser extent, language.

educational programs and services

early intervention/preschool

During the late 1960s, it became widely recognized that hearing-impaired children can benefit from educational efforts before the normal school-entry age. Early intervention can take advantage of the ''critical period'' of language development (see Chapter 5). Most early intervention programs emphasize parental involvement in the educational process. Programs are typically carried out through home visits by a clinician, parental visits to the clinic/demonstration home, or a combination thereof (see Chapter 8). After this type of early, home-based training the child may be placed in a variety of preschool and later primary/secondary educational settings.

school placement alternatives

It is a mistake to think of the educational options as being limited to segregated vs. integrated placement. In general, the most common types of programs for hearing-impaired children may be classified as follows:

1. *Residential schools.* In most such programs a majority of students reside in the school. However, in areas accessible to large populations, substantial numbers of children live at home and commute daily. The pattern is for children within commuting distance to attend on a day basis, with those living farther away staying at school at least during weekdays. Most classes are self-contained. Growing numbers of residential schools are developing cooperative programs with local public schools for integrated education for some of their students.

2. *Day schools.* These programs are established in some of the larger metropolitan areas in separate schools for the deaf to which children commute daily. Students with normal hearing do not attend these schools.

3. *Day classes.* Day class programs have traditionally been differentiated from day schools in that the latter refer to classes for the hearing impaired in a public school building where the majority of students have normal hearing. Classroom instruction may range from completely self-contained classes for the hearing impaired to children spending most of their time in a regular classroom. In the past, children having some hearing and better oral communication skills were integrated. Now many programs, especially at the secondary level, utilize manual interpreters in regular classes thereby enabling many profoundly deaf children to attend.

4. *Resource rooms.* Most resource rooms are planned so that children spend most of their day in regular classes, returning to the teacher of the hearing impaired for special attention, usually in language and in academic areas of concern. Whereas day class programs typically contain several classes with homogeneous groupings of hearing-impaired children, there may be only one or two resource rooms in a building with the teacher providing individualized services to children who vary in age, hearing loss, and academic achievement.

5. *Itinerant programs.* Under this type of program, a child attends regular classes full time and receives service on an ''itinerant'' basis periodically. This may vary from daily to weekly lessons, depending on a child's needs. In these situations one teacher might work with children from several schools.

6. *Team teaching.* The authors have worked with programs in which a class of hearing children and a class of hearing-impaired children are merged and taught cooperatively by a regular classroom teacher and a teacher of the deaf. In several such cases simultaneous oral/manual communication has been employed. The results of these efforts have been encouraging, and it is hoped that a trend toward this type of placement will develop over the next several years.

present patterns

Rawlings and Trybus (1978) sent questionnaires to 1,020 programs identified as serving hearing-impaired children and received 809 responses. A total enrollment of 60,231 students was obtained, from which the authors estimated that the total national enrollment in special education programs for hearing-impaired children is about 69,000. The disparity between this figure and that of 111,000 reported by BEH may be explained by the large number of children receiving speech and hearing services only.

Of the students identified, almost 50% were enrolled in part-time or full-time classes in public school programs. Another 32% were enrolled in residential schools for the deaf. The remainder attended public day schools for the deaf separate from schools for children with normal hearing or separate day or residential programs for the multiply handicapped. The median enrollment was 256 for residential schools, 17 for school districts with full-time classes, and 25 for school districts with part-time classes. As might be expected, the support services varied tremendously across categories. For example, 97% of the residential schools reported having the services of an audiologist or audiometrist, as opposed to 37% of the school districts with full-time classes and 50% of the districts with part-time classes. On the other hand, the latter programs had available services of public school personnel representative of most school districts. Thus, we find that the services of speech-language pathologists are available in more than 80% of the school districts, but only 63% of the residential schools.

educational placement, public law 94-142, and mainstreaming

The placement of hearing-impaired children has received growing attention in recent years, an attention that was magnified in November, 1975, with the passage of PL 94-142, the Education of all Handicapped Children Act. The major goal of PL 94-142 is to assure that all handicapped children from ages 3 through 21 receive appropriate special educational services. In 1986, PL 99-457 was enacted, which basically mandates these same services to children from birth through two years of age (see Chapter 8). In order to meet this goal, states are mandated to develop plans by which handicapped children must be served. As a result of a series of court decisions, the impetus has been to develop appropriate educational programs for those children demonstrating the most severe handicaps and children who previously have not received special services. Much of the activity has also been related to the concept of "least restrictive environment," that is, the idea that it is preferable to educate handicapped children together with nonhandicapped children to the greatest extent possible. In some areas, this has been tied with the *mainstreaming movement*. Until recently mainstreaming consisted essentially of moving children classified as mildly mentally retarded out of special classes and back into regular classrooms. Essentially, these are children who never should have been segregated in the first place (Kirk, 1975). Educators of the hearing impaired never committed the sin of mislabeling and segregating children with mild and moderate handicaps. Our sin was one of omission. We never identified the children in the first place. Over the generations these children have tended to sit in the regular classrooms without services. As previously noted, 80% of all hard-of-hearing children receive no special services. For these children, mainstreaming is irrelevant—they have always been mainstreamed—the objective now is to provide them the services they never have received in their neighborhood schools. It is anticipated that the mandate of PL 94-142 and PL 99-457 to provide special services to children who have been without services in the past will be of special benefit to children who fall under the classification of *hard of hearing*

For children currently receiving services, the question of segregated and integrated placement cannot be answered adequately because the characteristics of the children in different settings are variable. For example, in an extensive study of over 49,000 children, Karchmer and Trybus (1977) reported that nearly two-thirds of the children in residential schools were classified as profoundly deaf (91 dB loss or greater in the better ear) as contrasted to only 18% of children in integrated programs. In addition, the percentage of postlingually deafened children was three times as great in integrated programs (13% to 4%). Karchmer and Trybus continued:

> The integrated programs enroll the highest proportion of children from high income families (i.e., over $20,000 annually) and the lowest proportion of

> very low income families (under $5,000 annually) . . . Children in integrated
> programs have the highest proportion of college educated fathers (36%) while
> children in day schools have the lowest (19%). (p. 3)

As might be expected, integrated programs enroll a higher proportion of children with "intelligible" or "very intelligible" speech. Karchmer and Trybus expressed surprise at their finding that this group did
not report the highest levels of hearing aid use—it was exceeded in this
regard by children in segregated day schools and in segregated full-time
classes. The authors speculated that this may be related, in part, to the
high proportion of very mild hearing losses in the integrated group.
Also, the children in residential schools tend to be older. Specifically,
47% of the residential students were 15 years or older, compared to 36%
of the integrated students, 23% of the day school students, and 18%
of the segregated day class students. These figures represent a tendency
for children to move from a day to a residential education as they reach
adolescence—a tendency likely to decline as the impact of PL 94-142
is felt in years to come.

Karchmer and Trybus (1977) summarized their data as follows:

> This is where mainstreaming is at the present time. It will be interesting
> and of critical importance to trace the changes in this picture over the next
> few years under the influence of PL 94-142. For the present, however, it
> is clear that the integrated programs are generally serving a group of hear-
> ing impaired children who are very different on many educationally critical
> dimensions from those children who attend other types of special educa-
> tional programs. (p. 3)

In an attempt to chart the impact of PL 94-142 and examine its
influence on mainstreaming since 1977 (the law was passed in 1975 but
implementation was scheduled for 1977-78), the present authors analyzed enrollment data from the Directory of Services issues of the *American Annals of the Deaf*. Enrollments were compared from the 1971-72
academic year, five years before implementation of PL 94-142, to enrollments for 1982-83, the latest date for which data were available and five
years after implementation. The first important finding is that enrollment was similar for the two academic years: 46,075 in 1971-72 (Craig
& Craig, 1972) and 46,257 in 1982-83 (Craig & Craig, 1983). The same
sources report that enrollment in residential schools for the deaf declined
4.7% during the same period, from 18,767 in 1971-72 to 17,887 in 1982-83.
Put another way, children enrolled in public residential schools
represented 41% (18,767 of 46,075) of children identified in 1971-72 and
39% (17,887 of 46,257) in 1982-83. Thus, in spite of extensive attention

to mainstreaming of deaf students, the impact on enrollments in public residential schools appears to be surprisingly small.

The real impact, therefore, appears to have been not on public but on private residential school enrollment. Specifically, during the same period there was a 74% decline in private residential school enrollment, from 1,847 in 1971-72 (Craig & Craig, 1972) to 475 in 1982-83 (Craig & Craig, 1983). This means that for 1972-73, approximately 4% of students were enrolled in private residential schools for the deaf (1,847 of 46,075). By 1982-83 this number had dropped to 1% (475 of 46,257). Further evidence of the decline is found in reports by private residential schools that 69 students graduated in 1972 (Craig & Craig, 1972), only 20 in 1982 (Craig & Craig, 1983).

To date, therefore, the free appropriate public education and least restrictive environment mandates of PL 94-142 in general have had only moderate impact on public residential school educational programs for the deaf while having tremendous implications for private residential school educational programs, where enrollments have declined precipitously.

In turning to the hard of hearing it should be noted that educators of hard-of-hearing students are more restrained in their enthusiasm about mainstreaming than other educators. For example, Ross (1977) stated,

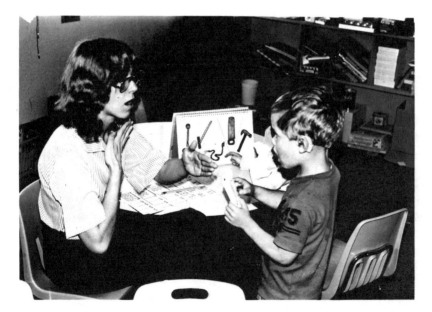

Figure 7.1. Therapy conducted outside the classroom for mainstreamed children.

"Although physically present in the mainstream, they [hard-of-hearing children] have been, more often than not, if one can forgive the cliché, simply drowning there" (p. 5). In a similar vein, Davis (1977) noted that hard-of-hearing children are the most "mainstreamed" of all handicapped children, but that they have not received the special help they need:

> The result of these facts is such that few educators point with pride toward the results of mainstreaming as they are demonstrated in the achievements of hard of hearing children. For one thing very little is known about the children's educational achievements, the types of problems they face in regular classrooms, their acceptance or non-acceptance by normally hearing peers, the relation between the support services offered them and their achievements, or the extent of those support services in the average school system. . . . It is painfully evident that, for the hard of hearing, at least, mainstreaming is a very mixed blessing when the children are not provided with special services. (p. 13)

In sum, changes toward mainstreaming have not been as dramatic as some educators have assumed. However, the trends are clear and should continue. The growing range of options for an increasing number of hearing-impaired children is impressive. Different issues now have to be addressed, including curriculum modification, socialization, and participation in extracurricular activities. The situation presents both interesting and exciting challenges.

student characteristics

As we move toward individual educational programs based on the unique characteristics of a particular child, a plethora of factors must be considered. Particularly educationally relevant characteristics might include extent of hearing loss, type of loss, age at onset, potential hearing status, presence of other handicapping conditions, ethnic background, and parental education. Given the pluralistic nature of American society children enter the educational system with a variety of backgrounds and expectations.

Information provided the authors by the Center for Assessment and Demographic Studies at Gallaudet College indicates that approximately 30% of children in programs for the hearing impaired are of minority status, with Blacks accounting for more than 20%, Hispanics for almost 10% of the total. These figures are higher than for the general school-age population. It is possible that the incidence of hearing loss for Black and Hispanic children is higher because of less adequate medical care. In a study of the needs of Black deaf children, Moores and Oden (1978) concluded that: (a) there was a higher rate of acquired hearing loss in Blacks because of a lack of medical services; (b) there was a scarcity of Black professionals, both hearing and deaf, in the field; (c) there were inadequate early identification programs and preschool services; and (d) there was a tendency to classify Black deaf children inappropriately as deaf/retarded.

Data also indicate a rapid increase in the numbers of Hispanic children receiving services in programs for the hearing impaired. For example, 26% of the children in programs for the hearing impaired in Texas were identified as Hispanic (Trybus, Rawlings, & Johnson, 1978). Spanish was spoken in the homes of 19% of all children in programs for the hearing impaired in Texas. While it is unclear to what extent the situation in Texas can be generalized to other states and regions in the country, there is little doubt that substantial numbers of Hispanic hearing-impaired children come from monolingual Spanish or bilingual Spanish/English environments.

There is a great need for a substantially increased number of Black and Hispanic professionals to work with hearing-impaired children. At the same time, there is an equally great need for all professionals to develop a sensitivity toward the multicultural nature of American society. This is especially true of hearing and speech specialists working with hearing-impaired children whose reference group may employ a dialect or language different from that of the specialist, with distinctions in phonology, morphology, syntax, semantics, and even social and pragmatic functions of language. Any program of aural habilitation or rehabilitation must take such considerations into account if it is to be successful (Maestras y Moores, 1983).

academic achievement

As in other areas, the academic problems of deaf children have been documented much more extensively than those of hard-of-hearing children. In general, deaf children of normal intelligence suffer from severe academic retardation caused primarily by difficulties in understanding and expressing standard English. Achievement, then, tends to be highest in the areas with relatively little reliance on English skills and lowest in areas highly dependent on English. Thus, in typical achievement test batteries, scores on subtests like arithmetic computation, spelling, and punctuation are relatively high. On the other hand, scores on subtests requiring proficiency in English (e.g., paragraph meaning, science, and word meaning) are relatively low.

Working with data on more than 16,000 deaf students, Gentile (1973) compared paragraph meaning and arithmetic computation grade-equivalent scores on the *Stanford Achievement Test* at ages 8, 11, 14, and 17. As illustrated in Figure 7.2, essentially no difference was found between males and females on either subtest at any age—an interesting finding since normal-hearing females tend to be superior to males in paragraph meaning with males superior to females in arithmetic computation (Moores, 1982).

Figure 7.2 also illustrates the differential growth in achievement between the subtests. At age 8, the scores are similar, slightly less than Grade 2. By 17 years of age the average deaf student achieves a 6.03 grade-equivalent score in arithmetic achievement and 4.02 in paragraph meaning, a differential of two years.

Although arithmetic computation scores are relatively high compared to paragraph meaning, they are far below what should be achieved. Thus, an average 17-year-old should achieve at the 12th-grade level. There-

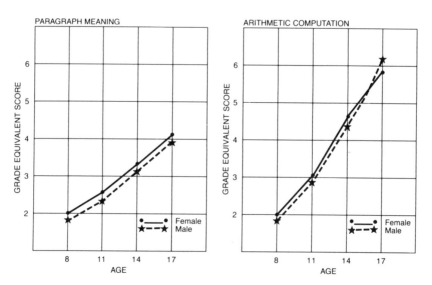

Figure 7.2. Grade-equivalent scores for deaf males and females at four ages. (From *Additional Handicapping Conditions among Hearing Impaired Students, United States, 1971–1972* (p. 5) by A. Gentile and B. McCarthy, 1973, Washington, DC: Gallaudet College Office of Demographic Studies, Series D., No. 13.)

fore, based on these data, deaf 17-year-olds are six years behind in arithmetic computation and eight years behind in paragraph meaning. Given the evidence that deaf children have normal intellectual abilities, the results illustrate glaring weaknesses in traditional educational programs for the deaf.

Table 7.1 lists the achievement of 1,439 hearing-impaired students, primarily of high-school age, who were tested on the Intermediate II Battery of the *Stanford Achievement Test*. Although the scores are somewhat higher than those reported by Gentile (1973), the problem is similar—the more dependent achievement is on knowledge of the English language, the more difficulty hearing-impaired children will encounter. Thus, spelling and arithmetic computation are relatively high, with reading (word meaning and paragraph meaning) and science scores low. The challenge for educators of the hearing impaired, therefore, is to work constantly on improving their students' expressive and receptive communication skills while exposing them to appropriate academic content in areas like the natural and behavioral sciences. Frequently, given the intellectual capacity of deaf students, course content may be the same as that for students with normal hearing. Teachers must strive to present the material at appropriate intellectual levels while working within the constraints of the students' limitations in complex English grammar and vocabulary.

TABLE 7.1
Average Grade Equivalent for Hearing-Impaired Students.
Intermediate II Battery, *Stanford Achievement Test*

Subtest	Average Grade Equivalent
Spelling	7.71
Arithmetic Computation	7.12
Arithmetic Applications	6.26
Arithmetic Concepts	6.05
Social Studies	5.85
Language	5.77
Paragraph Meaning	5.29
Science	5.09
Word Meaning	4.83

Note. Students were primarily of high-school age.
From *Academic Test Results of a National Testing Program for Hearing Impaired Students* (p. 28) by S. DiFrancesca, 1972, Washington, DC: Gallaudet College Office of Demographic Studies, Series D., No. 9.

The research on hard-of-hearing children's academic performance is limited, but evidence suggests some academic retardation even with very mild hearing losses. Quigley and Thomure (1968), for example, found that children with losses as slight as 15 dB experienced academic difficulties. In dealing with otitis media, Ling (1972) noted that mild hearing losses were frequently accompanied by lowered academic performance and language disfluencies. Therefore, there is reason to believe that many children may be handicapped educationally by mild and moderate hearing losses. The reader is referred to Ross and Giolas (1978) and Roeser and Downs (1988) for an extensive summary of studies on this question, as well as to Chapter 5 in this text.

oral, manual, and total communication programs

Historically, hearing-impaired children have been educated using either an oral, manual, or a total communication approach. The oral approach emphasizes the use of speech, hearing, and speechreading to communicate, while the manual method utilizes a form of signs (see Chapter 4). Total communication involves the use of speech, hearing, speechreading, and manual communication in a combined, simultaneous manner.

With the exception of the move to integrate hearing-impaired children with normal-hearing peers, the greatest trend in education of the hearing impaired since the late 1960s has been a massive shift from oral-only or manual-only instruction—especially in the preschool and elementary grades—to combined oral-manual instruction, or total communication. Most of the research in the area has been conducted with children having severe to profound losses. Therefore, the extent to which results can be generalized to the entire hearing-impaired population is unclear.

The present chapter touches only lightly on issues related to use of manual-only communication, as this approach has not been utilized much by itself in recent years. (For an extended treatment of structural characteristics and educational research in manual communication, see Moores, 1974, 1979, 1987.) In the 1960s a move away from oral-only education began to gain momentum based on several empirical findings. First, a growing body of research showed that deaf children of deaf parents demonstrated superior academic achievement and English skills compared to deaf children of hearing parents, with oral-aural skills being equivalent. These results seriously challenged traditional beliefs that manual communication would detract from speech, speechreading, use of residual hearing, academic achievement, and acquisition of English. In contrast, it seemed to facilitate English, academic achievement, and speechreading, while having little or no effect on speech or use of residual hearing. Second, the claims of Soviet educators that use of fingerspelling improved language and academic skills received wide attention. Third, educators in the United States were frustrated over the apparent shortcomings of the oral-only techniques in use, a frustration that was intensified by the failure of so many of the preschool programs established in the 1950s and 1960s to document any lasting benefits. In fact, deaf children of deaf parents exhibited higher English and academic achievement without preschool than deaf children of hearing parents having had intensive preschool experience.

The shift in communication modes was strongly substantiated by the results of a study by Jordan, Gustason, and Rosen (1976), who reported that total communication was used in a majority of programs for the deaf by 1975. The term *total communication* (TC) was used to describe the use of all types of communication: speech, speechreading, residual hearing, fingerspelling, signs, and print. From 1968 to 1975, 302 programs had changed from oral-only methods to some form of simultaneous oral-manual instruction, only five had changed from oral-manual to oral-only. A followup investigation (Jordan, Gustason, & Rosen, 1979) revealed a continuation of the trend over a 10-year period from 1968 to 1978. During that time 481 programs discontinued oral-only instruction while 538 turned to total communication. At every level—preschool, elementary, junior high, and senior high—total communication was emphasized in a majority of programs. One interesting sidelight is the finding by Jordan et al. that more than 30% of programs reporting some form of mainstreaming provided sign interpreters in the regular classrooms.

At present, many programs are developing more flexibility toward children's communication needs. Thus, more and more programs are providing options depending on the needs of a particular child at a particular period of time. For example, in a large number of programs classified as total communication programs, students receive oral-only instruction. This situation suggests a growing adaptability among educators and a movement away from highly charged controversial stands on the issue of methodology. (See Chapter 11, Case 4, as an example of such flexibility.)

In a five-year evaluation of preschool programs for the severely hearing impaired, Moores and associates (Moores, 1985; Moores, Weiss, & Goodwin, 1978) found that the most successful programs implemented cognitive academic and simultaneous oral-manual components from the

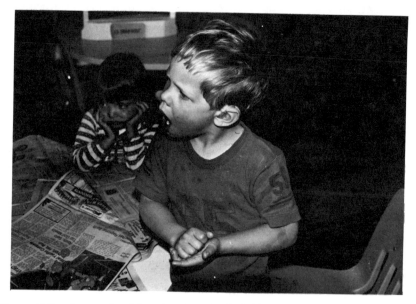

Figure 7.3. A preschool hearing-impaired child using total communication.

beginning. Evidence suggested that it was harmful to delay either cognitive-academic training or use of manual communication. Children who did not receive such training and communication at an early age did not catch up by 8 years of age. In fact, in some cases, the gap widened. The least beneficial approach for the children studied included an aural-only methodology within a traditional, socially oriented nursery school framework. In contrast, the most beneficial approach incorporated aural-oral-manual components with a wide degree of flexibility, depending upon the needs of the individual child.

In spite of documented improvements including the use of different communication systems, more placement options, early intervention programs, qualitative improvements in individual hearing aids, and so forth, there is not reason for sanguinity over either the current situation or projections for the near future. Large numbers of deaf adolescents still possess minimal speech, linguistic, academic, and vocational skills. Progress has been incremental, with no real qualitative breakthroughs, with the possible exception of the expansion of postsecondary programs.

The emergence of total communication programs has raised a number of issues. First, since it is clear that many hearing-impaired children perform adequately without recourse to manual communication, there is a need to develop an effective way to determine whether total communication or an oral-only approach is the most appropriate for a given child. Philosophically, this represents a break from previous approaches, in which the superiority of one method or another was argued for *all* children. Concern with the education of a *particular* child at a *particular* stage of development may move educators away from simplistic either/or dichotomies.

postsecondary education

The development of postsecondary educational programs for the deaf since the 1960s has been an unquestioned success. Gallaudet College, established in 1864, remained the only postsecondary institution for the deaf in the world up to the early 1960s. During that decade the federal government established the National Technical Institute for the Deaf as well as three regional vocational technical programs in St. Paul, Minnesota, Seattle, Washington, and New Orleans, Louisiana. Another cluster of programs developed out of federal legislation which specified that states were obligated to spend significant portions of federal money in support of vocational education to provide training for the handicapped. The growth of these programs has been so rapid that 102 postsecondary programs for the deaf in the United States were identified for the 1982-83 academic year (Rawlings, Karchmer, & Decaro, 1983). The majority of programs were established within facilities for students with normal hearing and ranged from vocational training programs through four-year degree programs. The programs offer a wide range of support services including interpreting (98% of the programs), notetaking (95%), vocational counseling (92%), and speech and hearing services (72%). For complete information the reader is referred to *College and Career Programs for Deaf Students: 1983 Edition* (Rawlings et al., 1983).

Finally, the tremendous growth in postsecondary enrollment may be illustrated by the fact that prior to 1960 Gallaudet College had an enrollment of less than 400 deaf students. Rawlings et al. identified 5,567 students in 102 programs in 1983; of these 1,142 attended Gallaudet and 993 were enrolled at NTID. Armstrong and Schneidmiller (1983) estimated that the college participation rate of young deaf adults is now roughly equivalent to that of the general young adult population—about 40%. To date, this virtual revolution has not received the attention it deserves.

summary

Educational alternatives for hearing-impaired children do not follow a clear pattern. For children with severe to profound hearing losses, great strides have been made in recent years. Thus, more children now have a wide range of placement options available, from residential schools to self-contained classrooms, to resource rooms, to services from an itinerant professional. Emotionally charged debates over the use of manual communication also appear to be on the wane, with a range of program options available in most settings. Also, there is a slow, but steady, increase in the quality of services available to children from ethnic minorities. Finally, evidence is accumulating to suggest that preschool programs are achieving greater success than those of even 10 years ago. Although many problems continue to exist, significant improvements have been made in education of the deaf in recent years.

The educational situation for those classified as hard of hearing provides less cause for optimism, however. A minority of these children receive special educational services at present. There is no clear understanding of their linguistic, social, or academic problems. Neither American Speech-Language-Hearing Association requirements for speech-language pathologists and audiologists nor Council on Education of the Deaf certification requirements for teachers of the hearing impaired differentiate between deaf and hard-of-hearing students. As a result, the more obvious needs of deaf children have received priority (Davis & Murphy, 1977). With the mandates of PL 94-142 and the recent PL 99-457 perhaps the situation will begin to change. The law stipulates that special attention be given to children not currently served and that all children must have an individualized education program (IEP). If, indeed, the intent of the law is carried out, hard-of-hearing children will begin to receive the attention often denied them in the past.

recommended readings

Meadow, K. (1980). *Deafness and child development*. Berkeley: University of California Press.

Moores, D. (1987). *Educating the deaf: Psychology, principles and practices*. Boston: Houghton Mifflin.

Roeser, R., & Downs, M. (Eds.). (1988). *Auditory disorders in school children* (2nd ed.). New York: Thieme-Stratton.

Ross, M. (1982). *Hard of hearing children in regular schools*. Englewood Cliffs, NJ: Prentice Hall.

organizations and journals for further information

Alexander Graham Bell Association for the Deaf, 3417 Volta Place, NW, Washington, DC 20007 (Organization for teachers and other professionals interested in deaf education.) Publication: *Volta Review*.

American Deafness and Rehabilitation Association, 814 Thayer Avenue, Silver Spring, MD 20910 (Organization for rehabilitation and human service delivery personnel serving deaf adults.) Publication: *Journal of Rehabilitation of the Deaf*.

Convention of American Instructors of the Deaf, 814 Thayer Avenue, Silver Spring, MD 20910 (Organization for teachers and other professionals interested in deaf education.) Publication: *American Annals of the Deaf*.

International Association of Parents of the Deaf, 814 Thayer Avenue, Silver Spring, MD 20910 (An organization by and for parents of deaf children.) Publication: *The Endeavor*.

John Tracy Clinic, 806 W. Adams Blvd., Los Angeles, CA 90007.

National Association of the Deaf, 814 Thayer Avenue, Silver Spring, MD 20910 (National organization of, by, and for deaf persons.) Publication: *The Deaf American*.

Public Service Programs, Gallaudet College, Washington, DC 20002.

references

Armstrong, D., & Schneidmiller, K. (1983). *Hearing impaired students enrolled in U.S. higher education institutions*. Washington, DC: Gallaudet College Office of Planning.

Chaves, T., & Solar, J. (1974). Pedro Ponce de Leon, first teacher of the deaf. *Sign Language Studies, 5*, 48-63.

Craig, W., & Craig, H. (Eds.). (1972). Directory of services. *American Annals of the Deaf, 116*.

Craig, W., & Craig, H. (Eds.). (1982). Directory of services. *American Annals of the Deaf, 126.*

Craig, W., & Craig, H. (Eds.). (1983). Directory of services. *American Annals of the Deaf, 127.*

Davis, J. (Ed.). (1977). *Our forgotten children: Hard of hearing pupils in the schools.* Minneapolis: University of Minnesota.

Davis, J., & Murphy, L. (1977). Personnel preparation for services to the hard of hearing. In J. Davis (Ed.), *Our forgotten children: Hard of hearing pupils in the schools* (pp. 43-52). Minneapolis: University of Minnesota.

DiFrancesca, S. (1972). *Academic test results of a national testing program for hearing impaired students.* Washington, DC: Gallaudet College Office of Demographic Studies, Series D, No. 9.

Frisina, R. (1974). *Report of the committee to redefine deaf and hard of hearing.* Washington, DC: Conference of Executives of American Schools for the Deaf.

Gentile, A. (1973). *Further studies in achievement testing.* Washington, DC: Gallaudet College Office of Demographic Studies, Series D, No. 13.

Gentile, A., & McCarthy, B. (1973). *Additional handicapping conditions among hearing impaired students, United States, 1971-1972.* Washington, DC: Gallaudet College Office of Demographic Studies, Series D, No. 14.

Jordan, I., Gustason, G., & Rosen, R. (1976). Current communication trends of programs for the deaf. *American Annals of the Deaf, 121,* 527-531.

Jordan, I., Gustason, G., & Rosen, R. (1979). An update on communication trends in programs for the deaf. *American Annals of the Deaf, 124,* 527-531.

Karchmer, M., & Trybus, R. (1977). *Who are the deaf children in "mainstream" programs?* Washington, DC: Gallaudet College of Demographic Studies, Series R, No. 4.

Kirk, S. (1975, August). *Labelling, categorizing and mainstreaming.* Paper presented at International Conference of Special Education, Kent, England.

Ling, D. (1972). Rehabilitation of cases with deafness secondary to otitis media. In A. Glorig & K. S. Gerwin (Eds.), *Otitis media* (pp. 249-253). Springfield, IL: Charles C. Thomas Publisher.

Maestas y Moores, J. (1983). Status of Hispanics in special education. In G. Gelgado (Ed.), *The Hispanic deaf* (pp. 14-27). Washington, DC: Gallaudet College Press.

Moores, D. (1974). Non-vocal systems of verbal behavior. In R. Schiefelbusch & L. Lloyd (Eds.), *Language perspectives: Acquisition, retardation, and intervention* (pp. 377-417). Baltimore, MD: University Park Press.

Moores, D. (1979). Hearing impairments. In S. Lily (Ed.), *Children with special needs: A survey of special education.* New York: Holt, Rinehart & Winston.

Moores, D. (1985). A longitudinal evaluation of early intervention programs for the deaf. In K. Nelson (Ed.), *Children's language* (pp. 159-186). Englewood Cliffs, NJ: Erlbaum.

Moores, D. (1987). *Educating the deaf: Psychology, principles, and practices.* Boston: Houghton Mifflin.

Moores, D., & Oden, C. (1978). Educational needs of Black deaf children. *American Annals of the Deaf, 122,* 313-318.

Moores, D., Weiss, K., & Goodwin, M. (1978). Early education programs for hearing impaired children. *American Annals of the Deaf, 123*, 925-936.

Quigley, S., & Thomure, R. (1968). *Some effects of hearing impairment on school performance.* Urbana, IL: University of Illinois, Institute for Research on Exceptional Children.

Rawlings, B., & Trybus, R. (1978). Personnel, facilities and services available in classes for hearing impaired children in the United States. *American Annals of the Deaf, 123*, 99-114.

Roeser, R., & Downs, M. (Eds.). (1988). *Auditory disorders in school children* (2nd ed.). New York: Thieme-Stratton.

Rosen, M., Clark, G., & Kivitz, M. (Eds.). (1976). *The history of mental retardation, vols. I and II.* Baltimore, MD: University Park Press.

Ross, M. (1977). Definitions and descriptions. In J. Davis (Ed.), *Our forgotten children: Hard of hearing pupils in the schools* (pp. 5-19). Minneapolis: University of Minnesota.

Ross, M., & Giolas, T. (1978). Introduction. In M. Ross & T. Giolas (Eds.), *Auditory management of hearing-impaired children: Principles and prerequisites for intervention* (pp. 1-13). Baltimore, MD: University Park Press.

Schein, J., & Delk, M. (1974). *The deaf population of the United States.* Silver Spring, MD: National Association of the Deaf.

Seguin, E. (1866). *Idiocy and its treatment of the physiological method.* New York: Wilbur Ward.

Sontag, E., Smith, J., & Certo, N. (Eds.). (1977). *Educational programming for the severely and profoundly handicapped.* Reston, VA: Council for Exceptional Children.

Trybus, R., Rawlings, B., & Johnson, R. (1978). *Texas state study of hearing impaired children and youth.* Washington, DC: Gallaudet College Office of Demographic Studies, Series C, No. 2.

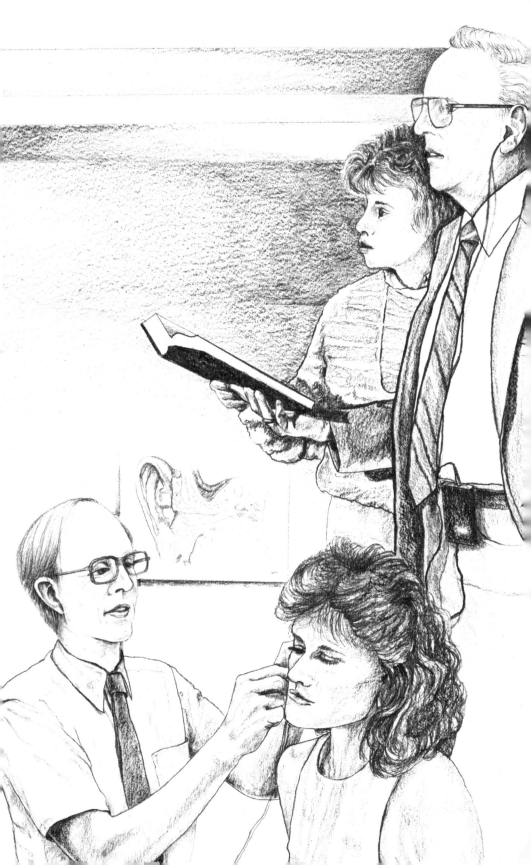

parttwo

comprehensive approaches
to aural rehabilitation

Rehabilitation of the hearing impaired has been an ongoing
concern for centuries. During this time, therefore, an extensive,
almost overwhelming variety of approaches and alternatives
to aural rehabilitation for persons of all ages and degrees of
impairment has been developed. This section will
describe past and present procedures and
their use with three major age groups.

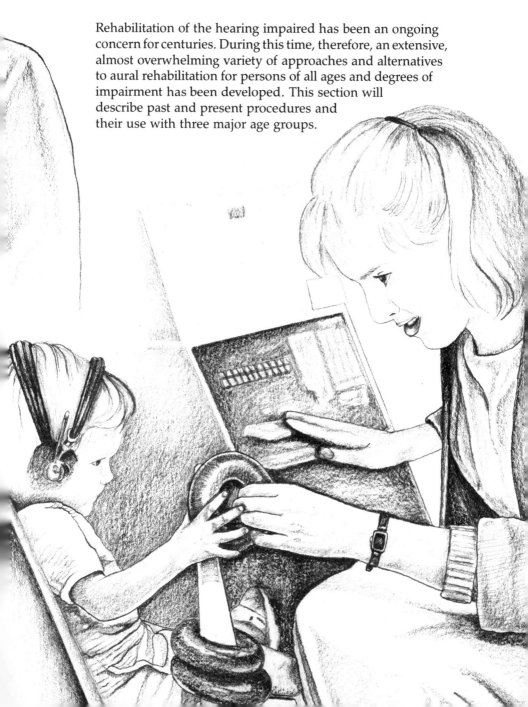

chaptereight

AURAL REHABILITATION FOR CHILDREN

SUSAN WATKINS

RONALD L. SCHOW

contents

introduction

This chapter will provide a comprehensive discussion of aural rehabilitation for children as provided at two major levels: (a) parent-infant and preschool and (b) the school years. Before the specific components that constitute the rehabilitation process at various stages of a child's development are addressed, however, the reader will get a brief overview of prevalence and service delivery statistics, applicable definitions and terms, a general profile of the client, typical rehabilitation settings at various age levels, and the identification/evaluation process.

prevalence of loss and level of service

Of all aural rehabilitation efforts, those focusing on the child are probably the most frequently applied. While numbers vary depending on the criteria used, it is estimated that there are approximately 50,000 deaf youngsters in the United States' educational system and that about 90% of them receive special services (*American Annals of the Deaf*, 1987; Ries, 1986). Further, Ross, Brackett, and Maxon (1982) estimated that there are 16-30 times more hard-of-hearing children than profoundly impaired. This estimate would suggest that one million or more youngsters are hard of hearing. This latter figure agrees with estimates developed by Berg (1976), and reflects a much poorer rate of service for the hard of hearing, since only about 400,000 are usually reported as receiving services.

The estimate of one million hard-of-hearing youngsters appears to be too conservative. Eagles, Wishik, Doerfler, Melnick, and Levine (1963) sampled the prevalence of hearing impairment in the Pittsburgh schools during a thorough longitudinal study. Their findings suggest an incidence of 50 per 1,000 children who have hearing levels outside the normal range in one or both ears. Thus, if both unilateral and bilateral losses are included, the prevalence of various kinds of hearing loss may be 2¼ million in school children across the United States (50/1000 × 45 million = 2,250,000; Plisko & Stern, 1985). Inclusion of the younger population (0-5 years) would put the total at over 3 million. General confirmation of this 3 million figure is derived from the Health Examination Survey of 6- to 11-year-olds (Roberts, 1972). Roberts found that 4% of the children were reported to have difficulty hearing, and this report was closely associated with actual hearing thresholds. Based on the number of children within these ages, this percentage suggests that 1 million have hearing trouble, comprising about ⅓ of all children.

Shepherd, Davis, Gorga, and Stelmachowicz (1981) studied hearing impairment in Iowa and found a relatively constant rate of mild-to-moderate sensorineural and mixed losses in school children from grades K-12. These losses included about ⅔ bilateral and ⅓ unilateral losses. About 13% of the children presented some other handicap such as noncorrectable visual problems, mental retardation, or motor coordination difficulties. These sensorineural losses did not include youngsters with high-frequency losses limited to 4,000 Hz and above, which affect a similar proportion as the sensorineural losses, nor did it include conductive losses of 10 dB or more found on the most recent audiogram of another group of almost equal size. These high-frequency and conductive losses may be transient or have limited impact, but they indicate that several million children not included in some estimates are at risk for hearing difficulties. Jerger (1980) confirmed this general estimate when he reported that 2½ million youngsters 0-6 years old suffer seriously from otitis media (which often causes conductive loss).

These numbers are in line with estimates in the Rand Report (1974) that 8-13 million children in the United States need services if those with unilateral and conductive losses are included. Thus, the prevalence of hearing loss in children affects up to 3 million children in this country in a substantial way and possibly three times that number in various minor ways.

The level of services (the percentage of youngsters receiving rehabilitation help) reported by Shepherd et al. (1981) for youngsters having sensorineural and mixed losses varies by the degree of loss. Specifically, there is only a 27% level of service for the mildest losses, but up to a 92% level for the worst losses. Although Iowa is considered to be providing exemplary services (70 school audiologists, 500 speech-language pathologists, 100 teachers of the hearing impaired) to its hearing-impaired school-age children, the state was found to be serving only 46% of all hearing-impaired youngsters with some kind of special placement or itinerant service. Further, slightly less than 50% of the overall sensorineural/mixed group were amplified. These data indicate a clear need to address, in a more comprehensive fashion, the needs of children with hearing impairments of all types and degrees.

terms/definitions

As noted in Chapter 1, a rigid distinction between habilitation and rehabilitation is not being made in this book. Although some prefer to use the word *habilitation* when dealing with children having prelingual hearing impairments, we use the term *aural rehabilitation* because of its generic usage in the profession.

Aural rehabilitation for the child may be viewed best as an advocacy, in which the rehabilitation professional works with the parents and the child to identify needs in relation to the hearing loss and subsequently arranges to help meet those needs. Needs resulting from hearing loss are detailed in the chapters on amplification (Chapter 2), speech/language communication (Chapter 5), psychosocial (Chapter 6), and educational issues (Chapter 7)—all of which are contained in the first section of this book. Aural rehabilitation (AR) includes both evaluation and remediation (see discussion in Chapter 1). While all these AR services are important, they are applied differently to various children depending, among other things, upon the degree and time of onset of the hearing loss and the age of the child. Consequently, a discussion of aural rehabilitation must be based on a profile of the client in order to be meaningful. The following section specifically focuses on severity and type of hearing loss, age of child, and other handicaps.

profile of the client

hearing loss

Deafness categories for children include *congenital* (present at birth), *prelingual* (onset before age 5), and *postlingual* (onset at or after age 5). Youngsters with congenital deafness should generally be served through early intervention programs which include parent-infant and preschool programs. As soon as the loss is identified (preferably by 1 year of age or before) the parent-infant program should start. Preschool programming typically begins when the child is at least 2½ years of age and may run concurrently with parent-infant programming. Ideally, children continue with such programs until AR services are provided in connection with school placement. Youngsters with prelingual deafness, with onset after birth, will generally receive similar treatment. Children with postlingual deafness, however, will most likely be served only in the schools.

A variety of hard-of-hearing children also participate in aural rehabilitation. Youngsters with milder losses are sometimes identified early and receive AR through early intervention. Other youngsters with slight or mild losses are not identified and/or do not receive assistance until after they start school. Indeed, some losses are progressive and only reach significant dimensions as the child gets older. One type of slight/mild loss involves middle ear infections, which result in conductive hearing problems. Frequently, such losses are of a transient nature, but in other cases they persist over a long period and require rehabilitation assistance. These conductive problems can have an educational impact on children even if the loss is only on the order of 15 dB hearing level (HL) (Rand Report, 1974; Roeser & Downs, 1988).

There are many more hard-of-hearing than deaf children. Thus, although aural rehabilitation may be performed with more severe forms of hearing impairment, most AR work involves the hard-of-hearing child. Involvement with the deaf may be more intensive because of the greater problems caused by the severity of the hearing loss. The child with more pronounced hearing loss tends to experience more language, speech, and educational difficulties and more remedial efforts will, therefore, be necessary (see Table 1.2; Chapter 7; Allen, 1986). In this chapter we describe the various types of rehabilitative efforts, without precisely distinguishing between service models for the deaf and the hard of hearing. Although this approach involves some loss of specificity, it is necessary to avoid excessive duplication. There is, naturally, much that is common in AR services regardless of the degree of hearing loss or the mode of communication. Thus, the reader must selectively apply AR techniques consistent with the individual child's needs.

age

If the assumption is made that children become adults somewhere between 18 and 21 years of age, graduation from high school provides a natural line of demarcation. In that case we may separate the years from birth to 18 into two basic divisions: those before elementary school years (0-5) and the school years themselves (5-18). In addition, we may make a number of other subdivisions, including the years of infancy and toddler (0-3), the preschool years (3-5), and the kindergarten, grade-school, junior-high, and high-school years (5-18).

In this chapter, we use the two-way division (0-5 and school years), since hearing-impaired children generally undergo a major adjustment of rehabilitation services when they enter regular school programming. Before that, aural rehabilitation includes parent-infant and preschool programs. When kindergarten begins, the school personnel will generally take over rehabilitation responsibilities from the early intervention/preschool professional. These age ranges are general; consequently, some children progress through intervention programs more quickly than others. Services are not time-locked, but sequential, depending on the child's progress.

other handicapping conditions

Hearing-impaired youngsters often have other handicapping conditions such as visual impairments, motor handicaps, or retardation. As noted earlier, 13% of all hearing-impaired students in Iowa have additional handicaps (Shepherd et al., 1981). The percentage could be even higher, on the order of 26%–30%, based on data from national surveys of young hearing-impaired children (Watkins & Parlin, 1987; see also Chapter 7). Improvements in medical science have resulted in the survival of more multiply handicapped children. This underscores the need for a multidisciplinary approach to rehabilitation in which important professionals coordinate all services to ensure integrated treatment of the child. (See Chapter 11, Case 1, for an example in working with such a youngster.)

rehabilitation settings and providers

AR settings and providers are determined to a great extent by the child's age, the severity of the hearing loss, and the presence of other handicapping conditions. Typically, services start as parent-infant programs in the home coordinated by a parent advisor and progress through preschool programs up through the formal school years. Throughout the rehabilitation process, the services of many professional disciplines are called upon in addition to continued strong parental involvement. As seen in the remainder of this chapter, an effective parent advisor is needed to ensure continued and consistent implementation of the various elements of the AR process.

early intervention: parent-infant programming

Parent-infant programming has only recently been recognized as a crucial rehabilitation tool for the hearing-impaired child. A pioneering effort was begun in 1942 by Mrs. Spencer Tracy who established the John Tracy Clinic in Los Angeles. Mrs. Tracy developed this program because of her difficulties in finding help for her deaf son. The clinic, named in his honor, helped provide much needed services for parents of hearing-impaired youngsters during the early years of development. The Tracy clinic staff developed a correspondence course which is widely available to parents and professionals. Parents follow therapy activities which are discussed in a clinic newsletter. The clinic also provides daily services to local residents and sponsors short-term programs for parents and their children willing to visit the area for intensive evaluation and remediation efforts (John Tracy Clinic Correspondence Course, 1983).

The Tracy clinic program has served as a prototype for a number of others. The earliest intervention efforts emphasized the development of oral communication skills. Visual training activities were also used to promote speechreading skills (Harris, 1963). Later, with advances in amplification, more stress was placed on the development of auditory skills, and a few programs abandoned emphasis on vision in favor of a unisensory auditory approach (Pollack, 1985). At first, programs were initiated in educational settings and were generally staffed by teachers of the hearing impaired. Later, programs with demonstration homes were established. Examples of these programs include the Bill Wilkerson Hearing and Speech Center in Nashville, Central Institute for the Deaf in St. Louis, and the Lexington School for the Deaf in New York City (Bess & McConnell, 1981; Downs & Hemenway, 1969; Horton, 1975; Northcott, 1973). Other programs provided visits to the home to take advantage of the natural atmosphere and language events in the home (Clark & Watkins, 1978). Most of these early programs have continued up to the present and a number of new ones have been added. Ling (1984a, 1984b) reviewed several programs, emphasizing that both oral (auditory-verbal and auditory-visual) and total communication approaches to early intervention are espoused.

Considerable impetus was given to these early intervention efforts in the 1960s when the rubella epidemic and frustrations with programs for hearing-impaired children caused professionals to redouble their efforts in early identification of hearing impairment. Specifically, early identification of children with hearing loss was promoted and developed through neonatal screening and high-risk registers (Downs & Sterritt, 1967; Tell, Levi, & Feinmesser, 1977). Programs were prompted by the recognition that the crucial language-development years from 0 to 4 or 5 are lost to the hearing-impaired child unless the loss is identified as early as possible. With early identification, rehabilitation efforts may begin immediately, and the devastating effects of the loss may be minimized.

One of the most successful of the early intervention programs is the SKI-HI Model (Clark & Watkins, 1984), which began in Utah in 1972 through funding from the United States Office of Education. The SKI-HI program includes a screening component whereby children are identified as being at risk for hearing impairment at birth and are followed until hearing loss is either confirmed or ruled out. Thus, hearing-impaired children—both deaf and hard of hearing—are identified early, often before 1 year of age.

AURAL REHABILITATION FOR CHILDREN

Besides early screening and followup audiologic assessment, the SKI-HI program provides for early intervention specialists (parent advisors) to begin extensive programming as soon as the hearing-handicapped youngsters are identified. Parent advisors visit the homes of the hearing-impaired children and help parents learn about amplification and how to communicate with their youngsters. Language development and psychologic adjustment are also stressed. (See schematic of SKI-HI Home Visit Program, Table 8.1.) All of this is designed to help parents through the first difficult years, and to give the child the necessary early help. Parent advisors coordinate their efforts with those of physicians, audiologists, psychologists, hearing aid dispensers, and later with school personnel. To date, the SKI-HI Model has been implemented in over 190 agencies in 45 states throughout the United States and in Canada.

TABLE 8.1
SKI*HI Home Visit Program

1. *Home Visit Component*

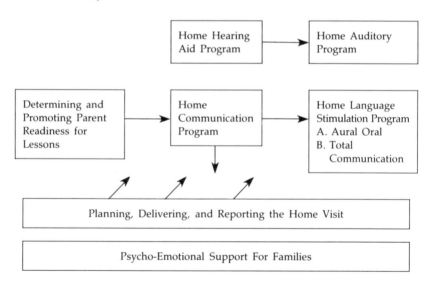

2. *Administrative Component* (child identification and processing, program management, etc.)

3. *Supportive Service Component* (audiological and hearing aid services, psychological support services, parent groups, child development services, etc.)

Most of these states now have state and locally funded programs, based on the original model, that provide early identification and intervention for hearing-impaired children. The basic intervention component is provided by the parent advisors, a network of individuals who are scattered throughout the states in reasonable proximity to the children and their parents. Idaho, for example, has six regions with a parent advisor in each. Originally trained as audiologists or teachers of the hearing impaired, parent advisors receive supplemental training in how to conduct effective home visits. In certain states, speech/language pathologists are called upon to make these home contacts in communities where they are employed full time by a school or some other agency. For these individuals the aural rehabilitation work is, therefore, a part-time job which allows service delivery to hearing-impaired children living in remote locations. In larger cities a full-time parent advisor may serve a larger patient population.

With the SKI-HI program serving as a model for more and more states, the dream of early effective help for the hearing-impaired child is becoming a reality. As noted earlier, similar programs are also achieving success. For example, many hospitals and clinics sponsor early identification programs. Children thus recognized are, in turn, served by state agencies, which arrange for services from a variety of public and private sources. In many states the Division of Services for Crippled Children acts as an advocate for the hearing-impaired child. Although they may not directly serve the needs of the parent and child, these agencies make appointments and pay for hearing aids and other services, if needed. In some states, summer institutes provide a setting for training of parents and children; for example, the summer programs of the John Tracy Clinic.

Research on the impact of early intervention programs for the hearing impaired is scanty and somewhat controversial. Criticism of the research has centered on the lack of control in research design. However, ethical concerns arise when services are denied to children in order to satisfy the demands of an experimental design. In support of early intervention programs, Balow and Brill (1975) reported that hearing-impaired children who previously attended a center-based early intervention program scored higher on several academic achievement measures than did children who received no treatment. Similarly, Horton (1976) noted that hearing-impaired children whose parents participated in a demonstration home intervention program scored higher than no-intervention children on Lee's *Developmental Sentence Types*.

Watkins (1987) studied the long-term effects of early home intervention programs on hearing-impaired children. The home-intervention children scored significantly higher than the no-home-intervention children on the outcome variables of receptive language, expressive language, communication, academic achievement, speech, and social-emotional adjustment. Factors that could confound treatment effects were selected and controlled by using analysis of covariance techniques. These factors included the child's age and hearing loss, existence and severity of other child handicaps, number of childhood middle ear infections, family index of social position, and mother's age. Further, Watkins and Parlin (1987) found that hearing-impaired children who participated in SKI-HI home visit programs showed significant language progress during an average 13 months of treatment.

Throughout the United States, then, the early intervention aspect of aural rehabilitation is being successfully implemented for the young hearing-impaired child. It is our recommendation that professionals in communities where no such program exists should assist in initiating early identification and early intervention efforts. Likewise, when programs do exist, efforts should be made to improve their quality and comprehensiveness. Through such efforts, in time, perhaps all hearing-impaired children requiring intervention will be identified at an early age and served.

early intervention: preschool

Preschool intervention alternatives are available for the hearing-impaired child. According to the Education for All Handicapped Children Act, Public Law (PL) 94-142, a free public education is to be provided for all hearing-impaired children beginning at 3 years of age, effective September, 1978. The passage of Public Law 99-457 by the United States Congress in 1986 amended PL 94-142, mandating extension of services to preschool populations. Many states have had preschool programs for younger (0–2) hearing-impaired children for several years. Thus, these children have received educational programming at age 3 instead of 5 like most of their normal-hearing peers. Preschool programs for even younger deaf children can increase the learning of language, social, emotional, and school-readiness skills. For deaf children, social contact with peers and adults outside the family is often an important experience that prepares them for regular school placement.

Preschool programs may be sponsored by private agencies or religious groups, public agencies such as schools for the deaf, groups of parents, or day care centers. The preschool teacher usually assumes responsibility for the child's aural rehabilitation and coordinates diagnostic and ancillary services. However, if the child is still in a parent-infant program, the parent advisor and the preschool teacher should work closely together in managing the child's complete aural rehabilitation program. Preschool programs usually last for 2-4 hours each day and serve children until they are 4 or 5 years old.

The earliest research on the efficacy of preschool programming did not reveal sustained positive effects. Thus, children who attended preschool did not score higher on academic achievement than did controls (Craig, 1964; Phillips, 1963; Vernon & Koh, 1970). More recent research, however, shows positive effects of preschool programming. Balow and Brill (1975) compared 264 graduates of the John Tracy Preschool Program with students at the Riverside School for the Deaf who had not had preschool programming. The John Tracy graduates scored significantly higher on the *Wechsler Adult Intelligence Scale* and the *Stanford Achievement Test* than the control children.

Watkins (1984) compared hearing-impaired children who had received formal preschool programming to those who had not. Significant group differences were found for 1/3 of the variables tested, all of which favored the preschool over no-preschool children.

school programs

In kindergarten or grade school aural rehabilitation is generally managed by school personnel. A few school districts or multidistrict units employ educational audiologists, who provide a combination of diagnostic and rehabilitative services for the hearing impaired (Garstecki, 1978; Wilson-Vlotman & Blair, 1986). Some hearing-impaired children are in special classrooms taught by teachers of the hearing impaired. Others are integrated into regular classes to varying degrees depending upon their hearing loss and other factors. Whenever possible, children with hearing loss are educated along with their normal-hearing peers as dictated by PL 94-142. Nevertheless, as indicated in Chapter 7, special classes or individual aural rehabilitation therapy generally supplement regular class instruction. Many of the children served by educational audiologists have temporary, conductive losses. Such losses do have an educational impact, and, since they can persist over long periods of time, it is important that these children and their parents be assisted in obtaining medical and other help until the hearing is restored. Children may manifest auditory perceptual disorders in connection with conductive loss or independent of any peripheral hearing loss. In either case the educational audiologist may assist in remediation (Lasky & Katz, 1983).

Children with more severe losses are often educated in day schools or residential schools for the deaf where teachers of the hearing impaired and audiologists jointly provide rehabilitation assistance. A distinction can be made between the academic, classroom work and rehabilitation work. The latter focuses on amplification, supplemental communication therapy, and coordination of all services needed by the child. Ideally, these latter matters, although important to the teacher, are the primary concern of the AR professional, leaving the teacher free to deal with the difficult demands of classroom teaching and management.

Depending upon their training as well as available facilities, aural rehabilitation therapists may handle the diagnostic aspects of audiology in the schools. Outside agencies and clinics can perform the audiology diagnostic services, but may not be in a position to participate actively in the total aural rehabilitation program. When educational or school audiologists are not available, however, some of the AR duties must be met by a speech/language pathologist, the nearby clinical audiologist, or the classroom teacher. Figure 8.1 contains an overview of the AR process as it relates to the roles of clinical audiologists, educators, and medical personnel.

identification/evaluation procedures with children

Early identification of children who are hearing impaired or who are at risk for hearing impairment is critical for successful rehabilitation. Further, proper diagnosis requires precise and appropriate screening and evaluation instruments administered, scored, and interpreted by skilled professionals. The following sections will present prevailing trends in these areas as well as implications for amplification and the overall AR process.

early identification

As indicated previously, aural rehabilitation personnel are frequently involved in early identification of hearing loss. Naturally, early aural rehabilitation efforts cannot be initiated until the presence of hearing loss is known. The status of these identification efforts is in a stage of rapid development and refinement, and methods are constantly being updated (Mahoney, 1984). For example, high-risk registers and diagnostic tests are used in locating infants with hearing loss as advocated by the *Third Joint Committee on Infant Hearing Screening* (1983). High-risk

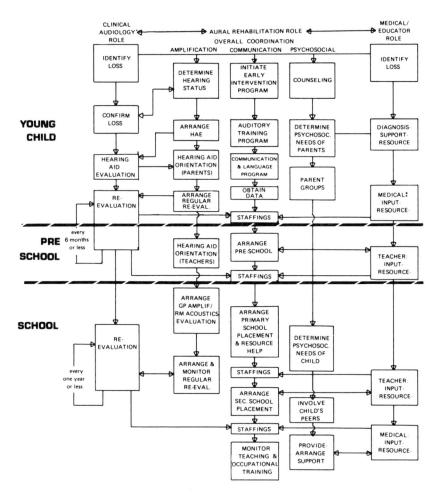

Figure 8.1. An overview of the AR process.

registers are connected with the birth and hospital stay of newborn children. Thus, children with a high risk of hearing impairment are identified based on seven risk factors including (a) family history, (b) congenital perinatal infections such as rubella or cytomegalovirus, (c) deformity of head or neck, (d) low birthweight, (e) hyperbilirubinemia requiring transfusion, (f) meningitis, and (g) severe asphyxia. Either the mother will check a maternal questionnaire indicating the presence of these high-risk factors or the mother and physician will note high-risk factors on the birth certificate. A list of high-risk infants can be extracted from the form or from the birth certificate by computer and be sent to the sponsoring agency for followup screening. About 15%-20% of all infants are designated as high risk as a result of these processes (Clark & Watkins, 1985; Gerkin & Downs, 1984; Mahoney, 1984). Once children with a high risk are identified, diagnostic screening is used to determine whether or not a hearing loss actually exists. When it is established that a loss exists, early intervention efforts can begin.

Diagnostic screening procedures which can identify youngsters at an early age include behavioral or electrophysiological (e.g., Auditory Brainstem Response, ABR) methods used in the newborn nursery. With these techniques it is possible to determine if the baby's responses are consistent with those seen in normal-hearing youngsters. When responses are not normal, the child is rescheduled for full audiological diagnostic testing. This retest should occur preferably by 3 months of age, but not later than 6 months. The advantage of this early hospital screening is that no other occasion or place prompts such universal participation until the child enters school, when it is too late to be looking for congenital hearing loss.

In addition to ABR, another test—the Crib-o-gram—has received increased attention of late. These two procedures can be costly and both require specialized equipment and personnel. For this reason, they have received mixed reviews as to feasibility and effectiveness (Cevette, 1984; Miller & Simmons, 1984; Northern & Downs, 1984; Simmons, 1980; Stein, 1984). Nevertheless, these newer procedures hold considerable promise when they are fully utilized in neonatal intensive care units (NICUs), where the percentage of high-risk infants is much higher than in a normal nursery. (Consider cautions from Case 5, Chapter 11.)

Beyond these early screening efforts, some hearing losses in very young children are identified by physicians. Usually such identification is based upon the report of alert parents who notice that their child does not respond appropriately to sound or fails to develop speech and language at the expected time. When organized screening or high-risk programs are not available, attentive physicians and parents are the major sources for hearing-loss identification. The dimensions of the loss can subsequently be established through testing in an audiology clinic.

school screening

Most children with severe hearing losses and some with milder losses are identified before entrance into school. A number of children, however, are not identified until they reach school age. Nearly all schools in the United States conduct a pure-tone hearing screening program beginning with kindergarten children or first graders. Although the specifics of these programs vary, a good model has been recommended by the American Speech-Language-Hearing Association (ASHA, 1985). Guidelines have also been published for the use of impedance audiometry in school screening (ASHA, 1978). Most children identified in school hearing conservation programs demonstrate conductive hearing loss. The rehabilitation efforts, therefore, involve coordination with parents, medical practitioners, and teachers. Some children with previously unidentified sensorineural losses may also be identified in these school programs. In such cases, medical referral is indicated to clarify the medical aspects of the loss, followed by aural rehabilitation assistance provided by educational audiologists or other personnel.

medical and audiologic evaluations

Before aural rehabilitation is initiated the child should undergo a medical examination as well as a basic hearing evaluation. Complete, definitive results are not always available on very young children. When the child is old enough, results from such evaluations should include information on both ears, giving: (a) otoscopic findings, (b) degree and configuration of loss, (c) type of loss and cause, (d) clarity of hearing (speech identification), (e) most comfortable level (MCL), and (f) threshold of discomfort (TD). Functional skills in the areas of academic achievement, language, and amplification systems should also be evaluated (Erber & Alencewicz, 1976; Madell, 1984). As Madell (1984) and Matkin (1984) pointed out, sometimes there is a tendency to omit certain aspects of testing as, for example, speech identification on youngsters with severe to profound losses, and sometimes there is a failure to consider functional hearing aid gain measures at all frequencies.

Medical clearance becomes necessary when decisions about amplification are made. After initial hearing aid fitting, regular medical evaluations should take place even for children with sensorineural losses since temporary conductive loss may occur and complicate the hearing situation, especially in young children (Ross & Tomassetti, 1988). Audiologic data should be obtained on a regular basis so that, if necessary, amplification or other dimensions of the rehabilitation program can be changed. In the early and preschool years, children should be seen for audiologic evaluation at least every 6 months. After that they should be clinically tested at least once a year.

aspects of aural rehabilitation: early intervention/ parent-infant and preschool

rehabilitation evaluation

With children, the extensive rehabilitative evaluations that generally precede remediation (see model in Chapter 1) are integrated with remediation more than with adult clients. Thus, we outline here an ongoing evaluation approach to the aural rehabilitation of the young hearing-impaired child, beginning at the confirmation of the loss and continuing through the child's school years. Throughout the aural rehabilitation process the dimensions and implications of the child's disability require constant diagnostic scrutiny. As suggested in the AR model (Chapter 1), the rehabilitation evaluation includes (a) consideration of communication status, (b) associated variables including psychosocial and educational issues, (c) related physical conditions and developmental landmarks, and (d) attitudes, especially of parents, toward remediation.

remediation

For the very young hearing-impaired child, the parents are usually in the best position to act as the primary educators as they spend the greatest amount of time with the child. Thus, through daily interactions as well as more formally structured activities, the parent-child relationship assumes an important role in the overall remediation program. To be effective and successful for both parents and child, home-based efforts must be coordinated and monitored as part of a comprehensive, long-term AR plan. To ensure such coordination, the aural rehabilitation therapist plays a vital part. In addition to overall coordination, the other three major aspects of remediation (i.e., amplification, communication rehabilitation, and psychosocial aspects) will be discussed in the following pages.

Overall Coordination. The major roles of the AR therapist should be: (a) to provide training for the parents so they can effectively teach the child and (b) to ensure appropriate amplification, diagnostic evaluations, and ancillary services for the child (Ross, 1986). Thus, the AR therapist serves as a team manager who either arranges for or provides appropriate rehabilitative services. The person who assumes this aural rehabilitation role is often called the *parent advisor*. Other designations include *counselor-tutor, instructional home teacher, teacher clinician, teacher counselor, pediatric educational audiologist* or *parent-infant facilitator* (Clark & Watkins, 1985; Grant, 1987; Horton, 1974; Ling & Ling, 1978).

Regardless of the term used, someone must assume the team manager role of making provisions for parent training and ancillary assistance to the child. Training the parents of the hearing-impaired infant is vital because of: (a) the critical period for language development during the child's first few years of life and (b) the importance of optimizing the home as the child's primary educational setting.

Critical period for language development. Evidence suggests that a critical period for language learning is the first two to three years of life (Boothroyd, 1982; Northern & Downs, 1984). After this time, language learning becomes increasingly difficult. Referring to this critical period, Harris (1981) stated: "There is no way that any hearing impaired child identified at a later age can, even with the best of follow-up services, compensate for that from which they have been unnecessarily deprived" (p. 59).

Several years ago it was not uncommon for clinics and schools to assume that rehabilitative work with a child could not begin until 3 or 4 years of age. However, if the aural rehabilitationist does not make provisions for amplification and effective language simulation during the early critical period, the child's language development will be severely delayed or will not develop naturally at all.

Early amplification and language stimulation, on the other hand, lead to positive effects on the language growth of hearing-impaired children. A few studies have compared hearing-impaired children who received early rehabilitation treatment with hearing-impaired children who received late treatment. For example, Covert and Clark (1984) compared children in four states who received SKI-HI intervention before 30 months to subjects who received intervention after 30 months. The children in the early treatment group scored significantly higher on measures of expressive and receptive language than children in the late treatment group. Similarly, Greenstein, Greenstein, McConville, and Stellini (1976) reported that children who received treatment before 16 months of age at the Lexington School for the Deaf Infant Center obtained significantly higher language scores than children who received treatment after 16 months. Greenberg (1980) compared children who received home intervention before age 3 to youngsters who did not receive early home intervention services. The early-intervention children were found to demonstrate more advanced social communication and pre-academic skills than the comparison group.

Parents as primary intervention agents and home as primary education setting. Considerable evidence points to the importance of involving parents as key intervention agents for their young handicapped children. In a comprehensive review of child-oriented and parent-oriented early intervention programs, Bronfenbrenner (1974) found that parent-involvement programs resulted in greater child gains during treatment as well as longer sustained effects after treatment than did the child-oriented programs. Early intervention programs that involve parents as the key educators of their children prepare them to continue training procedures after program termination. Since parents typically spend more time with their young child than anyone else, maximizing their interactive effectiveness, in turn, maximizes the child's communication growth. Several researchers have determined that hearing-impaired youngsters make significant gains in early communication development as a result of their parents having been trained to serve as the primary intervention agents (Herzog, 1985; Simmons-Martin, 1983; Watkins & Parlin, 1987). Parental involvement is critical, then, and should be arranged in either a center-based or a home-based intervention program. We prefer the latter model since the home is widely recognized as an ideal place for language stimulation of the hearing-impaired infant (Bradley, 1987; Shearer & Shearer, 1976). In the home, the parents and the hearing-impaired child are in their natural environment, and daily experiences that are ideal for language stimulation happen there, such as mealtime, changing the baby's diaper, and putting the child to bed. The home, therefore, should be the primary educational setting of the very young hearing-impaired child, and the aural rehabilitationist (parent advisor) living in the immediate geographic area should make regular visits to the home. It is recommended that the visits occur once weekly for about one hour.

The additional advantages of the home as the primary intervention setting include:

1. Visits can be arranged so that many or all family members can be involved. Of course, this promotes maximum language stimulation for the child during the week.

2. Family members do not need to get "dressed up" and drive to a center. Home visits seem to result in a higher rate of parent participation. For example, during a 3-year period in Utah's home visit program, over 90% of the parents were present when sessions were scheduled in their homes.

3. Interested friends and relatives can join in the sessions.

4. Home visit programs may be more cost-effective than center-based programs. Portage program costs for 9 months of home visit services average $1553 per child compared to $3031 for 9 months of ½ day, center-based services (Shortingas, 1980). In the Utah Parent Infant Program, the cost per child for 11 months of home visit treatment averages about $1500. This can be compared to an average $12,000 treatment cost per child per year at the Utah School for the Deaf (Clark, 1984).

Assessment and staffing.   It is helpful if both the parents and the parent advisor regularly collect data on the infant in the following areas: hearing aid usage, vocabulary acquisition, expressive and receptive language levels based on normative language development data, and auditory development. Also, the parent's ability to manage the hearing aid and conduct auditory and language activities should be recorded. Periodically administered language evaluations strengthen the program and provide additional data. Appropriate evaluations are described in Chapter 5; others are listed as recommended materials in Chapter 13.

With such information as a basis, staffings can be held every 3 to 6 months to facilitate the child's advancement. At these meetings data on the child's progress need to be discussed in conjunction with information from the pediatrician, the audiologist, psychologist, preschool teacher, and other professionals involved with the rehabilitation of the hearing-impaired child. The goals of staffing are to match programs to individual children, not children to programs.

Preschool placement.   Discussion of relevant data is important not only for parent-infant programming, but in decisions for preschool placement. Various alternatives are available, but no one placement is best for all children.

Preschool placement alternatives for the hearing-impaired child include (a) self-contained classrooms, (b) integration into public or private preschools, and (c) preschools for the multiply handicapped. As indicated by PL 94-142, the child should be educated in the least restrictive environment to the maximum extent possible. That is, the child should be educated with nonhandicapped children, and the removal of the child from a regular classroom should occur only when the severity of the handicap is such that removal would be appropriate (DHEW, 1977).

In addition to placement, curricular emphasis should also be carefully investigated for each child. Two major types of preschool curriculum are:

a. *pre-academic:* structured programs which typically emphasize school readiness skills such as phonics and visual-motor coordination; read-

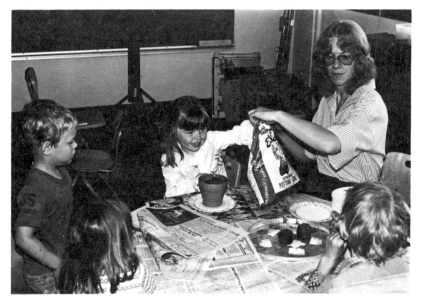

Figure 8.2. Preschool classroom of hearing-impaired youngsters.

iness workbooks are often used where children write numbers, the alphabet, simple words, and so forth;

b. *social-interaction:* less structured programs which emphasize such activities as free play, toys, and story time (Davis & Hardick, 1981).

Specific curriculum content should also be carefully considered. The following are typical, curricular options at the preschool level:

(a) *cognition awareness:* child learns about properties of things (color, size, shape, etc.) and learns how to match, categorize, sequence, generalize, etc.

(b) *vocabulary development:* child learns new words

(c) *perceptual training:* child learns how to watch and listen (auditory-visual training)

(d) *speech training:* child learns how to produce correct speech sounds and combine them into connected speech

(e) *language comprehension and use:* child learns how to understand and use new language structures

(f) *social development:* child learns about such things as cooperative play, roles in society, and responding to implied conversational meanings

(g) *writing training:* child learns how to write letters

(h) *reading readiness:* child learns letter and word identification.

Each preschool program emphasizes different curricular areas depending upon the philosophies or theories upon which it is based.

For example, an excellent preschool program at the Boys Town Institute (Moeller & McConkey, 1984) utilizes a cognitive-oriented curriculum based on the theories of Piaget with two major considerations for hearing-impaired children. First, since the hearing-impaired child has nonverbal intellectual abilities that exceed his language skills, the child's underlying knowledge of the world should be capitalized on to promote language learning. Second, since language can play an increasingly important role in the child's ability to interpret, evaluate, and integrate, the child should be helped to linguistically organize what he is experiencing. With these considerations as a conceptual framework, a number of teaching strategies are used.

For example, children are taught to interpret and discuss a key concept (such as the concept of "in") in a variety of situations (let's go "in" the closet; let's get "in" the box). Language is used which goes beyond the labeling of objects to include terms which reinforce the key concept. Children also learn to associate and describe many attributes of objects, manipulate pieces of information to understand the concept in its rational sense (get the flower and put it in the vase), and answer increasingly difficult comprehension questions.

If preschool placement is decided as appropriate for the child, parents and professionals should then select a program with particular curricular emphases using the following guidelines:

1. *Child skills needs:* Determine if the child needs particular help in specific areas (speech, auditory training, socialization, cognition). Based on data gathered during the parent-infant program, parents and professionals can make this determination.

2. *Parental values:* Determine what value parents place on specific curricular areas. For example, do parents desire an academic skill emphasis or a socialization emphasis, or do they feel a speech training emphasis is more important than a cognition emphasis?

3. *Accessibility of programs:* Determine what programs are available in particular geographical areas. This can be done by consulting the *American Annals of the Deaf* annual index to determine what preschool programs are available in a particular area.

We feel that, in general, children should remain in their own homes during the preschool years if the only other choice is a residential setting. In the home, the child is more likely to be exposed to an accepting, affectionate atmosphere and more natural, meaningful learning experiences which lead to affective, cognitive and language growth. The Report to the Secretary of HEW (1969) by the Advisory Committee on the Education of the Deaf indicated that the young deaf child, if placed in a residential school, is deprived of the natural family attention that living at home affords. However, some studies reveal no detrimental effects of institutional placement if the programs provide a warm atmosphere and relevant learning experiences (Clarke & Clarke, 1977; Quigley & Kretchmer, 1982).

Individualized programs (IEP and IFSP). In addition to educating the preschool child in the most appropriate, least restrictive educational environment, PL 99-457 establishes the use of the Individualized Family Service Plan (IFSP) for infants and toddlers, birth through 2 years, and requires the development of the Individualized Educational Program (IEP) for 3-, 4-, and 5-year-old children. The IFSP must be in writing, and contains the following components: (a) a statement of the infant's/toddler's present levels of development; (b) a statement of the family's strengths and needs; (c) a statement of major outcome objectives expected to be achieved for the child and family; (d) a statement of specific early intervention services needed to meet the needs of the child and family; (e) projected dates for initiation of services; (f) name of the case manager; and (g) steps to be taken to support the transition of the child to services provided under PL 94-142. The IEP must also be in writing and include the child's present level of educational performance, annual goals, short-term instructional objectives, specific educational services needed, dates services will begin and length of time services will be given, extent to which the child will participate in the regular classroom, and names of individuals responsible for providing the recommended services. Further, a meeting must be held annually on each child to develop, review, or revise the IEP. Participants in the meeting must include a representative of the public agency (school), such as an educational audiologist, special education director, or another individual who is assuming the AR therapist role. Also included in the meeting would be the child's teacher, one or both parents, the child (as appropriate), and other individuals deemed necessary, such as evaluation personnel

(DHEW, 1977). Evaluation of the preschool child must include such areas as language and communication skills, preacademic skills, and psychosocial skills. (Specific evaluations are described later in this chapter and in Chapters 6 and 11.) In addition, it is helpful for the preschool teacher to keep child competency data on hearing aid usage, vocabulary acquisition, and so on, similar to the information gathered by parents and the parent advisor.

Even if the child is placed in the preschool program, the family should continue to provide appropriate language stimulation. If this does not occur, the parent advisor should maintain home visits or other appropriate contact. As the family becomes increasingly proficient in language stimulation, contact can be terminated or kept up on a limited basis. In many situations, telephone contact may be sufficient.

Amplification/Assistive Device Aspects

Hearing aid evaluation. Once preliminary medical and audiologic findings are available on the child, the selection of amplification, when appropriate, becomes an early goal in the rehabilitative program. Ling (1984a) underscored the importance of this step: "Hearing aids are the most useful tools that can be used in early intervention programs" (p. 3). Other authorities have also supported this emphasis since the use of amplification has assisted many children in developing their residual hearing and their speech and language abilities (Bess, Freeman, & Sinclair, 1981; Ross, Bracket, & Maxon, 1982). Unfortunately, as previously noted, many hearing-impaired youngsters are not presently using amplification (Matkin, 1984; Shepherd et al., 1981); consequently, the efforts of the aural rehabilitationist may need to be directed toward achieving that goal. The hearing aid evaluation will be performed by an audiologist who may also be providing other rehabilitative services (see Figure 8.1). If the AR therapist does not perform the evaluation, he or she will want to review its adequacy (Bess & McConnell, 1981). Although hearing aid fitting is a first priority, other assistive amplification devices should also be considered such as auditory training equipment for the older child.

Type and arrangement of aid. The type of aid (ear-level or body) and the arrangement (monaural, binaural or other special fittings such as CROS, direct input feature) need careful attention and review in the AR process.

Matkin (1984) detailed the trend toward increased, and sometimes near-total, use of ear-level instruments by some groups of hearing-impaired youngsters. Percentage of use ranged from 63% to 98% in the groups he sampled. Ear-level instruments allow a binaural advantage and the elimination of clothing noise, but sometimes they are subject to severe feedback problems. According to Matkin, body-type aids should be reserved for use with youngsters having such feedback problems or with certain children having profound impairments, infants and toddlers with small pinnas or congenital atresia, or children with major motor deficits who cannot manage aids by themselves. In-the-ear/canal aids are used by some children, especially teenagers. While requiring special adjustment, these are feasible for use by certain individuals. In a survey of audiologists' amplification recommendations Curran (1985) found that for most children, in-the-ear (ITE) aids were recommended for 13- to 18-year-olds with mild hearing losses. However, Madell (1984) reported that at the New York League for the Hard of Hearing it was found that for young children with severe and profound losses, body-worn aids "are the best initial hearing aids for almost all children" (p. 358). It was also observed that (a) speech identification scores were significantly better for many children with body aids, (b) they liked the flexibility body aids allow in bringing the microphone closer to the speaker in auditory training, and (c) feedback problems were nonexistent. Matkin (1984) also offered cautions to those who seem overly enthusiastic about the use of only ear-level aids.

If an ear-level aid is utilized, evidence should justify the selection of the ear(s) to be aided and the reasons for a monaural or binaural fitting. In the case of a body aid, evidence or rationale should be given for the choice of a binaural, monaural, or Y-cord fitting. (See a discussion of these factors in Chapter 2, which covers hearing aid fitting procedures, and in Ross et al., 1982.) From a rehabilitative standpoint binaural fittings are nearly always the rule, since hearing-impaired children require every educational advantage possible. Sometimes this goal is contraindicated in cases requiring high-powered amplification (saturation levels of $120-132+$ dB SPL). In such instances, the danger of additional hearing loss from noise exposure sometimes prompts monaural fittings with the aid being alternated from ear to ear (Rintelmann & Bess, 1977). However, nearly all authorities agree that monaural fittings should be a rare choice. Unfortunately, the minority of hearing-impaired children with bilateral losses are using binaural aids. Recent reports place this minority at somewhere between 20-40% (Karchmer & Kirwin, 1977; Shepard et al., 1981). Even after a careful analysis to eliminate the children with bilateral losses who were not candidates for a second aid, Matkin (1984) found that only 38% of the children who could use two aids were doing so.

If children are found to have no usable residual hearing, cochlear implants may be considered. There has been controversy about whether this is appropriate for children who are too young to participate in making a choice which is possibly irreversible. Initial promising results with children who have been implanted are leading to an increased use of implants. Implant device surgery is very expensive, and when children are implanted extensive aural rehabilitation followup is needed.

Hearing aid features. Several features of the aid should be specified in the evaluation/fitting process. These include: (a) frequency response, (b) gain, (c) saturation sound pressure level (SSPL), (d) battery to be used, and (e) provision of a telephone switch and/or direct audio input. The last item is generally advisable for hearing-impaired youngsters since they may be placed in a situation or use equipment where induction-loop amplification is utilized, necessitating reception to come through the telephone mode.

Hearing aid adjustment. In the traditional hearing aid evaluation, the audiologist will specify the type of instrument to be procured along with the desired features of the aids. The hearing aid dispenser then supplies and fits the specified instruments. This approach can be modified by giving the child an extended trial with several different hearing aids that meet the general specifications of the audiologist. In the meantime, careful observations can be made by parents and the professional who visits the home on a weekly basis. This approach can be useful in selecting aid features and fitting arrangements.

In connection with hearing aid adjustment it may be helpful for the AR therapist to use the five-sound test described by Ling (1978). According to Ling the sounds /u/, /a/, /i/, /ʃ/, and /s/ can be used to determine how effective an aid is. With the infant, visually reinforced audiometry can be used to determine if the child can hear these sounds. Older children can simply indicate they hear the sounds. According to Ling, if the child has measurable residual hearing up to 1,000 Hz, he should be able to hear all three vowel sounds when they are spoken in a quiet voice at a distance of 5 yards. If the child has measurable hearing up to 2,000 or 4,000 Hz, he should be able to hear the /ʃ/ and /s/ sounds, respectively, at a distance of 1-2 yards. This test can also facilitate adjustment of the aid's frequency response.

Ling (1978) also recommended that children have amplification that provides some gain below 300 Hz so that they can hear suprasegmental information (intensity, duration, pitch, stress, rhythm) and some important vowel formants. He cautioned that the amount of gain at 200-300 Hz should be 30-40 dB less than provided at 2,000-3,000 Hz to avoid masking effects of low-frequency environmental noise.

After the aid has been obtained or after the fitting process just described, the child should be seen again by the clinical audiologist. The AR provider should encourage such hearing aid rechecks and ask the audiologist to provide him with the following information at both hearing aid rechecks and periodic reevaluations.

Earmold fit and gain setting of aid. With very young or fast-growing children, the earmold will need to be changed frequently to ensure a well-fitting mold and to provide adequate gain without feedback. Turning the gain down will help eliminate the feedback, but it is an unacceptable long-term solution. The therapist should not rely entirely on the clinical audiologist or the dispenser for this assessment, but should personally monitor the earmold condition on each rehabilitation visit. In some situations, the aural rehabilitationist is trained to make ear impressions. This can be a valuable asset to the program, especially considering the frequency of mold changes in an adequate program (see Table 8.2).

Sound-field evaluation of aid. Testing the child in a sound field, with his own aid(s) at the normal use setting as well as other settings, gives practical information about the performance of the amplification. Sound field data usually include unaided and aided findings on speech reception threshold, speech identification, warble tone thresholds, and thresholds of discomfort. Unfortunately, Matkin (1984) found that many clinics do very little aided testing with young children; this is a deplorable situation which should be reversed.

Real-ear measures. Recent developments in real-ear measurement of canal sound pressure beyond the aid have provided an alternative method for obtaining information roughly equivalent to sound field warble-tone thresholds (see Skinner, 1988, and Chapter 2). Real-ear measures can be made with and without the aid in place, and they make it possible to evaluate the benefit from the aid without requiring more than passive

TABLE 8.2

Average Months per Set of Earmolds for Children Whose Molds Were Replaced at the First Evidence of Feedback Difficulty[a]

	Average months per mold	
Degree of Loss	<2½-year-old child (N=25)	2½- to 5-year-old child (N=27)
Mild (30–55 dB)	3.0	5.2
Moderate (56–75 dB)	2.7	4.1
Severe (76–90 dB)	2.5	5.6
Profound (91–110 dB)	2.0	4.6

Reprinted by permission.
[a] Also included are average loss and gain values for children in total project (N=52) with properly fitting molds. Mean loss pure tone average (PTA), 75 dB; mean aided loss, 44 dB; mean gain, 31 dB.

cooperation from the child. Although the equipment to conduct these measurements is expensive, more and more audiologists are making this service available to their patients.

Electroacoustic evaluation of aid. An electroacoustic check of the aid should provide information on the frequency response, the gain, the SSPL, and the distortion of the instrument (see Chapter 2 for a description of this process). These data can help uncover inadequacies in the amplification that can otherwise be devastating to the child's progress in the rehabilitation program. Electroacoustic checks are particularly helpful in the case of distortions, which are not obtained in the sound-field or real-ear tests, and when biologic listening checks do not reveal a distortion problem (Bess, 1977; Schell, 1976). Additional information that may come from the electroacoustic evaluation includes the degree of nonlinearity of the gain control (each notch on the control usually will not produce an equal increment of gain) and the instrument's internal signal-to-noise ratio (S/N). This is also called *equivalent input noise* (Ln).

Hearing aid orientation. It is helpful for parents, teachers, school personnel, and other involved professionals to be knowledgeable about the auditory mechanism and hearing. This information can be provided in home visits, in clinic counseling sessions, in parent groups, and through inservice training in the school setting. The following subjects could be discussed:

1. Function, anatomy, and measurement of hearing

2. Type of loss and effect on child; need for hearing aid

3. Parts and function of hearing aid

4. Care, placement, and volume setting of hearing aid

5. Daily listening checks and earmold checks; troubleshooting of malfunctioning aid

6. Obtaining loaner aids, batteries, hearing aid parts, new earmolds, repairs.

Abundant printed material is available for use in giving such instruction (see Chapter 2 and Resource Materials in Chapter 13). Both parents and professionals may need several exposures to certain aspects of the presentation. Thus, studies have shown that parents often complain that they were never instructed about hearing aid use, even though dealers and clinical audiologists claim to have given such instruction (Blair, Wright, & Pollard, 1981; Gaeth & Lounsbury, 1966).

The benefit of hearing aid use may not be readily obvious to parents, especially in cases where auditory communication is minimal. The purposes for hearing aid use may include some or all of the following: verbal communication, signal or warning function, and environmental awareness (Ramsdell, 1978). Parents must recognize why their child is wearing an aid, since with younger children, they have the major responsibility for maintaining the aid and ensuring that it is used regularly. If parents understand hearing aids, they will be encouraged to help their child form good habits of use.

The aid will be more acceptable to the child when functioning properly, but the procedures for obtaining hearing aid accessories, repairs, or loaners will vary with local conditions. The AR provider should be aware of these conditions in order to be an effective resource person.

Communication Rehabilitation. The most important role of the aural rehabilitationist during the child's early intervention years is to facilitate communication between the child and his family. In order for communication to develop, the child needs effective stimulation in the areas of audition, communication-language, and speech. For the hearing-impaired infant, the aural rehabilitation therapist (parent advisor) works directly

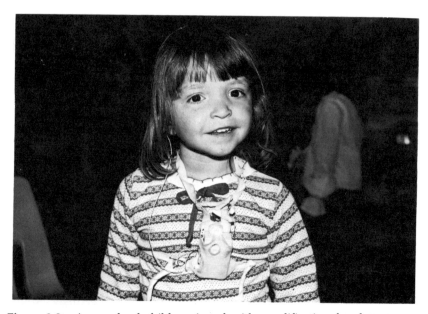

Figure 8.3. A preschool child equipped with amplification for classroom activities.

with the parents to teach them how to communicate effectively with their child. In a preschool setting, the preschool teacher interacts directly with the child and encourages parents to reinforce at home the skills and concepts taught in the classroom.

Auditory stimulation. As children are fitted with amplification they will be exposed to auditory stimuli in their environment. If systematically introduced to the child during the early years, environmental and vocal sounds will have a positive effect on language development. In contrast, children who receive such auditory training after 6 years of age will probably not learn to use their hearing for speech and language (Boothroyd, 1982; Wedenberg, 1981). Furthermore, early exposure and training provide an opportunity to determine the child's auditory potential. Early auditory training programs should consist of observing and promoting the child's listening skills in many meaningful daily activities. As Marlowe (1984) recommended "stress listening to people sounds rather than environmental sounds unless the latter are incorporated in meaningful experiences" (p. 6).

A variety of materials have been developed that describe auditory skills. Erber (1982) developed a particularly useful model which distinguishes between detection, discrimination, identification, and comprehension. (A discussion of Erber's system may be found in Chapter 3.) Table 8.3 contains a related conception of auditory skill development as well as a description of sequential listening skills. Parents need not focus on each step sequentially; however, it is helpful for them to be aware that there is a general hierarchy and that some skills develop sooner than others. Detailed suggestions for how to help children develop auditory skills can be found in Clark and Watkins (1985), Erber (1982), Hasenstab and Horner (1982), Ling and Ling (1978), and Stein et al. (1980).

If the AR therapist is working with parents, he or she should demonstrate all auditory stimulation skills that parents are asked to use with the child. The therapist and parent can discuss where, when, and how specific auditory stimulation skills can be effectively used in the home during the week.

Communication/language stimulation. At the same time auditory training is being initiated in the home, the therapist needs to help parents develop communication with their child. Effective interaction between parent and child is of utmost importance if language is to develop in the hearing-impaired child. The child should be viewed not simply as a language learner, but as a dynamic partner in a two-way communication system. (See Case 3, Chapter 11.)

Several authors (Kretschmer & Kretschmer, 1978; McAnally, Rose, & Quigley, 1987; Phillips, 1963; Snow, 1984) have described this interaction as involving unique ways that parents (mothers, typically) address

TABLE 8.3
Auditory Skill Development Sequence

Auditory Skills	Child Behaviors	Stimulation Skills
1. Attending/detection	Child attends to environmental sounds and voices. Child attends to distinct speech sounds.	Use auditory clues, show child sources of sound and reinforce child's responses to sound.
2. Recognizing	Child recognizes objects and events from their sounds.	Point out sounds and reinforce child's recognition of sound sources. Allow sound to be child's first source of information.
3. Locating	Child locates sound sources in space.	Create localization opportunities and reinforce all child attempts to localize.
4. Distances and Levels	Child locates sound sources at increased distances and above and below.	Create opportunities for child to hear sounds above and below and at distances; reinforce child's responses.
5. Environmental Discrimination, Identification and Comprehension	Child discriminates, identifies, and comprehends environmental sounds.	Repeatedly stimulate the child with environmental sounds and reinforce child's discrimination, identification and comprehension of sounds.
6. Vocal Discrimination, Identification and Comprehension	Child discriminates, identifies, and comprehends gross vocal sounds, words, and phrases.	Provide opportunities for child to discriminate, identify, and comprehend onomatopoeic sounds, words, and phrases.
7. Speech Discrimination, Identification and Comprehension	Child discriminates, identifies, and comprehends fine speech sounds: vowels then consonants.	Provide stimulation of vowel, then consonant sounds in meaningful words. Create opportunities for child to demonstrate discrimination, identification and comprehension of these words.

the infant. "Motherese" includes exaggerated intonation, gestures, higher pitched voice, redundancies, syntactic simplicity, special lexical items (baby talk), longer and more regular pauses, warm, accepting facial expressions, discussion of the "here and now," slower rate, and fewer disfluencies. This type of language stimulation serves an important purpose in communication development because it gets and holds the child's attention (Snow, 1976). Mothers of hearing-impaired children often use, inappropriately, many of the features of motherese. For example, they use atypical intonation patterns, few, if any gestures, and anxious, nonaccepting facial expressions (Greenstein et al., 1976; Goss, 1970; Quigley & Kretchmer, 1982). These parents may need help in learning to use motherese appropriately. Parents also need to become aware of their infant's attempts to communicate through a variety of verbal and nonverbal means (gestures, facial expressions, vocalizations) and react in ways that will get the child to respond again (such as imitating or waiting expectantly). If parents are sensitive to these expressed intentions and respond to them, the child will develop a communication system. If the child does not develop a communication system, he or she will not develop normal language. The AR therapist should help parents recognize the child's communication intents and encourage the child to continue the interaction. A list of specific suggestions that will facilitate communication between parents and their hearing-impaired child can be found in Table 8.4.

Closely related to early communication growth is early development of cognition. Several important thinking skills will enhance early communication development in the child. The AR therapist should help parents learn how to promote cognition development in the hearing-impaired child. Table 8.5 lists several early sensorimotor cognitive skills, how they enhance early communication development and suggestions for how parents can promote development of these skills in their hearing-impaired child.

After a communication system has been established between parent and child, a formal language development program can begin. Parents can be taught to provide constant language input, use natural activities in the home for language stimulation, increase the use of selected vocabulary and phrases, and apply expansion and reinforcement effectively. These skills are described in Table 8.6 and in Case 1, Chapter 11.

The question as to what language system is best for a family (total communication, aural-oralism) needs to be discussed from the outset. Parents should be informed about the various language methodology options and be told that the options represent a continuum (see Table 8.7)—not a dichotomy (aural-oralism vs. total communication). The intent of parent-infant programming should be to help parents and their child

TABLE 8.4
Methods for Parents to Establish Effective Communication with Their Hearing-Impaired Child

Objectives	Method
Establish an Effective Communication Setting	1. Keep background noises at a minimum when communicating with child.
	2. Allow child freedom to explore and play. Child must have chance to explore objects and learn what they are and do if he is to understand communication about them.
	3. Serve as a "communication consultant." Place child near you so you can frequently communicate with him.
	4. Use interactive turn-taking. Encourage child to "take turns" in a variety of activities and situations.
	5. Get down on child's level, as close to him as possible. Speech is most intelligible 3-4 feet from child.
	6. Occasionally provide *ad concham* stimulation (talk directly into child's ear).
	7. Maintain eye contact and direct conversation to child.
Establish Effective Nonverbal Communication	1. Use interesting, varied facial expressions.
	2. Use varied intonation and rhythm patterns.
	3. Use natural gestures.
	4. Touch child in stimulating way while vocalizing.
Establish Effective Verbal Communication	1. Regard child's cry as communicative and respond accordingly.
	2. Imitate and expand child's babbling and vocal play. Imitate and expand child's motions and add vocalizations. Introduce a few new babbling sounds each week for the child to hear.
	3. Identify and respond to child's verbal and nonverbal intents (vocalizing, pointing, tugging, stretching, looking, playing) with simple language.
	4. Use conversational turn-taking (wait expectantly for a response, signal the child to take a turn, use prods, chains, questions, etc., to keep conversation going).
	5. Talk about obvious objects and events. Talk about child's meaningful daily activities and emotional experiences.
	6. Talk about fun topics that interest child. Take advantage of child's curiosity.
	7. Use short, simple sentences and expressions rather than long, complicated ones.
	8. Communicate to child in ways he can understand (match child's communication level).
	9. When child is ready, encourage a more mature communication level.

find the appropriate position on the continuum. Several issues need to be carefully considered when deciding what language system is most appropriate. First, child characteristics and skills must be observed, documented, and discussed. Such factors as age of the child, intelligence, amount of aided residual hearing, other handicaps, and auditory or visual orientations need to be considered, since they will affect what communication system is best suited for the child. Parent interests, skills and values must also be discussed. For example, what are the parents' interests in learning and using a multimodality total communication approach? What are the parents' interest in using a unisensory auditory approach such as Acoupedics (Pollack, 1985)? What are the parents' natural interaction styles—gestural, demonstrative, verbal? What are the parents' values about their child developing oral communication skills compared to total communication/sign skills? All these considerations must be monitored throughout early parent-infant programming while the parents are establishing an interactive base with their child. During regular parent-infant program staffing, the most appropriate communication method for the family should be discussed and decided upon by parents, parent-infant program personnel, audiologists, and other professionals involved with the family. Various rating scales have been proposed to assist in this decision (Downs, 1974; Rupp, 1977). Once the best language system for the family has been selected, a specific language stimulation program can then be emphasized.

For many children, language based on listening is the most appropriate communication methodology. With proper training these children will learn to respond appropriately to meaningful sounds and communication and will make linguistic attempts. During this auditory programming with the young child, attention is not drawn to the speaker's lips in order to enhance and accelerate the acquisition of auditory-based communication. We believe that speechreading develops naturally in the hearing-impaired child as a supplement to listening; therefore, training efforts should at first be primarily directed toward establishing listening skills. Some initial speechreading skills will generally be learned without any particular emphasis (Wedenberg, 1981). Later, after auditory skills are better established, speechreading can be encouraged to varying degrees in order to supplement the auditory clues. The eventual importance of speechreading skills for a particular child will depend on the amount of hearing loss, background noise, and speaker position.

For many other children, total communication is the most appropriate communication methodology. A recommendation for total communication should be based on such variables as the child's auditory and language abilities, his/her aided hearing levels and age, and parents'

TABLE 8.5
Sensorimotor Cognitive Skills: Importance and Promotion

Early Sensorimotor Cognitive Skills	Importance for Communication Development	Promoting Early Cognitive Skills

1. *Assimilation and accommodation*: Child acts on environment, interprets and adapts to it	Environment must be acted on (interpreted and adjusted to) before it can be labeled and described	1. Promote bonding so child will feel free to explore environment instead of being preoccupied with safety and security
		   a. provide love and affection
		   b. avoid negative restrictive communication
		   c. avoid infant isolation and stillness
		   d. respond to child's actions
		   e. avoid expressions of anxiety
		2. Avoid overcorrecting child's expressed interpretations of reality so child's ability to interpret (assimilate) and correct self (accommodate) will not diminish

2. *Goal direction*: Child uses means to acquire goals	Child learns that "means" will result in goals and tries a variety of different means (including communication means such as gesturing, babbling and jabbering) to achieve goals	1. Respond to child's goal-directed actions 2. Provide toys and objects that can be acted on 3. Model goal-directed play 4. Encourage child's individual play patterns 5. Respond to child's goal-directed communication

Note. For a program on how to promote these early sensorimotor skills as well as later skills such as symbolic thought and play, ordering, concept formation, classification, and generalizing, see "Developing Cognition in Young Hearing Impaired Children" by S. Watkins, SKI*HI INSTITUTE, Utah State University, UMC 10, Logan, Utah 84322.

TABLE 8.5 (Continued)
Sensorimotor Cognitive Skills: Importance and Promotion

Early Sensorimotor Cognitive Skills	Importance for Communication Development	Promoting Early Cognitive Skills
3. *Object permanence*: Child learns objects exist even when out of sight	Child must be able to form mental images of objects and hold them in mind (even if objects are absent) so images can be referred to by labels (language)	1. Give child practice seeing objects disappear and reappear 2. Point out sound sources (especially distant ones child may have difficulty hearing) to teach child existence of these objects and their continual existence (even if not seen or heard)
4. *Causality and space functions*: Child learns that (a) certain objects or events cause others and (b) relationships exist between persons and objects	Child must understand cause-effect and space relationships in order to organize environment and later describe it (example: agent-action-object-forms; prepositional forms)	1. Respond to child's communication so child will realize that communication has consequences (causality) 2. Encourage child to explore environment so child discovers cause-effect and space relationships 3. Provide home routines and respond predictably to the child 4. Point out objects (especially distant ones) that will help child learn his relationships to them
5. *Sensorimotor integration*: Child learns how to integrate all characteristics of an object (smell, taste, sound, sight, touch)	Child needs to learn that environment can be described in terms of all five senses	1. Direct communication about child's experiences in *all* five sense areas

TABLE 8.6
Language Skills

1. Parents use conversation in four language activity areas: (a) child care activities, (b) parent task activities, (c) child-initiated activities, and (d) parent-directed activities. Parents encourage child to converse by: (a) structuring activities for "give and take;" (b) waiting for child to respond; (c) responding in a way that encourages child to continue the conversation (such as signaling the child to take a turn, showing that a response is expected, or imitating the child); (d) sharing activity choice; and (e) responding on a level the child understands and enjoys.

2. Parents select and use target words and phrases that (a) are what the parents want the child to learn; (b) are appropriate for the ideas the child is trying to express; (c) are natural to the family; (d) are appropriate for the child's developmental level; and (e) relate to the child's current experiences.

3. Parents reinforce child's language attempts positively, promptly, and frequently.

4. Parents expand child's language attempts to more mature forms.

5. Parents maintain naturalness in their conversations with child.

TABLE 8.7
Continuum of Language System Options

Pantomime/Gestures
Predominant Use of American Sign Language and Fingerspelling
Predominant Use of Signed English
Predominant Use of a S.E.E. System (Manually Coded English)
Use of Both Aural-Oralism and Total Communication
Predominant Use of Speech, Speechreading and Listening with a Lot of Animation and Gesturing
Predominant Use of Cued Speech
Predominant Use of Speech, Speechreading, and Listening
Predominant Use of Speech and Listening (Acoupedic)

skills and attitudes. The recommendation occurs at a professional staffing and needs the support of the parents in order to be successful.

For those children who begin using a sign system, it is critical that all family members learn it. A videocassette tape program is an effective way of teaching families signs. Such a program was developed by the SKI-HI Institute. The videocassette program allows parents to slip a cassette into a playback unit, turn on their family television, and view a lesson of their choosing. The lessons can be observed as often as desired. (This and other materials associated with the SKI-HI program can be obtained by writing to Home Oriented Program Essentials, 1780 North Research Park Way, Utah State University, Logan, UT 84321.) The therapist can also teach the family signs in the home or arrange for the family to attend a signing class.

Families using total communication need to learn the same communication- and language–stimulation skills as those described for families using an auditory approach. However, cautions are in order (see cases 2–5, Chapter 11) and additional skills may be necessary:

1. using sign with simplicity (total communication telegrams)

2. using sign emphasis (meaningful signs appropriate to child's language and visual development)

3. signing consistently (even when not communicating directly to the child)

4. using animation effectively in total communication

5. getting the child to watch the signer

6. using increasing numbers of affixes and non-content signs

7. avoiding overcorrection of the child's signing, shaping signs when appropriate, and

8. involving extended family and neighbors in learning total communication.

Speech stimulation. We believe the child in parent-infant programs should not receive formal speech training, which typically involves drill and correction. Instead, we believe parents and professionals should be aware of the general sequence in which speech sounds emerge and then provide extensive modeling of speech just above the child's production level. An excellent source on the sequence of speech sound emergence is the Phonetic Level Test in "Speech and the Hearing Impaired Child" (Ling, 1976).

Parents can encourage their child's initial speech sound production by vocalizing animatedly during active play with the child. For example, as the child is being gently bounced on the parent's knee, the parent can say ma-ma-ma-ma. Or the parent can say ah-boo, boo ah-boo during a game of peek-a-boo. Parents should warmly reinforce the child's initial accidental production of sounds. At the vocal play and babbling stage the young infant can be reinforced by imitating the child's vocal sounds, especially in interesting syllable chains. "You said bub! Yes, bub, bub, bub, bub!" For the older infant, new sounds can be imitated in repeated syllable chains and then used in simple words and phrases.

Parents should encourage the infant's development of early suprasegmental aspects of speech. Breath control can be developed in blowing activities such as blowing up balloons or blowing out candles. Intensity and pitch control can be developed in play where the child is encouraged to make soft and loud, and high and low sounds. Speech rhythms can be learned by encouraging the child to participate in play activities in which speech tempos are produced slowly and then quickly.

Some children in preschool classes may require formal speech training. We recommend Ling's approach which involves the following: (a) Assess the child's phonological and phonetic speech production. (b) Select target phonemes to use in training (based on what phonemes the child can already produce and the sequence of speech sound development). (c) Determine if the target sound is audible to the child; if not, visual cues and possibly tactile cues should be used. (d) Attempt to evoke the target speech sound through imitation in a variety of contexts. (e) Reinforce the child's correct productions. (f) If the child produces a consonant, train the child to repeat it in syllables. (g) Combine the new target sound with established sounds and use in linguistic context (Ling, 1976).

A thorough discussion of speech training procedures is beyond the scope of this chapter. (See Osberger, 1983; and Chapter 5 for an evaluation of various speech remediation methods.)

Psychosocial Aspects. During the early years of the hearing-impaired child's life, the psychosocial aspects of the hearing deficit are, for a great part, related to the parents as the primary caregivers and teachers. Parenthood is a great challenge for all fathers and mothers. The added responsibility of having a hearing-impaired child enhances this challenge in various ways, not the least of these being the emotional toll on parents.

Needs of parents. Psychosocial support is vital for the parents of hearing-impaired infants. Thus, many writers have discussed the importance of psychological assistance (see Chapter 6; Moses, 1985; Phillips, 1987). For instance, Lillie (1969) commented:

The birth of a child does not automatically turn two human beings into understanding and informed parents. Nor does the birth of a hearing handicapped child mean that his parents are endowed with all the understanding and acceptance necessary for them to help their child develop into a whole person. Those parents need guidance. (p. 2)

Mindel and Vernon (1987) wrote: "unless parents' emotional needs are attended to, the programs for young hearing handicapped children have limited benefit" (p. 23).

The AR therapist cannot provide effective psychosocial support for parents of hearing-impaired children unless the parents' basic psychosocial needs are understood. We will discuss these basic needs, and then explore how the therapist can provide or arrange effective psychosocial support.

The need for psychosocial support begins the day a child is diagnosed as having a hearing loss. For the parents this is a time of shock, confusion, denial, and misunderstanding. Grant (1987) referred to it as follows:

> The first reaction to the initial diagnosis is shock. Parents have wished for and expected a "normal" child. Now their dreams are shattered, and they feel devastated and helpless. The shock has numbed them into a state of docility. They are unable to assimilate what information is given them, as they are not functioning in a normal manner. It has been reported that sometimes after learning the diagnosis for the first time, parents are utterly and literally lost, unable even to locate their cars in the parking lot. (Luterman, 1987, p. 63)

After the initial shock, denial and confusion stage, parents usually experience anger, depression and guilt: "Why me?" Luterman (1987) noted: "Anger comes from a violation of expectations. Parents have many expectations about their unborn children not the least of which is that they will be normal. When they find that the child does not hear normally and cannot be cured, they feel cheated and wonder why they were singled out" (p. 42).

Anger also results from loss of control of personal freedom. Parents may experience a kind of aesthetic disavowel of the hearing-impaired child as they envision the restrictions the child may impose on their plans for the future. Anger also results from not knowing how to help the child. In addition to anger, parents often experience strong guilt feelings, manifested by overindulging the hearing-impaired child or placing excessive demands on him. If these feelings of guilt and despair are not resolved, parents begin an unending search for a "magic cure" by a doctor who will deny the difficulty, or the "best" school so they can remove themselves from parental responsibility.

This period of anger, depression and guilt is often followed by a time of withdrawal, solitude, and introspection. Parents begin to see that many handicapped people reside, work, produce, and lead normal lives in society. Grant (1987) remarked that arrival at this stage does not preclude continued problems and adjustments. Arrival at this stage does not mean that the adjustments parents of handicapped children must make are completed. On the contrary, as new crises surface, as new programs, new medical problems arise, parents must go through additional emotional adjustments.

Gradually parents come to see that their child has a future and they begin to accept the handicap. Acceptance of the handicap leads the parents back to the feelings they were experiencing toward their child before the diagnosis of deafness. The duration of each stage depends upon the parents. Some stages may pass in a matter of minutes, others may last for months or years, and, as indicated, the parents may re-experience some of the stages at later times in their lives. Generally, however, parents go through the stages just described. (See Chapter 6 for additional detail. There, this period is divided into five stages—denial, anger, frustration, mourning, and constructive coping.)

Support for parents. It is the responsibility of the AR therapist to help parents deal with the psychosocial stages discussed above. The therapist is not to hurry parents through the stages or encourage avoidance of them; rather, the therapist should skillfully, but gently, help parents progress from one stage to the next. The following discussion describes how this may be accomplished. (See also case examples, Chapter 11.)

During the first stage, which is characterized by confusion and denial, the aural rehabilitationist establishes contact with the family. This is done immediately after the diagnosis of a hearing loss. The professional's role is to offer emotional support and realistic hope. The therapist explains programs that will involve all family members and how these programs will help the hearing-impaired child.

During the next stage, anger and depression, the therapist may erroneously try to counteract the parents' emotions by helping them feel less depressed. At this period, the therapist (parent advisor) needs to exhibit genuine understanding and good listening skills rather than attempt to talk the parents out of their feelings (Moses, 1985).

The effective therapist contributes greatly to the third stage of quietude and introspection. It is during this time that parents usually open up and ask questions about the future of their child, educational considerations, and society's perception of them and their handicapped youngster. The professional needs to introduce discussion concerning unrealistic expectations the parents may have for the child, which may be based upon their own needs rather than those of the child. The therapist should assist the parents in avoiding overprotection of the child. Parents need to know that their hearing-impaired child can laugh and cry and run and play just like any other child. The aural rehabilitationist needs to be able to answer questions about educational placement, keeping in mind that such placement depends upon the child's skills and needs. As a caution, Northern and Downs (1984) suggested that professionals may err by giving too much advice about educational methods without due consideration of the child's individualized needs. A variety of professionals including audiologists, educators, and psychologists should help in these decisions. Perhaps the most important contribution the therapist can make during this stage is to give the parents constructive activities to do to develop their child's listening, communicative, and language abilities. When the parents see the child responding, growing, and learning, acceptance occurs. They realize they have a child who can be taught and loved just like any other child.

Consultation between psychologist and AR therapist. Many parents do not move easily through the stages just outlined. On the way they may have problems: unrealistic expectations for the child, overprotection, rejection, or confusion over conflicting information about educational methods. They may have problems with general child-rearing practices, such as discipline and sibling rivalry. The therapist may need special help from psychologists or social workers in dealing with these problems. However, parents often do not desire direct psychological counseling and respond to offers for counseling by saying, "I don't have a problem; I don't need a psychologist. My child has the problem." When this is the case, sessions can be set up between the AR therapist and a psychologist. The therapist meets with the psychologist and discusses the problems of the hearing-impaired child and his family. The psychologist, in turn, offers suggestions for what to do, what to say, or which professionals to contact if the problems are severe or continue. The aural rehabilitationist proceeds to implement these suggestions during his contact with the family. (See Case 2, Chapter 11.)

For parents who want psychological counseling, the AR therapist should act as facilitator and ensure such therapy is arranged.

Support group meetings. Another invaluable way of giving psychosocial support to parents is to arrange parent group meetings. "There is probably no greater gift that a professional can give to families than to provide them with a support group. Groups are marvelous vehicles for learning and emotional support. . ." (Luterman, 1987, p. 113). Support group meetings are part of many early intervention programs. Usually eight or nine meetings are held, once a week, with a psychologist or social worker in charge. The first part of each meeting often consists of a presentation by a professional. Such topics as "Language Development," "Communication Methods," "Development of Self-Concept," and "Making the Home Environment Responsive" can be discussed. The last part of each meeting is devoted to group interaction. Luterman (1987) described the benefits of support group interactions: (a) They enable members to recognize the universality of their feelings; members come to appreciate that others in the group have similar feelings. (b) They give participants the opportunity to help one another. (c) They become a powerful vehicle for imparting information.

Parents are great sources of help and comfort to other parents. In attending support group meetings we have been constantly impressed with the amount of help and moral support parents give each other. Often one of the highlights of parent group meetings is called "Meet the Deaf Night." This session generally occurs about halfway through the series. Deaf adults are invited to attend, tell about themselves, and answer questions about being deaf. The deaf adults are invited to return to the remaining meetings and contribute to the group discussions. By the end of the series, the parents genuinely care for the deaf adults. They emotionally accept the realization that their child can lead a happy, fulfilling life as a deaf adult.

Parents can also share their experiences and feelings with each other in newsletters or informal, voluntary groups. For example, "Pop-in Parents" have been tried in some states. As part of this program, parents who are having psychosocial problems are visited by "veteran" parents who have resolved their problems. Lasting friendships are often formed and valuable experiences are shared.

Needs of and support for the child. Successful resolution of parental anxieties, warm acceptance of the handicapped child, and establishment of communication with the hearing-impaired child promote normal psychosocial development. However, the child may also present social, emotional, or psychological problems. Consequently, the therapist must have a knowledge of what to expect from the hearing-impaired child in these developmental areas.

Development scales established by Vincent et al. (1986), Shearer and Shearer (1976), and others enable professionals to know what behaviors a child should exhibit at a particular age (see Materials Lists in Chapter 13). The aural rehabilitationist observes the child's behaviors and determines what age levels they typify. In addition to developmental scales, the therapist should arrange for appropriate developmental and psychosocial evaluations for the child. These tests should be administered by competent psychologists who are familiar with hearing-impaired children. According to Davis (1977), this may be difficult since ''most psychologists receive little or no training in testing or working with hearing impaired children'' (p. 36). (See Chapter 6 for suggestions on how to resolve this dilemma.)

If the child is lagging in a specific area, the aural rehabilitationist can seek help from other professionals such as child-development specialists, psychologists, social workers, occupational and physical therapists, pediatricians, and nurses.

aspects of aural rehabilitation: school years

rehabilitation evaluation/IEP meeting

PL 94-142 stipulates that primary– and secondary–school placements must be based on evaluations of the child which are reviewed in an individualized education program (IEP) meeting. The IEP meetings serve to develop, review, or revise annual educational programs for the elementary and secondary student. The AR therapist is responsible for arranging for appropriate assessment before the IEP meeting. The AR therapist of primary– and secondary-school-age children may be an educational audiologist, special education teacher, speech-hearing therapist, or some other professional charged with the responsibility of supervising the child's education. Assessment of the school-age child includes the four general areas mentioned in the AR model introduced in Chapter 1:

1. Communication status including audiologic and amplification issues;

2. Associated variables of academic achievement, psychosocial adaptation, prevocational and vocational skills;

3. Related physical conditions; and,

4. Attitude of child and parents.

This model is consistent with the four evaluation need areas described by Ross et al. (1982): area 1: audiologic, amplification and communication matters; area 2: academic achievement, psychological testing; area 3: classroom observations; and area 4: parental observations. A member of the evaluation team or a representative of the team who is familiar with the results of the evaluation must attend the IEP meeting (often the aural rehabilitationist) along with the teacher, parents, and child, as appropriate. Based on the educational recommendation from the child's IEP, the AR therapist proceeds to arrange for or provide needed services.

remediation

For older hearing-impaired children, remediation of their deficit continues to be a prime consideration. Hence remediation must be continually monitored and adjusted according to the results of both short- and long-range assessments and screenings. In addition to adjusting the typical remediation efforts of early childhood to the specific needs of the growing child, other considerations come to assume importance, including social skills, and college or occupational training. Although the hearing-impaired child/adolescent gradually becomes able to assume responsibility for some aspects of the AR program, the services of a capable coordinator will continue to be required to ensure consistent and appropriate programming. The four major remediation areas (overall coordination, amplification, communication rehabilitation, psychosocial aspects) are discussed below:

Overall Coordination. As a part of the overall coordination, the therapist is responsible for maximizing the child's learning environment (classroom), assisting in securing ancillary services, promoting development of social skills, and arranging for special college preparation or occupational training. If the primary educational programming is delivered by someone other than the AR therapist (e.g., the teacher), the therapist needs to assume a supporting role and assist the teacher in these areas.

Child's learning environment (classroom management). School placement alternatives are necessary so that the best educational setting can be selected. For the older child, additional placement options are available beyond those listed for the preschool child. Thus, the range of options includes: (a) residential school placement; (b) day school or day classes for the hearing impaired; (c) resource rooms where the hearing-impaired child learns communication skills and is integrated into regular classrooms for less language-oriented subjects, such as math and physical education; (d) integration into public schools with ancillary services like speech therapy; and (e) team-taught combined classes of normal and hearing-impaired youngsters. (See Johnson, 1987, and Chapter 7 on School Placement Alternatives for a discussion of these options.)

The aural rehabilitationist is responsible for informing the child's teachers of the conditions that will optimize learning, that is, seating, lighting, visual aids, and reduction of classroom noises. Helpful guides for teachers who have hearing-impaired children in their classrooms have been written (Birch, 1975; Davis, 1977; Gildston, 1973; see also Appendix 8A). In addition, the therapist should ensure that an appropriate student-teacher ratio is maintained. Flint (1971) suggested that a class size for the hearing impaired must not exceed seven, stressing that a class size of five or less greatly improves learning. It is estimated that one hearing-impaired pupil adds the equivalent of three hearing pupils to regular classes in terms of demand on a teacher's time (Rafferty, 1970).

The AR therapist should also promote home and school coordination. Cooperation can be facilitated by regular conferences between parents and teachers, periodic visits to the home by the teacher, notes, newsletters, and special student work sent home to the parents, telephone conversations, and allowing parents to participate in classroom activities.

Ancillary services. The therapist may also need to help set up ancillary services required for the hearing-impaired child. Services like otologic evaluations and treatment, occupational or physical therapy, medical exams and treatment, social services, and neurologic, ophthalmologic, and psychological services are important components of a hearing-impaired child's welfare (Rafferty, 1970). Finally, hearing-impaired secondary students in public school programs may require the services of notetakers or interpreters.

Development of social skills. Social activities are very important for the adolescent. Therefore, the therapist should ascertain what activities are available in the school and in the community and encourage the hearing-impaired student to become involved.

Occupational or college preparation. Secondary hearing-impaired students need special help in occupational training. Even though the percentage is steadily dropping, it is estimated that 66% of all jobs now available need no more preparation than a high-school education (BOL Statistics, 1975, 1977). It is necessary to provide vocational training and occupational guidance for those high-school students who want to enter the work force. Likewise, college preparation courses and guidance counseling are needed for those who desire a college education.

Amplification/Assistive Device Aspects. If children obtain their hearing aids during the early intervention period and go through the adjustment and orientation steps described earlier in this chapter, they have a good start on dealing with amplification concerns. However, this area requires a continued focus since new amplification needs or problems may arise when children enter school. Regular hearing aid reevaluation at 6-month to 1-year intervals and daily monitoring of the aid by school personnel should occur. Unfortunately, such regular monitoring is often neglected. Therefore, aural rehabilitation personnel need to be vigilant in this area (Bess & Logan, 1984). The major deficit for these children is their impaired hearing. Therefore, the most obvious remediation is to restore as much of that hearing through amplification devices and excellent acoustic listening conditions as possible. In this manner, we may remove the need for some therapy that would otherwise be required.

Hearing aids. Some hearing-impaired children will not be identified until they reach school, and some of them will receive their first amplification attention at this time. As indicated in the section on early intervention, when children with hearing losses are identified they should also be evaluated medically and audiologically. After specific assessment information has been obtained, the way is cleared for carefully evaluating the place of amplification in the overall remediation program. Children with mild or severe losses in the speech frequencies should proceed with a hearing aid evaluation, and additional aural rehabilitation can assist them in hearing aid adjustment and/or orientation aspects, as described previously.

Children with slight losses, high-frequency losses, or chronic conductive losses present a more difficult problem in terms of amplification. A careful assessment of such children's language and speech status and a report on their ability to function in the classroom will help determine whether they can function successfully without amplification. Preferential seating can provide some help, but, at best, it is an imperfect and perhaps only a temporary solution. Some have recommended fitting hearing aids on children with chronic conductive losses and shown that it is a feasible alternative (Mathiesen, 1985; Northern & Downs, 1984). Another possible solution is temporary use of FM amplification devices until the hearing problems are resolved. Such units may also be used for children with slight sensorineural losses. However, when a hearing aid can be fitted comfortably, it is generally better to fit children with sensorineural losses with aid(s) while they are younger. As they get older, they tend to become more concerned about the unfortunate social stigma associated with amplification devices. In contrast, children who use amplification from an early age know how much it can help them and are less likely to part company with it as they get older. Nevertheless, getting children to use their hearing aid(s) on a regular basis may be one of the greatest challenges faced by the AR therapist.

Teachers and parents and, later, the child himself/herself can provide information on how regularly the hearing aid is used. The therapist should seek out this information and try to modify behavior when necessary (Hanners & Sitton, 1974). Young children will often respond to methods like public charting of their daily hearing aid use. The child can be made responsible for the charting. Older children should understand the purpose for amplification. When they are old enough, therefore, they need to receive the same instruction and information about their hearing loss as their parents were given previously. (See Amplification/Assistive Devices under Early Intervention in this chapter.)

Full-time use of an aid is preferable because the child is less likely to forget or lose the instrument. With older children, however, it is sometimes unrealistic. In the case of mild loss, the aid may provide little, if any, benefit in many play or recreational circumstances. The teenager, therefore, may elect not to use the aid during these times. The aural rehabilitationist may help the young person identify the situations where the aid should be used.

As the child gets older, she can begin to assume the responsibility for the care and management of the hearing aid. At that point, the AR therapist should teach the child about hearing aid function, repair, and use (see Chapter 2). Maintenance of children's hearing aids is often neglected as shown in a series of studies starting with Gaeth and Lounsbury (1966). These writers found that approximately half of the hearing aids in their study were not in working order and parents were generally ill informed about the rudiments of aid care. Unfortunately, that situa-

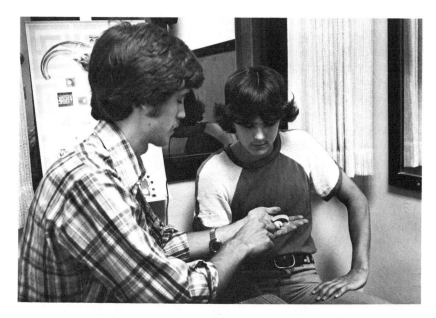

Figure 8.4. Orienting a teenager about the use of his behind-the-ear hearing aid.

tion has not improved appreciably as reflected in subsequent studies, nearly all of which have shown 50% poor function among children's aids (Bess, 1977; Blair et al., 1981; Coleman, 1972; Porter, 1973; Robinson & Sterling, 1980; Zink, 1972). Furthermore, school programs have been similarly negligent about maintaining children's aids (Rawlings & Trybus, 1978; Sinclair, Bess, & Riggs, 1981) even though some projects have demonstrated that children's aids may be substantially improved by regular maintenance (Bess, 1977; Hoverstein, 1981; Kemker, McConnell, Logan, & Green, 1979).

In cases where the child's management skills are deficient due to age or length of experience with the aid, help and instruction should be provided (see Hoverstein [1981] for suggestions).

Assistive listening devices/classroom acoustics. Other aspects of amplification that become important in the school years include use of group amplification systems and the concern for quiet classroom environments. While no knowledgeable person would dispute the importance of quiet conditions for the hearing impaired, there has been some controversy about whether school-age youngsters should use educational (FM) auditory systems instead of personal hearing aids. Data from nearly 1900 classrooms for the hearing impaired suggest that about one third of children use personal hearing aids. Most students in these classes, therefore, use various types of group amplification. Specifically, one fourth use FM systems, another third use a combination of FM and personal aids, while the remainder ($\frac{1}{12}$) use loop or desk amplification systems (Sinclair & Freeman, 1981).

Personal hearing aids have improved appreciably over the past years so they now provide good fidelity, wearing comfort, and cosmetic appeal. In addition, they allow good student–to–student communication, self-monitoring by the child, and in small groups they provide satisfactory amplification for teacher–to–student communication purposes.

Consequently, personal hearing aids may be a reasonable choice in small classes made up entirely of hearing-impaired children when there is excellent acoustic treatment. However, whenever the class is large enough or noisy enough to create adverse signal-to-noise ratios, or when a child is mainstreamed, personal hearing aids present a major disadvantage. Specifically, when a person using a personal aid is not close to the speaker, the speaker's voice will not be as loud nor will the signal-to-noise ratio be as favorable as when a microphone can be placed close to the speaker. (See Case 6, Chapter 11.)

Chapter 2 contains a description of the different types of group amplification equipment in use. *FM radio-frequency* systems, used almost exclusively now, allow teacher and students more freedom and flexibility than other systems. FM systems may also be used with hearing aids by direct audio hookup and by induction loop transmission. The older forms of classroom amplification, the *standard* or *hard-wire* systems, and *induction loop amplification* (ILA) systems are still used for some special applications. One other device is the *infrared system*, which utilizes light rays for transmission. The infrared system is usable in auditoriums and in many public buildings and for personal use and TV watching by some hearing-impaired persons.

The aural rehabilitationist must be knowledgeable about the various types of equipment and must be able to instruct others in daily operation and monitoring. Occasionally, AR professionals will also be asked to recommend the best arrangement for a particular setting. More frequently, they will simply be responsible for regularly evaluating, or getting someone else to evaluate, the function of existing systems. Several sources (Bess et al., 1981; Bess & Logan, 1984; Ross, 1987) contain thorough discussions of factors that should be considered when evaluating amplification equipment. Suffice it to say that attention should be given to: (a) electroacoustic considerations, (b) auditory self-monitoring capability of the units, (c) child-to-child communication potential, (d) signal-to-noise ratios, (e) binaural reception, and (f) simplicity and stability of operation.

Other assistive devices. It is important that the hearing-impaired youngster be introduced to other available accessory devices. Such devices include amplifiers for telephone, television, radio; decoders for television; signal devices for doorbells, alarm clocks, and so forth. These devices are described in Chapters 2 and 13. In addition, therapy materials are available to help in familiarization (Castle, 1984).

Sound treatment. Well-functioning group amplifying systems will be more effective if used in an acoustically treated environment. In this regard, hearing-impaired youngsters with sensorineural losses will have more serious difficulties than the normal-hearing child when noise is present (Ross & Giolas, 1971). When all sounds are amplified, it is important to avoid excessive reverberation in the amplified environment. Reverberation occurs when reflected sound is present and added to the original sound. In an unbounded space (anechoic chamber) there is no reverberation. A sound occurs, moves through space, and is absorbed. However, in the usual listening environment like a classroom, sound hits various hard surfaces as it fans out in all directions, and it is reflected back. Consequently, not only the original unreflected sound, but a variety of reflected versions of the sound are present at once. This results in less distinct signals since signals are "smeared" in the time domain.

Reverberation Time (RT) is a measure of how long it takes before a sound is reduced by 60 dB once it is turned off. In an anechoic chamber RT is near 0 seconds. In a typical classroom it is around 1.2 seconds.

However, in a sound-treated classroom, one with carpets, acoustical tile, and solid-core doors the RT can be on the order of .4 seconds. Finitzo-Heiber and Tillman (1978) showed the effect of RT and environmental signal–to–noise (S/N) ratio. The S/N ratio is a measure of how loud the desired signal (such as a teacher's voice) might be, compared to other random classroom noise. A +12 S/N ratio is considered acceptable for hearing-impaired children while +6 S/N and 0 S/N ratios are more typical of ordinary classrooms. As seen in Table 8.8 the speech identification of normal and hard-of-hearing children is adversely affected when S/N ratios are poorer and RTs are increased. The hard-of-hearing child's performance is more adversely affected by poor conditions than is the normal child.

In the ordinary classroom, noise levels tend to be about 60 dBA, but in an open classroom they rise to 70 dBA. Gyms and cafeterias have noise levels of 70-90 dBA, with high amounts of reverberation. A carpeted classroom with five hearing-impaired students and a teacher generates about 40-45 dBA of random noise. According to Finitzo-Heiber (1981), since voices at close range average 60-65 dBA, the S/N ratio in sound-treated classrooms may be +20 dB if the listener is close to the teacher. If the listener is further away from the teacher, the signal will get weaker and the S/N ratio will be poorer. In view of poor performance by hard-

TABLE 8.8
Mean Word Identification Scores of Normal-Hearing and Hearing-Impaired Children under a High-Fidelity (Loudspeaker) and through an Ear-Level Hearing Aid Condition for Various Combinations of Reverberation and S/N Ratios

Reverberation Time (RT) Sec	S/N Ratio in dB	Mean Word Identification Score (%)		
		Normal Group (PTA = 0 – 10 dB) Loudspeaker	Hearing-Impaired Group (PTA = 35 – 55 dB)	
			Loudspeaker	Hearing Aid
0.4	+12	83	69	60
	+ 6	71	55	52
	0	48	29	28
1.2	+12	69	50	41
	+ 6	54	40	27
	0	30	15	11

Adapted from "Room Acoustics' Effects on Monosyllabic Word Discrimination Ability for Normal and Hearing Impaired Children" by T. Finitzo-Heiber and T. Tillman, 1978, *Journal of Speech and Hearing Research, 21,* pp. 440-458.

of-hearing youngsters in noisy conditions (see Table 8.8), it is recommended that class noise levels be 45 dBA for gym and arts/crafts classes, but 30-35 dBA in the classrooms where these students spend most of their time (Bess & McConnell, 1981). Others have suggested that noise levels of about 50 dBA may be more feasible (Berg, 1986; Gengel, 1971). This would allow minimally acceptable S/N ratios of 15-20 dB. Reverberation times are easier to reduce than noise levels. Thus, carpeting, acoustical tile, and even commercially available foam sheets may be placed in classrooms to help absorb noise. A feasible goal may be to reduce the RT to .3-.4 seconds. In addition, provisions should be made to keep the hearing-impaired child close to the speaker (teacher). This can be accomplished through use of group amplification (FM) equipment since the location of the microphone is, in effect, the position at which listening occurs. Extensive rationale and methods for providing sound treatment are available elsewhere (Berg, 1986; Crum & Matkin, 1976; Finitzo-Heiber & Tillman, 1978; Olsen, 1977).

To summarize, the aural rehabilitationist plays a crucial role in providing and encouraging both routine and extensive checks of group amplifying systems and in obtaining adequate sound treatment.

Communication Rehabilitation. As indicated previously, children may be educated in a wide range of school placements. Consequently, they will receive communication rehabilitation through various combinations of the important professionals who serve them. Speech pathologists, audiologists, and special educators (teachers of the hearing impaired) will provide the bulk of this service. The degree of involvement for each specialist is likely to be different for a child in a residential school compared to a student who is mainstreamed with daily resource-room participation. Furthermore, the interest, availability, and skills of participating professionals may dictate the degree of their involvement in the child's program. Nevertheless, what is needed is *not* a series of disjointed, separate therapeutic efforts. Rather, a coordinated, cohesive program should be achieved in which language remediation, speech therapy, and auditory/visual training are integrated and related to academic and other important aspects of the child's life (Erber, 1982; Esterbrooks, 1987; and Johnson, 1987). (See Case 6, Chapter 11.)

Each professional tends to possess specialty skills. The audiologist should be skilled in auditory areas (measuring hearing, monitoring and maintaining amplification, and auditory/visual training). The speech-language pathologist should be able to assess language and speech skills and provide effective remediation. The special educator, in turn, generally is able to assess academic skills and deficits, including those that are language related such as reading and writing. It is rare that one professional can provide high-quality assistance in all these areas. Furthermore, some professionals will not have had prior experience with hearing-impaired children (Simmons-Martin, 1978). When key professionals are inexperienced, certain resources may be recommended. Specifically, the speech-language therapist and teacher of the hearing impaired may be referred to excellent indepth texts like Ling (1976) and Kretschmer and Kretschmer (1978), while audiologists may consult Ross, Brackett, and Maxon (1982) as well as other sources listed as recommended reading at the end of this chapter. Regardless of experience, however, coordinated efforts among professionals will enhance service to the child and provide important interaction between professionals.

One professional should also be monitoring the full range of AR services available to the child (i.e., he should be the child's advocate). This person generally leads interdisciplinary coordination on communication aspects. We recommend that the aural rehabilitationist be the school audiologist, but in many cases the speech-language therapist or the special educator assumes this role. As the team works together, the AR coordinator (AR therapist) must monitor a number of communication aspects, including auditory training, language and vocabulary development, visual attentiveness, speech skills, writing skills, and reading skills.

Auditory (language) training. There is general agreement that audition is a natural modality for language learning (Boothroyd, 1978; Fry, 1978; Kretschmer & Kretschmer, 1984). Based upon this premise, Kretschmer and Kretschmer (1978) stated:

> The content of auditory training programs for young hearing-impaired children should be predominantly linguistic in character to assure that the acquisition of spoken language is achieved through the sense best designed for this mastery . . . It would be a mistake for the reader to conclude that this strategy is reasonable or possible for every child with significant hearing loss. On the other hand, however, it may be an alternative for many more children than in previous years because of improvements in early identification procedures, infant management programs, and the consistent application of personal amplification. (p. 234)

When using language as the basis for auditory training, a careful language assessment should first be made. (Suggestions on how to conduct this assessment and a variety of materials that may be used for this purpose are listed in Chapter 5 and under Resources and Materials List–Children in Chapter 13.) After the assessment is completed, the therapist can begin to work with the child at his or her current language level. The therapist may also help the child expand his language skills in connection with an extensive language remediation program.

A determination can be made on whether language problems reflect an inherent deviance or a developmental delay, or both. According to Kretschmer and Kretschmer (1978), language remediation should focus first on deviant patterns to prevent greater deviations in the future. Language activities should then proceed with an emphasis on the simplest, yet most powerful, language forms and should follow a well-documented developmental sequence of the sort presented by Kretschmer and Kretschmer. These authors offer suggestions for how to use this remediation approach for both young and older hearing-impaired youngsters. In using such a language-based approach to auditory training, clinicians, either singly or in combination, must bring to therapy a good understanding of language disorders and their remediation.

Many discrimination activities that have historically been performed in the name of auditory training have limited utility for the school-age child. Ling (1978) cited evidence that supports this position. Often extensive therapy time has been spent with these youngsters requesting that they listen to recorded environmental sounds or perform discrimination tasks based on phonemes in isolation or contrived sentences. Based on our professional experience, a heavy emphasis on this type of formal auditory training may have limited value for both therapist and client. Instead, the therapist should be concerned with encouraging and reinforcing the hearing-impaired child's listening techniques. Pointing out environmental sounds to hearing-impaired youngsters may at times be appropriate and is more meaningful than using recorded sounds, but more relevant listening experiences can be provided each day in connection with language/speech therapy, academic subjects, and in social situations. In other words, language-related auditory training should be stressed. This type of therapy applies to children who have auditory-based language. In addition, children who use total communication rely on listening in conjunction with their sign system. For them, too, natural, communication-based listening experiences are much more meaningful than short, isolated listening sessions. Erber (1982) suggested three general types of auditory (language) training activities. These include:

1. a natural conversational approach

2. a moderately structured approach, and

3. practice on specific tasks.

He gives some useful, practical suggestions on when to apply each one of these strategies. Also, a comprehensive program of auditory training activities is found in Stein et al. (1980). New developments with interactive computer-based laser videodisk systems may eventually be perfected and be available for general use in auditory/visual communication rehabilitation. At present, only experimental forms of such systems are available (Tye-Murray & Tyler, 1988; see also Chapter 3).

Vocabulary development. The preceding discussion has emphasized language-based activities that may utilize the child's present skills or expand his language abilities through a solid language-remediation program. Such a program will incorporate training in syntax and semantics. In connection with this, the therapist will want to ascertain the status of the child's functional vocabulary. A baseline measure of each child's receptive and expressive vocabulary may be obtained through language samplings; parent logging; and observation by teachers and therapists. After such an initial assessment the professional can begin adding the necessary vocabulary for use in educational and home settings. The Dolch Basic Word List (Dolch, 1945) is one of many tools used in teaching functional vocabulary. Most normal-hearing children should master the words on this list by the third grade.

Kretschmer and Kretschmer (1978) offered suggestions on how to establish a core lexicon (vocabulary), which may be as small as 35 words for the very young child. They stressed that the words selected should permit frequent usage and be associated with ideas that are commonly

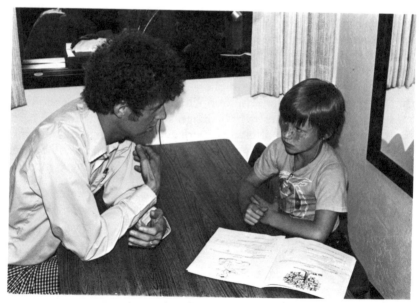

Figure 8.5. Individual therapy combining attention to language acquisition and auditory training.

expressed at the child's developmental level. New vocabulary should be taught effectively and should be familiar to the hearing-impaired child before he or she encounters the words in reading. Further, parents, teachers, and others involved with the child's education must be aware of the vocabulary words and use them in meaningful situations as frequently as possible. It is recommended that vocabulary lists be sent home to parents. The words should probably not be taught in isolation or through a dictionary or synonym approach; instead, they should be used in sentences and in conversational or interpersonal exchanges. Even though it is advisable that only one meaning per word be introduced at a time, the child should learn that many words have more than one meaning.

Visual attentiveness.   We believe that effective use of speechreading is mainly achieved by encouraging visual attentiveness in academic training, rather than through formal speechreading drill. Some may wish to carry out extensive speechreading therapy activities. However, our preference is to initially allow the child to receive the visual information without drawing undue attention to it. Later, visual attentiveness may be more directly encouraged and, when audition is inadequate for the task of recognition, the child can specifically be taught place of articulation through visual information. At these times we may say that an analytic approach is used (Ling, 1976, 1978). This approach is most frequently used in cases of severe or profound deafness, and requires that the clinician be familiar with visemes and the acoustic aspects of speech.

Even children with severe and profound losses can gain most of their speechreading skill synthetically or globally in connection with ongoing language-based therapeutic activities (Simmons-Martin, 1978). When such children are trained using an oral-aural method, visual attentiveness is very important. Children trained in this manner also need considerable ability in processing auditory information. For children who use a linguistically based total communication system, speechreading also serves as a natural source of supplementary information, and should, therefore, be encouraged.

Speechreading training, which frequently omits the auditory signal, is unrealistic since the hearing-impaired child can almost always make use of residual hearing to some extent. There are times when the therapist or teacher may wish to reduce voice intensity briefly to encourage visual attentiveness. At other times, for example, when a child is learning a new vocabulary word or when he is having difficulty with reception of auditory cues that can be effectively supplemented by vision, it may be necessary to present key words and ideas auditorily, visually, and then bimodally. However, if the child possesses adequate language, we are in agreement with many writers that bimodal stimulation results in more effective communication and greater visual and auditory recognition of familiar language (Erber, 1982; Griffith, 1969).

Speech skills. The AR therapist is responsible for monitoring the type of speech remediation that is provided to the hearing-impaired child. For instance, the services of a speech therapist will be indicated for articulation and voice therapy. In evaluating the need for therapy, overall intelligibility, as well as voice and articulation, should be assessed. Based on the results of such assessments, speech rehabilitation programs can be designed and initiated. It may be noted that both theorists and clinicians (Fry, 1978; Ling, 1978) believe that production serves an important role in auditory language remediation. That is, children can often learn more easily to perceive different auditory stimuli after they have learned to produce the sounds correctly. This again emphasizes the importance of a coordinated approach in teaching speech, language (verbal or sign), and auditory training. For a description of speech evaluation materials and remediation strategies, see Chapter 5.

Writing and reading skills. A child's written language should be assessed primarily by informal evaluation procedures. It is important to focus on a limited number of objectives since overcorrection can destroy the language learning process. Depending on the child's language development stage, the emphasis may be on the *planning* stage (quantity, organization), the *translating* stage (making sense, interest and style devices) or the *reviewing* stage (paragraph or sentence structure, syntax, etc.). Once goals are established, youngsters are appraised of the objectives. The teacher should avoid neglecting the positive language-expansion objectives as well as more traditional corrective procedure objectives. For example, a youngster who is writing syntactically correct short sentences should be encouraged and directed to create more complex syntactically correct sentences (see Hayes & Flower, 1980; Pehrsson & Denner, 1988a).

The hearing-impaired child's reading abilities should also be ascertained. However, unless the child is linguistically near normal, standardized tests are not appropriate. Criterion-referenced tests may be more suitable since they allow for individual objectives to be established. In addition (and probably most useful), the informal approach based on curriculum materials in the classroom must not be overlooked. In selecting materials for reading instruction the focus should be on (a) whether the child will learn from reading the material or become frustrated; and (b) whether the child will be able to learn independently or what degree of direct instruction he or she requires.

A variety of approaches may be used to teach reading to hearing-impaired children; no one approach is appropriate for *all* children. In some cases, children learn best from a parts-to-whole approach with initial emphasis on phonics and word cards. Other children seem to do better with a whole-to-parts strategy such as a language experience approach ("Tell me a story and I'll write it down."). More recently, the use of graphic organizers has been incorporated into reading and writing lessons, which is a good strategy for use with the hearing impaired (Pehrsson & Denner, 1988b; Pehrsson & Robinson, 1985). Another approach which involves modeling the reading process is known as a *metacognitive approach* (Baker & Brown, 1984; Brown, 1980). The reader is referred to Pehrsson and Denner (1988a) for an excellent discussion and detailed suggestions on how to teach reading to the hearing-impaired child.

Efforts in reading and writing should not represent isolated therapy activities. Instead, they should be closely coordinated and related to an overall language acquisition and development plan which includes these two subjects as well as spelling, speech, and auditory training activities. Such efforts are needed to avoid fragmented, counterproductive learning experiences.

Adjustments for mild losses/auditory-language processing problems. Children with mild hearing problems (i.e., mild sensorineural loss, conductive loss) and those with auditory-language processing difficulties may require communication rehabilitation along with children who demonstrate more pronounced losses. Although the language-related problems may be minimized in the case of milder losses, they are apt to be present and require attention (Downs, 1988; Katz, 1978; Quigley, 1978; Webster, 1983). A careful multidisciplinary evaluation of the child's difficulties should be conducted consisting of reports from teachers, parents, the child, and others in addition to observation and diagnostic testing.

Most authorities agree that an auditory-language processing deficit involves a variety of difficulties either in one or all areas of (a) detection, (b) interpretation, or (c) categorization, as persons process mainly linguistic information received through audition. Such difficulties may involve a peripheral, central or general cognitive problem, or a combination thereof (Hasenstab & Schoeny, 1982; Keith, 1981; Lasky & Katz, 1983). Duchan and Katz (1983) raised the question whether children suspected of having auditory-language processing problems are primarily language disabled or primarily poor auditory processors. These authors urged a synthesis of views. In a simple model they suggested that sometimes there is a greater problem with language processing and a lesser problem with lower order auditory processing. In other cases, the reverse is true. At yet other times, there may be a more equal problem in the two areas.

One approach in a diagnostic workup on such a child involves an emphasis on both thorough evaluation of language skills and a variety of auditory manipulation tasks that focus on linguistic information presented (a) at differing rates of speed, (b) at various levels of linguistic complexity, (c) along with variable background noise levels, (d) with various rates/kinds of interruptions, (e) at various levels of familiarity, and (f) at differing levels of completeness/abstractness (Butler, 1983). However, Butler's approach puts most emphasis on informal, practical assessment and remediation (see Table 8.9 for various areas to be informally evaluated as suggested by Cole and Wood, 1978). Other writers use a more formal battery of tests or a combination of formal and informal procedures (Lasky & Cox, 1983; Matkin & Hook, 1983). (A variety of diagnostic tools have been developed for this purpose; see Chapter 13, List of Resources and Materials.) Regardless of the evaluation approach used, the effort to establish a diagnosis for these difficulties is not yet very exact.

Useful assistance can probably be rendered by identifying the specific difficulties the child experiences as determined from a list such as seen in Table 8.9 or as found in the questionnaire assessment procedure used

TABLE 8.9
Diagnostically Significant Behaviors of Children with
Nonsensory Auditory Disorders

Auditory reception
    Disregard of speech or all sounds
    Better responses in quiet than in noise
    Hypersensitivity to sound
    Echolalia
    Difficulty following verbal instructions unless accompanied by visual
        demonstrations
    Difficulty learning in group situations
    Failure to remember what people say
    Failure to generalize information from one experience to another

Verbal expression
    Reduced quantity of verbalization
    Inadequate vocabulary
    Defective sentence structure
    Inability to verbalize experiences using a series of utterances
    Incorrect pronunciation (articulation) of words
    Disorganized content within or among utterances
    Dependence on gestures to express information
    Unusually literal content in ideas expressed

TABLE 8.9 (Continued)

Social-emotional behaviors
  Problems in attention to pertinent tasks
  Inability to inhibit behavior
  Inability to cope with change
  Disorientation in space and time
  Immature self-help skills
  Perseveration
  Hyperactivity
  Inappropriate emotional reactions
  Social isolation
  Extreme aggression
  Limited interpersonal relationships

Academic behaviors
  Difficulty following verbal instructions or learning from verbal explanations
    in the classroom
  Difficulty learning phonics
  Inadequate reading or spelling
  Poor comprehension of what is read
  Disorganization in content of written material
  Poor sentence construction in written work
  Discrepancy between achievement level and potential for learning

Test behaviors
  Significant discrepancy between verbal and nonverbal scores
  Low scores on verbal tests
  Discrepancy between test-retest scores on same measure or on tests
    designed to measure similar abilities
  Low achievement test scores

From "Differential Diagnosis" by P. R. Cole and M. L. Wood. In *Pediatric Audiology* (pp. 306–307) by Frederick N. Martin (Ed.), 1978, Englewood Cliffs, NJ: Prentice-Hall. Reprinted by permission.

with the child's clinician, teacher, and/or parent. (See Appendixes 8B and 8C.) After identifying unusual auditory behaviors the therapist may assist teachers, parents, and children in becoming more aware of, and hence avoiding, situations that contribute to the child's difficulties. Boothroyd (1982) provided some useful suggestions for therapy with these youngsters, as do other authorities who summarize their methods in Lasky and Katz (1983). Sometimes a series of suggestions may be implemented to help the child cope with difficult listening situations (Rupp, 1979; Willeford & Billger, 1978). (See Appendixes 8D and 8E.)

Psychosocial Aspects. As the hearing-impaired child grows older, the aural rehabilitationist can help promote the child's psychosocial well-being.

The child and his peers. An essential psychosocial area relates to peer relations. Thus, the professional should determine if the child's peers are informed about their friend's hearing impairment and are empathically interacting with the child. Some ways of promoting this attitude include:

1. Involve the peers in home visits by the AR therapist. One mother invited the children in the community to meet with the AR therapist so the children could learn signs and communicate with the hearing-impaired child during play. The AR therapist also taught signs to the child's Sunday School teacher who, in turn, taught the other children in the Sunday School class basic signs for in-class communication with the child.

2. Involve the hearing-impaired child's friends in special family functions, such as birthdays, family trips, home movies.

3. Inform the leaders of peer groups (Sunday School, Scout troops) about the hearing impairment and how they can most effectively communicate with the child.

4. Arrange for school presentations (preferably by the hearing-impaired child himself) to inform peers about the hearing impairment, the hearing aid and how it works, and what it is like to perceive sounds with a hearing loss. (Records that simulate different types of hearing losses are available; see children's resources and materials in Chapter 13.)

5. Instigate a "buddy system." The therapist arranges for a friend of the hearing-impaired child to do special things for him like taking notes, telling the hearing-impaired child when something is said from a distance (or position) that the child cannot perceive, and making sure he understands assignments, etc.

Support for those working with the child. The professional needs to make sure that those who work with the hearing-impaired child are fostering a positive self-image for the child. In addition, the youngster needs to develop trust, independence, affection, purposefulness, and an appropriate sex role. If those individuals who work with the hearing-impaired child (parents, professionals, church and community leaders) are not promoting these characteristics in the child, the aural rehabilitationist should visit them and discuss these problems.

summary

This chapter has provided an introduction to aural rehabilitation, which should be available to hearing-impaired children in two major modes and in various settings: early intervention/preschool programming and school programming. Although the services in these settings are delivered by a variety of personnel, one professional—the parent advisor or AR therapist—should provide overall coordination and act as an advocate for the child. After early identification of the hearing loss the aural rehabilitation program is initiated. Evaluation efforts to prepare for remediation are followed by specific efforts in four major areas: overall coordination, amplification, communication rehabilitation, and psychosocial considerations. Remediation presents challenges to parents, children, and therapists. Nevertheless, if proper attention is given to all these aspects, prospects for effective remediation may be very good. If the hearing-impaired child's problems are partially or totally neglected, however, the youngster may be needlessly left to the devastation of hearing impairment. Therefore, the opportunity is great for each person involved in aural rehabilitation of children.

recommended readings

American Speech-Language-Hearing Association. (1980). *Guidelines for audiology programs in educational settings for hearing impaired children*. Rockville, MD: American Speech and Hearing Assoc.

Berg, F., Blair, J., Viehwig, S., & Wilson-Voltman, A. (1986). *Educational audiology for the hard of hearing child*. Orlando, FL: Grune and Stratton.

Bess, F., & McConnell, F. (1981). *Audiology, education and the hearing-impaired child*. St. Louis: C. V. Mosby Co.

Boothroyd, A. (1982). *Hearing impairments in young children*. Englewood Cliffs, NJ: Prentice-Hall.

Clark, T., & Watkins, S. (1985). *Programming for hearing impaired infants through amplification and home intervention* (4th ed.). Logan: Utah State University, SKI-HI Institute.

Martin, F.N. (Ed.). (1987). *Hearing disorders in children* (Chapters 9, 10, 11, 12, 13). Austin, TX: Pro-Ed.

Perkins, W.H. (1984). *Current therapy of communication disorders: Hearing disorders*. New York: Thieme-Stratton.

Roeser, R., & Downs, M. (1988). *Auditory disorders in school children* (2nd ed.). New York: Thieme-Stratton.

Ross, M., Brackett, D., & Maxon, A. (1982). *Hard of hearing children in regular schools.* Englewood Cliffs, NJ: Prentice-Hall.

references

American Annals of the Deaf. (1987). Educational programs and services. *American Annals of the Deaf, 132*(2), 124.

Allen, T.E. (1986). Patterns of academic achievement among hearing impaired students: 1974-1983. In A.N. Schildroth & M.A. Karchmer (Eds.), *Deaf children in America* (pp. 161-206). San Diego: College-Hill Press.

ASHA–American Speech and Hearing Association. (1978). *Guidelines for acoustic immittance screening of middle-ear function. Asha, 20*(7), 550-555.

ASHA–American Speech and Hearing Association. (1985). *Guidelines for identification audiometry. Asha, 28,* 49-52.

Baker, L., & Brown, A.L. (1984). Cognitive monitoring in reading. In J. Flood (Ed.), *Understanding reading comprehension* (pp. 21-44). Newark, DE: International Reading Association.

Balow, I.H., & Brill, R.G. (1975). An evaluation of reading and academic levels of sixteen graduating classes of the California School for the Deaf. *Volta Review, 77,* 255-266.

Berg, F.S. (1976). *Educational audiology: Hearing and speech management.* New York: Grune & Stratton.

Berg, F.S. (1986). Classroom acoustics and signal transmission. In F. Berg et al. (Eds.), *Educational audiology for the hard of hearing child* (pp. 157-180). Orlando, FL: Grune and Stratton.

Bess, F. (1977). Condition of hearing aids worn by children in a public school setting. In *The condition of hearing aids worn by children in a public school program.* (DHEW Publication (OE) 77-05002). Washington, DC: U.S. Government Printing Office.

Bess, F., Freeman, B., & Sinclair, J.S. (1981). *Amplification in education.* Washington, DC: Alexander Graham Bell Association for the Deaf.

Bess, F.H., & Logan, S.A. (1984). Amplification in the educational setting. In F. Bess & J. Jerger (Eds.), *Pediatric audiology* (pp. 147-176). San Diego: College-Hill Press.

Bess, F., & McConnell, F. (1981). *Audiology, education, and the hearing impaired child.* St. Louis: Mosby.

Birch, J. (1975). *Hearing impaired children in the mainstream.* Reston, VA: Council for Exceptional Children.

Blair, J., Wright, K., & Pollard, G. (1981). Parental understanding of their children's hearing aids. *Volta Review, 83,* 375-382.

BOL Statistics. (1975). *Monthly labor review reader.* (Bulletin 1868). USDL Bureau of Labor Statistics. Washington, DC: U.S. Government Printing Office.

BOL Statistics. (1977). *Education attainment of workers, special labor force report 209.* USDL Bureau of Labor Statistics. Washington, DC: U.S. Government Printing Office.

Boothroyd, A. (1978). Speech perception and sensorineural hearing loss. In M. Ross & T. Giolas (Eds.), *Auditory management of hearing-impaired children* (pp. 117-144). Austin, TX: Pro-Ed.

Boothroyd, A. (1982). *Hearing impairments in young children.* Englewood Cliffs, NJ: Prentice-Hall.

Bradley, R.H. (1987). The home environment: Providing a stimulating and supportive home environment for young children. *Early Childhood Update, 3*(1), 1,6.

Bronfenbrenner, U. (1974). *Is early intervention effective? A report on longitudinal evaluations of preschool programs* (Vol. II). (Department of Health, Education and Welfare, Office of Human Development, Office of Child Development, Children's Bureau, Department of Health, Education, and Welfare Publication No. OHD-76-30020). Washington, DC: U.S. Government Printing.

Brown, A.L. (1980). Metacognitive development and reading. In R.J. Spiro, B.B. Bruce, & W.F. Brewer (Eds.), *Theoretical issues in reading comprehension* (pp. 453-481). Hillsdale, NJ: Erlbaum.

Butler, K.G. (1983). Language processing: Selective attention and mnemonic strategies. In E. Lasky & J. Katz (Eds.), *Central auditory processing disorders* (pp. 297-315). Austin, TX: Pro-Ed.

Castle, D. (1984). *Telephone training for hearing-impaired persons: Amplified telephones, tdd's, codes.* Washington, DC: Alexander Graham Bell Association for the Deaf.

Cevette, M.J. (1984). Auditory brainstem response testing in the intensive care unit. In J. Northern & W. Perkins (Eds.), *Seminars in Hearing, 5*, 57-70.

Clarke, A., & Clarke, A. (1977). *Early experiences: Myth and evidence.* New York: Free Press.

Clark T., & Watkins, S. (1978). *Programming for hearing impaired infants through amplification and home intervention* (3rd ed.). Logan: Utah State University: Project SKI-HI.

Clark, T., & Watkins, S. (1985). *Programming for hearing impaired infants through amplification and home intervention* (4th ed.). Logan: Utah State University: Project SKI-HI.

Coleman, R.F. (1972). *Stability of children's hearing aids in an acoustic preschool.* (Final report). Washington, DC: HEW, U.S. Office of Education, National Center for Educational Research and Development, 522466.

Covert, R., & Clark, C. (1984). *Recertification program statement: Project SKI-HI.* Logan: Utah State University, SKI-HI Institute.

Craig, W.N. (1964). Effects of preschool training on the development of reading and lipreading skills of deaf children. *American Annals of the Deaf, 199*, 280-296.

Crum, M., & Matkin, N. (1976). Room acoustics: The forgotten variable? *Language, Speech and Hearing Services in the Schools, 7*, 106-110.

Curran, J.R. (1985). ITE aids for children: Survey of attitudes and practices of audiologists. *Hearing Instruments, 36*(4), 20-25.

Davis, J. (1977). Personnel and services. In J. Davis (Ed.), *Our forgotten children: Hard of hearing pupils in the schools* (pp. 27-42). Minneapolis: University of Minnesota Press.

Davis, J., & Hardick, E. (1981). *Rehabilitative audiology for children and adults.* New York: John Wiley and Sons.

DHEW. (1977). Department of Health, Education and Welfare. *Federal Register,* 42474-42518.

Dolch, E.W. (1945). *A manual for remedial reading* (2nd ed.). Champaign, IL: Garrard Press.

Downs, M. (1974). The deafness management quotient. *Hearing and Speech News, 42,* 8-28.

Downs, M. (1988). Contributions of mild hearing loss to auditory language learning problems. In R. Roeser & M. Downs (Eds.), *Auditory disorders in school children* (pp. 177-189). New York: Thieme-Stratton.

Downs, M., & Hemenway, W. (1969). Report on the hearing screening of 17,000 neonates. *International Audiology, 8,* 72-76.

Downs, M., & Sterritt, G. (1967). A guide to newborn and infant hearing screening programs. *Archives of Otolaryngology, 85,* 15-22.

Duchan, J.F., & Katz, J. (1983). Language and auditory processing: Top down plus bottom up. In E. Lasky & J. Katz (Eds.), *Central auditory processing disorders* (pp. 31-45). Austin, TX: Pro-Ed.

Eagles, E., Wishik, S., Doerfler, L., Melnick, W., & Levine, H. (1963). Hearing sensitivity and related factors in children. *Laryngoscope,* Special Monograph.

Easterbrooks, S.R. (1987). Speech/language assessment and intervention with school-age hearing impaired children. In J. Alpiner & P. McCarthy (Eds.), *Rehabilitative audiology: children and adults* (pp. 188-240). Baltimore, MD: Williams and Wilkins.

Erber, N. (1982). *Auditory training.* Washington, DC: Alexander Graham Bell Association for the Deaf.

Erber, N.P., & Alencewicz, C.M. (1976). Audiological evaluation of deaf children. *Journal of Speech and Hearing Disorders, 41,* 256-267.

Finitzo-Heiber, T. (1981). Classroom acoustics. In R. Roeser & M. Downs (Eds.), *Auditory disorders in school children* (pp. 250-262). New York: Thieme-Stratton.

Finitzo-Heiber, T., & Tillman, T. (1978). Room acoustics' effects on monosyllabic word discrimination ability for normal and hearing impaired children. *Journal of Speech and Hearing Research, 21,* 440-458.

Flint, W. (1971). Literacy: The keystone for providing more opportunities for deaf children. *Proceedings of the Forty-Fifth Meeting of the Convention of American Instructors for the Deaf.*

Fry, D. (1978). The role and primacy of the auditory channel in speech and language development. In M. Ross & T. Giolas (Eds.), *Auditory management of hearing-impaired children* (pp. 15-44). Austin, TX: Pro-Ed.

Gaeth, J., & Lounsbury, E. (1966). Hearing aids and children in elementary schools. *Journal of Speech and Hearing Disorders, 31,* 283-289.

Garstecki, D. (1978). Survey of school audiologists. *Asha, 20*(4), 291-296.

Gengel, R. (1971). Acceptable speech-to-noise ratios for aided speech discrimination by the hearing impaired. *Journal of Audiological Research, 11,* 219-222.

Gerkin, K.P., & Downs, M.P. (1984). The high risk register for newborn hearing programs. In J. Northern & W. Perkins (Eds.), *Seminars in Hearing, 5,* 9-16.

Gildston, P. (1973). The hearing impaired child in the classroom: A guide for the classroom teacher. In W.H. Northcott (Ed.), *The hearing impaired child in a regular classroom: Preschool, elementary, and secondary years* (pp. 37-43). Washington, DC: Alexander Graham Bell Association for the Deaf.

Grant, J. (1987). *The hearing impaired: Birth to six.* Boston: College Hill Press.

Greenberg, M.T. (1980). Social interaction between deaf preschoolers and their mothers: the effects of communication method and communication competence. *Developmental Psychology, 16,* 465-474.

Greenstein, J.B., Greenstein, K., McConville, K., & Stellini, L. (1976). *Acquisition in deaf children.* New York: Lexington School for the Deaf.

Griffith, J. (Ed.). (1969). *Persons with hearing loss.* Springfield, IL: Charles C. Thomas.

Goss, R. (1970). Language used by mothers of deaf children and mothers of hearing children. *American Annals of the Deaf, 115,* 93-96.

Hanners, B.A., & Sitton, A.B. (1974). Ear to hear: A daily hearing aid monitor program. *Volta Review, 76,* 530-536.

Harris, G.M. (1963). *Language for the preschool deaf child.* New York: Grune & Stratton.

Harris, G.M. (1981). Growths, gaps and future obligations: Keynote address Winnipeg conference on early management of hearing loss. In G.T. Mencher & S.E. Gerber (Eds.), *Early management of hearing loss.* New York: Grune & Stratton.

Hasenstab, M.S., & Horner, J.S. (1982). *Comprehensive intervention with hearing impaired infants and preschool children.* Rockville, MD: Aspen Systems.

Hasenstab, M.S., & Schoeny, Z.G. (1982). Auditory processing. In M.S. Hasenstab & J.S. Horner (Eds.), *Comprehensive intervention with hearing impaired infants and preschool children* (pp. 69-89). Rockville, MD: Aspen Systems.

Hayes, J., & Flower, L. (1980). Identifying the organization of writing processes. In W. Gregg & R. Steinberg (Eds.), *Cognitive processes in writing.* Hillsdale, NJ: Lawrence Erlbaum Associates.

Herzog, J.E. (1985). A study of the effectiveness of early intervention for hearing handicapped children. *Dissertation Abstracts International, 46,* 121A.

Horton, K.B. (1974). Infant intervention and language learning. In R.L. Schiefelbusch & L.L. Lloyd (Eds.), *Language perspectives—Acquisition, retardation, and intervention* (pp. 469-492). Austin, TX: Pro-Ed.

Horton, K.B. (1975). Early intervention through parent training. *Otolaryngologic Clinic of North America, 8,* 143-157.

Horton, K.B. (1976). Early intervention for hearing impaired infants and young children. In T.D. Tjossem (Ed.), *Intervention strategies for high risk infants and young children.* Baltimore, MD: University Park Press.

Hoverstein, G. (1981). A public school audiology program: Amplification maintenance, auditory management, and inservice education. In F. Bess et al. (Eds.), *Amplification in education*. Washington, DC: Alexander Graham Bell Association for the Deaf.

Jerger, J. (1980). Dissenting report: Mass impedance screening. *Annals of Otology, Thinology, and Laryngology, 89* (Suppl. 69), 21-22.

John Tracy Clinic Correspondence Course. (1983). *For parents of young deaf children: Part A and B*. Los Angeles, CA: John Tracy Clinic.

Johnson, C.D. (1987). Educational management of the hearing impaired child. In J. Alpiner & P. McCarthy (Eds.), *Rehabilitative audiology: children and adults* (pp. 241-268). Baltimore, MD: Williams & Wilkins.

Katz, J. (1978). The effects of conductive hearing loss on auditory function. *Asha, 20*(1), 879-886.

Keith, R.W. (1981). *Central auditory and language disorders in children*. San Diego, CA: College-Hill Press.

Kemker, J.F., McConnell, F., Logan, S.A., & Green, B.W. (1979). A field study of children's hearing aids in a school environment. *Language, Speech and Hearing Services in the Schools, 10*, 47-53.

Kretschmer, R., & Kretschmer, L. (1978). *Language development and intervention with the hearing impaired*. Austin, TX: Pro-Ed.

Kretschmer, R., & Kretschmer, L. (1984). Habilitation of language of deaf children. In W.H. Perkins (Ed.), *Current therapy of communication disorders: hearing disorders*. New York: Thieme-Stratton.

Lasky, E.Z., & Cox, L.C. (1983). Auditory processing and language interaction: Evaluation and intervention strategies. In E.Z. Lasky & J. Katz (Eds.), *Central auditory processing disorders* (pp. 243-368). Austin, TX: Pro-Ed.

Lasky, E.Z., & Katz, J. (1983). *Central auditory processing disorders*. Austin, TX: Pro-Ed.

Lillie, S.M. (1969). *Management of deafness in infants and very young children through their parents*. Address at the 47th Annual International Convention, Council for Exceptional Children, Denver.

Ling, D. (1976). *Speech and the hearing impaired child: Theory and practice*. Washington, DC: Alexander Graham Bell Association for the Deaf.

Ling, D. (1978). Auditory coding and recoding: An analysis of auditory training procedures for hearing-impaired children. In M. Ross & T. Giolas (Eds.), *Auditory management of hearing-impaired children: Principles and prerequisites for intervention* (pp. 181-218). Austin, TX: Pro-Ed.

Ling, D. (1984a). *Early intervention for hearing-impaired children: Oral options*. San Diego: College-Hill Press.

Ling, D. (1984b). *Early intervention for hearing impaired children: Total communication options*. San Diego: College-Hill Press.

Ling, D., & Ling, A. (1978). *Aural habilitation: The foundations of verbal learning in hearing-impaired children*. Washington, DC: Alexander Graham Bell Association for the Deaf.

Luterman, D. (1987). *Deafness in the family*. San Diego, CA: College-Hill Press.

Madell, J.R. (1984). Audiological management of the hearing-impaired child in the mainstream setting. In J. Northern & W. Perkins (Eds.), *Seminars in Hearing, 5,* 353-365.

Mahoney, T. (1984). High-risk hearing screening of large general newborn populations. In J. Northern & W. Perkins (Eds.), *Seminars in Hearing, 5,* 25-38.

Marlowe, J.A. (1984). The auditory approach to communication development for the infant with hearing loss. In W. Perkins (Ed.), *Current therapy of communication disorders: Hearing disorders* (pp. 3-9). New York: Thieme-Stratton.

Mathiesen, C.J. (1985). *Hearing aid applications in young children with recurrent otitis media.* Unpublished master's thesis, Idaho State University.

Matkin, N.D. (1984). Wearable amplification: A litany of persisting problems. In J. Jerger (Ed.), *Pediatric audiology: Current trends* (pp. 125-145). San Diego, CA: College-Hill Press.

Matkin, N.D., & Hook, P.E. (1983). A multidisciplinary approach to central auditory evaluations. In E.Z. Lasky & J. Katz (Eds.), *Central auditory processing disorders* (pp. 223-242). Austin, TX: Pro-Ed.

McAnally, P.L., Rose, S., & Quigley, S.P. (1987). *Language learning practices with deaf children.* San Diego, CA: College-Hill Press.

Miller, K., & Simmons, F.B. (1984). A retrospective and an update on the Crib-o-gram neonatal hearing screening audiometer. In J. Northern & W. Perkins (Eds.), *Seminars in Hearing, 5,* 49-56.

Mindel, E.D., & Vernon, M. (1987). *They grow in silence: The deaf child and his family* (2nd ed.). Silver Spring, MD: National Association of the Deaf.

Moeller, M.P., & McConkey, A.J. (1984). Language intervention with preschool deaf children: a cognitive/linguistic approach. In W.H. Perkins (Ed.), *Current therapy of communication disorders: Hearing disorders.* New York: Thieme-Stratton, Inc.

Moeller, M.P., Osberger, M.J., & Morford, B.A. (1987). Speech-language assessment and intervention with preschool hearing impaired children. In J. Alpiner & P. McCarthy (Eds.), *Rehabilitative audiology: Children and adults* (pp. 163-187). Baltimore, MD: Williams & Wilkins.

Moses, K.L. (1985). Infant deafness and parental grief: Psychosocial early intervention. In F. Powell et al. (Eds.), *Education of the hearing impaired child* (pp. 85-102). San Diego, CA: College-Hill Press.

Northcott, W. (1973). Implementing programs for young hearing impaired children. *Exceptional Child, 38*(1), 455-463.

Northern, J., & Downs, M. (1984). *Hearing in children* (3rd ed.). Baltimore, MD: Williams & Wikins.

Olsen, W. (1977). Acoustic and amplification in classrooms for the hearing impaired. In F. Bess (Ed.), *Childhood deafness: Causation, assessment, and management* (pp. 251-266). New York: Grune & Stratton.

Osberger, M.J. (1983). Development and evaluation of some speech training procedures for hearing-impaired children. In I. Hochberg, H.J. Levitt, & M.J. Osberger (Eds.), *Speech of the hearing impaired—Research, training and personnel preparation.* Austin, TX: Pro-Ed.

Pehrsson, R., & Denner, P. (1988a). *The semantic organizer approach to writing and study strategies.* Rockville, MD: Aspen Publishers.

Pehrsson, R., & Denner, P. (1988b). Semantic organizers: Implications for reading and writing. *Topics in Language Disorders.*

Pehrsson, R.S., & Robinson, H.A. (1985). *The semantic organizer approach to writing and reading instruction.* Rockville, MD: Aspen Publishers.

Phillips, A.L. (1987). Working with parents. A story of personal and professional growth. In D. Atkins (Ed.), Families and their hearing-impaired children. *Volta Review, 89*(5), 131-146.

Phillips, J. (1963). Syntax and vocabulary of mothers' speech to young children: Age and sex comparisons. *Child Development, 44,* 182-185.

Plisko, V.W., & Stern, J.D. (1985). *The condition of education. Statistical report.* Washington, DC: National Center for Educational Statistics, U.S. Department of Education.

Pollack, D. (1985). *Educational audiology for the limited hearing infant and pre-schooler* (2nd ed.). Springfield, IL: Charles C. Thomas.

Porter, T.A. (1973). Hearing aids in a residential school. *American Annals of the Deaf, 118,* 31-33.

Quigley, S. (1978). Effects of early hearing impairment on normal language development. In F. Martin (Ed.), *Pediatric audiology* (pp. 35-63). Englewood Cliffs, NJ: Prentice-Hall.

Quigley, S.P., & Kretschmer, R.E. (1982). *The education of deaf children: Issues, theories, and practice.* Baltimore, MD: University Park Press.

Rafferty, M. (1970). *Report of the study committee on state wide planning for the education of the deaf and severely hard of hearing in California state schools.* Sacramento: California State Department of Education.

Ramsdell, D. (1978). The psychology of the hard-of-hearing and the deafened adult. In H. Davis & R. Silverman (Eds.), *Hearing and deafness* (4th ed., pp. 499-510). New York: Holt, Rinehart & Winston.

Rand Report. (1974). *Improving services to handicapped children.* Santa Monica, CA: The Rand Corporation.

Rawlings, B., & Trybus, R. (1978). Personnel, facilities, and services available in schools and classes for hearing impaired children in the United States. *American Annals of the Deaf, 123,* 99-114.

Report to the Secretary of Health, Education and Welfare. (1969). Washington, DC: U.S. Department of Health, Education and Welfare Advisory Committee on the Education of the Deaf.

Ries, P. (1986). Characteristics of hearing impaired youth in the general population and of students in special educational programs for the hearing impaired. In A.N. Schildroth & M.A. Karchmer (Eds.), *Deaf children in America* (pp. 1-31). San Diego, CA: College Hill Press.

Rintelmann, W., & Bess, F. (1977). High level amplification and potential hearing loss in children. In F. Bess (Ed.), *Childhood deafness: Causation, assessment and management* (pp. 267-293). New York: Grune & Stratton.

Roberts, J. (1972). *Hearing and related medical findings among children. Race, area and socioeconomic differentials.* DHEW Publication No. (HMS) 73-1604. USDEH. Rockville, MD: National Center for Health Statistics.

Sinclair, S., Bess, F.H., & Riggs, D.E. (1981). *A field study of FM-wireless amplification in hearing impaired classrooms*. Paper presented at ASHA Convention, Los Angeles.

Skinner, M.W. (1988). *Hearing aid evaluation*. Englewood Cliffs, NJ: Prentice Hall.

Snow, C.E. (1976). The development of conversation between mothers and babies. *Journal of Child Language, 41*, 1-22.

Snow, C.E. (1984). Parent-child interaction and the development of communication ability. In R.L. Schiefelbusch & J. Pickar (Eds.), *The acquisition of communicative competence* (pp. 69-107). Baltimore, MD: University Park Press.

Stein, D., Benner, G., Hoversten, G., McGinnis, M., & Thies, T. (1980). *Auditory skills curriculum*. North Hollywood, CA: Foreworks.

Stein, L.K. (1984). Evaluating the efficiency of auditory brainstem response as a neonatal hearing screening test. In J. Northern & W. Perkins (Eds.), *Seminars in Hearing, 5*, 71-78.

Tell, L., Levi, C., & Feinmesser, M. (1977). Screening of infants for deafness in baby clinics. In F. Bess (Ed.), *Childhood deafness: Causation, assessment and management* (pp. 117-126). New York: Grune & Stratton.

Third Joint Committee of Infant Hearing Screening. (1983). Joint committee on infant hearing position statement. (1982). *Ear and Hearing, 4*(1), 3-4.

Tye-Murray, N., & Tyler, R. (1988). *Using laser videodisk technology to train speechreading and assertive listening skills*. Academy of Rehabilitative Audiology Summer Institute, Winter Park, CO.

Vernon, M., & Koh, S.D. (1970). Effects of early manual communication on achievement of deaf children. *American Annals of the Deaf, 115*, 527-536.

Vincent, L., Davis, J., Brown, P., Broome, K., Funkhouser, K., Miller, J., & Gruenewald, L. (1986). *Parent inventory of child development in non-school environment*. Madison: University of Wisconsin, Department of Rehabilitation Psychology and Special Education.

Watkins, S. (1984). *Longitudinal study on the effects of home intervention on hearing impaired children*. Unpublished doctoral dissertation, Utah State University.

Watkins, S. (1987). Long term effects of home intervention with hearing impaired children. *American Annals of the Deaf, 132*, 267-271.

Watkins, S., & Parlin, M. (1987). *SKI-HI 1986-87 national data report*. Logan: Utah State University, SKI-HI Institute.

Webster, D.B. (1983). Effects of peripheral hearing losses on the auditory brainstem. In E. Lasky & J. Katz (Eds.), *Central auditory processing disorders* (pp. 185-199). Austin, TX: Pro-Ed.

Wedenberg, E. (1981). Auditory training in historical perspective. In F. Bess et al. (Eds.), *Amplification in education* (pp. 1-25). Washington, DC: Alexander Graham Bell Association for the Deaf.

Willeford, J., & Billger, J. (1978). Auditory perception in children with learning disabilities. In J. Katz (Ed.), *Handbook of clinical audiology* (2nd ed., pp. 410-425). Baltimore, MD: Williams & Wilkins.

Wilson-Vlotman, A.L., & Blair, J.C. (1986). A survey of audiologists working full-time in school systems. *Asha, 28*, 11, 33-38.

Zink, G.D. (1972). Hearing aids children wear: A longitudinal study of performance. *The Volta Review, 74*, 41-51.

Robinson, D.O., & Sterling, G.R. (1980). Hearing aids and children in schools: A follow-up study. *The Volta Review, 82,* 229-235.

Roeser, R., & Downs, M. (1987). *Auditory disorders in school children* (2nd ed.). New York: Thieme-Stratton.

Ross, M. (1986). *Principles of aural habilitation.* Austin, TX: Pro-Ed.

Ross, M. (1987). Classroom amplification. In W. Hodgson & P. Skinner (Eds.), *Hearing aid assessment and use in audiologic habilitation* (3rd ed., pp. 231-265). Baltimore, MD: The Williams & Wilkins Co.

Ross, M., Brackett, D., & Maxon, A. (1982). *Hard of hearing children in regular schools.* Englewood Cliffs, NJ: Prentice-Hall.

Ross, M., & Giolas, T. (1971). Effects of three classroom listening conditions on speech intelligibility. *American Annals of the Deaf, 116,* 580-584.

Ross, M., & Tomassetti, C. (1987). Hearing aid selection for preverbal hearing-impaired children. In M.C. Pollack (Ed.), *Amplification for the hearing impaired* (3rd ed., pp. 213-253). New York: Grune & Stratton.

Rupp, R.R. (1977). Feasibility scale for language acquisition routing for young hearing impaired children. *Language, Speech and Hearing Services in Schools, VIII,* 222-233.

Rupp, R. (1979). A review of the audiology processing skills of fifty children and recommendations for educational management. *Journal of the Academy of Rehabilitative Audiology, 12*(2), 62-85.

Schell, Y. (1976). Electroacoustic evaluation of hearing aids worn by public school children. *Audiology and Hearing Education, 2,* 7-15.

Shearer, D.E., & Shearer, M.S. (1976). The portage project: A model for early childhood intervention. In T.D. Tjossem (Ed.), *Intervention strategies for high risk infants and young children* (pp. 335-350). Austin, TX: Pro-Ed.

Shepherd, N., Davis, J., Gorga, M., & Stelmachowicz, P. (1981). Characteristics of hearing impaired children in the public schools: Part I—Demographic data. *Journal of Speech and Hearing Disorders, 46,* 123-129.

Shortingas, C. (1980). *Cost effectiveness of home program.* First Annual Cost Effectiveness Workshop, HCEEP Rural Network, Nashville, TN.

Simmons, F.B. (1980). Diagnosis and rehabilitation of deaf newborns: Part II. *Asha, 22,* 475-479.

Simmons-Martin, A. (1978). Early management procedures for the hearing impaired child. In F. Martin (Ed.), *Pediatric audiology* (pp. 356-385). Englewood Cliffs, NJ: Prentice-Hall.

Simmons-Martin, A. (1983). Salient features from the literature, with implications for parent-infant programming. *American Annals of the Deaf, 128* (No. 2), 107-117.

Simpson, J.G., Schow, R.L., & Deputy, P.M. (1983). *Comparison of two behavioral screening scales for auditory processing disorders.* American Speech-Language-Hearing Association Western Regional Conference, Honolulu.

Sinclair, J.S., & Freeman, B.A. (1981). The status of classroom amplification in American education. In F. Bess et al. (Eds.), *Amplification in education.* Washington, DC: Alexander Graham Bell Association for the Deaf.

APPENDIX EIGHT A

the hearing-impaired child in the regular classroom

GENERAL SUGGESTIONS

1. The hearing-impaired child should be encouraged to watch the teacher whenever she is talking to the class.

2. The teacher should use natural gestures when they complement, not substitute for speech.

3. Whenever reports are given or during class meetings, have the children stand in the front of the class so the hard-of-hearing child can see lips.

4. During class discussions, let the hard-of-hearing child turn around and face the class so he can see the lips of the reciter.

5. To help the child follow instructions accurately, assignments should be written on the board so he can copy them in a notebook.

6. As other children with sensory defects, the child with impaired hearing needs individual attention. The teacher must be alert to every opportunity to provide individual help to fill gaps stemming from the child's hearing defect.

7. Ask the hearing-impaired child if he understands after an extensive explanation of arithmetic problems or class discussion. Write key words of an idea or lesson on chalkboard or slip of paper.

8. Enlist class cooperation in understanding the hearing-impaired student's problem. Designate a student to be his helper in assignments, someone who notes that he is on the right page and doing the right exercise. However, do not let the hearing-impaired child become too dependent on his "helper."

9. The child with impaired hearing should be seated no farther than 5-8 feet from the teacher. He should be allowed to shift his seat in order to follow the change in routine. This position will enable him to see the teacher's face and to hear her voice more easily.

10. If the child's hearing impairment involves only one ear or if the impairment is greater in one ear than the other, seat the child in the front with the poorer ear toward the noisy classroom and the better ear turned to the teacher or primary signal. When both ears have the same loss, center placement is recommended.

11. Seat the hearing-impaired child away from the heating/cooling systems, hallways, playground noise, etc.

12. If a choice of teachers is possible, the child with a hearing loss should be placed with the teacher who enunciates clearly. Distinct articulation is more helpful than raising one's voice.

13. The hearing-impaired child should be carefully watched to be sure he is not withdrawing from the group or that he is not suffering a personality change as a result of his hearing impairment. Make him feel like "one of the gang."

14. Be natural with the hard-of-hearing child. He will appreciate it if he knows you are considerate of his handicap.

15. In the lower grades, watch particularly that the hearing-impaired student does his part and is not favored or babied.

16. Use visual aids in your presentation of lessons. Visual aids provide the hearing-impaired child with the association necessary for learning new things.

17. Encourage the hearing-impaired child to accept his handicap and inspire him to make the most of it. Maintain his confidence in you so he will report any difficulty.

18. Parents should know the truth about their child's achievement. If marking is lenient because of the handicap, the parents should know that the child is not necessarily equaling the achievement of a normal-hearing child.

19. Hearing-impaired students need special encouragement when they pass from elementary to junior-high school and later into senior high. The pace is swifter. There is much more discussion. Pupils report to five or more teachers instead of one.

20. As the hearing-impaired youngster approaches the age of 16, be especially watchful. He may want to give up. Explain that he needs much preparation to enjoy a life of success and happiness.

HOW TO HELP A HEARING-IMPAIRED CHILD
USE SPEECHREADING SKILLS MORE EFFECTIVELY

1. Don't stand with your back to the window while talking (shadow and glare make it difficult to see your lips).

2. Stand still while speaking and in a place with a normal amount of light on your face.

3. Keep your hand and books down from your face while speaking.

4. Don't talk while writing on the blackboard.

5. Be sure you have his attention before you give assignments or announcements.

6. Speak naturally. Do not exaggerate or overemphasize. It is to be expected that it will be more difficult to hold the attention of the hard-of-hearing child. Never forget that the hard-of-hearing child gets fatigued sooner than other children because he not only has to use his eyes on all written and printed work, but also has to watch the lips.

7. Particular care must be used in dictating spelling. Use the words in sentences to show which of two similar words is meant (i.e., "Meet me after school" and "Give the dog some meat"). Thirteen words look like "meat" when spoken, such as been, bead and beet. The word "king" shows little or no lip movement. Context of the sentence gives the child the clue to the right word. Have the hard-of-hearing child say the words to himself before a mirror as he studies his spelling lesson.

8. If the hard-of-hearing child misunderstands, restate the question in a different way. Chances are you are using words with invisible movements. Be patient and never skip him. Be sure that things do not get past him.

HOW TO HELP THE HEARING-IMPAIRED CHILD
USE HIS SPEECH SKILLS MORE EFFECTIVELY

1. A severe hearing impairment that lasts over a period of time tends to result in a dull, monotonous voice and inaccurate enunciation. Therefore, a child with such hearing loss should be encouraged to speak clearly. Keeping the child "speech conscious" will help him resist the usual damage to the voice that a severe hearing impairment produces. Do not let the child get the habit of shaking his head or speaking indistinctly instead of answering in complete sentences.

2. Encourage him to participate in musical activities. This will stimulate his residual hearing and add rhythm to his speech.

3. Since a hearing impairment affects the language processes, the child should be encouraged to compensate by a more active interest in all language activities: reading, spelling, original language, etc.

4. If the young hard-of-hearing child is poor in reading, chances are he needs basic phonics to improve both reading and speech.

5. Teach the child to use the dictionary with skill, to learn the pronunciation system so he can pronounce new words.

6. Build up his vocabulary by assigning supplementary materials.

7. Give him a chance to read ahead on the subject to be discussed. Make sure he is familiar with the vocabulary so he can follow along better.

8. Praise and encourage the hearing-impaired child, where justified, to give him a feeling of success which he needs in order to build up his confidence in his speaking abilities.

APPENDIX EIGHT B

clinician scale of auditory behaviors

After administering the receptive portion of the *Northwestern Syntax Screening Test*, please rate each item by circling a number that best fits the observed behavior of the child you are rating. At the top of the column of numbers there is a term indicating the frequency with which the behavior is observed. Please consider these terms carefully when rating each possible behavior. A description for each item is provided with this screening instrument to guide the user in making the ratings. A child may or may not display one or more of these behaviors. A high or low rating in one or more areas does not indicate any particular pattern. When rating a group of children, please refer to the description often. If you are undecided about the rating on an item, use your best judgment.

From *Comparison of Two Behavioral Screening Scales for Auditory Processing Disorders* by J. G. Simpson, R. L. Schow, and P. M. Deputy, 1983. Paper presented at American Speech-Language-Hearing Association Western Regional Conference, Honolulu, HI.

Name: _____ Age: ____ Grade: ____ Today's Date: _____

Clinician: _____ School: _____ Score: _____
        (Informant)

Frequently	Often	Sometimes	Seldom	Never	ITEMS
1	2	3	4	5	Impulsive
1	2	3	4	5	Inefficient in searching behavior
1	2	3	4	5	Forgets instructions
1	2	3	4	5	Needs confirmation
1	2	3	4	5	Exhibits consistent, significant delay
1	2	3	4	5	Has short attention span
1	2	3	4	5	Perseverates
1	2	3	4	5	Shows lack of precision in pointing response
1	2	3	4	5	Operates in a confusion set

Comments:

EXPLANATION FOR *CLINICIAN SCALE*

The following descriptions explain what might be characterized as a "number 1" child, or a youngster who shows these behaviors frequently. In contrast, a "number 5" child is one who shows none of these characteristics.

1. *Impulsive*

   An impulsive child is one whose responses are sudden, often appearing to be without prior thought or consideration. This child will attempt to make a response before instructions are complete. The clinician finds herself constantly reminding the child to wait until she has finished giving the cue.

2. *Inefficient in searching behavior*
A child who is inefficient in searching behavior will not systematically search a plate with four or five possible responses. The child may consider one or two items and ignore other possibilities. The clinician must frequently remind the child to look at all the pictures.

3. *Forgets instructions*
This child may learn the task and complete a few tasks. Then part way through the series, he seems to forget what he was expected to do and has to be retrained to complete the rest of the series.

4. *Needs confirmation*
This child does not appear to have confidence in his responses even if they are correct. He may start to point and just as he does, hesitate and look at the clinician as if to ask, "is this right?". The child may express this need for confirmation even on the simplest and most obvious of responses.

5. *Exhibits consistent, significant delay*
An occasional delayed response is normal. However, if the delay in responding occurs on many of the items, the delay may be considered consistent. The significance of the delay is judged by the clinician. Small, momentary delays may not be considered significant. An experienced clinician will have little trouble distinguishing a significant delay in responding.

6. *Has short attention span*
This youngster has difficulty attending to a task for any length of time. He may show an inability to sit still and pay attention. He may be considered as highly active. He may also seem unable to process or grasp information when auditorily presented, even in a face-to-face situation. Such a youngster may be judged to be unresponsive in these cases.

7. *Perseverates*
This type of a child may consistently point to one of the choices presented; for example, he may always point to the first choice or always to the last choice. The child may perseverate on concepts. For example, if preceding items have to do with color and then a dimension is added, the child may continue to try to respond to the task as a color task. The child may have difficulty changing when the format of the task or the desired response changes.

8. *Shows lack of precision in pointing response*
This child may not point directly with the index finger. Instead, he may bang his hand down on the picture or use several fingers to point. The child may place his fingers so that the indicated response is not clear to the clinician, or he may use his forearm or elbow to try to point. Responses are often ambiguous and the clinician frequently says, "Which one did you mean?".

9. *Operates in a confusion set*
This child appears to be confused about the simplest instructions or tasks. Even after he has learned a task, he appears to be confused when he is completing it. The child seemingly expects to be confused although he can do the task, or the instructions are simple. When the clinician changes tasks, the child may indicate an inability to understand the new instructions.

APPENDIX EIGHT C

teacher scale of auditory behaviors

Please rate each item by circling a number that best fits the behavior of the child you are rating. At the top of the column of numbers there is a term indicating the frequency with which the behavior is observed. Please consider these terms carefully when rating each possible behavior. A description for each item is provided with this screening instrument to guide the user in making the ratings. A child may or may not display one or more of these behaviors. A high or low rating in one or more of the areas does not indicate any particular pattern. When rating a group of children, please refer to the description often. If you are undecided about the rating on an item, use your best judgment.

From *Comparison of Two Behavioral Screening Scales for Auditory Processing Disorders* by J. G. Simpson, R. L. Schow, and P. M. Deputy, 1983. Paper presented at American Speech-Language-Hearing Association Western Regional Conference, Honolulu, HI.

Name: _____ Age: ____ Grade: ____ Today's Date: _____

Teacher: _____ School: _____ Score: _____
(Informant)

Frequently	Often	Sometimes	Seldom	Never	ITEMS
1	2	3	4	5	Fails to complete task
1	2	3	4	5	Inattentive in group situations
1	2	3	4	5	Inattentive in individual situations
1	2	3	4	5	Fails to understand and follow oral instructions
1	2	3	4	5	Compulsive, rigid, perseverative
1	2	3	4	5	Extremely active, impulsive
1	2	3	4	5	Exhibits behavioral problems
1	2	3	4	5	Has poor interpersonal skills
1	2	3	4	5	Has learning difficulties
1	2	3	4	5	Has problems telling about experiences
1	2	3	4	5	Disorganized

Comments:

EXPLANATION FOR *TEACHER SCALE*

The following descriptions explain what might be characterized as a "number 1" child, or a youngster who shows these behaviors frequently. In contrast, a "number 5" child is one who shows none of these characteristics.

1. *Fails to complete task*
   A child who fails to complete a task will stop doing the task for some reason. He may often get side tracked or become distracted and for-

get to go back to the task. He may resist doing the task and fail to do it in spite of frequent adult encouragement. He may be responding to his own lack of confidence in being able to do tasks and give up many times with only half-hearted attempts. These behaviors are accentuated when the child is working independently. Whatever the reason, this is a child that fails to complete different kinds of tasks in many different situations.

2. *Inattentive in group situations*
Youngsters with this symptom will have unusually poor attending behaviors when part of a group. In fact, this child will have difficulty learning in a group situation. The inattentive behavior may be related to a low tolerance for the noise generated in the group, but may also be present in a general classroom situation where the distractions are visual or auditory.

3. *Inattentive in individual situations*
These youngsters have difficulty in attending when they are receiving individual instructions. They may show an inability to sit still and pay attention. They may be considered by those involved with them as highly active. They may also seem unable to process or grasp information when auditorily presented, even in a face-to-face situation. They may be judged to be unresponsive in these cases.

4. *Fails to understand and follow oral instructions*
This youngster will have a hard time following directions. Often this behavior is the first to be mentioned by a teacher or parent. The child may be able to follow simple one-stage instructions but breaks down when the instructions get more complicated. He may only remember or complete a portion of the instructions. He may be easily confused or misunderstand the instructions such as bringing an object to the adult instead of putting it on the table. These children may understand an initial instruction but lose the idea of the instruction halfway through a series of tasks. The child may impulsively try to complete an instruction before the adult finishes giving it. He may consistently delay his attempt to complete an instruction while trying to think through the instruction. Some of these children are observed repeating the instruction over to themselves. They may often request that the instruction be repeated.

5. *Compulsive, rigid, perseverative*
This child may insist verbally and behaviorally on completing some behavior. For example, he may be looking out the window and when

directed away from the window may repeatedly go back to it or resist direction. He may seem to be compulsive in other behaviors. Change may be difficult for this child. A change in schedule or routine may seem to be hard for him to comprehend. He may repeat an action or behavior over and over such as drawing the same picture or throwing a bean bag to the same box. When completing a series of tasks with three or more choices he may always select the item on the left or right. He may be known for insisting on doing things his way.

6. *Extremely active, impulsive*

This child seems to be in constant motion. He may or may not be medically diagnosed as hyperactive, but many adults involved with him may use that term. Often parents state ''maybe he is hyperactive.'' Whenever there are materials out in preparation for an activity, this child is reaching for them and manipulating them before the adult is ready to begin the task. This child's overall activity level may be described as impulsive. For example, when told it is time to go he may suddenly jump up and leave the room. An adult may hand him an object and prepare to instruct the child about the object and he may grab the object and try to manipulate it before receiving the instruction. When receiving verbal instructions the child often attempts to complete the item before the instructions are completed. He may be thought of as a child who often ''jumps the gun.''

7. *Exhibits behavioral problems*

A behavioral problem is defined as consistent action or behavior which interrupts a child's ability to function smoothly and learn in the classroom. The child may be anxious, moody or depressed. He may display poor self-esteem and often overtly or covertly express feelings of inadequacy. Often in attempting to complete a task there is an overt display of frustration and aggression. He may exhibit frequent inappropriate emotional reactions such as uncontrollable laughing and over-excitement when experiencing or anticipating pleasure. He may show excessive loudness, shouting or temper tantrums when frustrated or angry. His behavior may be considered disruptive and/or destructive. He may express aggression towards other children, even hitting them. His general behavior may be described by teachers and parents as obstinate and hard to handle.

8. *Has poor interpersonal skills*

This child may be experiencing social problems in the classroom and at home. He may be a loner and be socially isolated. He may seek companionship with older or younger people. Eye contact may be poor. Responses to individuals may be characterized by inappropriate intonation and gestures accompanying verbal responses. Some of his behavior may appear strange or weird. He may be the child that is teased and ostracized by others. He may exhibit anti-social behavior and reject others' attempts to make friends with him.

9. *Has learning difficulties*
The child who has learning difficulties may display this difficulty in many different ways. He may have more trouble with pre-academic learning skills like arranging objects or pictures in an appropriate sequence (sequencing problems). He may have difficulty learning phonics or associating sounds with letters (sound-symbol). He may have difficulty with other learning tasks such as matching or rhyming. He may not retain what he learns or not generalize from one experience to the other. He may have a great deal of difficulty with abstract concepts. He may be learning or working below expected levels in one or more areas for no apparent reason.

10. *Has problems telling about his experiences*
This problem can show up in one of two ways. First, the child might be limited in the amount of verbalization he uses to describe and explain situations. The child may use short, even if well-constructed sentences. His descriptions and explanations are not considered full or elaborate. Often an adult has to question further in order to elicit enough explanation of a situation to be able to understand it.

The second form of expression problem is exhibited by a child who is highly verbal. This child talks constantly. However, this child seems to be talking around the topic instead of saying specifically what is on his mind. He uses a lot of verbalization to express the intent of his communication. He may often leave the listener and himself confused as to the purpose of the communication. Both types of children may get the sequence of events mixed up when trying to tell something. There may be some hesitancies, interjections and word-finding problems. Overall, this is a child who, although capable of verbalizing, does not do it effectively.

11. *Disorganized*
The child who is disorganized demonstrates this characteristic in many ways. His appearance may not be neat. His desk and/or work area may always be messy. He carries out tasks in a haphazard manner even though he may complete them. He often loses small items. At times during group class activities he may appear to be disoriented.

APPENDIX EIGHT D

suggestions for children who have difficulty with auditory memory

For the child with shortened sequential auditory memory, the family and teacher should consider the following modifications or suggestions:

1. Directions or instructions to the child should be reduced in length, and the length should be in keeping with the upper limit of the child's syllable recall ability.

2. Ideally, if the child can read, detailed work assignments should be written out, so the child can visually double check his auditory input. Saturday work assignments at home could be aurally given and then supplemented with a written list (which could be marked off by the child as he/she completes each item). Similarly, the teacher may wish to write crucial assignments on the board so that the special child can visually check on himself.

3. As a support process, the teacher may quietly assign a "friend" to help the child on directions, if written or special aid cannot be given.

4. If the child cannot read, then home and school directions can be modified by lists of key drawings or sketches to help the child keep the outline in correct order.

5. In discussions at home and at school, silent intervals may help this child to "catch up" with the topic.

6. When the parent or teacher is not sure the child has understood the process, a request for a verbal review may clarify whether the youngster is ready to follow through on the assignment appropriately.

7. There are commercially available programs to help the child strengthen his sequential memory skills as well as other auditory processing abilities. These have been reviewed by Rupp et al. (1978). These "packaged" programs are available to assist the teacher, the audiologist, the speech and language pathologist or the resource teacher to expe-

From "A Review of the Audiology Processing Skills of Fifty Children and Recommendations for Educational Management" by R. Rupp, 1979, *Journal of the Academy of Rehabilitative Audiology*, 12(2), pp. 62–85. Reprinted by permission.

dite the therapeutic programs for children with specific auditory processing problems. Three such representative programs that are available to help the clinician work through a habilitative process are the *Lindamood and Lindamood Auditory Discrimination in Depth*, the *Semel Auditory Processing Program*, published in 1970, and the *Auditory Perceptual Training Program* published by Witkin and her colleagues in 1976. Obviously, the skilled clinician will not simply run one of these programs with a child, but will design a therapeutic program and use portions of available programs as they fit the needs of a specific child. In the present discussion, the intervention goal would be to lengthen the child's auditory sequential memory.

APPENDIX EIGHT E

suggestions for children who have difficulty in noisy environments

For the child who cannot listen effectively in noisy environments, a series of monitor and modification approaches may be employed:

1. Preferential or roving seating can be instituted within the classroom so that a more favorable signal-to-noise ratio can be established with the child in closer proximity to the teacher. Additionally, such an arrangement also places the ambient classroom noises behind the child, and if our findings support that performance improves with separation of noise spatially from the desired speech signal, then this signal will be doubly benefited for the child gets a stronger speech signal and is able to "tune out" the background noise more easily.

2. Realistically, the family should realize that stereos, television, and noisy siblings also have a negative effect on ease of attending in the home environment. Therefore, when it is important that this child listen at home most easily, the other noises in the environment should be suppressed or turned off. Important listening would be at mealtime, when discussing family issues involving the participation of the

From "A Review of the Audiology Processing Skills of Fifty Children and Recommendations for Educational Management" by R. Rupp, 1979, *Journal of the Academy of Rehabilitative Audiology*, 12(2), pp. 62–85. Reprinted by permission.

child, and when one parent may be helping the child with necessary (and catch-up) homework. In these instances, unnecessary "noise" should be abolished for meal and discussion times. Homework discussions should be done in the child's quiet room as far away as possible from the bustling activity of the home.

3. Recognition should be given that this child may not respond appropriately if mother calls to him from another room as he listens to a favorite television show. Important conversations need to come during a commercial or after the set has been turned off.

4. Annual principal-parent conferences should be scheduled prior to the assignment of the child to the next grade. Such childen function optimally in a quiet classroom with an articulate teacher. If there are three possible teachers available for the next year's classroom assignment (and all are assumed to be equally effective), then the student will perform best in the most quiet classroom.

5. There will be times when the family and school cannot control the noise levels which interfere with easy listening. When this occurs, the expectations on the child should be modified and reduced because of the adverse environment.

6. A summary suggestion is to maximize the desirable speech signal and to suppress the noise.

chapternine

AURAL REHABILITATION FOR ADULTS

JEROME G. ALPINER

DEAN C. GARSTECKI

contents

introduction

The vast majority of hearing-impaired persons in the United States are adults who have acquired hearing loss due to etiologies such as illness, accident, noise exposure, and the aging process (Santore, Tulko, & Kearney, 1983). Most of these individuals have maintained some residual hearing which enables them to communicate. The effect of hearing loss on these adults varies greatly depending on time and circumstances of loss as well as extent of loss. Many hearing-impaired persons benefit from aural rehabilitation procedures which include hearing/sensory aids/assistive devices, communication training (speechreading, auditory training), and counseling. Perhaps the most significant development in aural rehabilitation is amplification, which now affords the hearing-impaired person the opportunity to communicate more effectively than ever before, particularly in conjunction with other rehabilitation measures.

profile of the adult client

Although the age of 65 is often referred to as the beginning of "old age," hearing loss due to aging may occur well before. Chapter 10 focuses on the special problems of the adult elderly in the retirement years. The present chapter deals primarily with those adults who could be classified as hard of hearing and who experience hearing-related problems during their working years. Much of what is said here also applies to the adult with congenital deafness.

Remediation for adults with hearing loss must be tied to concomitant problems in social, familial, and vocational relationships. These relationships are tied to communication situations in which most persons find themselves daily. Hearing loss in adults usually develops gradually and the progression of loss is slow, that is, the hearing impairment "sneaks up." Ordinarily, the higher frequencies diminish first, so the person hears speech but does not always understand clearly what is said. In the early stages, the hearing-impaired person blames others for mumbling or not speaking sufficiently loud. Ultimately, these situations lead to frustrations and tensions due to breakdown in the communication process. Soon difficulties begin to emerge with spouses, children, employers, and friends. Although these persons may suspect a hearing problem, this suggestion may not be accepted by the hearing-impaired person. A hearing problem is often not easily accepted because it involves the acknowledgment of a physical disability. Consequently, aural rehabilitation becomes an appropriate therapeutic consideration to help alleviate problem areas.

Goldstein and Stephens (1981) indicated that the nature and sequencing of treatment as well as the degree of success depend on four attitude types:

1. **Attitude Type I** - The patient has a strongly positive attitude toward hearing aids and audiological care. Both auditory and psychological factors are amenable to therapeutic solutions.

2. **Attitude Type II** - The patient has an essentially positive attitude toward hearing aids and aural rehabilitation but some complications are present. There may have been an unfavorable previous therapy experience or social, educational, or vocational factors which preclude the use of simple solutions. Also included in this group are clients with difficult-to-fit audiometric configurations, or mild impairment for which both the client and the audiologist want assurance of benefit to warrant the cost of treatment. About two-thirds to three-quarters of clients fitted with hearing aids fit into Type I, the remainder into Type II (Goldstein & Stephens, 1981).

3. **Attitude Type III** - The patient has a fundamentally negative attitude although there exists a shred of cooperative intent. The negative attitude towards hearing aids may arise from a variety of situations and comes in many forms. It may reflect the stigma of a hearing aid or a generalized inability to cope with change in status.

4. **Attitude Type IV** - The patient belongs to a small group who reject hearing aids and the entire rehabilitation process. A total discharge from the therapy process is likely, but a last-ditch effort to salvage a thread of remediation potential should be attempted.

To describe how patients may react upon recognizing the presence of hearing loss, a recent case study of one 50-year-old male client is presented. This man has a moderate sensorineural loss of hearing bilaterally with a greater deficit in the higher frequencies. Recognition ability for understanding speech is 80% in quiet and 65% in noise. It was determined, after medical examination by a physician, that the cause of the hearing loss was unknown. The physician referred the patient back to the center for hearing aid evaluation and aural rehabilitation. The client had been seen for speechreading therapy about five years earlier. The loss was in a mild to moderate category at that time, and he did not want a hearing aid. During the past five years, the client had remarried and purchased his own business. He reported that he was having both family and business difficulties with regard to communication. He stated that he really did not want to take the time to involve himself in the rehabilitation process. After considerable conversation and counseling, however, he admitted that he had to do something or his marital and business difficulties would increase. He agreed to amplification on a trial basis; he would not agree to other aural rehabilitation procedures including speechreading and auditory training. The patient stated that he just did not have time if his business was to succeed. He was willing to return for three post-hearing aid followup sessions as of the writing of this chapter. His attitude is not unique. He probably fits into Attitude Type II.

It is not always easy for individuals to accept the limitations of a sensory system that was once normal. Acceptance is a requisite to engaging in hearing aid evaluation and rehabilitation, however. Unless the hearing-impaired person fully realizes the problem, there always will be a tendency to shy away from rehabilitation. Thus, hearing loss represents more than a set of numerical measures. There is also a psychologic aspect that affects the person's ego. Unfortunately, it may be easier for many adults to withdraw socially from the mainstream than to accept hearing aids or hearing therapy. This general profile of one type of adult may help increase our awareness of the complexities involved in providing aural rehabilitation.

rehabilitation settings

Hearing-impaired adults seek rehabilitative care when they experience the need for better use of their residual hearing and/or hearing aid. They also may seek care to improve their social or vocational communication skills, or to increase their ability to manage hearing-loss-related problems. Rehabilitative care is delivered in a variety of settings. Some are full-service centers staffed by communication specialists. However, most are partial-service centers staffed by professionals, sales people, and/or lay persons. Popular service centers include university speech and hearing clinics, community hearing societies, hospitals, otologic clinics, senior citizen centers, vocational rehabilitation offices, and hearing aid sales offices.

University Programs. The first adult aural rehabilitation centers were university training programs for speech-language pathologists and audiologists and military hospitals for hearing-impaired World War II veterans. The focus of rehabilitation in these settings was, and still is, directed toward improvement of the adult's communication skills through use of appropriate amplification and communication remediation exercises, and by counseling and educating hearing-impaired adults and their families.

This early model continues to influence present-day programs. For example, Hardick (1977) described the Ohio State University program that centers on use of amplification, modifying the communication environment, consumer information, building a support system among the hearing-impaired adult's friends and family members, and developing a better understanding of factors that influence the everyday communication process.

Kirby and Rogan (1981) reported on a 4-week program for new hearing aid users at Purdue University. Program participants are oriented in ways to use and maintain their hearing aid and other communication devices. The nucleus of the program's weekly activities is built on consumer issues which include demonstration, discussion, and exercise in improving communication skills.

At Northwestern University, first consideration is given to motivating the adult toward hearing aid use through exercises that demonstrate how amplification can improve communication skills (Garstecki, 1984). Hearing aid candidates wear appropriate aids in contrived listening tasks. After four 1-hour sessions of "auditory training" involving interacting with successful users and discussing the pros and cons of hearing aid use, clients are able to make informed decisions regarding purchase of the aid. Beyond the fitting of an appropriate aid, major program emphasis is on improvement of auditory and auditory-visual communication skills. This is done through systematic manipulation of message variables inherent in everyday conversation such as amount of message information, type of competing noise, signal-to-noise ratio, and relevance of situational cues. In addition, clients are helped to develop strategies which enhance their communication skills. Finally, the client and family member or friend receive information on hearing loss and its treatment, hearing aids, factors influencing everyday communication, hearing conversation, assistive devices, warning systems, and community services for hearing-impaired individuals.

Military. In the military and in Veterans Administration Hospitals, aural rehabilitation services are available for current and former military personnel. Inpatients are scheduled for intensive blocks of service at the Walter Reed Army Medical Center, for example (Sedge, 1979), and those with high-frequency hearing loss are evaluated and rehabilitated in speech recognition and production skills, problem awareness, situation control skills, and social-vocational-emotional adjustments to hearing loss. The San Francisco Veterans Administration Medical Center applies a progressive approach to adult rehabilitation in which the emphasis is on creating an understanding of where and how communication breakdowns occur and removing hearing loss as a crutch (Fleming, 1972). The clients join one of two groups: (a) hearing-impaired individuals only, or (b) hearing-impaired individuals and family members or friends. An audiologist and a psychologist function as members of each group.

Community Centers and Agencies. Community hearing societies, such as those in San Francisco, Chicago, Milwaukee, and other large cities, provide rehabilitation settings where participants are usually highly motivated and well directed toward management of their problems. In San Francisco the Hearing Society for the Bay Area, for example, provides a program of two 6-hour sessions on successive weekends. Concentrated programs such as this draw people with a high interest in improving their ability to compensate for their loss. Attrition is considerably less under this concentrated meeting format, than when sessions are spread over longer periods of time (A. Grimes, personal communication, 1988).

Vocational rehabilitation offices provide hearing-impaired adults with access to a network of evaluation and remediation services often important for optimizing their potential for gainful employment and for helping them function as contributing members of a community. The vocational rehabilitation office can be an important setting in the aural rehabilitation process for hearing-handicapped adults in the work force.

Private Practice Audiologists and Hearing Aid Dealers. With some exceptions, services offered by private, practicing audiologists affiliated with otologic medical groups often do not extend beyond the fitting of a hearing aid, orientation to its use, and counseling regarding management of hearing problems. The advantage of services provided in this setting is that otologic and audiologic needs, sometimes including the fitting of a hearing aid, can be met in one place. For some hearing-impaired adults, this satisfies all their rehabilitative needs. Others, however, have additional concerns related to knowing how to deal effectively with their hearing loss. Once hearing-impaired adults know they have a hearing loss, they usually want to learn how to effectively compensate for the problems such a loss creates.

Most hearing aids are dispensed in hearing aid sales offices; therefore, sales people in these settings play a critical part in the rehabilitation process. Hearing aid dispensers provide hearing aids and associated devices and assist in initial adjustment to hearing aid use. They also provide supplies and services to keep the aid in working order. Few dispensers are trained to provide other rehabilitative services. However, as additional audiologists dispense hearing aids, more comprehensive aural rehabilitation service should be expected.

Consumer Helping Groups. An emerging hearing rehabilitation source may be found in such groups as the Self-Help for Hard of Hearing People, Inc. (SHHH) and others who are concerned about quality care from competent service providers (Davis, 1980; Madell, 1980; Smaldino & Sahli, 1980; and Stream & Stream, 1980; see also Chapter 13, Resources and Materials List - Adults/Elderly). Wanting to increase public awareness of the problems associated with hearing loss, these organizations have successfully spearheaded solutions to such problems as use of public telephones by hearing aid wearers and installation of group amplification systems in theatres, churches, lecture halls, and other public meeting places. Consumer groups provide a vehicle by which hearing-impaired adults can improve their ability to self-manage their problems. However, in some instances, important questions have gone unanswered, been incorrectly answered or answered from experience rather than from a data-base, thereby creating problems for some well-meaning groups and those they purport to serve. The value of the rehabilitative service provided in consumer meeting settings often depends on the input from professional hearing health care consultants.

The hearing-impaired adult should undergo a thorough audiologic/communication assessment in order to benefit from a rehabilitative program in any setting. The various aspects and procedures associated with the assessment process will be described in the following section.

rehabilitation evaluation of communication impairment and handicap with adults

Procedures used in audiometric and nonaudiometric evaluation of potential rehabilitation program participants are described in this section. *Hearing impairment* refers to limitations in hearing ability while *hearing handicap* refers to the effects of these limitations on everyday life.

While we have extensive audiometric methods for measuring hearing impairment, Schow and Nerbonne (1982) emphasized that little has been done to perfect and standardize methods for assessing the overall communication abilities (impairment plus handicap) of individuals who are hearing impaired. The need to combine audiometric measures with nonaudiometric assessment for determining hearing impairment and hearing handicap is a priority for clinicians and researchers. Unfortunately, the vast majority of audiologists in the United States, for whatever reason, have given scant attention to handicap and the self-assessment tools generally used to measure handicap.

Assessment of *communication function* in the aural rehabilitation process is important for several reasons. First, there is a need to obtain information that will contribute to a change or a manipulation of the hearing-impaired person's family, work or social environment. Second, an assessment of the psychological manifestations of the hearing handicap is needed. Emotional and psychologic problems may be extensions of the organic hearing problem and often create a greater handicap than the actual hearing loss. Client input is helpful in dealing with this aspect of aural rehabilitation. Finally, it is important to assess the effectiveness of aural rehabilitation. Assessment procedures can be used in both pre- and posttherapy thereby allowing a measure of improvement in communication function. It is hoped that efforts in both impairment and handicap assessment will continue to expand and improve in order to provide more adequate information about overall communication ability.

audiometric impairment evaluation

According to Keith (1984), the audiometric evaluation has two purposes: to assist in (a) diagnosis and (b) rehabilitation. The diagnostic test battery consists of pure-tone air and bone-conduction audiometry, speech threshold tests, speech-recognition tests, and measures of tolerance. The basic audiometric battery results indicate whether a hearing loss exists, degree and type of loss, and if the loss is likely to be remedied medically or surgically or compensated for through amplification. A variety of test procedures may be added to the standard assessment battery to differentiate cochlear from retrocochlear problems, determine vestibular function, assess middle-ear function, and measure central auditory-processing ability.

To develop relevant goals and activities for improving communication skills, it may be desirable to extend the audiometric test battery to include identification of those circumstances under which speech-recognition ability changes. For example, test materials might be selected to help determine patterns of recognition difficulty. The *California Consonant Test* (Owens & Schubert, 1977) has been found to be sensitive to the phonetic confusions demonstrated by subjects with high-frequency sensorineural hearing loss (Schwartz & Surr, 1979). The results of such tests are helpful in designing remediation programs for adults who demonstrate phonetic confusions (see Chapter 3).

Since everyday conversation involves phrases and sentences, it may be of interest to measure a hearing-impaired adult's sentence recognition ability. Monosyllabic words provide phonetic and semantic cues to their perception and sentences provide syntactic and temporal cues. While the resolving power of sentence tests is lower than that of word tests, sentence recognition tests provide useful information for purposes of communication skill assessment and remediation. For example, *CID Everyday Speech Sentences* have been used for purposes of information evaluation. These sentences were developed by Grant Fairbanks and a working group of the Armed Forces (i.e., the National Research Council Committee on Hearing and Bio-Acoustics, in Davis & Silverman, 1970). Jerger, Speaks, and Trannell (1968) developed synthetic sentence materials. Kalikow, Stevens, and Elliott (1977) designed *Speech Perception in Noise* (SPIN) test materials to measure sentence recognition ability.

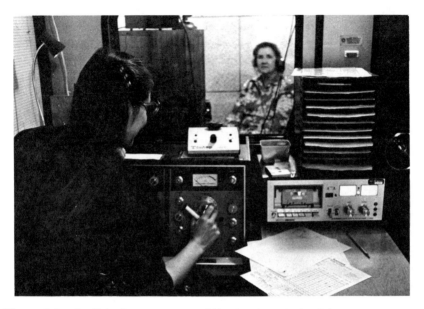

Figure 9.1. Audiologic assessment of hearing-impaired adult.

Preliminary research findings (Hutcherson, Dirks, & Morgan, 1979) suggest that SPIN test results provide a realistic estimate of speech-recognition ability under everyday listening conditions.

Auditory/Visual Testing. In addition to varying type of test materials used and presentation conditions (quiet or noise background), consideration should be given to alternate test materials. Alpiner (1978), Binnie (1973), Byman (1974), Erber (1971), Garstecki (1980) and others have suggested that since everyday message perception involves simultaneous processing of auditory and visual speech information, communication skills must be evaluated using materials presented in a way that utilizes both visual and auditory information. This would involve speechreading testing in conjunction with auditory identification tests.

nonaudiometric handicap evaluation

Hearing handicap is different from a hearing impairment. A loss of hearing is measured easily in terms of decibels on an audiometric grid or percent correct on a speech discrimination test thereby yielding numerical indicators of the amount of hearing impairment. Unfortunately, these numbers are not indicators of the human problems which may be manifested by hearing impairment. We know from experience, for example, that two individuals with the same numerical hearing loss may encounter entirely different difficulties as a result of their hearing impairment. A case history interview is one way of obtaining hearing handicap information on the extent of the human problems associated with hearing loss for a given person.

Case History. Some audiologists prefer to have a case history form completed before seeing the client. Others use an interview technique since there are times when a client's responses should be further explored. The interview form usually asks for information on general topics, such as the nature and onset of the problem, whether or not hearing is becoming poorer, the kinds of situations in which communication difficulties are experienced, the client's involvement with amplification, and a general case history (see Figure 9.2). The history, along with the audiogram, provides us with the opportunity to obtain an initial impression of the client.

Other Forms of Handicap Evaluation: Areas of Inquiry. It only has been within the past 20 years that significant efforts have been made to assess hearing handicap beyond the traditional case history. Various additional approaches used to assess hearing handicap are discussed in this chapter. Most of them involve self-assessment by questionnaire. Schow (personal communication, 1988) summarized the various kinds of handicap information assessed in connection with self-assessment inventories (see Table 9.1).

1. Speech communication: general speech; estimates of communication ability in varius settings: home, work, social, one-on-one, small and large groups.

2. Speech communication: special; while listening to TV, a telephone; with and without visual cues; and while in adverse listening situations.

3. Emotional reactions/feelings, behaviors, and attitudes about hearing impairment and hearing aids including response to auditory failure, acceptance of loss.

4. Reactions and behaviors of others/societal feedback with reference to the hearing loss.

5. Nonspeech communications; door and phone bell, warnings, traffic, localization.

```
┌─────────────────────────────────────────────────────────────────────────┐
│                      SPEECH AND HEARING CENTER                          │
│  Adult Case History            Date _____ │
│  Audiology                     Referral source _____ │
│                                Physician _____ │
│                                Informant _____ │
│  Name _____ Birth date _____ Age _____ │
│  Address _____ Phone _____ │
│            (Street)    (City)    (State)    (Zip)                        │
│  Occupation (if retired, former occupation) _____ │
│  Business address _____ Phone _____  │
│  Send reports to: _____ │
│  _____ │
│  Nature and onset of problem: _____ │
│  _____ │
│  Other evaluations (when, where) _____ │
│  _____ │
│  Does your hearing seem to be getting worse? _____ │
│  Does your hearing fluctuate? _____ Is one ear better than the other? ____ │
│  Client reports difficulty with hearing in:                             │
│      Groups _____ Individuals _____ │
│      Distance _____ │
│      Telephone: RE _____ LE _____ Both _____ │
│      Radio and TV _____ │
│      Direction of sound _____ │
│      Does hearing loss interfere with work? _____ │
│  Ever worn a hearing aid? _____ When? _____ How long? ___ │
│  Who recommended an aid? _____ Attitude toward use _____ │
│  Complaints _____ │
│  _____ │
│  Present aid: Make _____ Model _____ Receiver _____ Ear ___ │
│  Any bias toward a particular type or make of hearing aid? _____ │
│  _____ │
│  Special training in aural rehabilitation _____ │
│  _____ │
│  Medical History                                                        │
│  History of hearing loss in family _____ │
│  _____ │
│  Middle ear infections _____ │
│  Ear surgery _____ │
│  Other serious diseases or illnesses _____ │
│  _____ │
│  Concussion _____ │
│  Vertigo _____ │
│  Tinnitus _____ │
│  Nausea _____ │
│  Drug therapy _____ │
│  Noise exposure _____ │
│  Other factors that might have contributed to loss _____ │
│  _____ │
│  Latest medical examination _____ │
└─────────────────────────────────────────────────────────────────────────┘
```

Figure 9.2. General audiological case history.

TABLE 9.1
Summary of Various Handicap Aspects Assessed in Self-Assessment Inventories

Handicap Aspects	INVENTORIES/APPROACHES											
	HHS	HMS	SHI	DEN-VER	SAND-ERS	STEPH-ENS	HPI-A	SAC/SOAC	HHIE	M-A	HPI	CPHI
Speech Communication	X	X	X	X	X	X	X	X	X	X	X	X
General Speech		X	X	X	X	X	X	X	X	X	X	X
home/family				X	X							X
vocational/work				X	X					X	X	X
social				X	X				X	X	X	X
1 on 1, sm. grp, lg. grp.			X						X			
Special Communications	X	X	X		X	X	X	X	X		X	X
with and w/out visual cues	X				X						X	
avg. and adverse conditions	X										X	X
telephone/TV/radio	X										X	
Emotional/Personal/Psych. Rx.		X		X		X	X	X	X	X		X
response to auditory failure												X
acceptance of self/loss		X										X
use of hearing aid												
effect on activities/need												
discouragement/embarrassment												X
anger/stress/anxiety												X
withdrawal/introversion												X
neuroticism												X

TABLE 9.1 (Continued)

	INVENTORIES/APPROACHES											
Handicap Aspects	HHS	HMS	SHI	DEN-VER	SAND-ERS	STEPH-ENS	HPI-A	SAC/SOAC	HHIE	M-A	HPI	CPHI
Opinion/Behavior of Others				X		X	X	X				
family relations												
work performance												
societal response												
Nonspeech Communication	X	X				X	X	X			X	
intensity/localization	X	X									X	
doorbell/phone bell												
warnings/traffic												
Related Symptons		X				X		X				
tinnitus/fluctuation/tolerance												

6. Other related symptoms; fluctuating hearing loss, reactions to tinnitus and limited tolerance for loud sounds.

By considering these aspects of handicap, we are more fully relating to the total rehabilitation needs of the adult with hearing loss.

O'Neill and Oyer (1981) addressed the same areas from a slightly different perspective in connection with the communication process. Their categories include: (a) the speaker-sender, (b) the speechreader-receiver, (c) the environment, and (d) the code or stimulus (see Table 9.2). Consideration of all these aspects is important in aural rehabilitation.

Screening/Short-Scale Approaches. A variety of efforts have been made to measure hearing handicap. One of the earliest attempts involved the use of pure-tone and speech recognition information to derive a Social Adequacy Index (Davis, 1948). In a similar manner, the American Medical Association and the American-Speech-Language-Hearing Association (ASHA) have suggested that estimates of hearing handicap can be made from pure-tone findings (Colodzin et al., 1981). During the 1960s and

TABLE 9.2
Variables in Speechreading Process

Speaker-Sender	Speechreader-Receiver
1. Facial characteristics	1. Visual acuity and discrimination
2. Articulatory movements	2. Communication "set"
(a) Rate of speaking	3. Residual hearing
(b) Distinctness of speaking	4. Personality
3. Gesture activity	(a) Intelligence
4. Amount of voice used	(b) Behavior patterns
5. Feedback characteristics	(c) Past communicative experience
	(d) Visual feedback

Environment	Code or Stimulus
1. Lighting conditions	1. Visibility
2. Physical arrangements	2. Familiarity
3. Number of senders	3. Structure
4. Physical distractions	4. Rate of transmission
	5. Auditory-visual aspects

From *Visual Communication for the Hard of Hearing* (p. 39) by J. J. O'Neill and H. J. Oyer, 1981, Englewood Cliffs, NJ: Prentice-Hall. Reprinted by permission.

early 1970s several small, screening-type scales were introduced for use in national interview surveys including the *Rating Scale for Each Ear* (RSEE) and the *Health, Education, and Welfare Expanded Hearing Ability Scale* (HEW-EHAS—sometimes called the *Gallaudet Scale*; Schein Gentile, & Haase, 1970). These two scales were used as substitutes for pure-tone testing to estimate prevalence of hearing loss. Therefore, they are more related to estimates of hearing impairment rather than handicap.

In the 1970s and 1980s several new techniques were proposed. For example, Koniditsiotis (1971) introduced a 7-item scale to look at handicap. Habib and Hinchcliffe (1978) recommended a subjective rating scale in which subjects select a number between 1 and 100 to estimate their hearing handicap (100 = handicap from complete deafness). Stephens (1980) suggested an open-ended questionnaire in which persons list all their hearing difficulties in order of importance.

Two companion scales for screening handicap were introduced by Schow and Nerbonne (1982)—the *Self-Assessment of Communication* (SAC) and the *Significant Other Assessment of Communication* (SOAC). The SAC (see Figure 9.3) is a 10-item, self-assessment screening test with items drawn from longer, diagnostic instruments. Items assess communication difficulties in various situations, the clients' emotional feelings about their handicap, and the clients' perception of how their hearing is viewed by others (societal response). The SOAC (see Appendix 9A) contains the same 10 items, except now the behaviors are rated by a significant other. Both scales are undergoing refinement and adjustment as additional use data are gathered. Also, other handicap screening tools have been proposed for use with the elderly (see Chapter 10 and Ventry and Weinstein, 1983).

Intermediate-Length Inventories. More detailed inventories of handicap were developed during the 1960s and 1970s including the *Hearing Handicap Scale*, the *Hearing Measurement Scale*, the *Denver Scale*, and the *Social Hearing Handicap Index* (Alpiner et al., 1974; Ewertsen & Birk-Nielsen, 1973; High, Fairbanks, & Glorig, 1964; Noble & Atherley, 1970). Those receiving most frequent use are discussed below.

The *Hearing Handicap Scale* (HHS) was the first major self-assessment inventory for measuring handicap (High et al., 1964). The HHS consists of 20 formalized questions with a 5-point closed-set answering arrangement. Two forms of the test are available, both assessing four content areas: speech perception, localization, telephone communication, and noise situations. The HHS has been used widely since its introduction. Schow and Tannahill (1977) proposed a range of hearing handicap categories allowing for interpretation of HHS scores in measuring the effect

SELF-ASSESSMENT OF COMMUNICATION (SAC)

Name _____ Date _____

One of the following 5 descriptions should be assigned to each of the statements below.
Fill in a number from 1 to 5 next to each statement (do not answer with yes or no).

1) Almost Never   **2)** Occasionally   **3)** About Half of   **4)** Frequently   **5)** Practically
(or Never)   (About ¼ of   the Time   (About ¾ of   Always
the Time)   the Time)   (or Always)

circle
number
below

VARIOUS COMMUNICATION SITUATIONS

1. Do you experience communication difficulties in situations when
speaking with one other person? (For example, at home, at work, in a
social situation, with a waitress, a store clerk, with a spouse, boss, etc.)   1 2 3 4 5

2. Do you experience communication difficulties in situations when
conversing with a small group of several persons? (For example, with
friends or family, co-workers, in meetings or casual conversations,
over dinner or while playing cards, etc.)   1 2 3 4 5

3. Do you experience communication difficulties while listening to a large
group? (For example, at church or in a civic meeting, in a fraternal or
women's club, at an educational lecture, etc.)   1 2 3 4 5

4. Do you experience communication difficulties while participating in
various types of entertainment? (For example, movies, TV, radio,
plays, night clubs, musical entertainment, etc.)   1 2 3 4 5

5. Do you experience communication difficulties when you are in an
unfavorable listening environment? (For example, at a noisy party,
where there is background music, when riding in an auto or bus, when
someone whispers or talks from across the room, etc.)   1 2 3 4 5

6. Do you experience communication difficulties when using or listening to
various communication devices? (For example, telephone, telephone
ring, doorbell, public address system, warning signals, alarms, etc.)   1 2 3 4 5

FEELINGS ABOUT COMMUNICATION

7. Do you feel that any difficulty with your hearing limits or hampers your
personal or social life?   1 2 3 4 5

8. Does any problem or difficulty with your hearing upset you?   1 2 3 4 5

OTHER PEOPLE

9. Do others suggest that you have a hearing problem?   1 2 3 4 5

10. Do others leave you out of conversations or become annoyed because
of your hearing?   1 2 3 4 5

Raw Score _____ × 2 = _____ − 20 = _____ × 1.25 _____%

Figure 9.3.   Self-assessment of communication (SAC). (From ''Communication
Screening Profile: Use with Elderly Clients'' by R. L. Schow and
M. A. Nerbonne, 1982, *Ear and Hearing, 3,* 135–147.)

of hearing loss on everyday communication activities. (The HHS [Form A] is found in Appendix 9B.)

The *Hearing Measurement Scale* (HMS) by Noble and Atherley (1970; Noble, 1972) was developed within a few years after the HHS. Although this scale was devised for assessing the degree of auditory handicap exhibited by persons in industrial settings who were exposed to noise, it may be used with most persons. The scale is valuable in that it emphasizes the importance of assessing client attitudes toward hearing loss. Seven general areas are assessed:

1. Speech-hearing

2. Acuity of nonspeech sounds

3. Localization

4. Reaction to handicap

5. Speech distortion

6. Tinnitus

7. Personal opinion of hearing loss

The authors stress that client reactions to hearing loss should have a definite place in the overall evaluation of each individual's problem.

The *Denver Scale of Communication Function* (DSCF) (Alpiner et al., 1974) was designed to assist clinicians in making a subjective assessment of adult attitudes and feelings toward their hearing loss. The scale was originally designed to measure pre- and postaural rehabilitation therapy or pre- and posthearing aid selection. The scale allows comparison of hearing-impaired adults with themselves, not with their therapy counterparts or any norm. The authors felt that speechreading tests fail to assess communication difficulties, and therefore, were not appropriate pretest measures. The DSCF allows a client to judge himself in communication function using a semantic differential-type continuum for each of 25 separate items. A profile form is used for plotting client responses (see Figure 9.4). The form allows seven responses which range from "agree" to "disagree" including a "midpoint". The 25 questions within the questionnaire have been grouped into four categories: family communicative situations (items 1-4); client's personal feelings (items 5-9); perception about social-vocational situations (items 10-20); and client's general communication experience (items 21-25) (see original questions in Appendix 9C).

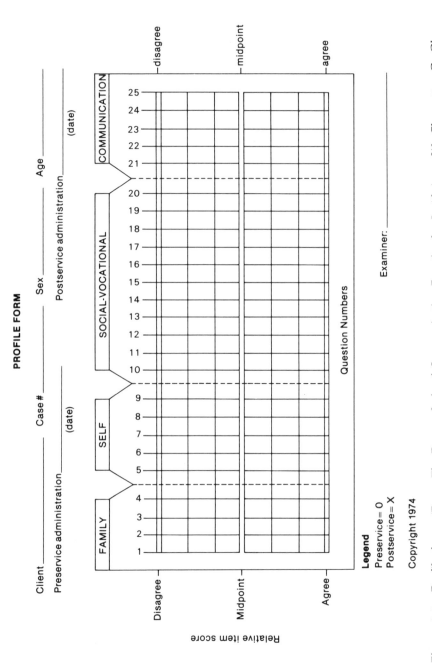

Figure 9.4. Profile form. (From *The Denver Scale of Communication Function* by J. Alpiner, W. Chevrette, G. Glascoe, M. Metz, and B. Olsen, 1974, Denver: University of Denver.)

Schow and Nerbonne (1980) modified the original *Denver Scale of Communication Function* into the *Quantified Denver Scale (QDS)*. The QDS yields an estimate of handicap that allows comparison of scores with other persons having similar or different losses (see Appendix 9C).

By the late 1970s, a new flurry of activity in handicap assessment had begun which has continued into the 1980s. Specifically, Sanders (1975) designed scales for special situations like vocational and home environments. Other scales were developed for special populations, including two for nursing home residents. (These are discussed in Chapter 10.) Jerger and Jerger (1979) proposed a method involving visual and auditory tasks for quantifying auditory handicap (QUAH). A new scale for assessing hearing aid users was also introduced, the *Hearing Profile Inventory* (HPI-A) (Hutton, 1980). In 1983 an improved scale was published by McCarthy and Alpiner (1983), the M-A Scale. In England a variety of handicap scale items were introduced in connection with the National Study of Hearing (Davis, 1983). And most recently, in Denmark, a new handicap scale was proposed (Salomon & Parving, 1985). Several of these newer intermediate-length scales are discussed below.

Sanders (1975) developed three profile questionnaires which enable adults to rate their communicative performance in the home as well as in occupational and social environments. The major emphasis is on assessing specific communication breakdowns in the three environmental situations. Questionnaires do not assess client feelings and attitudes. However, they do incorporate an interesting feature—the importance of the situation is rated along with how well the person gets along in that situation.

The *Hearing Problem Inventory* (HPI-A) was developed for use with a veterans population (Hutton, 1980) (see Appendix 9D). The HPI-A is a 51-item, self-administered instrument, designed for individuals with hearing aids. Pre- and postdata were obtained from 329 clients representing initial fittings and replacement fittings. Results indicated that older individuals had increased problems along with decreased wearing time. Employed persons had slightly higher problem scores but also reported longer hours of hearing aid use. Pre- and post-test comparisons revealed reduction in self-assessed problems by persons receiving counseling and orientation training along with their initial fittings. For clients receiving replacement aids, both pre- and postdata indicated a decrease in wear time after age 54. A decrease in aid wear time of roughly one hour per day per decade above age 55 was reported. For all subjects, hours of wear time increased as hearing loss increased. Additional information gathered in this study points to the need for aural rehabilitation to ensure successful hearing aid use.

Hearing Performance Inventory (Revised Form).

Name _____ Age _____ Date _____

Address _____ Phone _____

Test Location _____ Marital Status _____

Employed _____ Education _____ Sex _____ Hearing Aid Wearer: Yes ☐ No ☐

Prior Aural Rehabilitation Course Experience? _____ If Yes, When? _____

	Practically Always	Frequently	About Half The Time	Occasionally	Almost Never		Does Not Apply
1.	☐	☐	☐	☐	☐	—	☐
2.	☐	☐	☐	☐	☐	—	☐
3.	☐	☐	☐	☐	☐	—	☐
4.	☐	☐	☐	☐	☐	—	☐
5.	☐	☐	☐	☐	☐	—	☐
6.	☐	☐	☐	☐	☐	—	☐
7.	☐	☐	☐	☐	☐	—	☐
8.	☐	☐	☐	☐	☐	—	☐
9.	☐	☐	☐	☐	☐	—	☐
10.	☐	☐	☐	☐	☐	—	☐
11.	☐	☐	☐	☐	☐	—	☐
12.	☐	☐	☐	☐	☐	—	☐
13.	☐	☐	☐	☐	☐	—	☐
14.	☐	☐	☐	☐	☐	—	☐
15.	☐	☐	☐	☐	☐	—	☐
*16.	☐	☐	☐	☐	☐	—	☐
17.	☐	☐	☐	☐	☐	—	☐
18.	☐	☐	☐	☐	☐	—	☐
19.	☐	☐	☐	☐	☐	—	☐
20.	☐	☐	☐	☐	☐	—	☐
21.	☐	☐	☐	☐	☐	—	☐
*22.	☐	☐	☐	☐	☐	—	☐
23.	☐	☐	☐	☐	☐	—	☐
24.	☐	☐	☐	☐	☐	—	☐
25.	☐	☐	☐	☐	☐	—	☐
26.	☐	☐	☐	☐	☐	—	☐
*27.	☐	☐	☐	☐	☐	—	☐
28.	☐	☐	☐	☐	☐	—	☐
*29.	☐	☐	☐	☐	☐	—	☐
30.	☐	☐	☐	☐	☐	—	☐
31.	☐	☐	☐	☐	☐	—	☐
*32.	☐	☐	☐	☐	☐	—	☐
33.	☐	☐	☐	☐	☐	—	☐
34.	☐	☐	☐	☐	☐	—	☐
35.	☐	☐	☐	☐	☐	—	☐
36.	☐	☐	☐	☐	☐	—	☐
37.	☐	☐	☐	☐	☐	—	☐
38.	☐	☐	☐	☐	☐	—	☐
*39.	☐	☐	☐	☐	☐	—	☐
40.	☐	☐	☐	☐	☐	—	☐
41.	☐	☐	☐	☐	☐	—	☐
*42.	☐	☐	☐	☐	☐	—	☐
43.	☐	☐	☐	☐	☐	—	☐
44.	☐	☐	☐	☐	☐	—	☐
45.	☐	☐	☐	☐	☐	—	☐

	Practically Always	Frequently	About Half The Time	Occasionally	Almost Never		Does Not Apply
46.	☐	☐	☐	☐	☐	—	☐
47.	☐	☐	☐	☐	☐	—	☐
48.	☐	☐	☐	☐	☐	—	☐
*49.	☐	☐	☐	☐	☐	—	☐
50.	☐	☐	☐	☐	☐	—	☐
51.	☐	☐	☐	☐	☐	—	☐
52.	☐	☐	☐	☐	☐	—	☐
53.	☐	☐	☐	☐	☐	—	☐
54.	☐	☐	☐	☐	☐	—	☐
55.	☐	☐	☐	☐	☐	—	☐
56.	☐	☐	☐	☐	☐	—	☐
57.	☐	☐	☐	☐	☐	—	☐
58.	☐	☐	☐	☐	☐	—	☐
59.	☐	☐	☐	☐	☐	—	☐
60.	☐	☐	☐	☐	☐	—	☐
61.	☐	☐	☐	☐	☐	—	☐
*62.	☐	☐	☐	☐	☐	—	☐
63.	☐	☐	☐	☐	☐	—	☐
64.	☐	☐	☐	☐	☐	—	☐
65.	☐	☐	☐	☐	☐	—	☐
66.	☐	☐	☐	☐	☐	—	☐
67.	☐	☐	☐	☐	☐	—	☐
*68.	☐	☐	☐	☐	☐	—	☐
69.	☐	☐	☐	☐	☐	—	☐
70.	☐	☐	☐	☐	☐	—	☐
71.	☐	☐	☐	☐	☐	—	☐
*72.	☐	☐	☐	☐	☐	—	☐
73.	☐	☐	☐	☐	☐	—	☐
74.	☐	☐	☐	☐	☐	—	☐
75.	☐	☐	☐	☐	☐	—	☐
76.	☐	☐	☐	☐	☐	—	☐
*77.	☐	☐	☐	☐	☐	—	☐
*78.	☐	☐	☐	☐	☐	—	☐
79.	☐	☐	☐	☐	☐	—	☐
80.	☐	☐	☐	☐	☐	—	☐
81.	☐	☐	☐	☐	☐	—	☐
82.	☐	☐	☐	☐	☐	—	☐
83.	☐	☐	☐	☐	☐	—	☐
84.	☐	☐	☐	☐	☐	—	☐
85.	☐	☐	☐	☐	☐	—	☐
*86.	☐	☐	☐	☐	☐	—	☐
87.	☐	☐	☐	☐	☐	—	☐
*88.	☐	☐	☐	☐	☐	—	☐
89.	☐	☐	☐	☐	☐	—	☐
90.	☐	☐	☐	☐	☐	—	☐

* Items to be reversed before scoring.

Figure 9.5. Hearing performance inventory (HPI)—revised form. (From *Hearing Performance Inventory—Revised Form* by S. W. Lamb, E. Owens, E. D. Schubert, and T. G. Giolas, 1984, San Diego: College-Hill Press.)

The *McCarthy-Alpiner Scale of Hearing Handicap* (the M-A Scale, 1980) assesses the psychologic, social, and vocational effects of adult hearing loss. (The M-A Scale is found in Appendix 9E.) It is administered to both the individual with hearing loss and another close person in the client's environment, usually a spouse. The following important findings emerged in the initial M-A study for aural rehabilitation:

1. Hearing-impaired individuals may fail to accept, understand, or deal with hearing problems while members of the family are keenly aware of the handicapping effects.

2. Some family members are unable to recognize, understand, or deal with the individual's hearing impairment.

3. The impaired person and family members often fail to agree on what the problem areas are.

Diagnostic Full-Length Inventories. Two major efforts were launched in the recent past to develop detailed diagnostic-type questionnaires. One of these, the *Hearing Performance Inventory* (HPI), was developed by Giolas, Owens, Lamb, and Schubert (1979) and subsequently revised and shortened (Lamb, Owens, Schubert, & Giolas, 1984). The HPI consists of six sections: (a) understanding speech; (b) intensity; (c) response to auditory failure; (d) social; (e) personal; and (f) occupational.

The revised HPI consists of 90 questions with five response choices plus a "does not apply" response (Figure 9.5 shows the response form). Examples of items from the HPI follow:

1. You are watching your favorite news program on television. Can you understand the news reporter (female) when her voice is loud enough for you?

2. Does your hearing problem interfere with helping or instructing others on the job?

3. You are in a room with music or noise in the background. Can you hear a person calling you from another room?

4. Does your hearing problem discourage you from attending lectures?

5. Does your hearing problem tend to make you feel nervous or tense?

The other long inventory, the *Communication Profile for the Hearing Impaired* (CPHI), was developed in connection with rehabilitation programs at the Walter Reed Army Medical Center by Demorest and Erdman (1986). Twenty-five scales are incorporated in this inventory.

In designing these latest inventories considerable stress was placed on careful development and attention to psychometric properties including reliability, validity, item-total correlations, and factor analysis (Demorest & Walden, 1984).

Differences and Similarities in Handicap Inventories. Through the years various scoring procedures have been tried. Most inventories have used a 5- or 7-item scaling technique. Ewertson and Birk-Nielsen (1973) and Ventry and Weinstein (1982), however, recommended a smaller 3-point scaling. Most inventories include subsections which focus on special aspects like family-home, social environments, and work-vocational settings (*Denver*, HPI, HHIE, CPHI, SAC/SOAC, M-A Scale). Many also yield one overall score (HHS, Q-*Denver*, SHI, SAC/SOAC, HHIE) for summarizing the total inventory. All instruments with the exception of the CPHI indicate more handicap with higher scores; in this way, they are similar to pure-tone audiometric data.

It is hoped that, with time, advantages and specific uses for various protocols will become clearer. Issues of validity, reliability, and careful scale development continue to require attention. Nevertheless, a variety of options for handicap assessment are now available to the audiologist engaged in aural rehabilitation. The successful use of any assessment tool (auditory or nonauditory) depends on the skill and experience of the audiologist who administers it. With careful interpretation, however, many of these self-assessment tools can be useful in rehabilitation planning.

summary profile for rehabilitation planning

Several rehabilitative audiologists have emphasized the need for a profile to summarize the communication ability of hearing-impaired adults to facilitate rehabilitation planning. Thus, various approaches to collecting assessment information for a profile of rehabilitative needs have been proposed. Garstecki (1980) developed a Speech Communication Profile (see Figure 9.6). This is a form for recording a hearing-handicapped adult's communication ability in her/his normal listening mode, that is, with or without a hearing aid. This profile is not intended to serve the purpose of a diagnostic evaluation or interview form. Instead, it may be useful for establishing a hierarchy of goals and activities in an aural rehabilitation program. Under Section 1.0 (see Figure 9.6), the hearing loss description is entered as described in otologic or audiologic reports or as obtained in audiologic assessment. The description of the hearing handicap is obtained through the client's self-report. Speech audiometry results (Section 2.0) reflect performance using a standardized test administered to the client under his/her most natural listening mode (aided or unaided). Section 3.0 alerts the examiner to consider an individual's ability to compensate for an auditory deficit through use of vision. Together, these three sections contain information pertaining to the client's sensory capability.

Section 4.0 asks the client to rate the influence of message redundancy on understanding speech. Tasks may be presented across the various conditions listed in grid 5.3 to answer questions of primary concern to the client. For example, if the question pertains to differences in performance under auditory (A) versus auditory-visual (AV) reception modes, parallel tasks can be presented (i.e., same noise condition, same cue condition, same stimulus material conditions) to determine the effect of input mode on message perception. The same procedure could be used to isolate other variables. In this way, the Speech Communication Profile can be used to portray specific problem areas that might be resolved in a rehabilitation program as well as providing some direction on how to organize the remediation material. This battery provides information about an individual's communication ability that cannot be obtained from limited, traditional audiometric tests alone.

Similar approaches have been proposed to look at hearing/communication ability in the deaf and the hard of hearing. A procedure has been developed for the deaf called the Communication Performance Profile (CPP) (Johnson, 1976). In this profile information is used to determine medical and nonmedical rehabilitation intervention needs. The profile incorporates results of tests of speech discrimination, speechreading with and without sound, manual language reception, simultaneous spoken and signal language reception, and comprehension of written English. In addition, test results of written and spoken English intelligibility are recorded. Recently another profile was proposed for use with the hard of hearing, the Communication Assessment Profile (CAP) (Schow & Nerbonne, 1982).

Use of a screening profile (CPP or CAP) followed by more detailed, diagnostic self-assessments (HPI or CPHI), and summarized as proposed by Garstecki in the Speech Communication Profile appears feasible for the aural rehabilitation process. These approaches represent a new generation of assessment instruments designed to help audiologists evaluate hearing-impaired adults' need for aural rehabilitation. By reporting results of audiometric and nonaudiometric assessment in profile form, isolated and interacting factors that contribute to communication problems can be identified and solutions to these problems can be planned taking into account the dynamics of the problem situation.

Name _____ Age _____ Date _____

1.0 Introductory Remarks
   1.1 Description of hearing loss:

   1.2 Description of hearing handicap:

2.0 Speech Audiometry
   2.1 Test Equipment and Conditions
      2.1.1 Audiometer:
      2.1.2 Test Stimulus:
      2.1.3 Stimulus presentation: _____ Tape _____ MLV
      2.1.4 Primary signal: _____ Rt. Spkr. _____ Left Spkr. _____
           R & L Spkrs. _____
      2.1.5 Competing message: _____Multi-Speaker babble _____
           Other _____
                              (specify)
      2.1.6 P/CM: _____ O dB HL _____
           Other-specify _____
      2.1.7 Primary signal presentation level: _____60 dB HL _____
           Other-specify _____
      2.1.8 Listening condition: _____ Sound Field _____
           Other-specify _____
      2.1.9 Listening Mode: _____ Unaided _____ Aided
          2.1.9.1 Aid make:
          2.1.9.2 Aid model/style:
          2.1.9.3 Receiver type:
          2.1.9.4 Settings:
          2.1.9.5 Battery:
          2.1.9.6 Earmold:
          2.1.9.7 Aided Ear: _____Right _____Left _____Both
   2.2 Test Findings
      2.2.1 SAT:A = _____
      2.2.2 SRT:A = _____
      2.2.3 Discrim.-Q:A = _____ A/V = _____
      2.2.4 Discrim.-N:A = _____ A/V = _____

3.0 Vision
   3.1 Binocular visual acuity: _____ (Snellen Chart)
   3.2 Description of vision problem:

Figure 9.6. Speech communication profile. (From "Auditory–Visual Training Paradigm for Hearing-Impaired Adults" by D. C. Garstecki, 1981, *Journal of the Academy of Rehabilitative Audiology, 14,* pp. 223–238.)

4.0 Sensory Input Channel Efficiency Rating
4.1 Auditory Channel

	low (Intelligibility Rating) high					
4.1.1 Telephone conversation	1	2	3	4	5	NA
4.1.2 CB Radio conversation	1	2	3	4	5	NA
4.1.3 Walkie-Talkie/Intercom	1	2	3	4	5	NA
4.1.4 Public address system	1	2	3	4	5	NA
4.1.5 Radio broadcast	1	2	3	4	5	NA
4.1.6 Other _____	1	2	3	4	5	NA

4.2 Auditory-Visual Channel

	low (Intelligibility Rating) high					
4.2.1 One-to-one conversation	1	2	3	4	5	NA
4.2.2 Group conversation	1	2	3	4	5	NA
4.2.3 Lecture/Oral presentation	1	2	3	4	5	NA
4.2.4 Movie	1	2	3	4	5	NA
4.2.5 Theater	1	2	3	4	5	NA
4.2.6 Television program	1	2	3	4	5	NA
4.2.7 Other _____	1	2	3	4	5	NA

5.0 Auditory Message Perception
5.1 Description of problem:

5.2 Evaluation procedure (including description of test stimuli, competing message type, P/CM level, situational cues, etc.):

5.3 Estimated level of message perception

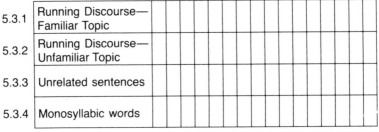

5.3.1	Running Discourse—Familiar Topic	
5.3.2	Running Discourse—Unfamiliar Topic	
5.3.3	Unrelated sentences	
5.3.4	Monosyllabic words	

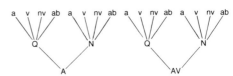

KEY: A = Auditory Channel; A/V = Auditory-Visual Channels; Q = Quiet Condition; N = Noise Condition; SC = Situational Clues (a = auditory; v = visual/picture; nv = non-verbal; ab = absent)

Figure 9.6. Continued.

interpretation of rehabilitation evaluation

Rehabilitation Recommendation. After gathering audiometric and nonaudiometric data and summarizing these in a profile, the audiologist is in a position to determine the need for aural rehabilitation and how to approach the resolution of remediable problems. There is no formula or guaranteed indicator of the need for aural rehabilitation. It is the audiologist and the hearing-impaired adult who decide whether to embark on such an effort, and it is the audiologist's responsibility to lead in designing and implementing a client-centered program. To determine the need for aural rehabilitation, consideration should be given to:

1. *The nature of the hearing loss.* If medical information suggests that the loss is not medically or surgically reversible, the hearing-impaired adult should be considered a candidate for rehabilitation.

2. *The adult's ability to compensate for hearing loss.* If use of a hearing aid does not fully restore auditory communication ability in all situations important for the hearing-impaired person, additional rehabilitation should be considered. Also, if use of residual hearing (aided or unaided) and natural visual-perception skills (speechreading) does not enable the adult to communicate successfully in important situations, additional aural rehabilitation is advised.

3. *The nature of the hearing handicap.* If the hearing-impaired adult experiences difficulty understanding speech without or with speechreading cues, understanding low-intensity speech or speech presented in a noise background, appropriately and successfully stage-managing his/her communication situations (social-vocational-family), or accepting responsibility for self-management of hearing problems, he or she should be considered as a candidate for aural rehabilitation.

the remediation process

Since most hearing-impaired adults have acquired their hearing loss at some point during their lives, they tend to have some residual hearing, which will enable them to communicate. The rehabilitation process for adults, therefore, differs somewhat from that described previously for children. However, with adults as with the younger age groups, individual AR programs must be based on thorough evaluation and screening and coordinated in its various phases by competent, dedicated staff.

overall coordination

Alpiner (1978) devised a service delivery model to show the complexities of the total aural rehabilitation process (Figure 9.7). This model assists the audiologist in making determinations about individual needs for clients:

1. Is remediation necessary after completion of the audiologic examination?

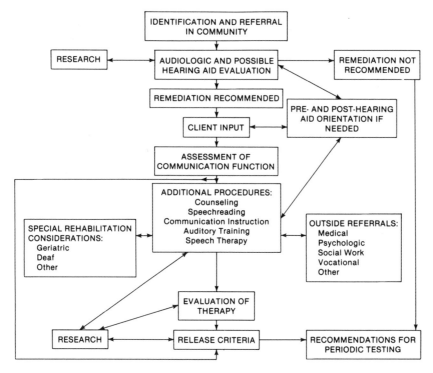

Figure 9.7. Flow chart of the rehabilitative audiology process. (From *Handbook of Adult Rehabilitative Audiology* (p. 13) by J. G. Alpiner (Ed.), 1978, Baltimore, MD: Williams & Wilkins. Reprinted by permission.)

2. Should amplification be considered to determine if the hearing impairment can be minimized? Consideration of amplification is the point at which aural rehabilitation usually begins. The model demonstrates the importance of this aspect by indicating that pre- and posthearing aid orientation is inherent throughout the process, relating to all its components. For example, it may relate to client input, assessment of communication function, counseling, and release criteria.

3. Is additional remediation necessary after completion of the hearing aid evaluation? Here and in item 1, remediation is recommended if, on the basis of the audiologist's information and judgment, the client is unable to communicate effectively without assistance. Conversely, on the same basis, additional remediation is recommended when the client needs assistance to improve communication ability or to minimize any concomitant problems resulting from hearing loss.

4. What are the client's communication needs? In the initial stages of rehabilitation, client input helps provide significant information regarding his communication. At the same time, pre- and posttest hearing aid orientation may be necessary if amplification is being considered.

5. Should the client be released? An assessment of communication function is considered in the process of determining if remediation is necessary. At this point, on the basis of established criteria, the audiologist and/or client may determine that therapy is no longer indicated. When therapy is terminated, recommendations are made for periodic diagnostic testing and continual assessment of rehabilitative needs.

6. Which additional rehabilitation procedures should be recommended? Further remediation may include procedures like counseling, speechreading, communication instruction, auditory training, and speech therapy.

7. Should referrals be made? The client's condition may call for referral to other professionals, such as physicians, psychologists, social workers, vocational counselors, and family counselors. Generally, professionals in other disciplines will refer directly back to the audiologist or work with the client concurrently.

8. Are special therapy considerations necessary? Additional procedures may be necessary when dealing with geriatric clients, deaf clients, mentally retarded clients, and individuals with additional physical problems. Sometimes it is desirable to include family members in the therapy session so they better understand the client's situation.

9. Has therapy succeeded? During the course of rehabilitation, periodic evaluation will measure the client's success and readiness for therapy termination. Release from therapy will be made on the basis of the criteria established by the audiologist in items 4 and 6. Periodic diagnostic testing and rehabilitative needs assessment should be recommended for the client. The time frame in item 5 applies to all clients.

Goldstein and Stephens (1981) developed a model of the rehabilitative process that incorporates instrumental and noninstrumental components while also considering sequencing and interaction of various procedures. The model is depicted as a computer flow chart (see Figure 9.8). As one reads from left to right each column in the figure is another presentation of the same process, only depicted in a greater detail. Thus, the evaluation component considers measurement of communication skills along a variety of communication modes. In addition, variables that potentially influence communication status are weighed and related conditions are considered. Attitude toward or acceptance of the hearing loss conditions and expectations which interact favorably with the prospects for rehabilitation are viewed as critical ingredients feeding into the remediation process. Data gathered and stored in evaluations are reviewed, analyzed, and integrated into decisions on the sequence of events, devices or procedures, and goals to be incorporated into a remediation plan. Then, amplifying device, sensory aid, and warning system need and use are considered. Communication strategies are developed. The role of ancillary professionals is reviewed. Finally, communication training is provided, consisting of providing information, building communication skills, successful use of an amplification system, and counseling.

These models clearly demonstrate that aural rehabilitation is a broad, interrelated series of events. It is a dynamic process, not merely audiologic evaluation, hearing aid fitting, and speechreading instruction.

amplification

This section will deal with a major component of adult aural rehabilitation—amplification. The discussion will include issues related to hearing aid evaluation, adjustment and orientation for adults with special emphasis on the importance of the client's motivation for successful rehabilitation.

Hearing Aid Evaluation and Adjustment. Ross (1978) maintained that most hearing-impaired individuals are prospective hearing aid candidates. Many current and potential hearing aid users are unaware that

Enter		Enter			Enter	
I		C	Communication Status	1	Auditory	
				2	Visual	
				3	Language	
				4	Manual	
	E			5	Pre Rehab	
	V			6	Overall	
	A	A	Associated Variables	1	Psychological	
	L			2	Sociological	
	U			3	Vocational	
	A			4	Educational	
	T					
	I	R	Related Conditions	1	Mobility	
	O			2	Upper Limb	
	N			3	Aural Pathology	
		A	Attitude	1	Type I	
				2	Type II	
				3	Type III	
				4	Type IV	
II		P		1	Interpretation	
				2	Information	
				3	Counseling/Guidance	
				4	Acceptance	
	R			5	Understanding	
	E			6	Expectation	
	M	A	Strategy	1	Hearing Aid Fitting	
	E			2	Alert Warning	
	D			3	Other Assistive Devices	
	I			4	Instruction/Orientation	
	A			5	Adjustment	
	T	C	Ancillary	1	Goals	
	I			2	Philosophy	
	O			3	Tactics	
	N			4	Skill Building	
		O	Communication Training	1	Vocational	
				2	Educational	
				3	Social Work	
				4	Medicine	
Discharge		Discharge			Discharge	

Figure 9.8. Outline of Goldstein and Stephens' (1981) model as adapted and presented in Chapter 1. (From "Audiological Rehabilitation: Management Model I" by D. P. Goldstein and S. D. G. Stephens, 1981, *Audiology, 20,* pp. 432–452.)

various kinds of help are available to assist them in adjusting to amplification. Kasten and McCroskey (1982) pointed out that amplification is only a first step in the total counseling process. The major aspects of the rehabilitation program should be carried out with the hearing aid user and those who interact regularly with the user.

In spite of counseling and information, the hearing-impaired person must be prepared for a period of adjustment during which increasing benefit from hearing aid use will become apparent. Garstecki (1983) outlined some of the questions which may be asked during the adjustment process including:

1. Why does my hearing aid amplify background noise?

2. Why do I experience a feeling of fullness in my ear when I wear my aid?

3. Why does my hearing aid whistle?

4. Why do I sound different when I am wearing my aid?

5. What can I do about wind noise?

6. Why does the earmold hurt my ear?

7. Will my aid create further hearing loss?

8. Why do others yell at me when they see that I am wearing an aid?

9. Why can't I understand others better with my aid?

The audiologist should be ready to answer these and other questions during the aural rehabilitation process. In addition, Beltone Electronics Corporation (1981) has developed a Listening Guide to assist clients in adjusting to their hearing aids. Some examples of suggestions in the guide include:

1. Listen to a familiar person talk or read aloud so you can hear the new sound of speech.

2. Listen to a new familiar sound each day.

3. Listen to a person talking with other sounds in the room.

4. Listen on a telephone with switch or microphone.

5. Listen and learn to respond to alarm systems.

Another technique was developed at the Hearing Society for the Bay Area several years ago (J.L. Darby, personal communication, 1978). In this program, the client uses a "Hearing Aid Usage Record" (see Appendix 9F) to record the times during the day at which the hearing aid is used and the situations in which it is used. The client is to note what she liked or disliked about the hearing aid.

Based on information gathered via such records, the audiologist will have data that may show the need for aural rehabilitation. Although this type of hearing aid adjustment process is effective, no one method should be imposed on all adult clients. Individual needs must be considered.

Hearing Aid Orientation. Winchester (1964) presented a comprehensive summary of hearing aid orientation issues which remains relevant for aural rehabilitation. Certain of these aspects follow:

1. *Patient's attitude:* Frequently the patient is unhappy because his hearing impairment is not correctable by surgery or he has been advised to wear an instrument which may suit his needs, but not his aesthetic values. The patient must be made to feel that he is being helped. He should be gently guided into recognizing that the selected instrument is the best one for him. Gentle guidance rather than high-pressure salesmanship makes for a better hearing aid clinician-patient relationship and for a more satisfied patient.

2. *Patient's motivation:* The extent of the need for hearing aid assistance and the circumstances of this need determine patient motivation. The greater the need for assistance, the greater the motivation and the chances for successful use of a suitable aid. Some persons do not respond with immediate success to hearing aid use, and consequently become sufficiently discouraged to discontinue its use. Patients with low motivation and a difficult hearing problem require considerable followup assistance to get them through the difficult initial adjustment period. By seeing the patient during this period, the clinician may provide psychological support as well as minor adjustments to the hearing aid. Some persons take as long as 6 months to achieve satisfactory adjustment to a hearing aid. For these patients, guidance and support are of paramount importance.

3. *Need for auditory rehabilitation:* For the person who continues to experience communication difficulties even after selection of a suitable hearing aid and the usual adjustment period, a program of auditory rehabilitation should be set up. Here, orientation to hearing aid use, auditory training, speechreading, and speech conservation should be stressed.

Alpiner and Steighner (1983) developed a hearing aid orientation manual for patients at Porter Memorial Hospital. A number of key components in the manual may be used for both pre- and posthearing aid orientation. Some of these components include:

1. An overview of the anatomy and physiology of the auditory system including a pictorial representation of the ear.

2. The different types of hearing including conductive and sensorineural with descriptions of each type.

3. General information about hearing aids including cost, monaural versus binaural selection, and various modifications.

4. Trouble-shooting including, feedback, "dead" hearing aid, hearing aid going "on and off."

5. General maintenance procedures to ensure proper functioning of the aid.

6. Communication suggestions for members of the family.

7. General overview of aural rehabilitation techniques.

The following information from Alpiner and Steighner's manual concerns general hearing aid maintenance:

Many times a simple maintenance schedule will help prevent problems from occurring.

EVERY DAY:	a. check to see that no wax is in the earmold
	b. test the battery
	c. dust aid off with tissue
EVERY EVENING:	a. turn aid off, open battery case, and place in dry location
EVERY YEAR:	a. receive a complete hearing test and hearing aid check
	b. check plastic tubing; replace if necessary
	c. have earmold checked
WHEN NECESSARY:	a. replace earmold
	b. wash earmold with mild soapy water
	c. change batteries
	d. have hearing aid cleaned

Even experienced hearing aid users can often profit from hearing aid orientation, although the degree of coverage is usually not as extensive as with the person utilizing amplification for the first time. (Further materials may be obtained from the Alexander Graham Bell Association in Washington, DC.)

communication rehabilitation

The traditional approach to communication remediation for adults emphasizes speechreading and auditory training. Exercises have been developed according to two methods—the analytic and the synthetic. The former is based on the premise that once an individual recognizes distinctive features of nonmeaningful message units (i.e., syllables) he can apply this information to the understanding of larger message units (i.e., sentences). The synthetic approach, in turn, is based on the premise that everyday messages are highly redundant, both linguistically and in terms of extralinguistic or situational cue information. According to the synthetic approach to message perception, therefore, the hearing-handicapped person is expected to focus on understanding the Gestalt, that is, draw conclusions by associating all available visible speech, and sender and situational cues, rather than depending on distinctive feature information alone.

Today, a combination of these approaches is incorporated in communication remediation. However, formal exercises in either speechreading or auditory training may vary across clinics. For example, Fleming (1972) described a "progressive" approach used with hearing-handicapped veterans in which speechreading and auditory training, as such, are deemphasized. Instead, Fleming develops these skills indirectly through discussion of other aspects of the communication process. As her clients discuss their communication problems they develop improved speechreading and listening skills. The focus, however, is on developing assertive behavior and personal adjustment to hearing loss.

The Walter Reed Army Hospital (Sedge, Walden, & Montgomery, 1978) offers a concentrated and comprehensive rehabilitation program which incorporates hearing aid evaluation and fitting; assessment of self-perceived hearing handicap; and evaluation of auditory, visual, and auditory-visual speech perception ability. The speech perception evaluation consists of measures of visual and auditory confusions in phoneme recognition, as well as assessment of ability to integrate auditory and visual cues in understanding everyday messages. Communication skill remediation activities combine speech perception drills with instruction on how to adjust to hearing loss.

Hardick (1977) and others have reported on programs for adults who require more than the use of a hearing aid. Most often these programs incorporate hearing aid management, communication skill assessment and remediation, and counseling. Emphasis is directed toward development of auditory communication skills. Visual communication of speech-reading skills is developed through combined auditory-visual training exercises, rather than in isolation. Most aural rehabilitation program candidates have some usable residual hearing, and there is no evidence to demonstrate that deprivation of auditory information will improve communication ability. As a result, speechreading in the traditional "no voice" form is not emphasized as an isolated form of message perception, but only as a component of auditory-visual communication.

Auditory Communication Training. Many times auditory communication problems remain after medical or surgical intervention and after the fitting of a hearing aid. Client interviews, self-reports, and responses to hearing handicap questionnaires provide information about clients' everyday communication problems that the audiologist may find useful in designing a practical, client-centered program. Experiences encountered by the client can be simulated in such a program, along with instruction on how to apply appropriate strategies to improve success in communication situations.

Auditory training procedures described in rehabilitation literature are typically based on Carhart's (1960) four levels of training: (a) development of sound awareness, (b) development of gross sound discrimination, (c) development of broad speech discrimination, and (d) development of fine speech discrimination (See Chapter 3.).

In clinical practice, hearing-impaired adults move quickly to focusing on how to improve their everyday communication skills. They are frustrated by the filtering and distorting effect that hearing loss has on message perception. They want immediate solutions to everyday problems.

Garstecki (1981) described an approach to auditory communication training based on improving message perception skills by means of a program where message redundancy is systematically controlled. The client's everyday communication situation is analyzed in terms of four parameters: (a) amount of message content, (b) type of competing background noise, (c) primary message to competing noise ratio, and (d) relevance of situational cues. Message redundancy is varied by changing parameters alone or in combination. For example, the amount of message information can range from syllables or words (low message content) to paragraphs or stories (high message content). The greater the amount of information provided, the more redundant the message. Background noise and level of background noise in comparison with the level of the primary signal also contribute to message redundancy. The less obtrusive and the lower the intensity of the background noise compared to the primary signal, the greater the potential for message perception. Finally, redundancy is increased when environmental or situational cues correspond with the topic of the message.

In Garstecki's auditory-communication training paradigm (see Figure 9.9), message types range from syllable to story materials, competing noise from a combination of cafeteria noise and multispeaker babble to quiet, primary to competing noise levels range from -6 dB to $> +12$ dB, and situational cues from distractions to descriptive cues. In order to determine a baseline level in the paradigm (see Figure 9.10), Garstecki recommends presenting monosyllabic words with multispeaker babble at a 0 dB signal-to-noise ratio. Situational cues are not provided. This is similar to the format used in standard speech discrimination testing. After baseline levels have been established, speech perception ability may be assessed at higher levels of redundancy until a predetermined criterion (usually 80%) is achieved. Mastery of criterion is regarded as the "ceiling level." The training implications of this procedure are that training will begin under the conditions determined to be the ceiling level and progress back to baseline level performance.

Theoretically, it would be necessary to progress below the baseline condition only in unusual circumstances. However, it may be necessary to probe at levels greater than level #17 (see Figure 9.10). In these instances, the first step is to change the primary-to-competing noise ratio from 0 dB to successively higher ratios (SN_1, or SN_2, or SN_3) while continuing to modify other message parameters according to the original training program paradigm. If necessary, this process may be expanded by changing both primary-to-competing noise ratio and noise type following the stages of increasing redundancy of information listed in Figure 9.10.

Garstecki's auditory communication exercises are designed to improve the client's ability to understand messages when the speaker is outside viewing range, as when in another room, speaking on the telephone, over a public address system, or on a radio broadcast. The exercise materials are selected based on the client's interests and needs. For example, a hardware store manager may be presented with newspaper or magazine articles relating to hardware store items, services, and topics of concern to customers. These listening exercises are accompanied by information and instructions on how to stage-manage the communication situation to the client's benefit. Thus, the hearing handicapped adult learns how to optimize listening conditions, ask appropriate questions, and predict messages from nonverbal and situational cues.

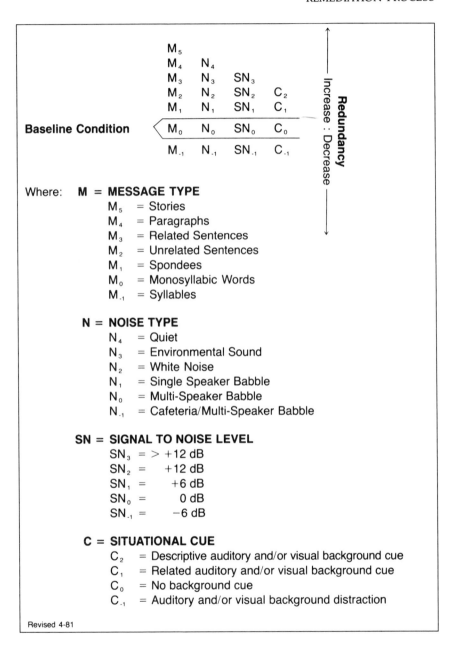

Where: **M = MESSAGE TYPE**
M_5 = Stories
M_4 = Paragraphs
M_3 = Related Sentences
M_2 = Unrelated Sentences
M_1 = Spondees
M_0 = Monosyllabic Words
M_{-1} = Syllables

N = NOISE TYPE
N_4 = Quiet
N_3 = Environmental Sound
N_2 = White Noise
N_1 = Single Speaker Babble
N_0 = Multi-Speaker Babble
N_{-1} = Cafeteria/Multi-Speaker Babble

SN = SIGNAL TO NOISE LEVEL
SN_3 = > +12 dB
SN_2 = +12 dB
SN_1 = +6 dB
SN_0 = 0 dB
SN_{-1} = −6 dB

C = SITUATIONAL CUE
C_2 = Descriptive auditory and/or visual background cue
C_1 = Related auditory and/or visual background cue
C_0 = No background cue
C_{-1} = Auditory and/or visual background distraction

Revised 4-81

Figure 9.9. Auditory communication training paradigm. (From ''Auditory–Visual Training Paradigm for Hearing-Impaired Adults'' by D. C. Garstecki, 1981, *Journal of the Academy of Rehabilitative Audiology, 14*, pp. 223–238.)

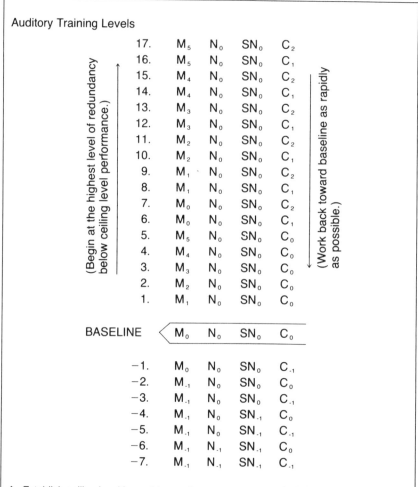

Auditory Training Levels

17.	M_5	N_0	SN_0	C_2
16.	M_5	N_0	SN_0	C_1
15.	M_4	N_0	SN_0	C_2
14.	M_4	N_0	SN_0	C_1
13.	M_3	N_0	SN_0	C_2
12.	M_3	N_0	SN_0	C_1
11.	M_2	N_0	SN_0	C_2
10.	M_2	N_0	SN_0	C_1
9.	M_1	N_0	SN_0	C_2
8.	M_1	N_0	SN_0	C_1
7.	M_0	N_0	SN_0	C_2
6.	M_0	N_0	SN_0	C_1
5.	M_5	N_0	SN_0	C_0
4.	M_4	N_0	SN_0	C_0
3.	M_3	N_0	SN_0	C_0
2.	M_2	N_0	SN_0	C_0
1.	M_1	N_0	SN_0	C_0

(Begin at the highest level of redundancy below ceiling level performance.)

(Work back toward baseline as rapidly as possible.)

BASELINE	M_0	N_0	SN_0	C_0
−1.	M_0	N_0	SN_0	C_{-1}
−2.	M_{-1}	N_0	SN_0	C_0
−3.	M_{-1}	N_0	SN_0	C_{-1}
−4.	M_{-1}	N_0	SN_{-1}	C_0
−5.	M_{-1}	N_0	SN_{-1}	C_{-1}
−6.	M_{-1}	N_{-1}	SN_{-1}	C_0
−7.	M_{-1}	N_{-1}	SN_{-1}	C_{-1}

A. Establish ceiling level by probing performance at successively higher levels of redundancy. Once the ceiling level has been determined, begin training at the next lowest level of redundancy, working back toward baseline.

B. If criterion cannot be met at the highest level of redundancy (#17), repeat baseline procedures first at higher signal-to-noise levels ($SN_{1,2,3}$), then at higher levels with "less effective" masking noises (i.e. $M_0 N_0 SN_1 C_0 \rightarrow M_0 N_0 SN_2 C_0 \rightarrow M_0 N_0 SN_3 C_0 \rightarrow M_0 N_1 SN_1 C_0 \rightarrow M_0 N_1 SN_2 C_0 \ldots M_0 N_4 C_0$).

Figure 9.10. Auditory training baseline levels. (From "Auditory–Visual Training Paradigm for Hearing-Impaired Adults" by D. C. Garstecki, 1981, *Journal of the Academy of Rehabilitative Audiology, 14,* pp. 223–238.)

Barker (1971) proposed that a listening quiz (see Figure 9.11) be presented in early auditory communication training to encourage the client to become aware of the importance of listening and various other factors involved in successful communication. (Answers to all the items are false according to the author of the quiz.)

Sims (1985) described an auditory training method used at the National Technical Institute for the Deaf. Training is individualized because of the wide range of speech-sound discrimination abilities among students. Programmed self-instruction is used in which sentence materials are incorporated from three nontechnical areas: (a) on-the-job social, (b) campus social, and (c) survival communication. The difficulty of the training task can be regulated by changing speaking rate, length of sentences, male vs. female voices, and levels of competing background noise.

Many methods are available for improving auditory communication. When selecting a training program, the following considerations should be met: (a) the client must first be evaluated to determine the level at which training should begin, (b) results should be quantifiable, and (c) instruction should focus on the client's everyday communication problems.

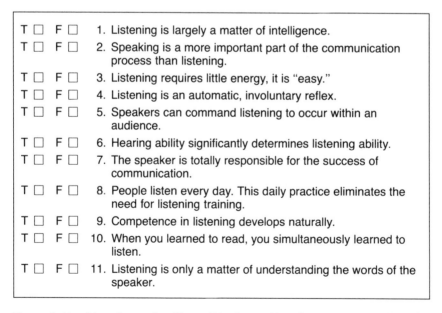

T ☐	F ☐	1. Listening is largely a matter of intelligence.
T ☐	F ☐	2. Speaking is a more important part of the communication process than listening.
T ☐	F ☐	3. Listening requires little energy, it is "easy."
T ☐	F ☐	4. Listening is an automatic, involuntary reflex.
T ☐	F ☐	5. Speakers can command listening to occur within an audience.
T ☐	F ☐	6. Hearing ability significantly determines listening ability.
T ☐	F ☐	7. The speaker is totally responsible for the success of communication.
T ☐	F ☐	8. People listen every day. This daily practice eliminates the need for listening training.
T ☐	F ☐	9. Competence in listening develops naturally.
T ☐	F ☐	10. When you learned to read, you simultaneously learned to listen.
T ☐	F ☐	11. Listening is only a matter of understanding the words of the speaker.

Figure 9.11. Listening quiz. (From "Auditory–Visual Training Paradigm for Hearing-Impaired Adults" by D. C. Garstecki, 1981, *Journal of the Academy of Rehabilitative Audiology, 14*, pp. 223–238.)

Auditory-Visual Communication Training. It is becoming more common to extend auditory communication training so as to incorporate visual information in combined auditory-visual training format. The purpose of this training is to improve the adult's ability to use visual cues to supplement auditory information as in face-to-face conversation where the speaker's lip movements, facial expression, body gesture, and the communication setting may complement perceived acoustic cues to message perception. Commonly encountered auditory-visual communication experiences include viewing/watching television programs, theatrical productions, and lectures.

As in auditory communication training, it is important that the client optimize his or her sensory capabilities through use of a hearing aid. For those who experience vision problems in everyday communication situations, corrective lenses or eyeglasses should be used. Hardick, Oyer, and Irion (1970) determined that binocular visual acuity poorer than 20/40 may contribute to visual speech perception or speechreading difficulty. Recent attention to changes in visual contrast sensitivity with age indicates another area of importance in trying to optimize the hearing-impaired adult's ability to succeed in auditory-visual communication.

Auditory-visual communication problems are unveiled in the same way as auditory communication problems. However, because information from one input modality may complement information from the other, problems in auditory-visual communication are encountered less frequently than in auditory-only communication. The organizational approach proposed by Garstecki (1981) for auditory-communication training applies to auditory-visual training, with the exception that the range of message types incorporated in this paradigm deemphasizes word and syllable information (see Figure 9.12). The baseline measure can be made using videotaped or face-to-face presentations of unrelated sentence materials, such as Utley Lipreading Test sentences or CID sentences, presented at a conversational speech level along with multispeaker babble at a 0 dB SN ratio. Situational cues are not provided. Ceiling levels are determined in the manner described for auditory communication training. Training procedures also parallel those described previously (see Figure 9.13).

Whenever possible, both auditory and auditory-visual training is incorporated into the rehabilitation program. Progress in one realm often expedites progress in the other during the early stages of remediation. Throughout the training program, individual and group activities are organized according to the proposed scheme. The major difference between the two types of activities is that message topics may be more generalized in group instruction; also, some participants will find some levels of group exercise more challenging than others. Roleplaying and

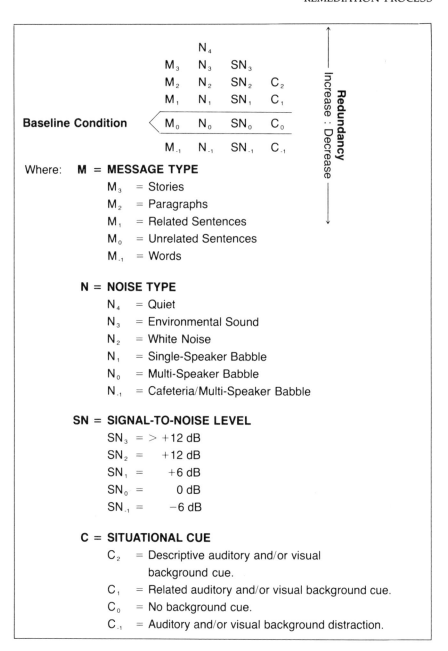

Figure 9.12. Auditory visual communication training program paradigm. (From "Auditory–Visual Training Paradigm for Hearing-Impaired Adults" by D. C. Garstecki, 1981, *Journal of the Academy of Rehabilitative Audiology, 14,* pp. 223–238.)

AV Training Levels

Begin at the highest level of redundancy below ceiling level performance. →

	M	N	SN	C
11.	M_3	N_0	SN_0	$C_?$
10.	M_3	N_0	SN_0	C_1
9.	M_2	N_0	SN_0	C_2
8.	M_2	N_0	SN_0	C_1
7.	M_1	N_0	SN_0	C_2
6.	M_1	N_0	SN_0	C_1
5.	M_0	N_0	SN_0	C_2
4.	M_0	N_0	SN_0	C_1
3.	M_3	N_0	SN_0	C_0
2.	M_2	N_0	SN_0	C_0
1.	M_1	N_0	SN_0	C_0

Work back toward baseline as rapidly as possible.

BASELINE	M_0	N_0	SN_0	C_0
−1.	M_0	N_0	SN_0	C_{-1}
−2.	M_{-1}	N_0	SN_0	C_0
−3.	M_{-1}	N_0	SN_0	C_{-1}
−4.	M_{-1}	N_0	SN_{-1}	C_0
−5.	M_{-1}	N_0	SN_{-1}	C_{-1}
−6.	M_{-1}	N_{-1}	SN_{-1}	C_0

A. Establish ceiling level by probing performance at successively higher levels of redundancy. Once the ceiling level has been determined, begin training at the next lowest level of redundancy, working back toward baseline.

B. If criterion cannot be met at the highest level of redundancy (#11), repeat baseline procedures first at higher signal-to-noise levels ($SN_{1,2,3}$), then at higher levels with "less effective" masking noises (i.e., $M_0 N_0 SN_1 C_0 \rightarrow M_0 N_0 SN_2 C_0 \rightarrow M_0 N_0 SN_3 C_0 \rightarrow M_0 N_1 SN_1 C_0 \rightarrow M_0 N_1 SN_2 C_0 \ldots M_0 N_4 C_0$).

Figure 9.13. Auditory visual training levels. (From "Auditory–Visual Training Paradigm for Hearing-Impaired Adults" by D. C. Garstecki, 1981, *Journal of the Academy of Rehabilitative Audiology, 14,* pp. 223–238.)

group discussion are incorporated into the program to facilitate application of new information in a controlled environment before carryover to everyday communication situations.

Case history. The following sample case illustrates an auditory-visual training program. The client is a 39-year-old sales executive who had a severe, bilateral, sensorineural hearing impairment resulting from scarlet fever. His unaided speech reception thresholds were 85 and 95 dB HL for his right and left ears, respectively. Unaided speech discrimination scores were 36% and 28%, respectively, for right and left ears. At 60 dB HL, his aided discrimination was 60% (measured using NU Test No. 6 stimuli presented in quiet). Interview and Hearing Performance Inventory results revealed that his greatest difficulties occurred in situations which restricted his stage-managing opportunities, such as when attending a theatrical production, lecture, or church service. He reported problems following one-on-one as well as group conversation, especially when it was impossible to ask for repetition, rephrasing, or further clarification of a message. This client wanted practical advice and immediate solutions to his communication problems.

In consideration of this client's poor auditory discrimination ability, regular procedures for establishing baseline-level performance were modified to provide an estimate of auditory-visual sentence perception under a +6 dB primary-to-competing signal condition. The result of this assessment is shown in Figure 9.14. With a baseline score of 50%, the client was expected to demonstrate improved performance under conditions of greater message redundancy. He attained a score of 100% when stimulus material consisted of short paragraphs with accompanying pictures of related visual background cues. Remediation goals progressed from this point back toward the baseline condition with materials designed to provide a progressively decreasing amount of linguistic content and situational cues.

Reassessment at the end of an 8–week training program resulted in an improvement from 50% to 90% in the client's ability to perceive unrelated sentences in noise. The client attributed his success to an improvement in his "problem-solving" ability. Problems created in training were resolved through discussion and systematic, logically progressing, message-perception exercises. He more consciously applied what he practiced in training to everyday social and work situations. By developing successful strategies under controlled training conditions, he felt more confident when facing difficult communication situations. This approach worked for this client because he could understand those communication parameters over which he had control and those for which he had to compensate. The remediation plan was logically organized,

Auditory-Visual Training Levels					Pretraining Score(s)	Posttraining Score(s)
11.	M_3	N_0	SN_1	C_2		
10.	M_3	N_0	SN_1	C_1	100	
9.	M_2	N_0	SN_1	C_2		
8.	M_2	N_0	SN_1	C_1		
7.	M_1	N_0	SN_1	C_2		
6.	M_1	N_0	SN_1	C_1	80	
5.	M_0	N_0	SN_1	C_2		
4.	M_0	N_0	SN_1	C_1	70	
3.	M_3	N_0	SN_1	C_0	75	
2.	M_2	N_0	SN_1	C_0		
1.	M_1	N_0	SN_1	C_0	60	
Baseline	M_0	N_0	SN_1	C_0	50	90

Figure 9.14. Example of auditory visual training levels. (From ''Auditory–Visual Training Paradigm for Hearing-Impaired Adults'' by D. C. Garstecki, 1981, *Journal of the Academy of Rehabilitative Audiology, 14*, pp. 223–238.)

and the procedures had direct bearing on the client's immediate communication concerns. Other examples of auditory-visual communication training procedures are provided by Garstecki (1981).

Some of the principles applied in traditional speechreading training are incorporated in auditory-visual communication training, with the addition that materials are presented with voice. Describing the importance of visual cues to communication, Ripley and Cummings (1977) stressed the value of training clients to recognize cues and become aware of body movements and gestures that accompany everyday conversation. For example, a simple shake of the head may indicate negation; clenched fists, anger; and so forth. It is to the client's advantage to become aware of these cues since they may offer a way of gaining additional meaning from a conversation. By heeding the speaker's facial expressions, the listener may gain additional insight into the mood of the conversation and the emotional state of the speaker. Raised eyebrows, a smile or a frown, a puzzled look, or an expression of surprise are just a few of the facial cues that contribute information to communication. A simple exercise can be utilized in therapy to teach awareness of facial expressions; each client may act out certain emotions, with other clients guessing what is meant.

Clients should also be taught to observe environmental cues. This means showing them how to take advantage of cues inherent in specific communication situations. By taking advantage of envionmental cues, the client may take an educated guess at the topic of conversation. Roleplaying activities can be used in the remediation situation to practice observation of environmental cues.

It is also helpful to demonstrate to hearing-impaired clients that some cues to message perception are provided by visible lipreading movements. Ripley and Cummings (1977) recommended that, during therapy sessions, groups of sounds be presented that are homophenous in nature, beginning with the most visible and proceeding to the least visible sounds. The order of presentation of homophenous sound groups may vary. The following was suggested by Binnie, Jackson, and Montgomery (1976):

1. /f,v/

2. /p,b,m/

3. /w/

4. /l,n/

5. /ʃ,z/

6. /r/

7. /ɝ,θ/

8. /t,d,s,z/

9. /k,g/

These sound groups or visemes are introduced using a traditional, analytic approach. Initially, they are presented in isolation, along with an explanation and demonstration of how they appear on the lips. As a visual aid, it may be helpful to write sounds in common script rather than in phonetics for the client.

In the synthetic approach to speechreading, sounds are incorporated into words and sentences. Thus, visual speech-perception skills can be developed through use of "quick recognition" and "quick identification" exercises (Jeffers & Barley, 1971). In quick recognition exercises, the client must visually discriminate between three similarly positioned phonemes (e.g., thin, fin, pin). Quick identification exercises provide an opportunity for the client to better understand word homopheneity through consideration of alternate word choices for a single speech movement pattern (e.g., fat, fad, fan, vat, van, fanned). By incorporating homophenous words in sentences, the client learns the importance of linguistic cues to message perception.

The current approach to communication remediation focuses on auditory-visual presentation of materials because this is the way clients usually process everyday conversation, and bisensory presentation improves message perception significantly. However, this focus does not preclude utilizing "visual-only" or "auditory-only" approaches to remediation or attempting to improve these modalities independently. In all efforts, however, major emphasis should be placed on improvement of the hearing-impaired client's everyday communication skills.

psychosocial and other rehabilitation considerations

Counseling. Recently, some audiologists have emphasized a counseling-oriented approach to adult aural rehabilitation. This *progressive approach* (Alpiner, 1982; Alpiner & McCarthy, 1987) attempts to deal with adjustment to and acceptance of problems concomitant with hearing loss (Alpiner, 1971; Fleming, 1972). Specifically, clients learn to cope with communication situations and reduce anxieties through counseling rather than speechreading techniques. Although traditional procedures may help improve communication ability, they do not necessarily eliminate other problems resulting from hearing impairment. The progressive approach is in consonance with the contemporary program described earlier.

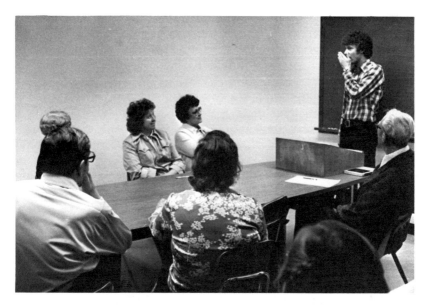

Figure 9.15. Presenting oral discourse with restricted visual cues.

Stressing the need for counseling Northern and Sanders (1972) suggested careful consideration of three factors:

1. The client's reaction to his hearing loss influences his success in achieving satisfactory communication.
2. The client's psychologic stability may be threatened due to increased problems resulting from the hearing loss.
3. A preoccupation with personal problems may hamper the hard-of-hearing client's progress in the aural rehabilitation process.

Ripley and Cummings (1977) asked how many "professional hats" the clinician must wear to become effective. Not only is the clinician expected to be an audiologist, but also a social, vocational, and family counselor. While audiologic training covers the prerequisites for the first role, it usually only introduces us to the others.

Common psychosocial problems of hearing-impaired clients stem from family, vocational, or social situations involving the client's communication, or, more likely, miscommunication. At times these problems are sufficiently severe to warrant referral to ancillary professionals. The audiologist may be the first person whom clients see with regard to their communication problems. If the audiologist feels uncomfortable about working with clients who appear to demonstrate problems beyond the need to improve communication function, it is recommended that appropriate referral be made to family counselors, social workers, psychologists, or others.

Group counseling sessions may be used effectively to improve communication. There clients often realize for the first time that they are not the only ones experiencing difficulties. Thus, the group situation may improve clients' willingness to discuss their problems openly. Group members also may make good counselors. They may be able to offer each other suggestions for how to cope with specific communication problems. (See sample group outline, Chapter 13.)

Problems relating to hearing impairment commonly occur in family communication situations. Clients may feel that their role as a family member has diminished and they are frustrated by an inability to participate effectively in family discussions. Complaints may include the perception that family members have neither the patience nor the courtesy to communicate with them. Family members may feel equally frustrated. Consequently, a vicious cycle can result and, until the cycle is broken, the client may isolate himself from his family. Under such circumstances, it often proves helpful to include family members in remediation sessions. Family members may reach a better understanding of the difficulties experienced by the client, as well as learn about the ramifications of hearing loss. Finally, this approach may help improve the lines of communication in the family setting.

Clients may also experience difficulties in their vocational role. In this connection, it may be necessary for the audiologist, with the client's permission, to contact the client's employer to educate him about hearing loss. A referral to a vocational rehabilitation counselor may also be in order. Vocational rehabilitation counselors are found in all states and are funded by state and federal appropriations. They work with both clients and employers to assess the appropriateness of specific vocations. Counselors will determine whether the client is overemployed, underemployed, or unemployed.

Communication difficulties in social situations are often another major concern. Group situations (meetings, parties, and so forth) and settings with high levels of background noise (e.g., factories, restaurants) may cause serious communication difficulties. These situations can cause the client to withdraw socially and take a less active role in everyday living activities. Participating in an aural rehabilitation program may be a first step in reestablishing social relationships. If rewarding, the program may provide the client with the motivation needed to remain in the mainstream. Some general goals for the client are:

1. Be willing to admit the existence of hearing loss and its handicapping effects.

2. Be willing to admit the hearing loss to others.

3. Be willing to take positive action to minimize communication difficulties by asking others to repeat, asking them to speak more clearly, and asking for selective seating.

Related to this, Wylde (1982) described three counseling areas important for audiologists to address in helping the hearing-impaired adult: (a) information, (b) rational acceptance, and (c) emotional acceptance (see Table 9.3). To assist the client in achieving success in self-management of problems covered by these counseling areas, Brammer (1973) discussed eight stages and goals for developing a helping relationship. All of them have been applied in rehabilitating hearing-impaired adults (see Table 9.4). Through application of these principles and approaches, audiolo-

TABLE 9.3
Counseling Areas for Audiologists

Informational	Rational Acceptance/ Adjustment	Emotional Acceptance/ Adjustment
Hearing loss	Hearing loss	Effect of hearing loss
Description	Permanency of	on self
Comparison with	Need for treatment	Feelings
normal	Need for additional	Attitude
Cause	testing	Image
Anatomy/function of ear	Need for hearing	Ability to
Availability of medical	aid(s)	communicate
assistance	Need to conserve	Ability to work
Hearing aids	residual hearing	Effect of hearing loss
Costs	Aural rehabilitation	on relationships
Where to purchase	Need to learn new	Family
Advantages/	communication skills	Friends
disadvantages	Need to improve	Associates
Care/use/function	communication	
Availability of other	habits	
technical devices	Family	
Availability of other	Friends	
services	Work place	

From "The Remediation Process: Psychologic and Counseling Aspects" by M. A. Wylde. In *Handbook of Adult Rehabilitative Audiology,* 2nd ed. (pp. 137–159) by J. G. Alpiner (Ed.), 1982, Baltimore: Williams & Wilkins.

TABLE 9.4
Eight Stages of the Helping Relationship

Stage	Goals
Entry	1. Open the avenue for assistance from the audiologist. 2. Lay the groundwork for trust. 3. Enable the patient to define his problems related to his hearing impairment.
Clarification	1. Define the client's specific problems as related to his hearing impairment. 2. Get a better feel for how the client sees his hearing impairment and its effect on his general life situation.
Structure	1. Determine if the audiologist has the skills necessary to meet the client's needs. 2. Identification of the agency and the type of help offered, the qualifications and limitations of the audiologist. 3. Acknowledgment of the time to be involved, any fees to be charged and any restrictions to be imposed.
Relationship	A turning point in the process. The client and audiologist either continue to build the relationship through mutual agreement or the relationship is terminated by either party.
Exploration	1. The strategies for intervention are outlined. 2. The client's feelings are explored. 3. The alternatives of action are outlined.
Consolidation	1. The client will decide on a course of action. 2. The client's feelings are clarified. 3. The client will practice new skills.
Planning	1. Plans for termination and continuing alone are formulated. 2. Plans for referral are completed (agencies are contacted, applications completed).

Termination	1. Accomplishments are summarized.
	2. The helping relationship is ended through:
	  a. Termination.
	  b. Referral.
	  c. The promise of follow-up.
	  d. The offer of "stand-by" help.

From L. Brammer as cited in "The Remediation Process: Psychologic and Counseling Aspects" by M. A. Wylde. In *Handbook of Adult Rehabilitative Audiology*, 2d ed., by J. G. Alpiner (Ed.), 1982, Baltimore: Williams & Wilkins.

gists will experience one of the most rewarding aspects of their professional practice, that of observing their clients develop the self-confidence and ability necessary to manage their own hearing problems.

Program Design, Goals, Format.   In designing an appropriate rehabilitation program, consideration should be given to the audiologist's approach to the client and the program, remediation goals, and overall program format. Clients must feel certain that the audiologist understands their problem and has their primary needs in mind in all rehabilitation procedures. The audiologist, in turn, should focus on solutions to major handicapping and remediable problems. Family members, spouses, or close friends should be part of the rehabilitation process. Also, both individual and group remediation activities should be provided.

Individual therapy permits intensive instruction, focusing only on the client's individual difficulties. Using this format fewer sessions may be required to reach the goals established for rehabilitation. Also, one-on-one sessions are sometimes more acceptable to an individual who does not want to or is unable to attend long-term therapy. Oyer (1966) cited several of the advantages afforded by group therapy, including peer evaluation, psychologic support from others with hearing loss, opportunity to compare and contrast individual efforts, and opportunity to perform socially in a practice environment. Finally, Sanders (1971) pointed out that economics may promote interest in a group remediation format.

Program goals should be practically oriented to motivate the adult to succeed. They should serve to inform the client about the dynamics of everyday communication, the communication cycle, and the impact that hearing loss has on this process. Barriers to effective communication should be identified and hints for how to stage-manage difficult situations should be discussed and practiced.

The program should be conducted in a pleasant, comfortable, functional environment. Efforts should be directed toward equipping a remediation facility in which environmental conditions can be manipulated and controlled to simulate various communication conditions. No helpful data exist regarding the appropriate length for a therapy term. It is not uncommon to find the length of a term dependent on the length of a quarter or semester if the setting is a university program. For other agencies, there appears to be no generally accepted timeframe; terms may be 3-day concentrated sessions (6 hours per day) or training may last 4 to 10 weeks or up to 6 months (1–1½ hours per week). Perhaps the best way to establish the length of a term is to consider the initial goals established. Eisenson, Auer, and Irwin (1963) stated that a listener cannot give continuous attention beyond 30 to 60 minutes. In group sessions clients would seem to realize their maximum benefit in 60 to 90 minutes.

Consumer Information. The impact consumers have on rehabilitation program design and services to the hearing-impaired population at large must be mentioned. When asked what their critical needs were, groups of hearing-impaired adults in Iowa City, New York, Duluth, and Galveston reported that they lacked opportunities to learn how to improve their communicative skill. They felt that the general public was not aware of the problems facing hearing-handicapped individuals. More importantly, professional resources and referral agents lacked information about their needs. Finally, these people wanted quality care from competent health care providers (Davis, 1980; Madell, 1980; Smaldino & Sahli, 1980; and Stream & Stream, 1980).

Such voicing of concerns has led to the development of consumer-oriented rehabilitation programs which direct great emphasis on meeting the practical, everyday needs of hearing-handicapped individuals. As a result, problems encountered in public meeting places, for example, have received greater attention, and group amplification systems are increasingly being installed and promoted for use by hearing-impaired individuals.

As mentioned earlier in the chapter, consumer groups have also been formed to raise the public's general level of consciousness about hearing impairment as well as to provide useful information to those concerned about living with hearing loss. For example, Self-Help for Hard of Hearing People,Inc. (SHHH) provides newsletters, periodical publications, national and local meetings, and service programs on topics of general interest to hearing-handicapped individuals. Through such actions, consumer groups may complement the efforts of audiologists and other hearing health professionals.

Computer Software. Computer-assisted rehabilitation is in its infancy. To date, computer programs have been developed for selecting amplification systems for speechreading instruction. Popelka (1983) described a computer program designed at The Central Institute for the Deaf for determining the most appropriate hearing aid characteristics for a given hearing loss. Similarly, Sims et al. (1979) developed DAVID: Digital and Visual Instruction Device for the presentation and analysis of a speechreading task (see Chapter 4). Kopra et al. (1984) found accessing of specific videoframes to be inordinately cumbersome and time-consuming, so they converted the DAVID concept to a laser videodisc interactive system. The laser videodisc system eliminated all the mechanical problems encountered with the videotape instructional systems. Traynor and Smaldino (1986) have prepared software to aid in rehabilitation planning. They used Goldstein and Stephens' (1981) aural rehabilitation model which makes their software useful as a companion study guide in the use of this text.

Tinnitus and Vertigo. Tinnitus is a condition in which individuals hear noises with varying characteristics. For example, tinnitus has been described as a ringing sound, as crickets chirping, as water rushing, and so forth. The etiologies for tinnitus are numerous including fluid in the middle ear and tumors along the auditory pathways.

Vertigo, in turn, is defined as the sensation of movement. It frequently occurs due to lesions in the inner ear, either auditory or vestibular. Meniere's disease is one of the more common causes of vertigo. Vertigo is common for individuals who have both conductive and sensorineural hearing losses.

It is not uncommon for persons to contact an audiologist because of tinnitus or vertigo, rather than hearing loss. In such cases it is the audiologist's responsibility to refer the person to a physician for a medical examination and possible dietary or surgical management. From an aural rehabilitation point of view, the audiologist's responsibility may be confined to counseling to help the client adjust to a condition which may not be medically remediated. The audiologist also may be asked to fit a tinnitus masker (see Chapter 2) on a patient whose tinnitus is very annoying. Also, some therapy efforts have involved biofeedback where patients learn they can control heart rate or blood pressure. They are then often able to develop control of the level and annoyance from tinnitus. In any of the above situations, it is mandatory that a medical evaluation take place prior to aural rehabilitation.

Cochlear Implants. Some profoundly hearing-impaired adults cannot be helped by hearing aids. After more than 10 years of experimental research, the cochlear implant is now available for carefully selected persons who have no other means available to them for communication.

By means of the cochlear implant, stimuli are delivered to the auditory nerve, which, in turn sends the stimuli to the brain. The profoundly hearing-impaired individual utilizes a microphone, a signal processor, and a transmitter. The stimulus from the transmitter allows electricity to go to a receiver implanted under the skin behind the ear. The auditory nerve sends electrical impulses to the brain where the sound is interpreted.

The implant offers the potential for perceiving environmental sounds like sirens, automobile horns, and so forth. In addition, individuals may be able to learn to distinguish between duration and intensity of auditory stimuli including monitoring their own voice. Some persons who have undergone a cochlear implant describe what they hear as synonymous to a radio that cannot be fine tuned. In essence, the individual learns a coding system for identification of selected stimuli. Aural rehabilitation emphasizes the learning of a new code to differentiate environmental sounds, loudness and duration. Training in speechreading also appears to be significant for improving communication. The procedures used are very similar to those employed in the typical aural rehabilitation process (see Chapter 12, Case 7).

It is important that candidates for cochlear implants understand that, unless they are one of the rare exceptions, they will not be able to understand speech and sounds in the way and with the precision that most persons with hearing aids do. Still, if they have virtually no hearing, it may be a dramatic improvement for them. Recent data on persons fitted with the newest devices suggest that speech perception with an implant can provide substantial benefits in speech understanding, making the future of this approach very promising.

---

summary

This chapter has provided an overview of aural rehabilitation procedures for the hearing-impaired adult. A profile of adult clients and the settings in which they may obtain assistance for their hearing impairment has been presented. Medical, audiometric, and nonaudiometric procedures have been outlined with regard to assessing communication difficulties and planning for individual rehabilitation needs. Specific rehabilitation procedures have been described, including hearing aid selection, adjustment and orientation; listening improvement; and auditory-visual communication therapy. Psychosocial and other aspects of the hearing-impaired client were also discussed in relationship to problems that may need attention during the remediation process. Most hearing-impaired adults can be assisted by a carefully managed AR program which emphasizes the client's individual needs.

recommended readings

Alpiner, J., & McCarthy, P. (1987). *Rehabilitative audiology: Children and adults.* Baltimore, MD: Williams & Wilkins.

Davis, J., & Hardick, E. (1981). *Rehabilitative audiology for children and adults.* New York: John Wiley & Sons.

Kaplan, H., Bally, S., & Garretson, C. (1985). *Speechreading: A way to improve understanding.* Washington, DC: Gallaudet College Press.

Luterman, D. (1986). *Deafness in perspective.* San Diego: College-Hill Press.

Orlans, H. (1985). *Adjustment to adult hearing loss.* San Diego: College-Hill Press.

Rezen, S., & Hausman, C. (1985). *Coping with hearing loss: A guide for adults and their families.* New York: Dembner Books.

Schwartz, A. (1984). *The handbook of microcomputer applications in communication disorders.* San Diego: College-Hill Press.

references

Alpiner, J.G. (1971). Planning a strategy of aural rehabilitation for the adult. *Hearing and Speech News, 39,* 21–26.

Alpiner, J.G. (1978). *Handbook of adult rehabilitative audiology.* Baltimore, MD: The Williams & Wilkins Co.

Alpiner, J.G. (1981). Communication assessment procedures in the aural rehabilitation process. *Seminars in Speech, Language and Hearing, 2,* 189–203.

Alpiner, J.G. (1982). *Handbook of adult rehabilitative audiology* (2nd ed.). Baltimore, MD: Williams and Wilkins.

Alpiner, J.G., Chevrette, W., Glascoe, G., Metz, M., & Olsen, B. (1974). *The Denver Scale of Communication Function.* Unpublished study, University of Denver.

Alpiner, J., & McCarthy, P. (1987). *Rehabilitative audiology: Children and adults.* Baltimore, MD: Williams & Wilkins.

Alpiner, J.G., & Steighner, R.L. (1983). *Hearing aid orientation manual.* Denver: Porter Memorial Hospital.

Barker, L.L. (1971). *Listening behavior.* Englewood Cliffs, NJ: Prentice-Hall.

Binnie, C.A. (1973). Bi-sensory articulation function for normal hearing and sensorineural hearing loss patients. *Journal of the Academcy of Rehabilitation Audiology, 6,* 43–53.

Binnie, C.A., Jackson, P.L., & Montgomery, A.A. (1976). Visual intelligibility of consonants: A lipreading test with implications for aural rehabilitation. *Journal of Speech and Hearing Disorders, 41,* 530–539.

Binnie, C.A., Montgomery, A.A., & Jackson, P.L. (1974). Auditory and visual contributions to the perception of consonants. *Journal of Speech and Hearing Research, 17,* 619–630.

Brammer, L. (1973). *The helping relationship: Process and skills.* Englewood Cliffs, NJ: Prentice-Hall.

Byman, J. (1974). Testing of auditory and audio-visual speech perception related to everyday communication. *Scandinavian Audiology Supplement, 4,* 58–66.

Carhart, R. (1960). Auditory training. In H. Davis & R. Silverman (Eds.), *Hearing and deafness* (2nd ed., pp. 368–386). New York: Holt, Rinehart & Winston.

Colodzin, L., Del Polito, G., Dickman, D., McLaughlin, R., & Sullivan, R. (1981). On the definition of hearing handicap. ASHA task force on the definition of hearing handicap. *Asha, 23,* 293–297.

Davis, A. (1983). Hearing disorders in the population: First phase findings of the MRC national study of hearing. In M.E. Lutman & M.P. Haggard (Eds.), *Hearing science and hearing disorders* (pp. 35–60). London: Academic Press.

Davis, H. (1948). The articulation area and the social adequacy index for hearing. *Laryngoscope, 58,* 761–778.

Davis, H., & Silverman, S.R. (1970). *Hearing and deafness.* New York: Holt Rinehart and Winston.

Davis, J.M. (1980). Advice from some satisfied consumers. *Journal of the Academy of Rehabilitative Audiology, 13,* 122–127.

Davis, J.M., & Hardick, E.J. (1981). *Rehabilitative audiology for children and adults.* New York: John Wiley and Sons.

Demorest, M.E., & Erdman, S.A. (1986). Scale composition and item analysis of the communication profile for the hearing impaired. *Journal of Speech and Hearing Research, 29,* 515–535.

Demorest, M.E., & Walden, B.E. (1984). Psychometric principles in the selection, interpretation, and evaluation of communication self-assessment inventories. *Journal of Speech and Hearing Disorders, 49,* 226–240.

Eisenson, J., Auer, J.J., & Irwin, J.V. (1963). *The psychology of communication.* New York: Appleton-Century-Crofts.

Erber, N.P. (1971). Auditory and audiovisual reception of words in low frequency noise by children with normal hearing and by children with impaired hearing. *Journal of Speech and Hearing Research, 14,* 496–512.

Ewertson, H., & Birk-Nielsen, H. (1973). Social hearing handicap index: Social handicap in relation to hearing impairment. *Audiology, 12,* 180–187.

Fleming, M. (1972). A total approach to communication therapy. *Journal of the Academy of Rehabilitative Audiology, 5,* 28–31.

Garstecki, D.C. (1980). Alternative approaches to measuring speech discrimination efficiency. In R.R. Rupp & K.G. Stockdall (Eds.), *Speech protocols in audiology* (pp. 119–143). New York: Grune & Stratton.

Garstecki, D.C. (1981). Auditory-visual training paradigm for hearing-impaired adults. *Journal of the Academy of Rehabilitative Audiology, 14,* 223–238.

Garstecki, D.C. (1981, November). *Communication skill evaluation and remediation in adult aural rehabilitation.* Paper presented at the American Speech-Language-Hearing Association Convention, Los Angeles.

Garstecki, D.C. (1983, January–February). Adjusting to the use of your hearing aid. *Shhh*, 9–11.

Garstecki, D.C. (1984). Aural rehabilitation of hearing-impaired adults. In W.M. Perkins (Ed.), *Current therapy for communication disorders*. New York: Grune & Stratton.

Giolas, T., Owens, E., Lamb, S.H., & Schubert, E.D. (1979). Hearing performance inventory. *Journal of Speech and Hearing Disorders, 44*, 169–195.

Goldstein, D.P., & Stephens, S.D.G. (1981). Audiological rehabilitation: Management model I. *Audiology, 20*, 432–452.

Habib, R.G., & Hinchcliffe, R. (1978). Subjective magnitude of auditory impairment. *Audiology, 17*, 68–76.

Hardick, E. (1977). Aural rehabilitation programs for the aged can be successful. *Journal of the Academy of Rehabilitative Audiology, 10*, 51–67.

Hardick, E.J., Oyer, H.J., & Irion, P.E. (1970). Lipreading performance as related to measurements of vision. *Journal of Speech and Hearing Research, 13*, 92–100.

High, W.S., Fairbanks, G., & Glorig, A. (1964). Scale for self-assessment of hearing handicap. *Journal of Speech and Hearing Disorders, 29*, 215–230.

Hutcherson, R.W., Dirks, D.D., & Morgan, D.E. (1979). Evaluation of the speech perception in noise (SPIN) test. *Otolaryngology and Head and Neck Surgery, 6*, 43–53.

Hutton, C.L. (1980). Response to a hearing problem inventory. *Journal of the Academy of Rehabilitative Audiology, 13*, 133–154.

Jeffers, J., & Barley, M. (1971). *Speechreading (lipreading)*. Springfield, IL: Charles C. Thomas.

Jerger, S., & Jerger, J. (1979). Quantifying auditory handicap: A new approach. *Audiology, 18*, 225–237.

Jerger, J., Speaks, C., & Trannell, J. (1968). A new approach to speech audiometry. *Journal of Speech and Hearing Disorders, 33*, 318–328.

Johnson, D. (1976). Communication characteristics of a young deaf adult population: Techniques for evaluating their communication skills. *American Annals of the Deaf, 12*, 409–424.

Kalikow, D.N., Stevens, K.N., & Elliott, L.L. (1977). Development of a test of speech intelligibility in noise using sentence materials with controlled word predictability. *Journal of the Acoustical Society of America, 61*, 1337–1351.

Kasten, R.N., & McCroskey, R.L. (1982). The hearing aid as related to rehabilitation. In J. Alpiner (Ed.), *Handbook of adult rehabilitative audiology* (pp. 79–98). Baltimore, MD: The Williams & Wilkins Co.

Keith, R.W. (1984). The basic audiologic evaluation. In J.L. Northern (Ed.), *Hearing disorders* (pp. 13–24). Boston: Little, Brown & Co.

Kirby, V., Rogan, S. (1981). A four-week group communication training program for adults. *Journal of the Academy of Rehabilitative Audiology, 14*, 8–16.

Koniditsiotis, C.Y. (1971). The use of hearing tests to provide information about the extent to which an individual's hearing loss handicaps him. *Maico Audiological Library Series, IX*, 10.

Kopra, L., Kopra, M., & Dunlap, R. (1984). *Computer-assisted instruction in lipreading*. Paper presented at the Summer Institute of the Academy of Rehabilitative Audiology, Watts Bar Dam, TN.

Lamb, S.W., Owens, E., Schubert, E.D., & Giolas, T.G. (1984). Hearing Performance Inventory. *Hearing Disorders in Adults*. San Diego: College-Hill Press.

A listening guide. (1981). Chicago: Beltone Electronics Corp.

Madell, J. (1980). Self-perceived needs of adults with hearing impairments. *Journal of the Academy of Rehabilitative Audiology, 13*, 116–121.

McCarthy, P.A., & Alpiner, J.G. (1983). An assessment scale of hearing handicap for use in family counseling. *Journal of the Academy of Rehabilitative Audiology, 16*, 256–270.

Noble, W.G. (1972). The measurement of hearing handicap: A further viewpoint. *Maico Audiological Library Series, X*, 5.

Noble, W.G., & Atherley, G.R.C. (1970). The hearing measurement scale: A questionnaire for the assessment of auditory disability. *Journal of Audiological Research, 10*, 229–250.

Northern, J.J., & Sanders, D.A. (1972). Philosophical considerations in aural rehabilitation. In J. Katz (Ed.), *Handbook of clinical audiology* (pp. 694–701). Baltimore, MD: The Williams & Wilkins Co.

O'Neill, J.J., & Oyer, H.J. (1981). *Visual communication for the hard of hearing.* Englewood Cliffs, NJ: Prentice-Hall.

Owens, E., & Schubert, E.D. (1977). Development of the California consonant test. *Journal of Speech and Hearing Research, 20*, 463–474.

Oyer, H.J. (1966). *Auditory communication for the hard of hearing.* Englewood Cliffs, NJ: Prentice-Hall.

Popelka, G. (1983). *Computer-assisted hearing aid evaluation and fitting program.* St. Louis: Central Institute for the Deaf, Publications Department.

Ripley, J., & Cummings, T. (1977). *A guide to teaching beginning lipreading groups.* Unpublished project, University of Denver.

Ross, M. (1978). Hearing and evaluation. In J. Katz (Ed.), *Handbook of clinical audiology* (pp. 524–544). Baltimore, MD: The Williams & Wilkins Co.

Saloman, G., & Parving, A. (1985). Hearing disability and communication handicap for compensation purposes based on self-assessment and audiometric testing. *Audiology, 24*, 135–145.

Sanders, D. (1971). *Aural rehabilitation.* Englewood Cliffs, NJ: Prentice-Hall.

Sanders, D. (1975). Hearing aid orientation and counseling. In M. Pollack (Ed.), *Amplification for the hearing impaired* (pp. 323–372). New York: Grune & Stratton.

Sanders, D.A. (1982). *Aural rehabilitation. A management model.* Englewood Cliffs, NJ: Prentice-Hall.

Santore, F., Tulko, C., & Kearney, A. (1983). Communication therapy for the adult with impaired hearing. *New York League for the Hard of Hearing Rehabilitation Quarterly, 8*(1), 5–7.

Schein, J., Gentile, A., & Haase, K. (1970). Development and evaluation of an expanded hearing loss scale questionnaire. *Vital and Health Statistics, 2*, 37.

Schow, R.L., & Nerbonne, M.A. (1980). Hearing handicap and Denver scales: Applications, categories, interpretation. *Journal of the Academy of Rehabilitative Audiology, 13*, 66–77.

Schow, R.L., & Nerbonne, M.A. (1982). Communication screening profile: Use with elderly clients. *Ear and Hearing, 3,* 135–147.

Schow, R.L., & Tannahill, C. (1977). Hearing handicap scores and categories for subjects with normal and impaired hearing sensitivity. *Journal of the American Audiology Society, 3,* 134–139.

Schwartz, D.M., & Surr, R.K. (1979). Three experiments on the California Consonant Test. *Journal of Speech and Hearing Disorders, 44,* 61–72.

Sedge, R.K. (1979, June). *Aural rehabilitation for individuals with high frequency hearing loss.* Paper presented at the annual meeting of the Academy of Rehabilitative Audiology, Brainerd.

Sedge, R., Walden, B., & Montgomery, A. (1978). *Aural rehabilitation for individuals with high frequency hearing loss.* Unpublished manuscript.

Sims, D.G. (1985). Visual and auditory training for adults. In J. Katz (Ed.), *Handbook of clinical audiology* (pp. 565–580). Baltimore, MD: Williams & Wilkins Co.

Sims, D., VonFeldt, J., Dowaliby, K., Hutchinson, K., & Myers, T. (1979). A pilot experiment in computer assisted speechreading instruction utilizing DAVID. *American Annals of the Deaf, 124,* 618–623.

Smaldino, J., & Sahli, J. (1980). A litany of needs of hearing-impaired consumers. *Journal of the Academy of Rehabilitative Audiology, 13,* 109–115.

Stephens, S.D.G. (1980). Evaluating the problems of the hearing impaired. *Audiology, 19,* 205–220.

Stream, R.W., & Stream, K.S. (1980). Focusing on the hearing needs of the elderly. *Journal of the Academy of Rehabilitative Audiology, 13,* 104–108.

Traynor, P., & Smaldino, J. (1986). *Computerized adult aural rehabilitation. Software Demonstration Disk.* San Diego, CA: College-Hill Press.

Ventry, I., & Weinstein, B. (1982). The hearing handicap inventory for the elderly: A new tool. *Ear and Hearing, 3,* 128–134.

Ventry, I.M., & Weinstein, B.E. (1983). Identification of elderly people with hearing problems. *Asha, 25,* 128–134.

Winchester, R.A. (1964). When is a hearing aid needed? *Maico Audiological Library Series, I,* 12.

Wylde, M.A. (1982). The remediation process: psychologic and counseling aspects. In J.G. Alpiner (Ed.), *Handbook of adult rehabilitative audiology* (2nd ed.). Baltimore: The Williams and Wilkins Co.

Zarnoch, J.M., & Alpiner, J.G. (1978). The Denver scale of communication function for senior citizens living in retirement centers. In J. Alpiner (Ed.), *Handbook of adult rehabilitative audiology* (Appendix 7-A). Baltimore, MD: Williams & Wilkins Co.

APPENDIX NINE A

significant other assessment of communication (soac)

Name _____

Form filled out with reference to _____ (client/patient)

Informant's relationship to client/patient _____ (wife, son, friend, etc.)

Date _____

One of the following 5 descriptions should be assigned to each of the statements below. Circle a number from 1 to 5 next to each statement (Do not answer with yes or no).

1) Almost Never (or never)	2) Occasionally (about ¼ of the time)	3) About Half of the Time	4) Frequently (about ¾ of the time)	5) Practically always (or always)

Various Communication Situations	Circle number below
1. Does he/she experience communication difficulties in situations when speaking with one other person? (For example, at home, at work, in a social situation, with a waitress, a store clerk, with a spouse, boss, etc.)	1 2 3 4 5
2. Does he/she experience communication difficulties in situations when conversing with a small group of several persons? (For example, with friends or family, co-workers, in meetings or casual conversations, over dinner or while playing cards, etc.)	1 2 3 4 5
3. Does he/she experience communication difficulties while listening to a large group? (For example, at church or in a civic meeting, in a fraternal or women's club, at an educational lecture, etc.)	1 2 3 4 5

From "Communication Screening Profile: Use with Elderly Clients" by R. L. Schow and M. A. Nerbonne, 1982, *Ear and Hearing, 3*, pp. 135-147. Adapted by permission.

Various Communication Situations **(Continued)**	Circle number below
4. Does he/she experience communication difficulties while participating in various types of entertainment? (For example, movies, TV, radio, plays, night clubs, musical entertainment, etc.)	1 2 3 4 5
5. Does he/she experience communication difficulties when you are in an unfavorable listening environment? (For example, at a noisy party, where there is background music, when riding in an auto or bus, when someone whispers or talks from across the room, etc.)	1 2 3 4 5
6. Does he/she experience communication difficulties when using or listening to various communication devices? (For example, telephone, telephone ring, doorbell, public address system, warning signals, alarms, etc.)	1 2 3 4 5

Feelings about Communication

7. Do you feel that any difficulty with his/her hearing limits or hampers his/her personal or social life?	1 2 3 4 5
8. Does any problem or difficulty with his/her hearing upset you?	1 2 3 4 5

Other People

9. Do others suggest that he/she has a hearing problem?	1 2 3 4 5
10. Do others leave him/her out of conversations or become annoyed because of his/her hearing?	1 2 3 4 5

Raw Score_____ × 2 = _____ − 20 = _____ × 1.25_____%

APPENDIX NINE B

hearing handicap scale (form a)

1. If you are 6 to 12 feet from the loudspeaker of a radio do you understand speech well?
2. Can you carry on a telephone conversation without difficulty?
3. If you are 6 to 12 feet away from a television set, do you understand most of what is said?
4. Can you carry on a conversation with one other person when you are on a noisy street corner?
5. Do you hear all right when you are in a street car, airplane, bus, or train?
6. If there are noises from other voices, typewriters, traffic, music, etc., can you understand when someone speaks to you?
7. Can you understand a person when you are seated beside him and cannot see his face?
8. Can you understand if someone speaks to you while you are chewing crisp foods, such as potato chips or celery?
9. Can you carry on a conversation with one other person when you are in a noisy place, such as a restaurant or at a party?
10. Can you understand if someone speaks to you in a whisper and you cannot see his face?
11. When you talk with a bus driver, waiter, ticket salesman, etc., can you understand all right?
12. Can you carry on a conversation if you are seated across the room from someone who speaks in a normal tone of voice?
13. Can you understand women when they talk?
14. Can you carry on a conversation with one other person when you are out-of-doors and it is reasonably quiet?
15. When you are in a meeting or at a large dinner table, would you know the speaker was talking if you could not see his lips moving?
16. Can you follow the conversation when you are at a large dinner table or in a meeting with a small group?
17. If you are seated under the balcony of a theater or auditorium, can you hear well enough to follow what is going on?
18. When you are in a large formal gathering (a church, lodge, lecture hall, etc.), can you hear what is said when the speaker does not use a microphone?
19. Can you hear the telephone ring when you are in the room where it is located?
20. Can you hear warning signals, such as automobile horns, railway crossing bells, or emergency vehicle sirens?

From "Scale for Self-Assessment of Hearing Handicap" by W. S. High, G. Fairbanks, and A. Glorig, 1964, *Journal of Speech and Hearing Disorders, 29*, pp. 215–230. Reprinted by permission.

APPENDIX NINE C

quantified denver scale

Name _____   Score: _____

Age _____   Raw Score: _____

Date _____

	Strongly disagree			Strongly agree	
1. The members of my family are annoyed with my loss of hearing.	1	2	3	4	5
2. The members of my family sometimes leave me out of conversations or discussions.	1	2	3	4	5
3. Sometimes my family makes decisions for me because I have a hard time following discussions.	1	2	3	4	5
4. My family becomes annoyed when I ask them to repeat what was said because I did not hear them.	1	2	3	4	5
5. I am not an "outgoing" person because I have a hearing loss.	1	2	3	4	5
6. I now take less of an interest in many things as compared to when I did not have a hearing problem.	1	2	3	4	5
7. Other people do not realize how frustrated I get when I cannot hear or understand.	1	2	3	4	5
8. People sometimes avoid me because of my hearing loss.	1	2	3	4	5
9. I am not a calm person because of my hearing loss.	1	2	3	4	5
10. I tend to be negative about life in general because of my hearing loss.	1	2	3	4	5
11. I do not socialize as much as I did before I began to lose my hearing.	1	2	3	4	5

From *Denver Scale of Communication Function* by J. C. Alpiner, W. Chevrette, G. Glascoe, M. Metz, and B. Olsen, 1974, as cited in "Hearing Handicap and Denver Scales: Applications, Categories, Interpretation" by R. L. Schow and M. A. Nerbonne, 1980, *Journal of the Academy of Rehabilitative Audiology, 13*, pp. 66–77. Modified by permission.

12. Since I have trouble hearing, I do not like to go places with friends.   1 2 3 4 5

13. Since I have trouble hearing, I hesitate to meet new people.   1 2 3 4 5

14. I do not enjoy my job as much as I did before I began to lose my hearing.   1 2 3 4 5

15. Other people do not understand what it is like to have a hearing loss.   1 2 3 4 5

16. Because I have difficulty understanding what is said to me, I sometimes answer questions wrong.   1 2 3 4 5

17. I do not feel relaxed in a communicative situation.   1 2 3 4 5

18. I don't feel comfortable in most communication situations.   1 2 3 4 5

19. Conversations in a noisy room prevent me from attempting to communicate with others.   1 2 3 4 5

20. I am not comfortable having to speak in a group situation.   1 2 3 4 5

21. In general, I do not find listening relaxing.   1 2 3 4 5

22. I feel threatened by many communication situations due to difficulty hearing.   1 2 3 4 5

23. I seldom watch other people's facial expressions when talking to them.   1 2 3 4 5

24. I hesitate to ask people to repeat if I do not understand them the fist time they speak.   1 2 3 4 5

25. Because I have difficulty understanding what is said to me, I sometimes make comments that do not fit into the conversation.   1 2 3 4 5

APPENDIX NINE D

hearing problem inventory (Atlanta)

The purpose of this set of statements and questions is to give the audiologists who will be working with you as much information about your hearing problem as you can tell us.

From "Response to a Hearing Problem Inventory" by C. L. Hutton, 1980, *Journal of the Academy of Rehabilitative Audiology, 13*, pp. 133–154. Reprinted by permission.

Try to ask yourself each question separately and answer them one at a time. Sometimes there are different questions about how your hearing problems affect your job. Try to answer each one separately as best as you can.

You may find that some of the questions do not apply to you. If so, please write in the reason why. For example, if the statement is "I understand what my boss says to me at work," and if you are not working, please write an answer that states you are not working. This will let us know that you do not have a problem in this area.

If the question is "How many hours a day do you wear your hearing aid?", and if you do not have a hearing aid at this time, please write an answer such as "I do not have a hearing aid."

We want to know about *you* and your problems. In this way we can do a better job of solving your specific problems. There is space at the end for you to write about problems you have which are not listed.

HEARING PROBLEM INVENTORY

1. I turn the radio or TV down before I try to carry on a conversation:
   _____ Almost always
   _____ Most of the time
   _____ Half of the time
   _____ Usually not
   _____ Unnecessary to

2. The telephone pickup on my hearing aid is good:
   _____ Understand almost all
   _____ Understand most
   _____ Miss half or more
   _____ Cannot use on my aid
   _____ No pickup on my aid
   _____ Do not have aid

3. I don't have a problem hearing over the telephone at work or at home:
   _____ Almost no difficulty
   _____ Usually hear enough to understand
   _____ I get some but miss a lot
   _____ I miss most of what is said
   _____ I cannot use at all
   I have a problem because: _____

4. I can understand the people that I talk with a lot, like family and friends:
   _____ Almost always
   _____ Most of the time
   _____ Half of the time
   _____ Not usually
   _____ Almost never
   Don't understand because: _____

5. I feel that listening to several people talk at the same time is too hard:
   _____ Almost always too hard
   _____ Most of the time too hard
   _____ Half of the time
   _____ Usually too hard
   _____ Almost never too hard

6. My hearing loss is embarrassing to my family, especially when we go out:
   _____ Almost never embarrassing
   _____ Half of the time
   _____ More than half
   _____ Almost always

7. My family steps in and makes decisions for me when I don't hear:
   _____ Almost always they step in
   _____ Most of the time
   _____ Half of the time they do
   _____ Usually they don't
   _____ Almost never

8. People have to talk slowly for me to understand them:
   _____ Almost everyone has to
   _____ Most people have to
   _____ About half need to
   _____ Some need to
   _____ Almost no one

9. I feel people avoid talking to me because of my hearing loss:
   _____ Everyone avoids talking to me
   _____ Most people avoid
   _____ Half of the people avoid
   _____ Most people don't avoid
   _____ Almost never avoid

10. I do not take part in social activities as much as I did before I began to lose my hearing:
    _____ Almost always I do not
    _____ Most of the time I do not
    _____ Half of the time I do not
    _____ Usually I do
    _____ Almost always I do

11. I have difficulty understanding what people say in a large room:
    _____ Almost never
    _____ Not usually
    _____ Half of the time
    _____ Most of the time
    _____ Almost always

12. I ask people to repeat when I cannot understand what they say:
   _____ Almost always I ask
   _____ Most of the time
   _____ Half of the time I ask
   _____ Not usually
   _____ Almost never

13. When I have difficulty understanding my family and friends, they go right on talking and leave me out. This happens to me:
   _____ Almost never
   _____ Several times a day
   _____ Half of the time
   _____ Most of the time
   _____ Almost always

14. I avoid meeting strangers because of my hearing problem:
   _____ Almost never avoid
   _____ Usually do not avoid
   _____ Avoid half of the time
   _____ Avoid most of the time
   _____ Avoid almost always
   Avoid because _____

15. Because I have difficulty understanding what is said to me, I say things that don't fit into the conversation. This happens to me:
   _____ Less than once a day
   _____ Several times a day
   _____ Half of the time
   _____ Most of the time
   _____ Almost always

16. My family gets annoyed when I don't understand what they say:
   _____ Almost never gets annoyed
   _____ Several times a day
   _____ Half of the time
   _____ Most of the time
   _____ Almost always

17. I wear my aid:
   _____ Almost all the time
   _____ Most of the time but have problems
   _____ Wear about half the time
   _____ Do not have an aid
   _____ Not able to wear it
   _____ Only a little bit because
   Explain problems: _____

18. I can control the noise level where I live:
    _____ Almost always I can't
    _____ Most of the time I can't
    _____ Half of the time I can
    _____ Most of the time I can
    _____ Almost always I can
    I can't control it because: _____

19. The person I talk with most is easy to understand:
    _____ Almost never
    _____ Usually not
    _____ Half of the time
    _____ Most of the time
    _____ Almost always
    This person is my: _____

20. The people I talk with a lot get my attention before starting to talk to me:
    _____ Almost always do
    _____ Most of the time
    _____ Half of the time
    _____ Usually do not
    _____ Almost never do

21. People at work get my attention before they start to talk to me:
    _____ Almost always
    _____ Most of the time
    _____ Half of the time
    _____ Usually do not
    _____ Almost never
    _____ Not working

22. Trying to talk with my family makes me nervous:
    _____ Almost never does
    _____ Usually doesn't
    _____ Half of the time it does
    _____ Most of the time it does
    _____ Almost always

23. My hearing loss keeps me from going out and doing many things I want to do:
    _____ Almost always prevents me
    _____ Most of the time
    _____ Half of the time
    _____ Usually doesn't
    _____ Almost never interferes
    Cannot do: _____

24. When lots of people are talking in a large room I can't carry on a conversation:
    _____ Almost always can't hear
    _____ Most of the time I can't

____ Half of the time I can't
____ Usually can
____ Amost always can

25. When there are several conversations going on and I can't follow what is being said to me I feel left out and uncomfortable:
    ____ Almost always feel left out
    ____ Most of the time
    ____ Half of the time
    ____ Usually don't feel left out
    ____ Almost never feel left out

26. When someone talks behind me, I miss the first part of what they say:
    ____ Almost always miss
    ____ Most of the time
    ____ Miss half of the time
    ____ Usually don't miss
    ____ Miss less than once a day

27. I watch other people's facial expressions when talking to them:
    ____ Almost always
    ____ Most of the time
    ____ Half of the time
    ____ Not usually
    ____ Less than once a day

28. Except at home, trying to talk with people makes me feel uncomfortable:
    ____ Makes me uncomfortable almost always
    ____ Most of the time
    ____ Half of the time
    ____ Bothers me sometimes
    ____ Almost never

29. When I don't hear a whole statement, I try to guess at the words I missed and figure it out:
    ____ Almost always figure it out
    ____ Most of the time
    ____ Half of the time figure it out
    ____ Usually can't figure it out
    ____ Almost never

30. Other people do not seem to understand what it is like to have a hearing problem:
    ____ Almost never understand
    ____ Usually do not
    ____ Half of the time do
    ____ Most of the time understand
    ____ Almost always understand

31. My family and friends complain that I turn up the radio and TV too loud:
_____ Almost always I do
_____ Most of the time
_____ Half of the time
_____ Less than half the time
_____ Almost never

32. Listening requires a lot of hard work and concentration for me:
_____ Almost always
_____ Most of the time
_____ Half of the time
_____ Not usually
_____ Hardly ever

33. I am not having problems with my hearing aid because it:
_____ Helps in almost all situations
_____ Helps in most situations
_____ Helps in half the places
_____ Helps in only a few places
_____ I can't wear an aid
_____ I don't have an aid
Describe problems: _____

34. I have difficulty understanding if I cannot see the speaker's face well:
_____ Have difficulty less than once a day
_____ Several times a day
_____ Half of the time
_____ Most of the time
_____ Almost always

35. My hearing loss causes problems for me at work:
_____ Less than once a day
_____ Several times a day
_____ Half of the time
_____ Most of the time
_____ Almost always
_____ Not working
What problems? _____

36. Noise is a problem at work:
_____ Less than once a day
_____ Usually is not
_____ Half of the time
_____ Most of the time
_____ Almost always is
_____ Not working
Describe: _____

37. I don't hear important sounds around me, like the phone ringing:
    _____ Almost always don't hear
    _____ Usually don't hear
    _____ Hear about half of the sounds around me
    _____ Usually hear sounds around me
    _____ Almost always hear
    Environmental sounds I miss: _____

38. Because of my hearing loss I do not enjoy my job like I used to:
    _____ Almost never enjoy it
    _____ Don't enjoy it most of the time
    _____ Like it half as much
    _____ Like it most of the time
    _____ Still like it as much
    _____ Not working

39. Not knowing which direction sound is coming from is a problem to me:
    _____ Almost always can't tell direction
    _____ Most of the time
    _____ Half of the time I don't know
    _____ Not usually a problem
    _____ Almost never a problem

40. When watching a speaker I should concentrate on:
    _____ His lips
    _____ The lower half of his face
    _____ His whole face and body
    _____ Should not concentrate
    _____ Don't know

41. How many hours a day do you wear your aid? _____

42. I don't understand when people try to talk with me from another room:
    _____ Understand nothing
    _____ Understand less than half
    _____ Understand about half
    _____ Understand most
    _____ Understand almost all

43. I have trouble with my earmold:
    _____ It is too loose
    _____ It hurts my ear
    _____ It is too tight
    _____ My hearing aid squeals
    _____ My earmold is OK
    _____ I don't have an earmold

44. I wash my earmold: _____ Do not have an earmold
    _____ Once a day
    _____ Once a week

    ____ Once a month
    ____ Once a year
    ____ Hardly ever

45. Check those items which might cause hearing loss:
    ____ Cold weather
    ____ Some medications
    ____ Loud noises
    ____ Certain foods
    ____ Circulation problems

46. The aid I am wearing now is:
    ____ The best I've ever had because:
    ____ One of the better ones, but needs:
    ____ About the same as most aids
    ____ Not as good as most aids
    ____ The worst aid I've had
    ____ I don't have an aid
    Explain: _____

47. I cannot carry on a conversation with people who talk softly:
    ____ Almost never can
    ____ Usually can't
    ____ Can half the time
    ____ Can most of the time
    ____ Almost always can

48. If eligible I will receive a spare aid:
    ____ In the mail in 6 months
    ____ Only if I apply for it
    ____ Don't know
    ____ Have working spare aid

49. All batteries and repair needs are handled by:
    ____ Atlanta VA Prosthetics
    ____ Local hearing aid dealers
    ____ The Denver VA Center
    ____ Don't know

50. I control the corrosion caused by moisture and perspiration by using a drying kit:
    ____ Dry out my aid regularly
    ____ Dry aid in summer
    ____ Dry it only when needed
    ____ My aid does not require
    ____ Don't know about this
    ____ Don't have an aid

51. I have learned how to adjust to and manage my hearing problems:
    ____ Successfully manage them almost always
    ____ Manage them most of the time
    ____ Manage them about half the time
    ____ Usually cannot
    ____ Almost never can
    Cannot manage these problems: _____

    _____

_____

NAME   SS#   DATE

HOME TELEPHONE NUMBER   OFFICE TELEPHONE NUMBER

APPENDIX NINE E

McCarthy-Alpiner scale of hearing handicap (M-A scale)

FORM A

Name: _____ Date: _____

Age: _____ Sex: _____ Time: _____

Occupation: _____ Phone: _____

Address: _____

Hearing Aid: Yes _____ No _____ Onset of

Type _____ Hearing Loss: _____

How Long _____

Satisfaction _____

Audiogram: Date of Examination _____

Examiner _____

Category of Hearing Loss _____

Right Ear

	250 Hz	500 Hz	1000 Hz	2000 Hz	4000 Hz	8000 Hz
Air						
Bone						

Left Ear

	250 Hz	500 Hz	1000 Hz	2000 Hz	4000 Hz	8000 Hz
Air						
Bone						

Speech Reception Threshold: Speech Discrimination:

Right Ear _____ dB HL   Right Ear _____ % @ _____ dB HL

Left Ear _____ dB HL   Left Ear _____ % @ _____ dB HL

DIRECTIONS

The following questionnaire will be used to help audiologists understand what it is like to have a hearing loss and the effects of a hearing loss on your life. You are asked to give your reaction to each of the statements included in the questionnaire. For example, you might be given this statement:

People avoid me because of my hearing loss.

_____	_____	____X____	_____	_____
Always	Usually	Sometimes	Rarely	Never

You are asked to mark your reaction to the statement with an X on the appropriate space. Please mark every item with only one answer as seen in the example.

In marking your answer, please keep in mind that ALWAYS means at all times or on all occasions. USUALLY refers to generally, commonly or ordinarily. SOMETIMES means occasionally or on various occasions. RARELY refers to seldom or infrequently. NEVER means not ever or at no time.

If you are not presently employed, please respond "N/A" for not applicable.

All answers will be kept strictly confidential and used to help audiologists to understand what it is like to have a hearing loss and the effects of hearing loss on your life.

1. I get annoyed when people do not speak loud enough for me to hear them.

| Always | Usually | Sometimes | Rarely | Never |

2. I get upset if I cannot hear or understand a conversation.

| Always | Usually | Sometimes | Rarely | Never |

3. I feel like I am isolated from things because of my hearing loss.

| Always | Usually | Sometimes | Rarely | Never |

4. I feel negative about life in general because of my hearing loss.

| Always | Usually | Sometimes | Rarely | Never |

5. I admit that I have a hearing loss to most people.

| Always | Usually | Sometimes | Rarely | Never |

6. I get upset when I feel that people are "mumbling".

| Always | Usually | Sometimes | Rarely | Never |

7. I feel very frustrated when I cannot understand a conversation.

| Always | Usually | Sometimes | Rarely | Never |

8. I feel that people in general understand what it is like to have a hearing loss.

| Always | Usually | Sometimes | Rarely | Never |

9. My hearing loss has affected my life in general.

| Always | Usually | Sometimes | Rarely | Never |

10. I am afraid that people will not like me if they find out that I have a hearing loss.

| Always | Usually | Sometimes | Rarely | Never |

11. I tend to avoid people because of my hearing loss.

| Always | Usually | Sometimes | Rarely | Never |

12. People act annoyed when I cannot understand what is being said in a group conversation.

| Always | Usually | Sometimes | Rarely | Never |

13. My family is patient with me when I cannot hear.

| Always | Usually | Sometimes | Rarely | Never |

14. Strangers react rudely when I do not understand what they say.

| Always | Usually | Sometimes | Rarely | Never |

15. I ask a person to repeat if I do not hear or understand what he said.

| Always | Usually | Sometimes | Rarely | Never |

16. My hearing loss has affected my relationship with my spouse.

| Always | Usually | Sometimes | Rarely | Never |

17. I do not go places with my family because of my hearing loss.

| Always | Usually | Sometimes | Rarely | Never |

18. Group discussions make me nervous because of my hearing loss.

| Always | Usually | Sometimes | Rarely | Never |

19. People in general are tolerant of my hearing loss.

| Always | Usually | Sometimes | Rarely | Never |

20. I avoid going to movies or plays because of my hearing loss.

| Always | Usually | Sometimes | Rarely | Never |

21. I avoid going to restaurants because of my hearing loss.

| Always | Usually | Sometimes | Rarely | Never |

22. I enjoy social situations with considerable conversation.

| Always | Usually | Sometimes | Rarely | Never |

23. I am not interested in group activities because of my hearing loss.

| Always | Usually | Sometimes | Rarely | Never |

24. I enjoy group discussions even though I have a hearing loss.

| Always | Usually | Sometimes | Rarely | Never |

25. My hearing loss has interfered with my job performance.

Always	Usually	Sometimes	Rarely	Never

26. I cannot perform my job well because of my hearing loss.

Always	Usually	Sometimes	Rarely	Never

27. My co-workers know what it is like to have a hearing loss.

Always	Usually	Sometimes	Rarely	Never

28. I try to hide my hearing loss from my co-workers.

Always	Usually	Sometimes	Rarely	Never

29. I do not enjoy going to work because of my hearing loss.

Always	Usually	Sometimes	Rarely	Never

30. I am given credit for doing a good job at work even though I have a hearing loss.

Always	Usually	Sometimes	Rarely	Never

31. I feel more pressure at work because of my hearing loss.

Always	Usually	Sometimes	Rarely	Never

32. My employer understands what it is like to have a hearing loss.

Always	Usually	Sometimes	Rarely	Never

33. I try to hide my hearing loss from my employer.

Always	Usually	Sometimes	Rarely	Never

34. My co-workers speak loudly and clearly.

Always	Usually	Sometimes	Rarely	Never

THE McCARTHY-ALPINER SCALE OF HEARING HANDICAP
by
Patricia McCarthy, Ph.D., University of Georgia, Athens
and
Jerome G. Alpiner, Ph.D., VA Medical Center, Birmingham, AL

Name: _____ SS#: _____ Age: _____

Date: _____ Sex: _____ Audiologist: _____

PROFILE FORM

PSYCHOLOGICAL										SOCIAL														VOCATIONAL									
N	N	N	P	N	N	P	N	N	N	N	N	P	N	P	N	N	N	P	N	N	P	N	P	N	N	P	N	N	P	N	P	N	P
1	2	3	4	5	6	7	8	9	10	11	12	13	14	15	16	17	18	19	20	21	22	23	24	25	26	27	28	29	30	31	32	33	34

(Rows numbered 1, 2, 3, 4, 5)

DIRECTIONS: Items are worded negatively & positively and scored from 1 point to 5 points with 5 points indicating maximum handicap. Negative items are coded as "N" and positive items are coded "P". For "N" items, calculate always = 5 pts., usually = 4 pts., sometimes = 3 pts., rarely = 2 pts., and never = 1 pt. For "P" items, calculate always = 1 pt., usually = 2 pts., sometimes = 3 pts., rarely = 4 pts., and never = 5 pts.

LEGEND: Responses of hearing-impaired individual = X
Responses of family member = O

APPENDIX NINE F

hearing aid usage record

(Use as many times as needed for each day)

Date	Hours used	Volume setting	Situations in which aid was used	What did you like or dislike about it?

Name: _____ Hearing Society for the Bay Area
San Francisco, California 94109

From HEARING SOCIETY for the Bay Area, John L. Darby, Executive Director, San Francisco, CA 94109. Reprinted by permission.

chapterten

AURAL REHABILITATION FOR ELDERLY ADULTS

JAMES MAURER

contents

introduction

Today there is greater need than ever for providing aural rehabilitation services to older persons. Approximately 11% of the general population in this country is 65 years and older (Ronch, 1982). These numbers are projected to increase to 39% by the year 2000 as medical technology continues to extend our lifespans and the post World War II "baby boom" becomes the 21st century's "geriatric boom" (Office of Human Development—DHEW, 1978). Currently, adults 75 years and older constitute the fastest growing segment in our society (see Table 10.1). Senior adults will continue to live longer and be more active in their advanced years. A major requisite for maintaining and enhancing the quality of their remaining lifespan will be to maintain communication skills. The audiologist plays a pivotal role in providing rehabilitative services specifically

TABLE 10.1
Percent Distribution of Population
65 Years and over, by Age: 1950-2020

Age	1950	1970	1976	1980	2000	2020
65-69	40.7	35.0	36.1	34.9	28.9	35.4
70-74	27.8	27.2	25.8	27.3	25.9	26.9
75-79	17.4	19.2	17.7	17.3	20.1	16.8
80-84	9.3	11.5	11.9	11.3	13.3	10.2
85 and over	4.8	7.1	8.6	9.2	11.8	10.6

From "America's Elderly in the 1980's" by B. J. Soldo, 1980, *Population Bulletin, 35* p. 11. Copyright 1980 by Population Reference Bureau. Reprinted by permission.

tailored to the older person's individual needs in such efforts to maximize the quality of life during this increased longevity.

Intervention of hearing impairment among older persons is among the most challenging pursuits for clinical audiologists. This chapter addresses that challenge, which includes (a) knowledge about aging clients and the environmental milieu which surrounds them and interacts in unique ways with hearing loss, (b) methods of identifying and assessing the handicapping condition, (c) techniques for rehabilitating amplification needs and receptive communication skills, and (d) counseling strategies aimed at both gaining acceptance of the intervention process and relieving the stress associated with a decline in auditory skills during the later years of life.

profile of the client

In order to provide the hearing-impaired senior citizen with appropriate aural rehabilitative treatment, the audiologist must understand the factors involved in the aging process which directly relate to the individual's ability and desire to communicate. For no other age group does the environment undergo so many changes as for the aging individual. These changes must be given special consideration when rehabilitation measures are planned and implemented.

An individual's lifetime generally pursues a course towards greater growth and development of physical, psychological, and social needs. If changes occur which impede the acquisition or continuance of these needs, the individual may be forced to readjust his lifestyle to accommo-date the change. A younger person who draws support from a large reservoir of both internal and external resources readapts to a new situa-tion more readily than an older individual who is more limited in availa-ble options. As the support system continues to decrease with age, the frequency and severity of significant lifestyle changes, described by Ronch (1982) and summarized below, continue to increase.

Although most aging persons undergo a certain degree of change in every area listed below, their capacity to adapt to these changes is highly individualized, depending upon genetic inheritance, life experi-ences, past and present environments, and traditional ways of dealing with life (Ronch, 1982).

1. The family of origin—parents, brothers, and sisters become ill or die

2. Marital relationship—death or illness of spouse, estrangement due to empty-nest syndrome, pressures due to retirement

3. Peer group—friends die or become separated by geographical reloca-tion for health, family, or retirement reasons

4. Occupation—retirement

5. Recreation—opportunities become scarce due to physical limitations or unavailability

6. Economic—income reduced by retirement, limited income tapped by inflation or medical costs not covered by insurance

7. Physical condition—loss of youth, changes in physiological and bio-logical aspects of the body causing poor health and its emotional consequences

8. Emotional/sexual life—loss of significant others through death, sepa-ration, and reduction in sexual activity due to societal expectations, personal preference, or death of partner.

variables of the aging process

The variability in responses older individuals apply to the increasing number of lifestyle changes they must confront results in a more heter-ogeneous population than any other age group. It is, therefore, impossi-ble to accurately assess the affects of aging based solely on a person's chronological age. Not all individuals of the same age experience aging in the same way. Some people appear youthful well into their eighties, while others manifest old-age behaviors by their early forties.

The apparent variability of each person's rate and degree of aging, regardless of chronological age, is attributed to the unique interaction of three aspects of the aging process: biological, experiential, and psychosocial. *Biological* aging is determined by genetic programming, which affects cellular deterioration within a predetermined time frame. *Experiential* aging, in turn, is shaped by life forces and the associated environmental insults which contribute to physical deterioration in later life. *Psychosocial* aging reflects maladaptive behaviors and reduced social output in which the individual may engage when confronted with the radical lifestyle changes associated with increasing chronological age (Maurer, 1982).

physical and mental health

Most geriatrics are in relatively good health, but as reported by the Office of Human Development, DHEW Report (1978), approximately 41% of adults 65 years or older suffer from chronic health problems that restrict their activities to some degree. Only a small proportion of the aging population have physical disabilities so severe as to interfere with successful rehabilitative treatment. In general, the aging process is characteristically manifested by a slowing down or reduction of the bodily systems. According to Brody (1973), a gradual attrition of brain cells in the older individual can significantly affect the neuronal conduction rate. As transmission speed decreases, response time to sensory input increases. Subsequently, an older person may need more time to perceive, process, organize, and react to sensory stimuli than younger individuals. This can be further exacerbated by gradual deterioration of sensory receptors, a decline in motor coordination, and increased fatiguability. Biochemical changes can lead to metabolic imbalances or endocrine insufficiencies followed by lowered resistance to disease and increased resistance to healing associated with injury.

To some degree, the senior adult is required to adjust to a certain amount of physical disability and reduced activity level. As each new physical problem becomes apparent, and further reinforced by the inevitable continuance of deterioration, the older person is confronted daily with his or her own mortality. Realization of the consequences of age can, therefore, significantly affect an individual's attitude towards self-fulfillment. That is why it is difficult to discuss the physical and mental factors contributing to the aging process as separate entities. The interaction between the two is symbionic, with changes in one almost certainly influencing the other.

Mental or psychological factors associated with aging have been delineated by Ronch (1982) as (a) intellectual-cognitive changes and (b) emotional-personality alterations.

Intellectual-Cognitive. Robertson-Thabo (1984) reported that longitudinal studies on intelligence and aging generally do not indicate significant changes in intelligence test performance until the late years of life. As the author indicated, however, some aging persons decline in some aspects of cognitive functioning, while others do not. Extra-aging factors may well account for individual differences.

Atchley (1972) proposed that intelligence is probably more affected by health than by age. Reduced neural efficiency with its associated latency in response at the central processor may contribute to a gradual decrement in certain aspects of memory, logic, and awareness (Hunter, 1960). Aging individuals were reported by Rabbitt (1965) to have greater difficulty in discriminating between relevant and nonrelevant stimuli. This may interfere with the older person's ability to accurately assess sensory input and, subsequently, make appropriate responses. Craik (1977) noted increasing deficits in short-term memory as age increased. While this may mean that it takes longer to learn new materials, it does not necessarily affect the quality of learning.

Emotional-Personality. The aging population has the highest incidence of mental illness (Butler, 1975) and accounts for 25% of all reported suicides in this country (Butler & Lewis, 1977). As senior adults confront lifestyle changes, not all can readily adapt. Concomitant declines in sensory/motor skills and increased risk of illness and injury create a loss of independence and personal control. Feelings of depression, anxiety, and even hostility may cause the individual to withdraw from stress-producing environments and situations. Thus, senility, long regarded as the inevitable consequence of growing older, is no longer attributed entirely to biochemical changes associated with aging, nor is it considered entirely unalterable. The influence of hearing impairment, for example, on behaviors otherwise described as "senile" (e.g., inattentiveness, inappropriate responding) may give justifiable cause for a second opinion.

economic status

Adjustments to radical lifestyle changes are made easier when economic factors are not a concern. A higher income allows greater mobility to seek better health care and continue supportive social contacts. The affluent, socially active older person is more inclined to compensate for the detrimental effects of age by purchasing necessary medications, eyeglasses, dentures, or hearing aids. Low-income persons, on the other hand, have fewer options.

Retirement is perhaps the primary factor for change in the senior adult's economic status. Loss of employment may not only alter financial security, but may reduce social interaction and erode self-esteem. The added burden of increased medical expenses, of which Medicare meets only 42% (Ronch, 1982), pushes 25% of the aging population below the poverty level (Butler, 1975).

Although most older individuals are not considered poor, many live on fixed incomes and have their prime financial asset tied up in the equity of their home. The decision to sell the house for financial stability is frequently offset by the emotional stress produced by the subsequent loss of neighborhood, territorial familiarity, and security (Ronch, 1982). Many of the aged will sacrifice food and medical care rather than give up their environmental surroundings.

The economic status of senior citizens who live in long-term extended care facilities is usually lower than that of their counterparts who reside in privately owned homes. According to a survey of 19 nursing homes in the Portland metropolitan area, only 10% of the residents were considered financially independent, with a median of 70% receiving public assistance (Moulton, 1981).

living environments and aural rehabilitation settings

Older adults may live independently, with family members, or in some type of health-care facility. Most live in their own residence, with 83% being less than an hour's distance from one of their children (Sussman, 1976). Private residences for older persons, particularly of low income, are usually located in heavily populated, noisy, and sometimes dangerous urban areas. Many elderly adults are confined to their homes due to financial and health considerations and are often cared for by their spouses or children. Almost 30% of the aging population live with their children (Sussman, 1976), but the number residing in family settings rapidly decreases with advancing age (Office of Human Development—DHEW, 1978).

The older individual is likely to require professional health care beyond the capabilities of the family environment. For some, this may only necessitate moving to an apartment complex which provides health care services when needed. Those recently hospitalized who are yet unable to return home may choose to temporarily stay in short-term care facilities designed to provide 24-hour intensive care services by a professionally trained staff.

Health-care facilities most often associated with the aging population are nursing homes which provide long-term care. Only 5% of this country's senior citizens reside in such institutions (Butler & Lewis, 1977), but those who do represent an older segment of the geriatric population with generally more advanced physical and mental deterioration. This group is more socially isolated, with 50% having no nearby relatives and 60% seeing no visitors at all. Additional data from the Office of Human Development Report (1978) indicate that only 20% of nursing-home residents leave their extended care facilities for reasons other than death.

hearing loss and aging

The prevalence of hearing loss increases as age increases, as reflected by Figure 10.1 and Table 10.2. Over half the persons in the United States with bilateral hearing losses are 65 years and older (Gentile & Ries, 1971). Thus, Glorig and Roberts (1965) reported the prevalence of hearing loss in the general population as 23% in the age range between 65 and 74 years and 40% for individuals 75 years and older. For nursing-home residents and the hospitalized elderly, this figure climbs even higher.

TABLE 10.2
**Prevalence Rates of Hearing Impairment, per 100 Persons,
in the Civilian, Noninstitutionalized Population of the U.S.**

Age Group in Years	Number	Prevalence Rate %
<5	96,034	0.63
5-14	592,595	1.63
15-24	922,012	2.32
25-34	1,380,760	4.29
35-44	1,344,130	5.82
45-54	2,269,974	9.79
55-64	3,095,322	15.35
65-74	3,430,852	24.10
75+	3,087,095	38.55
All	16,218,774	7.64

Note. Rates are based on 1977 interview data from the National Center for Health Statistics, 1982. From "The Prevalence of Hearing Impairment" by J. Punch, 1983, *Asha, 25,* p. 27.

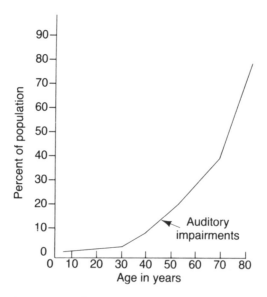

Figure 10.1. Percentage of persons in the U.S. with auditory impairments, ages 6–79 years. (From *Fact Book on Aging: A Profile of America's Older Population* (p. 100) by C. S. Harris, 1978, Washington, DC: The National Council on Aging.)

Schow and Nerbonne (1980) evaluated 202 nursing-home residents from five facilities and found that 82% of their sample demonstrated pure-tone threshold averages (PTAs) of 26 dB HL or greater, with 48% exhibiting PTAs of at least 40 dB HL.

Presbycusis. The aging process is perhaps the most common cause of hearing impairment. This type of deficit, *presbycusis*, was described by Schuknecht (1964) as an accumulation of age-related degenerative changes within the auditory system. In its most common form, presbycusis is a gradual process, initially affecting hearing sensitivity for the higher frequencies of a pure-tone audiogram. During its early stages, most individuals are unaware of the loss but as the deficit progresses, the ability to understand speech, especially in the presence of background noise, becomes increasingly impaired.

   Presbycusis is not the only cause of hearing loss in the geriatric population. Rarely does this type of impairment occur alone based solely on the effects of age. Cumulative effects of such factors as excessive noise exposure, ototoxic drugs, infectious diseases, head trauma, and genetic predisposition must also be considered. When superimposed upon a presbycusic hearing loss, these factors account for the wide variety of audiometric configurations and degrees of severity demonstrated by the aging population.

Phonemic Regression. In some older individuals, presbycusis is characterized by a more severe speech discrimination problem than expected on the basis of tone threshold configuration. This phenomenon, referred to as *phonemic regression* (Gaeth, 1948), causes perceptual confusions and distortions of the phonetic elements of speech and may not be overcome simply by amplification. Increasing the intensity of speech is not always helpful because phonemic regression is generally attributed to a dysfunction in the central auditory-processing system. Gaeth concluded a central auditory origin for phonemic regression when he found little relationship between this condition and age, duration of loss, educational or socioeconomic background, intelligence, or reaction time scores. When sensorineural pure-tone configurations of equal severity are compared for young and old persons, aging adults generally demonstrate greater difficulty with speech-discrimination ability than their younger counterparts.

identification/rehabilitation evaluation for elderly

A continuing need exists for auditory assessment protocols that present a meaningful profile of the older, hearing-impaired adult. Loss of hearing sensitivity is only one aspect of a complex set of interacting variables that cumulatively reflect the hearing handicap. As a number of authors (Davis, 1948; Ewertsen & Birk-Nielsen, 1973; Katz & White, 1982) have pointed out, because of the increased physical and mental limitations of older adults, the assessment process should focus on the communication breakdowns the individual is experiencing, thus aiming more realistically at understanding the handicap and ultimately arriving at an effective remediation plan. Such a combination of conventional audiologic test data with interview and self-assessment responses which are sensitive to attitudes, communication skills, and other life satisfaction indicators which interact with hearing loss is a relevant, if formidable, undertaking. The heterogeneity of the population defies any semblance of the standardized testing procedures used with infants, for example. Nonetheless, there are islands of progress in this ocean of clinical uncertainty (Schow & Nerbonne, 1982; Ventry & Weinstein, 1982).

audiologic testing of older persons

Changes in a number of conventional audiologic procedures may be necessary when assessing biologically older persons. These include longer-duration tonal presentations, increased delay between tone and word presentations, use of live-voice rather than recorded word lists, greater attention to client fatigue through use of speech recognition half lists and abbreviated test sessions, employment of assessment items with increased content redundancy, such as sentence tests, and an increased schedule of social reinforcement for responding. Modifications of test stimuli and response modes are particularly critical for the multiply handicapped, such as those with receptive and expressive language problems due to cerebral vascular accidents, Alzheimer's disease and other chronic brain syndromes, those who have been laryngectomized, and individuals afflicted with psychoses or depression. Even apparently healthy older persons may evidence memory-retrieval difficulties when the quality of the message is degraded (Jordan, 1977; Simon & Pouraghabagher, 1978).

Some studies of the slowing of reaction time during old age have indicated that delays in motor responding, as in a pure-tone hearing test, may be associated with the encoding process of decision making (Botwinick & Thompson, 1968; Nebes, 1978). These authors noted that older persons require a higher level of confidence before responding to certain tasks. However, Gordon-Salant (1986) questioned that poor performance on speech-recognition tasks was entirely attributable to caution in decision making. Her research suggested that older persons exhibit a high degree of confidence and guessing behavior in speech-recognition tasks. In social situations, communication breakdowns may occur because elderly listeners respond as if they understand the message, but really do not. Moreover, in speech-recognition testing, performance scores may be artificially inflated by correct guessing activity.

Some older persons do require allowances for increased response time during both pure-tone audiometry and speech testing. In some cases, reinstruction is necessary because of delayed responding, perseverative responses, and even memory-recall failure during the presentation of longer stimuli, such as sentences. Biologically younger aging persons who are in good physical condition may reveal none of these difficulties, in spite of subtle signs of neural depopulation during sensitized and degraded speech testing.

Determining performance skills for messages presented in noise seems to be a fruitful area of assessment for older persons, since one of their chief complaints regarding hearing is difficulty understanding a speaker in the presence of background noise. Propositional or meaningful noise, such as occurs in the background at a luncheon or meeting, is particularly disruptive. Differentiating between peripheral and central factors affecting speech perception would seem to be a worthwhile pursuit in diagnostic testing, since the prognosis for hearing aid performance is considerably poorer in instances of central auditory involvement (Hayes & Jerger, 1979). Since presbycusis represents a combined sensorineural dysfunction, audiologic test batteries should be designed to separate peripheral and central performance. Jerger and Hayes (1977) suggested the use of conventional speech-discrimination testing along with synthetic sentence identification (SSI). Performance-intensity functions on each of these two measures further differentiate between peripheral and neural involvement in the auditory system. Schow and Nerbonne (1982) added the dimension of visual/linguistic processing to speech perception in noise as a means of assessing the relative contribution of visual cues to message comprehension. The value of these sensitized tests extends beyond site of lesion testing. They offer a baseline for intervention in the sense that attending to primary messages while inhibiting background talkers and combining visual and auditory cues are learnable skills.

Young-old persons, those who are biologically younger than their years, seem to be well represented in the caseloads of audiology clinics; however, less mobile, biologically older individuals are measurably less conspicuous. The latter group represents one of the greatest challenges to the field of audiology, not only because of the increased incidence of hearing loss alluded to earlier, but also because they are less prone to do anything about it. They remain an invisible segment of the population unless the audiologist makes a special effort to seek them out. One method for accomplishing this is to conduct hearing screenings in nursing homes, convalescent hospitals, and low-income highrise apartment buildings, or outside the facility in a mobile testing van (Decker, 1974; Eisdorfer & Wilkie, 1972; McCartney, Maurer, & Sorenson, 1974). Project ARM (Auditory Rehabilitation Mobile) has conducted such a program at Portland State University since 1972, when a grant from the Kresge Foundation supported the construction of a mobile hearing testing van. Continued financial support for Project ARM activities has been sustained by the Lions' Sight and Hearing Foundation. Additional funding from Pacific Northwest Bell enabled the establishment of a hearing aid gift bank for the indigent elderly.

Hearing threshold data, followup testing, aural rehabilitative services, and interviewer assessment measures on this large population of elderly have yielded information which attests to the need for involvement among audiologists and aural rehabilitation specialists. The following summary statements reflect data on over 13,000 older persons (65–99 years) whose hearing deficits would be considered communicatively significant within a similar sample of younger persons.

1. Most did not seek professional assistance until the hearing difficulty became moderately impairing.

2. Lack of intervention by any discipline characterized the majority of the group.

3. The most common form of intervention cited among those obtaining assistance was from hearing aid representatives, with physicians and audiologists in second and third place, respectively.

4. The three most common reasons for not obtaining help were high cost of intervention (medical, prosthetic, etc.), lack of knowledge concerning the service available, and lack of transportation, in that order.

5. Black elderly persons were three times less likely to seek intervention than white elderly persons with the same hearing loss.

6. The most common complaint in receptive communication was difficulty hearing in noise, the incidence of which increased with each age decade.

7. The most common method of adjustment to stress associated with hearing impairment was denial by projection (i.e., "It's not that I can't hear, it's that the speaker mumbles!").

8. Most older persons judge their own hearing ability in relation to cohorts in their chronological age group, therefore underestimating the severity of the problem (i.e., "My hearing is good . . . [for my age]").

assessment of handicap

Traditional audiologic measures do not directly address the hearing handicap or loss of personal efficiency in daily living activities. An increasing number of assessment instruments have been reported which evaluate attitudes and feelings associated with hearing impairment. However, only a few are specifically in tune with the problems experienced by the aging population.

Widely used measures for adults and the elderly include the *Hearing Handicap Scale* (HHS) (High, Fairbanks, & Glorig, 1964), the *Hearing Measurement Scale* (HMS) (Noble & Atherley, 1970), and the *Denver Scale of Communication Function* (Alpiner et al., 1978). The 20-item HHS attempts to assess auditory difficulties encountered in everyday listening situations. The HMS probes more deeply into hearing-related problems, including perception for speech and nonspeech sounds, localization, speech distortion, tinnitus, and reactions and opinions concerning the loss and the handicap. The Denver Scale, a 25-item questionnaire, focuses on four areas of communication function: family, self, social-vocational, and general communication. A valid criticism of these popular assessment tools is their lack of relevance for the aging segment (see Chapter 9 for additional information on the scales).

A more recent attitudinal measure specifically designed for nursing home residents is the *Nursing Home Hearing Handicap Index* (NHHI) (Schow & Nerbonne, 1977). This assessment features brevity, relevance, and versatility in the sense that two separate test versions are provided, one that can be self-administered and one that permits response by nursing home staff. (These scales are found in Appendix 10A.) Similarly, the *Self-Assessment of Communication* (SAC) reliably measures perceived handicap as does the *Significant Other Assessment of Communication* (SOAC) (Schow & Nerbonne, 1982). The former provides a "reality" check on the older person's self-assessment, while the SOAC samples the impressions of those closest to the individual (e.g., wife, son, or friend), who may have valuable knowledge about the client (these scales can be found in Chapter 9).

Two other instruments merit discussion. The *Hearing Performance Inventory* (Giolas, Owens, Lamb, & Schubert, 1979), as revised in 1982 (Lamb, Owens, Schubert, & Giolas, 1982), is a self-assessment inventory of hearing skills ranging from speech understanding to response to auditory failure in a variety of daily listening situations. Items are situation specific and, therefore, provide a sensitive measure of life satisfaction as related to hearing skills. Ventry and Weinstein (1982) developed a scale specifically for elderly persons, *The Hearing Handicap Inventory for the Elderly* (HHIE) (see Appendix 10B). The inventory offers two subscales, one consisting of social-situational items, the other items measure emotional responses. The two subparts are scored along with an overall score. These scales identify problems related to hearing deficiency and measure attitudinal changes following intervention. A series of reports are available related to (a) issues of validity, (b) reliability, (c) comparison with audiometric measures, (d) use of a shortened form for screening, and (e) use of paper-and-pencil versus face-to-face administration (Weinstein, 1984a; Weinstein, Spitzer, & Ventry, 1986).

The need for interview questionnaires and self-assessment measures that reflect the presbycusic with a reasonable degree of validity is pressing for four primary reasons: (a) they provide a measure of the perceived handicap of the individual in his living environment; more objective test scores do not; (b) they open windows for counseling the older adult; (c) they may provide prognostic significance in the sense that particular score values may relate to the person's adaptability to overcome the ''handicap''; and (d) they may document the success of the aural rehabilitation program as a followup measure.

aspects of aural remediation

Following the rehabilitation-evaluation, remediation therapy is undertaken. The remediation process is presented in four major sections:

1. *Overall coordination* of the intervention program, which involves appropriate utilization of clinical sensitivity for hearing-impaired older persons to achieve realistic objectives in aural rehabilitation.

2. *Amplification aspects* of intervention in which the person, the prosthetic device, and the environment are examined as interdependent variables.

3. *Communication rehabilitation*, which focuses on factors that contribute to total life satisfaction through social communication and self-actualization.

4. *Psychosocial considerations*, which focus on attitudes among the elderly and methods of adjusting to stress related to hearing difficulties, as well as counseling strategies aimed at reducing the impairment associated with depressed hearing skills.

overall coordination

A well-coordinated aural rehabilitation program for older persons requires an organized body of knowledge about the clientele. This includes clinical sensitivity toward elderly persons in general, a thorough understanding of the older person in question, and prioritization of this information into a meaningful rehabilitative plan. In too many instances, failure or rejection during the intervention process is due to either lack of clinical sensitivity toward the client's needs, feelings, and priorities or insensitivity toward the aging population as a group. No segment of the world population of hearing impaired has more living experiences and well-established attitudes than the chronologically aged. To treat longevity lightly in this highly heterogeneous group is to open the door to failure.

Intake information, gleaned through interviews or formal assessment measures, is essential. Specific areas that are particularly useful among older persons are: (a) the hearing deficiencies, including: history, duration, and potential site(s) of lesion, as well as both a self-assessment of the handicap and assessments by significant other persons; (b) the history of previous attempts at intervention, medical or prosthetic; (c) knowledge about associated physical or mental difficulties, including arthritis, neuromuscular limitations, visual problems, tinnitus, and memory difficulties; and (d) an assessment of current life satisfaction.

Information on life satisfaction tends to surface during an informal, preintervention counseling session. The kinds of questions to be probed include: To what extent do physical, mental, or economic conditions

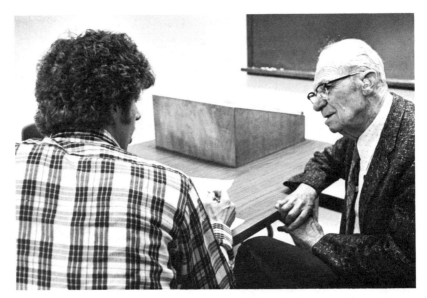

Figure 10.2. Thorough discussion about the use, adjustment to, and care of a hearing aid is particularly important for first-time users.

make this individual dependent upon others? What is the current activity level of this person? In what ways does this individual interact with the living environment and extended surroundings? Is the older person motivated to interact more in a social communicative sense? Is life satisfaction limited to vicarious pleasures, such as watching television in solitude, or is the self-imposed isolation a likely consequence of the hearing handicap?

The pervading question in this context is: Will the rehabilitation program make a significant, positive impact on the life satisfaction of this older person? A well-developed client profile substantially increases the probability of successful aural rehabilitation. Thus, the profile permits an educated focus on current aspects of the older person's lifestyle. It addresses and administers to client needs, rather than those of the clinic or the practitioner. It delineates whether the individual is a candidate for intervention, what particular plan should be tailored to meet the person's needs, what hypothetical objectives and terminal goals might be accomplished, what significant other persons should be involved, and where, when, and under whose auspices the program should be carried out.

The author is unimpressed by directive, informational counseling that includes "laundry lists" of questions aimed at elderly persons. While such an approach may be useful for time-oriented attendants at a hospital nursing station, the salience of the information sampled in this manner may be lost in the undertow of real needs and feelings that surface when the clinician simply listens to the client. Most of the complaints of older persons about their hearing difficulties, for example, are situation specific: "I can't hear in church." "I can't understand the speaker when there are people talking." "I don't watch the news on television, because the announcer talks too fast." Knowledge about such concerns provides for a practical, operational baseline from which positive rehabilitative changes can be measured.

The key to whether significant other persons should be included in the plan and subsequent coordination of the rehabilitation program is the extent of their present contribution toward the elderly individual's life satisfaction. Thus, observing interactions between the older person and others reveals the kind of support they will provide and whether they will be allies during intervention. Perhaps one of the paramount questions the clinician should ask on an intuitive level is whether significant others' support is based on a valid concern for the aging individual, or whether it is irregular or counterproductive. Relatives, friends, and staff members in the geriatric environment can constitute important links in the rehabilitative chain. Others who may act in concert with the audiologist to facilitate adjustive behaviors include members of the professional community who have knowledge about the client, the family support system, and the client's lifestyle. Relevant parties may include members of the clergy, physicians, welfare workers, and leaders of organizations and clubs in which the client holds membership.

Speechreading and Auditory Training: Groups. Aging individuals are generally understimulated. As alluded to earlier, their nucleus of cohorts is smaller than in previous years, and the opportunity to participate in a group experience is often welcomed. An important aspect of a small group is the opportunity to share information. Giolas (1982) suggested that the audiologist take the position of group leader and facilitate discussions by (a) bringing out those persons who are reluctant to share their experiences; (b) inhibiting those few who might dominate the group; (c) permitting the discussion topics to surface from the group rather than from the clinician; (d) acting as a resource person when expertise is needed; and, most importantly in the author's opinion, (e) acting as a good listener. Methods of achieving homogeneous grouping (i.e., bringing together persons who have similar perceived communication problems, as revealed in self-assessment profiles) are detailed by Giolas (1982).

Since older individuals are particularly ''value oriented'', the relevance of speechreading should be demonstrated to the group early. Providing the group with contrasting experience (e.g., communicating with optimal versus limited visual cues) may satisfy this objective. Specific activities aimed at accomplishing this, as well as group strategies for improving speechreading skills are documented by a number of authors (Erickson, 1978; McCarthy & Culpepper, 1987; Stephens & Goldstein, 1983). Further activities engineered to produce group cohesiveness may involve asking members to contact each other by telephone, the objective being to guess who the ''mystery caller'' is and report on the experience at the next group meeting (Maurer, 1979).

In the author's experience, a good group meeting is one that: (a) is primarily success– rather than problem-oriented, (b) provides an element of entertainment, (c) focuses on no more than three learning objectives, (d) incorporates sharing of ideas in a counseling medium, and (e) culminates with a clear understanding of how each member can take charge of his or her newly acquired learning through carryover activities.

The following is an example of a group meeting lesson devoted to developing good listening and speechreading skills.

Sample Lesson Plan Outline

Objective I: Microphone Location (Auditory Training)

Activity A: Each member must demonstrate to the group the location of the microphone on the hearing aid.

Activity B: Each member selects two aids from a box of consignment instruments, demonstrating to the group the location of the microphones.

Objective II: Microphone Distance and Lipreading Visibility (Auditory Training and Speechreading)

Activity A: The rehabilitation specialist reads at conversational level an abbreviated list of PB words that have highly visible initial consonants at a distance of 25 feet. Group members write down the words. The same list (randomized) is delivered from a distance of 6 feet. Group error scores are computed for each trial, announced, and the topics of microphone distance and speechreading visibility distance are discussed.

Activity B: Each client delivers an abbreviated word list to another client's offside (unaided) ear without visual cues at a distance of 3 feet. Randomized versions of the same list are delivered from the same distance to the aided ear, first without visual cues and then with visual cues. Error scores for the group are tallied for each condition and announced. Group discussion is directed toward (a) the importance of visual cues in speech intelligibility, (b) the effect of the head as an acoustic baffle, and (c) the need for both amplification and speechreading cues in understanding a message.

Activity C: Clients propose personal situations in which wearing only one hearing aid might produce listening difficulties (e.g., riding the bus, driving a car, conversing in a restaurant). Solutions are discussed.

Activity D: Clients propose personal situations in which distance is a factor in speechreading intelligibility (e.g., sitting at the back of a church, large auditorium). Solutions are discussed.

Carryover Activity: Each member is given five high-probability sentences from the *SPIN Test* (Kalikow, Stevens, & Elliot, 1977). Instructions are to mirror/ practice reading each sentence, except for the final word, which is delivered without audible cues. Names are drawn so that each reader will have a designated person to whom the list will be presented at the next session. Both the client achieving the highest score in comprehension and the reader delivering the list will receive prizes.

Additional help in planning group meetings can be found in Chapter 13, which contains a complete outline for a series of group meetings.

Individual Aural Rehabilitation. Some persons do not fit into a group training structure. For example, they may not be sufficiently mobile to meet regularly in the group environment; they may have personal problems or attitudes which do not lend themselves to group interaction; they may prefer meeting times that do not coincide with the group meeting time; or they may simply prefer the individual attention that is created by a one-on-one situation, or their intervention need is different from that of the group.

Although the goals and objectives are much the same for individual therapy as for group intervention, certain activities better lend themselves to a one-on-one situation. Whenever possible, it is important to have a significant other person in attendance during individual therapy to facilitate carryover to the residential environment.

A prime example of activities which require individualizing is the 10 Step Earmold Insertion Program (Maurer, 1979). Earmold and ITE (in-the-ear) hearing aid insertion is a common problem among the elderly. Lack of proper insertion may produce feedback and even physical pain. Use of this program among older persons with management problems has been highly successful as illustrated in Figure 10.3, which also contains the learning curve of the client who prompted the program.

An 83-year-old woman was observed to have difficulty inserting her silhouette earmold, which had been provided, along with her behind-the-ear hearing aid, by a salesman over a year earlier. A peer brought her into the audiology clinic because the woman had discontinued wearing her aid, and the two friends were having problems communicating. An observation of her repeated attempts at inserting the mold in her ear revealed: (a) she was capable of placing the aid appropriately on her ear; (b) having placed the aid, she engaged in trial-and-error attempts at locating the mold and grasping it "where the salesman showed me"; (c) her arthritic fingers invariably grasped the mold or tubing improperly

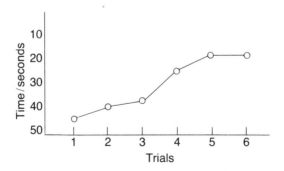

Figure 10.3. Time (seconds) required to achieve criterion over successive trials involving removal of amplification. (From "Aural Rehabilitation for the Aging" (p. 329) by J. F. Maurer. In *Hearing and Hearing Impairment* by L. J. Bradford and W. G. Hardy (Eds.), 1979, New York: Grune & Stratton.)

or her hand turned so that the mold was at an impractical angle for proper insertion; (d) her baseline for correct earmold placement in five trials was zero.

The woman acknowledged that she had received a 10-minute instruction following the sale of her aid. However, she had not received additional aural rehabilitation. Consequently, her various manipulative behaviors such as placing the aid on the table, opening the battery compartment, picking up the appliance, putting the mold in her ear, and so on, occurred in no methodical order. Analysis of the hearing aid showed that it was functioning properly and was reasonably appropriate for the client's needs.

A 10-step remediation program was designed around a time base. The terminal objective was to chain manipulative behaviors to respective stimuli in a serial order so that the complex act of establishing proper use of the prosthesis could be broken into discrete responses. It seemed more effective to work backwards from the point where the aid was operating in the ear (reverse chaining), since previous trials involving getting the mold in the ear had failed. In addition, the probability of error responding was reduced with the ear as a starting point; besides, the reinforcement of amplified sound was at a higher schedule early in the program when encouragement was most needed. With the exception of the first, each succeeding step was repeated until the behavior was deliberate and proficient. This was accomplished within five trials per step. Since Step 1 was a relative time base for estimating the terminal proficiency of the chaining program, it was timed and graphed. Social reinforcement was provided with each successful manipulation. It is also noteworthy that emphasis during the first half of the program was primarily tactile in the sense that stress was placed on how the earmold "feels" when it is properly seated, how it "feels to the fingers" when it is properly seated, and how it "feels to the fingers" when it is grasped properly. During the last half of the program, visual contact with the prosthesis was emphasized to reinforce the appropriate grasp of the mold and the precision of the chaining process.

Step 1

Gain turned down—earmold and aid removed—prosthesis placed in box—battery compartment opened.

Step 2

Gain turned down—earmold loosened by grasping heel near tubing insert—earmold reinserted—gain turned up.

Step 3

Gain turned down—earmold partially removed (1/4 inch)—earmold reinserted—gain turned up.

Step 4

Gain turned down—earmold completely removed from canal (1 inch)—earmold reinserted—gain turned up.

Step 5

Gain turned down—earmold completely removed—fingers release contact—fingers reestablish contact—earmold reinserted— gain turned up.

Step 6

Gain turned down—earmold completely removed—hand to lap—hand to aid and fingers reestablish contact with mold— earmold reinserted—gain turned up.

Step 7

Gain turned down—earmold completely removed—aid removed—visual inspection of finger placement on mold— earmold reinserted—aid replaced—gain turned up.

Step 8

Gain turned down—earmold completely removed—aid removed—prosthesis placed in box—hand to lap—hand to aid and fingers reestablish contact with mold—earmold reinserted— aid replaced—gain turned up.

Step 9

Gain turned down—earmold completely removed—aid removed—prosthesis placed in box—battery compartment opened—hand to lap—battery compartment closed—fingers reestablish contact with mold—earmold reinserted—aid replaced—gain turned up.

Step 10

Gain turned down—earmold completely removed—aid removed—prosthesis placed in box—battery compartment opened—box and prosthesis taken to another room by examiner—patient taken to the other room—battery compart- ment closed—fingers reestablish contact with mold—earmold reinserted—aid replaced—gain turned up.

It was deemed important to take time to encourage precise grasping of the earmold during the early stages; yet the entire program was com- pleted in less than 30 minutes. Moreover, the length of the second cycle of Step 10, involving replacement of amplification, was found to closely approximate the amount of time required for removal of amplification in Step 1, about 20 seconds. What appears most significant, however, is that a relatively simple application of behavioral engineering corrected a problem the client had been struggling with for months.

Individual speechreading instruction, rather than group activities, was deemed appropriate for a 62-year-old woman who had suffered loss of hearing in one ear due to Meniere's disease. Socially active in the community and vain about disclosing her impairment to others, the woman preferred the privacy of individual therapy. She was an avid bridge player; one activity that satisfied the five ingredients of a good group meeting described earlier consisted of "playing" bridge through a two-way mirror with only visual cues for statements such as "I bid three spades," "I pass," and so forth. The woman improved her ability to speechread the language of her favorite game. This proved fortuitous, since the signs of Meniere's (roaring tinnitus, vertigo, and nausea) signaled the eventual loss of hearing in her good ear.

amplification

While presbycusis currently is not a medically treatable disorder, the alternative choice—wearable amplification—is not highly regarded among many older persons. The present generation of aging is not far removed from the earlier stigmata of highly visible and clumsy hearing aid devices, unkind associations between deafness and dumbness, and uncharitable jokes about deafness and aging. Other factors which contribute to this vein of reticence include the initial high cost of hearing aids, continued lack of knowledge about the service-delivery system, and frequent lack of transportation to and from clinics and hearing aid dealerships.

Results of a questionnaire interview survey conducted among a random sample of 153 elderly, hearing-impaired individuals who had not purchased hearing aids tend to support this. Responding to the question, "What prevents older persons with hearing difficulties from getting help?", 47% of the respondents cited the high cost of appliances as the prime reason, 15% indicated lack of knowledge concerning where to go for assistance and what services were available, 11% attributed lack of transportation as the main problem, while 7% cited pride and vanity as the primary reasons for not seeking help. The remaining 20% described a variety of other problems, including fear of doctors and hearing aid dealers, lack of awareness of a hearing difficulty, projected determination to "get by" without assistance despite the handicap, and unfavorable reports about hearing aids from relatives and friends (Lundberg, 1979). Older persons tend to tolerate greater hearing impairment than younger persons before seeking audiologic assistance for their problems (Haggard, 1980).

Hearing Aid Evaluation and Adjustment. Although amplification is worn by individuals of all ages, most people who wear aids are beyond the sixth decade of life. A survey of 15,508 households in the United States revealed that 75% of the hearing aid wearers were between 60 and 100 years of age, compared with only 25% for persons under age 60 (Broenen, 1983).

Acknowledging the need for amplification represents considerably more than admitting to a sensory deficit within this age group. It represents an acquiescence to the reality of aging, an acknowledgment that another bodily system is failing. As one woman emphatically stated during a hearing aid counseling session, "Well, I suppose this thing will go along with my dentures, glasses, and support brace. It's getting so it takes me half the morning to make myself *whole!*" (Maurer, 1976, p. 72).

Nonetheless, most older persons can benefit from appropriately tested and fitted hearing aids, and the attitudes concerning amplification are gradually changing. In countries where hearing aids are provided at little or no cost by government programs, such as Denmark, evidence suggests that older persons can achieve life satisfaction benefits near equal to those of younger individuals wearing amplification (Birk-Nielsen, 1974). Contributing to a more positive acceptance of hearing aids are increased miniaturization and versatility of the devices, increased sophistication in hearing aid selection and fitting techniques, better consumer protection through FDA regulations, and increased professional awareness of the need for adequate rehabilitative followup among the aging.

Some hearing aid companies have conceded to the physical limitations of older persons by offering oversize volume controls, fool-proof battery compartments, and fingernail slots for easier removal of in-the-ear hearing aids. Earmold companies now offer "geriatric handles" on their devices and, as seen in Figure 10.4, certain manufacturers provide

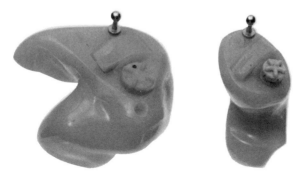

Figure 10.4. In-the-ear (ITE) and canal hearing aids with handles. (Courtesy of Starkey Northwest.)

handles on hearing aids. A few hearing aid manufacturers have grown concerned about the special needs of the elderly in nursing homes and convalescent hospitals, persons whose visual, tactile, neuromuscular, and memory difficulties contraindicate conventional forms of amplification. Therefore, Frye Electronics, for example, designed an inexpensive rechargeable body-type aid that features a large red volume control and accommodates a variety of hearing-loss candidates. While the cosmetic-conscious older person may reject the concept of a body-worn aid, Smith and Fay (1977) found in a long-term care facility in New York that body aids were more successfully accepted by the elderly than other forms of amplification. Out of 49 satisfied hearing aid users, 35 wore body systems while 14 used ear-level and eyeglass instruments. This finding is consistent with the author's experience among residents of a convalescent hospital for the aging. The popular aversion to body-aid "visibility" may be a blessing in disguise for nursing-home residents with poor management skills and visual limitations.

Biologically younger old persons generally accept amplification with fewer misgivings and adjustment problems. Those with physical limitations require substantially more assistance. In particular, the success of hearing aids depends to a great extent upon the individual's neurological state and his or her ability to physically manage the prosthesis. Those with central auditory-processing problems, such as post-stroke victims, often are not good candidates for hearing aids. In some instances, amplification of the speech message may further degrade the older person's ability to process the signal (Jerger & Jerger, 1971). This suprathreshold message distortion may not be apparent from the results of a conventional hearing test, but may be revealed during a comprehensive audiologic assessment. Nonetheless, Kricos, Lesner, Sandridge, and Yanke (1987) endorsed the need to counsel patients with central auditory deficits about the benefits and limitations of amplification. Hearing aids may not produce significantly improved speech discrimination scores, but may allow centrally impaired persons to maintain what these investigators describe as "a more natural auditory contact with the world" (p. 341). Certainly, the recommendation for amplification should not be ignored or contraindicated because of neurological impairment without a quantitative assessment of potential benefits during a reasonable trial period.

A number of modifications in conventional hearing aid evaluation techniques may be necessary for biologically older persons. First, early fatigue, lengthened reaction time, and a lower frustration threshold may mandate shorter sessions and the need for return visits to complete the evaluation. Although this recourse is often not desirable because of transportation problems, it may be necessary in view of other factors, including variability in performance scores, necessity for additional assessment, and perhaps most crucial, the need for concurrent counseling. Second, conventional word lists, sound-field procedures, real-ear measures, and master hearing aid techniques may need to be altered or abbreviated due to diminishing alertness and fatiguability. Also, during the hearing aid evaluation, for example, tests for sentence comprehension in cafeteria or propositional noise (intelligible background conversation) may provide a more valid indication of amplification success than monosyllabic word lists. Matthies, Bilger, and Roezckonski (1983) found that the age-related decrement in speech intelligibility in noise tended to disappear over a 90-day period as their subjects gained experience wearing amplification in noise. Third, the number of hearing aid choices may be restricted by the individual's lack of management skills, or by firmly entrenched attitudes as to what type of instrument will and will not be tolerated. Fourth, the biologically aging segment of the population requires more extensive rehabilitative followup, including counseling, supervised instruction, and hearing aid earmold modifications.

The hearing aid evaluation process among the elderly may encompass the entire 30- to 60-day trial period offered by the dealer, often taxing the patience of those whose primary interest is sale closure. However, the clinical audiologist must remain steadfast in terms of ethical responsibilities toward handicapped clients. Hardick (1977) utilized a number of hearing aids on the same individual during the aural rehabilitation process, rather than concentrating on hoped-for behavioral changes associated with the aid initially recommended in the hearing aid evaluation.

Another method of measuring the perceived benefit of amplification is the *Hearing Aid Performance Inventory* (HAPI), developed by Walden et al. (1984). This 64-item questionnaire assesses the helpfulness of hearing aids in different listening situations. Since perceived benefits are rated by the wearer of amplification, scale values have relevant prognostic value for the success or failure of remediation.

The question whether aging persons should wear one hearing aid or binaural amplification is an individual one, depending to a great extent upon prosthesis management and financial capabilities that must be weighed against perceived gains in social-receptive skills. An added variable is the attitudinal difference between wearing one instrument, as opposed to two. Thus, it is not uncommon to hear an elderly person comment, "I don't need two of these, do I? I'm not deaf!" Apparently, if one hearing aid represents a milestone in acquiescence to sensorineural aging, two become a millstone! However, life satisfaction is greater for those who can adjust to appropriately fitted binaural amplification. Birk-Nielsen (1974) noted in comparing monaural versus binaural amplification that two hearing aids reduced the amount of social hearing handicap among older persons. This two-ear advantage, which is discussed in Chapter 2, includes better speech discrimination in noise, reduced localized autophony (voice resonance), improved spacial balance and localization, and improved sound quality. Among those who have physical, financial, or cosmetic limitations, or whose quiescent lifestyles fail to support the need for two instruments, the choice of which ear to fit becomes an issue. Considerations that enter into this decision among geriatrics include: (a) earedness for social communication gain in quiet and in noise; (b) severity of arthritic or other physical involvements in the arms and hands as related to prosthesis manipulation; (c) handedness; (d) accustomed ear for telephone use; and (e) lifestyle factors affecting sidedness, such as driving a car or location of bed in a convalescent home. A more exhaustive treatise on the topic of hearing aid selection among older persons may be found in *Hearing and Aging: Tactics for Intervention* (Maurer & Rupp, 1979).

Audiologic Surveillance during the Trial Period. The first two weeks of the hearing aid trial period are critical. The audiologist should be ready for any problem that might occur between the client, the amplification system, and the environment. Counseling, either face to face or by telephone, is a continuing commitment that is based on the individual's adjustment needs. Schow, Christensen, Hutchinson, and Nerbonne (1978) discovered during a statewide nursing home survey that only 11% of potential hearing aid candidates were using amplification; another 20% of these responded that they had hearing aids, but were not using them. As pointed out earlier, the reasons for rejection of amplification devices are infinite, ranging from simple management difficulties to complex attitude adjustment problems. The clinician must allow these reasons to surface early in the trial period before rejection becomes ingrained. Another concept to be aware of during counseling is that rejection usually works in tandem with other age-related deficits. For example, rejection and reduced short-term memory may combine to become counterproductive, as summed up in the statement of an 89-year-old woman who, during a moment of exasperation, announced, ''I can never remember which way the battery goes in, and I hear better without this thing, anyway!'' Needless to say, she had the battery inserted backwards.

Attention given to the primary complaints of the client, family members, and friends during the pre-intervention phase should be re-addressed during the hearing aid trial period. Information from a case history illustrates the utility of this concept. The pre-intervention counseling session included the following list of complaints.

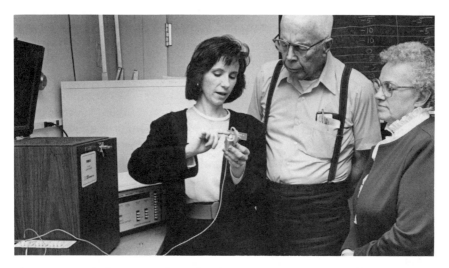

Figure 10.5. A clinician explains the electroacoustic properties of a hearing aid. Careful counseling throughout the aural rehabilitation process is critical for success with the elderly.

1. Difficulty understanding in church.

2. Daughter tired of repeating.

3. Unable to hear whispers, soft sounds.

4. Unable to hear driver on Senior Adult Center bus outings.

5. Difficulty understanding in dining room.

6. Turns TV set up too loud (daughter's complaint).

Consequently, audiologic surveillance during the first two weeks was aimed not only at prosthesis management, but at the environments where difficulties were noted. The above checklist of complaints became an immediate target for intervention. Each problem was investigated and appropriate measures were taken to reduce or eliminate it. For example, once the client was taught to compensate for listening difficulties encountered in the sanctuary, the recommended amplification device became an integral aspect of improved listening. Considered separately from the environment, the hearing aid would have been doomed to failure. Similarly, the overextended TV volume control was corrected by allowing the daughter to adjust the loudness to a "comfortable" level while the client was seated in her customary chair with her aids turned to half gain. This listening level was subsequently marked on the TV volume control with white fingernail polish.

The "Significant Other". The significant other person should understand the prosthetic device, its main components, the conditions under which it should be worn; should possess basic trouble-shooting information, warranty and repair information; and should be proficient at inserting, removing, and using the instrument. It is helpful to provide a written description of this information, as well as a list of special resources appropriate to the aging client. This would include the audiologist's phone number, the location and telephone number of a drug store providing low-cost batteries, special alerting, wake-up, and communication devices available, information on captioned films for television, if appropriate, and a time schedule for hearing aid checks, aural rehabilitation meetings, and annual audiologic assessment (see details on the above items in Chapter 2).

Advocacy in Restrictive Environments. The best method for encouraging aural rehabilitative assistance from the administration and staff of convalescent hospitals, nursing homes, high-rise facilities for the aging and senior adult centers is to offer them something in return. The hearing problems of their clientele rank low when compared to the sleeping, eating, cleaning, entertainment, and health needs within the facility. Sometimes it is difficult to gain entry into a restrictive environment on the basis of one client who has a hearing impairment and needs carryover assistance. A workable strategy for overcoming staff resistance is to seek out the activities director and explain that you are working with the client and his/her family. Offer to provide a slide session on hearing and aging as a staff inservice aimed at helping the staff understand and manage all clientele with hearing difficulties. Leaving the activities director with this public-service gesture and a copy of your professional credentials removes much of the suspicion associated with the doorstep intervention tactics of some commercial vendors.

A stimulating, solution-oriented talk nearly always produces advocates among residents and staff members—individuals who later may become allies in the rehabilitation plan. A nucleus is formed, and interest is maintained through a recognized need for further education as well as an open communication line to the audiologist's office. Weinstein (1984b) provided an effective 5-point plan for ensuring that the nursing staff will carry out their responsibilities with the hearing impaired:

1. Promote understanding of the structure of the auditory mechanism, the causes and effects (e.g., psychosocial) of hearing loss in the elderly.

2. Acquaint staff with the role of the audiologist in the hearing health care of the residents.

3. Provide suggestions for how to improve the staff's communication expressiveness (see Maurer & Rupp, 1979, pp. 159–160; Hull, 1982, pp. 383–407; Weinstein, 1984b, p. 267, for specific strategies).

4. Orient staff to maintenance, operation, and advantages and disadvantages of hearing aids and earmolds, emphasizing management of the prosthesis.

5. Offer suggestions for how to create/structure the institutional environment so that it facilitates interpersonal relationships among residents and staff (see Dancer & Keiser, 1980, p. 10; Bode, Tweedle, & Hull, 1982, pp. 101–117; Hepler, 1982, pp. 445–452, for specific recommendations).

Hurvitz et al. (1987) demonstrated an effective self-paced computer AR program designed to provide communication training to a nursing home population. Their software program covers content related to (a) mechanisms of the ear; (b) audiograms; (c) management of the hearing problem; (d) speechreading; (e) hearing aids; and (f) communication skills training. Short informational paragraphs are presented followed by multiple-choice questions in a user friendly format. Patients trained with this program showed more knowledge gains than in a conventional group classroom approach.

communication rehabilitation

In order for aural rehabilitation to be successful for the older person, positive changes must be brought about in the entire social-communicative milieu. The audiologist-counselor, acting in the multiple roles of diagnostician, hearing aid specialist, aural rehabilitation specialist, and gerontologist, becomes an integral part of this milieu, as expressed in Figure 10.6.

According to this model, the aging client is both a transmitter (XMTR) and a receiver (RCVR) of information in his daily interface with REALITY. Over the years, he has developed certain COMMUNICATION SKILLS with which he both expresses and receives information that contributes toward his KNOWLEDGE or understanding of his present

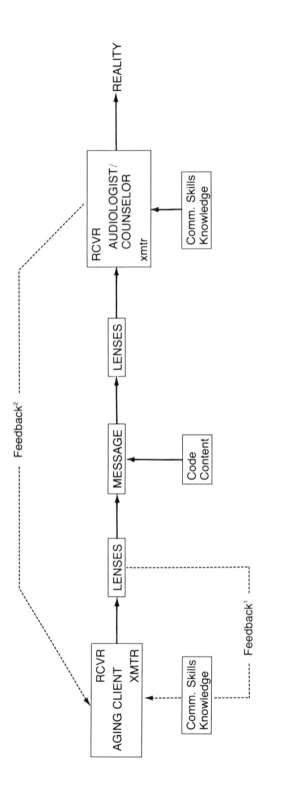

Figure 10.6. Role of audiologist-counselor in communication rehabilitation for the elderly.

living experiences, his lifestyle. He tends to view and interact with his reality through certain LENSES, or attitudes, that cumulatively reflect past experiences, lending a generous ingredient of uniqueness to both his personality and his abilities. The messages received or expressed have both code and content. The particular form that is revealed in this message transaction is represented by the client's CODE, what he does in the act of communicating. Does he utilize visual communication in the act of receiving? Does tactile stimulation (touching him on the arm) increase the likelihood of reception? Does his auditory reception skill agree with the quality, manner, and structure of the language being expressed?

Similarly, the code that is revealed in the client's expressive communication includes the quality, manner, and structure of his language system. The CONTENT of messages transmitted and received represents the judgments and inferences that he internalizes, his unique interpretation of the communication transaction that is channeled through two monitoring systems, FEEDBACK(1), his internal response to his own message, and FEEDBACK(2), his internal response to the messages of others.

Problems of audition, including loss of hearing sensitivity, slowing of neural processing of messages, increased difficulty understanding in noise, and deficits in short-term auditory memory storage, interact significantly in the communication model. A peripheral high-frequency hearing loss alters the code of the message received, thereby affecting the content and even influencing the outgoing response:

> Mr. Jacobson was helping his grandson paint the family shed. "Gramps," the younger person said, "let's quit for awhile and go get some thinner."
> The older man stared in amazement at his grandson. "Go get some dinner? Son, we just had lunch!"

Further, the message-delivery speed of the nightly television newscaster may alter the message code and content for older persons who simply cannot "keep up." As a result, maintaining intellectual currency with events in the world may slip in priority, affecting both general knowledge and the content of conversations with others. Increasing failure to inhibit background conversations and noises while attending to primary messages degrades the code and content to such an extent for some of the elderly that they retreat from such environments. The feedback of earlier communication may be tested severely by lapses in recent memory, not only altering the older person's trust in reality but even leading to a denial of it:

Mrs. Andrews' chief complaint about her new hearing aid was lack of battery life.

"Are you opening the battery case at night when you're not using the instrument?" the audiologist inquired.

"Heavens no. You didn't tell me to do that!"

"Yes, she did, mother," the daughter chimed in. "Don't you remember? It's even stated in that booklet in your purse."

"Well, this is the first time I've *heard* about it," the older woman retorted.

The critical implication of an auditory impairment on an aging individual is that it affects the lenses through which the client views reality. Thus, when the code and content of messages are altered, both Feedback 1 and Feedback 2 (see Figure 10.6) are affected so that the client comes to distrust what others say as well as his own interpretation of communicative events. Even continuing accumulation and expression of knowledge may stagnate as reality is restructured to avoid or escape from the stresses associated with growing older with a hearing impairment. This is reflected in such common disengagement statements as, "I don't go to church anymore.", "I've given up on the Senior Adult Center.", and ultimately, "Why should I go to lipreading classes and buy a hearing aid that lasts five years? I won't be around that long, anyway . . ."

A prime example of these forces at work in the expressive communication skills of the older person is the case of the laryngectomee. Most individuals who have undergone total laryngectomy surgery are within the senior adult age group. Most have hearing difficulties, and since esophageal speech generally has reduced intensity and less well defined vowel formants, laryngectomized persons are less intelligible to peers, who are also likely to be aging and hearing impaired. The esophageal speaker's increased tension and effort aimed at being understood are often undermined by an increase in noise from his tracheostoma, a surgically produced hole in the neck through which the laryngectomee breathes after the larynx is removed, causing further depreciation in speech intelligibility. For too many the frustrations arising from failure to communicate lead to extinction of esophageal speech and withdrawal from social situations.

The counselor-audiologist is positioned between the aging client and reality since his/her own communication skills and knowledge are called into play to assist the older person in restructuring his lifestyle to ameliorate or compensate for the hearing impairment. The model in Figure 10.6 depicts the audiologist-counselor as assuming a principal role in receiving rather than transmitting information. That is, the RCVR aspect of his/her communication skills must take precedence over the XMTR aspect, if the specialist is to arrive at a meaningful evaluation of the client and client adjustment during intervention. Dancer (1984) referred to this process as a "field of experience" surrounding the feedback mechanism. He suggested that effective communication takes place only to the extent that the counselor empathizes or shares common experiences with the aging client.

Sensitivity achieved through listening will have great effect on the outcome of the rehabilitation program. Slower in adapting to change and more fixed in their attitudes than younger hearing-impaired persons, the elderly demand more professional time for their feelings to surface. In some instances, the audiologist can bring about positive changes by simply permitting the client to register complaints and thereby achieve a more favorable polarity in the decision making:

> "My voice is so different with these aids on," Mrs. Gregory said, shaking her head. "I don't think I can get used to them . . ."
> "Uh huh."
> "Do I sound like this to others? My voice sounds so gravelly."
> "Hmm."
> "I wonder if I've been talking too loud to people . . . before I got these, I mean." Her eyes brightened. "Well, I certainly keep my voice down now."
> "Uh huh."
> "I can hear a whisper now . . . in a quiet room. But . . . Oh, the racket when I'm doing dishes! I took them off and put them on the window sill."
> "Uh huh."
> "I could hear the clerk in the checkout line yesterday. Heard everything he said . . ."
> "Hmm."
> "I suppose it's a matter of . . . getting used to them." She nodded her head. "They help . . . they really do."

In other instances, listening to the aging client permits the audiologist to orchestrate necessary changes in lifestyle which maintains the delicate balance between hearing for pleasure and adjusting to the perceived nuisances of a new prosthesis. For some individuals, communicative rehabilitation must concentrate on facilitating nonauditory channels:

> Mr. Stanley, a 77-year-old former steamfitter, had suffered a stroke which compounded the communication problems already associated with a severe high-frequency hearing loss. Amplification failed to improve his degraded speech discrimination skills. Individual speechreading training also failed to demonstrate any change in his ability to visually communicate. However, placement in a small-group speechreading program that also emphasized

group counseling produced a number of positive changes which cumulatively increased his life satisfaction. His self-tolerance and sense of humor returned as he listened to others openly discuss communicative "failures" with which he could identify. The frequency of his face-watching behavior increased, and despite the lack of progress noted in formal lipreading tests, there was a demonstrable improvement in his social-communicative skills. Moreover, his wife reported that a telephone amplifier had been installed in the home at his request and that her husband was starting to watch television again.

Listening to the elderly client can also effect changes in the audiologist's prescriptive statements:

One assertive client, returning for her first annual hearing test and hearing aid check, advised the clinician, "You shouldn't tell people not to wear their aids when sleeping. I sleep on my left side and wear my hearing aid in my right ear so I can hear the doorbell or the telephone ringing. It makes me feel more secure."

Assistive Listening Devices. A seemingly endless number of products and devices are now available for assisting older, hearing-impaired persons in a variety of environments. For a number of years, Vaughn (Vaughn & Lightfoot, 1983) and her colleagues have advocated considering clients' needs from the standpoint of social communicative devices rather than hearing aid appliances (see Chapters 2 and 13). Developed at the Birmingham Veterans Administration Hospital in Alabama, the Ecology of Human Communication encompasses testing and clinical investigation of a number of alternative listening and speaking devices, ranging from simple hardwire amplification systems for use in automobiles to infrared and FM systems for use in nursing homes, churches, and auditoriums. The VisiCom device (Vaughn, Gibbs, & Lightfoot, 1981), for example, displays information transmitted over telephone lines to a pocket-sized, portable, LED printout that is acoustically coupled to the mouthpiece of a touchtone-dial telephone. The VisiCom display enables hearing-impaired persons with relatively normal oral communication skills to converse on the telephone. Finally, computer-assisted aural rehabilitation is an active area of research and development by Vaughn and her colleagues. For example, her REMATE (Remote Machine-Assisted Treatment and Evaluation) system includes computerized intervention programs that can be transmitted through telephone lines to individuals in remote areas or others who lack mobility to travel to clinics. Various terminal devices, installed in the client's residence, can be made available, including telephone handsets, touchtone keyboards, teletype-

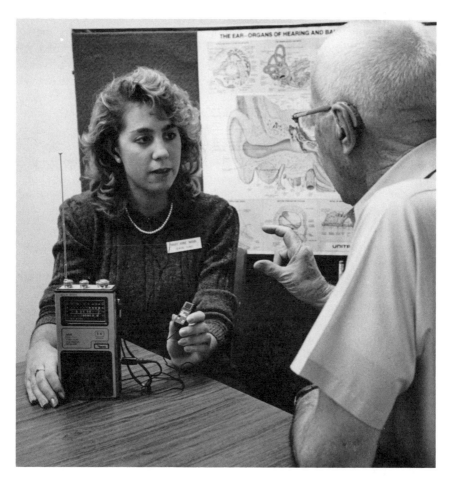

Figure 10.7. An elderly person learns about a simple assistive listening device system.

writers, telenote–writers, and others. The REMATE computer delivers the program, stores client responses, and reports them to the rehabilitation specialist.

psychosocial considerations

The varying degrees of adjustment to hearing loss within the geriatric population reflects the heterogeneity of the group. Lifestyles and subsequent need for oral communication differ widely. Some people are gregarious, socially active, and motivated to listen carefully and draw from nonverbal clues during difficult communicative situations. In general, these are the biologically younger aging persons, whose attitudes are less resistant to change and who evidence fewer emotional and physical problems. This group is more likely to take their hearing deficiencies in stride, require less aural rehabilitative followup, and compensate more successfully in a communicative sense. Others, who may exhibit the same extent of hearing deficiency, but who are not socially outgoing or adept at adjusting to new situations, may demonstrate greater handicap and poorer adjustive behaviors. They also may demonstrate more limited ability to integrate nonauditory stimuli, such as speechreading skills. These individuals tend to appear biologically older and more resigned to the aging process. Consequently, their communicative skills as well as attitudes toward intervention may be severely affected.

The aging individual with a hearing impairment often struggles through communication situations. Frequently, verbal messages are misinterpreted and inappropriate answers are given. Family and friends may attribute the older person's seeming inattentiveness and lack of appropriate social interaction to a number of descriptors, ranging from indifference to senility, any of which may lead to less and less social interaction between the aging individual and his support system.

When deprived of social interaction either due to a hearing loss and/or the attitudes of those around them, older persons become frustrated and reciprocate by avoiding those environments in which difficulties are encountered (i.e., family gatherings, church, movies, and other social activities previously enjoyed). Such a loss in close interpersonal communication can lead to decreased personal stimulation, resulting in depression and self-depreciation. Thus, many older, hearing-impaired persons exhibit what has been described as the ''geriapathy syndrome'':

> The individual feels disengaged from group interaction and apathy ensues, the product of the fatigue which sets in from the relentless effort of straining to hear. Frustration, kindled by begging too many pardons, gives way to subterfuges that disguise misunderstandings. The head nods in agreement with a conversation only vaguely interpreted. The voice registers approval of words often void of meaning. The ear strives for some redundancy that will make the message clearer. Finally, acquiescing to fatigue and frustration, thoughts stray from the conversation to mental imageries that are unburdened by the defective hearing mechanism. (Maurer, 1976)

In order to deal with the stresses associated with a hearing loss, the aging individual resorts to adjustive behaviors. These behaviors fall into two general categories (a) those that defend against the problem, and (b) those that offer stress reduction through escape from the problem. While anyone encountering stress may engage in defense and escape behaviors, it is propitious to reexamine these adjustment methods as they relate to hearing impairment and aging (Maurer & Rupp, 1979).

Defense Techniques. The elderly hearing-impaired resort to a variety of coping mechanisms to handle the challenges presented by their hearing loss. The techniques deemed to defend the patient against any stigma attached to the hearing impairment include: attention getting, identification, compensation, rationalization, and projection.

Attention getting. This method of adjustment is used to draw attention away from the hearing impairment by diverting concern to some other aspect of behavior or physical deficit. For example, the senior citizen who distracts the listener with a seemingly endless list of complaints, ranging from poor motor coordination to financial hardship, may be masking or devaluating the importance of the hearing impairment. The increased attention given to the older person's acting-out behaviors is reinforcing, and may sidetrack the listener's concern for the auditory problem.

Identification. Older individuals may reduce the stress accompanying a hearing impairment by assuming the identity or attributes of others whom they respect or admire. This defense technique is illustrated by the senior citizen who discounts the limitation of an auditory deficit by espousing the inherited keenness of her father's visual acuity.

Compensation. This method of adjustment is characterized by a substitution of activities to accommodate a hearing loss. Some people compensate successfully, as with the individual who acquires speechreading skills and learns to be more attentive in difficult communicative environments. Others choose to eliminate the aversiveness of difficult-to-hear situations by giving up previously enjoyed pastimes and decreasing social interactions. For the latter group, the hearing handicap is not so apparent if difficult listening situations never arise.

Rationalization. This defense mechanism relieves stress by providing invalid, but nevertheless logical and often socially acceptable reasons for auditory difficulties. For example, an older individual who is unable to adequately hear a lecturer may attribute the missed information to boredom or fatigue.

Projection. Perhaps the most common method of adjustment among aging persons with presbycusic hearing losses is projection. Characteristically, the older individual transfers his/her auditory difficulties to the behavior of others. This is exemplified by the senior citizen who denies a hearing handicap by attributing communication problems to the spouse, who supposedly does not "enunciate clearly."

Escape Techniques. As for defense mechanisms, the escape techniques some elderly hearing-impaired individuals resort to are intended to protect against or help them cope better with their hearing loss. The most common of these behaviors include insulation, negativism, regression, repression, and fantasy.

Insulation. Stress caused by hearing impairment may be lessened by simply retreating from the problem. Usually, the older person takes no rehabilitative action, showing little concern for possible alternatives and withdrawing completely to the security of the home, where there is less demand for receptive communication.

Negativism. This method of adjustment is characterized by aggressive, antagonistic behavior. The hearing-impaired senior citizen refuses any assistance towards aural rehabilitation, pessimistically offering reasons why treatment is not beneficial or possible to obtain.

Regression. By reverting to past, more dependent behaviors, an older person may effectively escape from the stress associated with a hearing loss. This is illustrated by the senior citizen who, when confronted with a difficult listening situation, turns to her spouse for repetition of the message. By readily assisting, the spouse, in turn, reinforces this dependency, thereby unwittingly encouraging further regressive behaviors, such as the constant need for physical assistance with the hearing aid.

Repression. This escape mechanism enables the hearing-impaired individual to avoid communicative difficulties by inhibiting or forgetting them. For example, the older person who consistently forgets to wear hearing aids cannot be held accountable for misunderstood messages by family and friends although that same individual never forgets to wear eyeglasses and earrings.

Fantasy. Escape from stress may be achieved by retreating from the adversities of reality into an imagined world where no physical deficits or social pressures exist. For the hearing-impaired geriatric, the continual frustration of listening to a confusing environment may lead to such inhibition, and subsequently be replaced by a more reinforcing fantasized world of daydreams.

The previously described adjustment methods are learned in childhood and utilized throughout one's lifetime to deal with the normal stresses of living. However, for the older individual these tension-reducing mechanisms may interfere with effective aural rehabilitative treatment if the stress-producing stimuli associated with the hearing loss are not recognized and dealt with during intervention.

The Geriatric Client's Attitude toward Aural Rehabilitation. In itself, growing older is not an obstacle towards successful participation in an aural rehabilitative program. Senior citizens who are in good physical and mental health, financially secure, and socially active often have the free time and desire to get involved in programs which will improve their communicative skills. Similarly, many older persons view a hearing loss as a minor inconvenience, and actively seek assistance so as not to allow the impairment to interfere with their lifestyles.

However, some senior adults are reluctant to participate in any aural rehabilitative treatment. According to Edwards and Klemmack (1973) and Neugarten, Havighurst, and Tobin (1961), the three most important factors associated with the older individual's self-fulfillment are (a) health status, (b) financial condition, and (c) activity level. When these are disrupted as a result of age, personal satisfaction may no longer be perceived as obtainable. Without an optimistic outlook towards the future, the older person's motivation can rapidly decline.

Changes in health status have perhaps the most significant effect on an individual's ability to actively participate in remediation. The senior citizen may not be enthusiastic about involvement in aural rehabilitation when other disabilities, unrelated to the hearing loss, are life-threatening and cause greater concern.

Difficulties with motor coordination, vision, memory, or general good health may also prohibit an aging person from initiating or sustaining interest in the intervention process. These disabilities are generally more severe among residents in extended health care facilities. Based on a survey of 62 nursing home residents who wore amplification, Smith and Fay (1977) concluded that almost 30% required daily assistance from staff.

When deteriorating health status is coupled with limited finances, older people often find themselves restricted to the confines of their own homes. Unlike their affluent peers, the aged poor have fewer options available to them in seeking aural rehabilitative assistance. Many cannot afford the necessary medical and clinical services, the purchase of hearing aids, or special amplification devices. Transportation costs can also be prohibitive. Similarly, travel to rehabilitative centers for speechreading classes or for hearing aid adjustments and repairs may be beyond their financial reach. Finally, the necessary encouragement often provided by family and friends may be restricted or nonexistent.

However, health or financial limitations are not always the basis for reluctance to participate in aural rehabilitative programs. In an investigation of 152 nursing home residents who were both physically and mentally capable of participating in a recommended remediation program, 35% refused all assistance (Alpiner, 1973). Schow et al. (1978) discovered during a nursing home screening program that 20% of residents who had hearing aids did not wear them.

A number of older people do not want to be a bother to relatives and friends, and some believe that nothing can be done to help them.

Some feel that a rehabilitation specialist's time is better spent with younger people, who have more productive years ahead of them to contribute to society. A number of aging individuals refuse remediation because they are reluctant to admit either the presence of a hearing loss or its severity. According to Alpiner (1973), lack of motivation was the primary reason given by 50% of the adults surveyed who decided against participation in a recommended aural rehabilitative program. Another 24% claimed they were not aware of the benefits or availability of such services, although all had been previously counseled on this issue.

The older person with a hearing deficit must come to believe in the importance of utilizing maximum auditory function. This can only be achieved through an environment in which communicative ability is considered essential and rewarding. Thus, a society which values good auditory skills is more likely to encourage its hearing-impaired members to seek aural rehabilitative treatment. If family, friends, and those who care for the aged demonstrate acceptance of amplification and express positive feelings towards remediation, the older person may learn to accept the same attitudes and come to value the same goals.

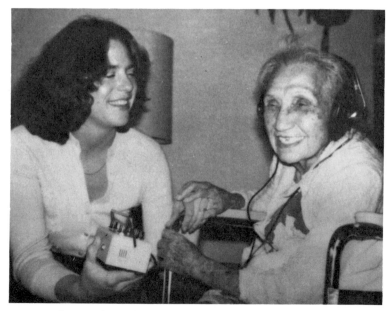

Figure 10.8. Devices like a hardwire auditory trainer can facilitate communication with some institutionalized elderly persons even when use of a hearing aid is not feasible.

summary

The aural rehabilitation specialist has a unique opportunity to provide services to the geriatric population. The complexity of changes occurring in advanced age together with the difficulties encountered due to auditory deficits requires that the audiologist become resourceful and willing to modify established techniques and protocols. The audiologist can significantly contribute to a positive future for hearing-impaired, aging persons—one that is more productive and less isolated. Better receptive communication skills may help lessen the stress caused by other disabilities, as well as facilitate social interaction between older persons and their living environments.

The need for specialized training in gerontology among graduate students specializing in speech and hearing sciences becomes increasingly apparent as the population of older persons expands and longevity increases. The current lack of commitment to training in gerontology among graduate programs in the United States must be radically reversed if audiologists are to maintain a leadership role in the care of the aging hearing impaired (Nerbonne, Schow, & Hutchinson, 1980; Raiford & Shadden, 1985). Addressing the problems of presbycusis is a professional challenge we must all face together.

recommended readings

Jacobs-Condit, L. (1984). *Gerontology and communication disorders.* Rockville, MD: American Speech-Language-Hearing Association.

Mauer, J., & Rupp, R. (1979). *Hearing and aging.* New York: Grune & Stratton.

McCarthy, P. (1987). Rehabilitation of the hearing impaired geriatric client. In J. Alpiner & P. McCarthy (Eds.) *Rehabilitative audiology: Children and adults* (pp. 370–427). Baltimore, MD: Williams & Wilkins.

Mueller, H.G., & Geoffrey, V.C. (1987). *Communication disorders in aging: Advances in assessment and management.* Washington, DC: Gallaudet University Press.

Schow, R., Christensen, J., Hutchinson, J., & Nerbonne, M. (1978). *Communication disorders of the aged.* Baltimore, MD: University Park Press.

Shadden, B.B. (1988). *Perspectives on communication behavior and aging: A sourcebook for clinicians.* Baltimore, MD: Williams & Wilkins.

Smith, C., & Fay, T. (1977). A program of auditory rehabilitation for aged persons in a chronic disease hospital. *Asha, 19,* 417–420.

references

Alpiner, J. (1963). Audiological problems of the aged. *Geriatrics, 18,* 19–26.

Alpiner, J. (1973). Aural rehabilitation and the aged client. *Audecibel, 22,* 102–104.

Alpiner, J., Chevrette, W., Glascoe, G., Metz, M., & Olsen, B. (1978). The Denver scale of communication function. In J.G. Alpiner (Ed.), *Adult rehabilitative audiology* (pp. 53–56). Balitmore, MD: Williams & Wilkins.

Alpiner, J., & McCarthy, P. (Eds.). (1987) *Rehabilitative audiology: Children and adults.* Baltimore, MD: Williams and Wilkins.

Atchley, R.C. (1972). *Social forces in later life.* Belmont, CA: Wadsworth Publishing Company.

Birk-Nielsen, H. (1974). Effect of monaural versus binaural hearing and treatment. *Scandinavian Audiology, 3,* 183–187.

Bode, D., Tweedle, D., & Hull R. (1982). Improving communication through aural rehabilitation. In R. Hull (Ed.), *Rehabilitative audiology* (pp.101–117). New York: Grune and Stratton.

Botwinick, J., & Thompson, L.W. (1968). Age differences in reaction time: An artifact? *Gerontology, 8,* 25–28.

Brody, H. (1973). In M. Rockstein & M. Sussman (Eds.), *Development and aging in the nervous system* (pp. 70 121–133). New York: Academic Press.

Broenen, J.A. (1983). Hearing aid population profile. *Hearing Instruments, 34,* 12–18.

Butler, R.N. (1975). *Why survive? Being old in America.* New York: Harper and Row.

Butler, R.N., & Lewis, M.I. (1977). *Aging and mental health: Positive psychosocial approaches.* St. Louis: C.V. Mosby.

Craik, F. (1977). Age differences in human memory. In J. Birun & K. Schail (Eds.), *Handbook of the psychology of aging* (pp. 394–420). New York: Van Nostrand Reinhold Co.

Dancer, J. (1984). General considerations in the management of older persons with communication disorders. In L. Jacobs-Condit (Ed.), *Gerontology and communication disorders* (pp. 172–184). Rockville, MD: American Speech-Language-Hearing Association.

Dancer, J., & Keiser, H. (1980). The hearing impaired elderly: Training others to help. *Hearing Aid Journal, 33*(4), 10.

Davis, H. (1948). The articulation area and the social adequacy index for hearing. *Laryngology, 58,* 761.

Decker, T. (1974). A survey of hearing loss in an older age hospital population. *The Gerontologist, 14,* 402–403.

Edwards, J.N., & Klemmack, D.L. (1973). Correlates of life satisfaction: A re-examination. *Journal of Gerontology, 26,* 497–502.

Eisdorfer, C., & Wilkie, F. (1972). Intellectual changes with advancing age. In L.F. Jarvic, C. Eisdorfer, & J.E. Blum (Eds.), *Intellectual functioning in adults* (pp. 21–30). New York: Springer.

Erickson, J.G. (1978). Speechreading: An aid to communication. Danville, IL: Interstate Printers and Publishers.

Ewertsen, H., & Birk-Nielsen, B. (1973). Social hearing handicap index: Social handicap in relation to hearing impairment. *Audiology, 12,* 180–181.

Gaeth, J. (1948). *A study of phonemic regression associated with hearing loss.* Unpublished doctoral dissertation, Northwestern University.

Gentile, A., & Ries, P. (1971). Population estimates of the number of deaf persons 65 years of age and over for the next 15 years. *Services for Elderly Deaf Persons* (pp. 15–18). New York: New York University, Deafness Research and Training Center.

Giolas, T. (1982). *Hearing handicapped adults.* Englewood Cliffs, NJ: Prentice-Hall.

Giolas, T.G., Owens, E., Lamb, S.G., & Schubert, E.D. (1979). Hearing performance inventory. *Journal of Speech and Hearing Disorders, 44,* 169–195.

Glorig, A., & Roberts, J. (1965). *Hearing levels of adults by age and sex, United States (1960–62).* National Center for Health Statistics, Series II, No. II. Washington, DC: U.S. Department of Health, Education and Welfare.

Gordon-Salant, S. (1986). Effects of aging on response criteria in speech recognition cases. *Journal of Speech and Hearing Research, 29*(2), 155–162.

Haggard, M.P. (1980). Six audiological paradoxes in the provision of hearing aid services. *Excerpta Medica,* 1–14.

Hardick, E.J. (1977). Aural rehabilitational programs for the aged can be successful. *Journal of the Academy of Rehabilitative Audiology, 10,* 51–67.

Hayes, D., & Jerger, J. (1979). Aging and the use of hearing aids. *Scandinavian Audiology, 8,* 33–40.

Hepler, J. (1982). The nurse in the aural rehabilitation process. In R. Hull (Ed.), *Rehabilitative audiology* (pp. 445–452). New York: Grune and Stratton.

High, W.S., Fairbanks, G., & Glorig, A. (1964). A scale for self-assessment of hearing handicap. *Journal of Speech and Hearing Disorders, 29,* 215–230.

Hull, R. (1982). Techniques for aural rehabilitation treatment for elderly clients. In R. Hull (Ed.), *Rehabilitative audiology* (pp. 383–407). New York: Grune and Stratton.

Hunter, W.F. (1960). The psychologist works with the aged individual. *Journal of Counseling Psychology, 7,* 120–126.

Hurvitz, J., Goldojorb, M., Walcek, A., & Manna-Levin K. (1987). *Comparison of two aural rehabilitation methods in a nursing home.* Paper presented at the ASHA National Convention, New Orleans.

Jerger, J., & Hayes, D. (1977). Diagnostic speech audiometry. *Archives of Otolaryngology, 103,* 216–222.

Jerger, J., & Jerger, S. (1971). Diagnostic significance of PB word functions. *Archives of Otolaryngology, 93,* 573–580.

Jordan, T.C. (1977). Response time to stimuli of increasing complexity as a function of aging. *British Journal of Psychology, 68,* 189–201.

Kalikow, D.N., Stevens, K.N., & Elliot, L. (1977). Development of a test of speech intelligibility in noise using sentence materials with controlled word predictability. *Journal of the Acoustical Society of America, 61,* 1337–1351.

Katz, J., & White, T.P. (1982). Introduction to the handicap of hearing impairment in the adult: Auditory impairment versus hearing handicap. In R. Hull (Ed.), *Rehabilitative audiology* (pp. 22–24). New York: Grune and Stratton.

Kricos, P., Lesner, S., Sandridge, S., & Yanke, R. (1987). Perceived benefits of amplification as a function of central auditory status in the elderly. *Ear and Hearing, 8,* 337–342.

Lamb, S.W., Owens, E., Schubert, E.D., & Giolas, T.G. (1982). Hearing performance inventory: Revised form. In T. Giolas (Ed.), *Hearing handicapped adults* (pp. 189–199). Englewood Cliffs, NJ: Prentice-Hall.

Lundberg, R. (1979). *Research survey.* Unpublished manuscript, Portland State University.

Matthies, M., Bilger, R., & Roezckowski, C. (1983). SPIN as a predictor of hearing aid use. *Asha, 25*(10), 61.

Maurer, J.F. (1976). Auditory impairment and aging. In B. Jacobs (Ed.), *Working with the impaired elderly* (p. 72). Washington, DC: National Council on the Aging.

Maurer, J.F. (1979). Aural rehabilitation for the aging. In L.J. Bradford & W.G. Hardy (Eds.), *Hearing and hearing impairment* (pp. 319–338). New York: Grune & Stratton.

Maurer, J.F. (1982). The psychosocial aspects of presbycusis. In R. Hull (Ed.), *Rehabilitative audiology* (pp. 271–281). New York: Grune & Stratton.

Maurer, J.F., & Rupp, R.R. (1979). *Hearing and aging: Tactics for intervention.* New York: Grune & Stratton.

McCarthy, J.P., & Culpepper, B. (1987). The adult remediation process. In J. Alpiner & J.P. McCarthy (Eds.), *Rehabilitative audiology: children and adults* (pp. 305–342). Baltimore, MD: Williams and Wilkins.

McCartney, J.H., Maurer, J.F., & Sorenson, F.D. (1974). A mobile audiology service for the elderly: A preliminary report. *Journal of the Academy of Rehabilitative Audiology, 7*(2), 25–35.

Miller, M., & Ort, R. (1965). Hearing problems in a home for the aged. *Acta Otolaryngologica, 59,* 33–44.

Moulton, C. (1981). *Aural rehabilitative needs for the elderly nursing home resident.* Unpublished research paper, Portland State University.

Nebes, R.D. (1978). Vocal versus manual response as a determinant of age differences in simple reaction time. *Journal of Gerontology, 33,* 884–889.

Nerbonne, M.A., Schow, R.L., & Hutchinson, J.M. (1980). Gerontologic training in communication disorders. *Asha, 22,* 404–408.

Neugarten, B.L., Havighurst, R., & Tobin, S. (1961). The measurement of life satisfaction. *Journal of Gerontology, 16,* 134–143.

Noble, W.G., & Atherley, G.R.C. (1970). The hearing measurement scale: A questionnaire for assessment of auditory disability. *Journal of Auditory Research, 10,* 229–250.

Office of Human Development. (1978). *Facts about older Americans.* National Clearing House on Aging Report, DHEW. Publication No. (OHD) 78-20006. Washington, DC: Administration of Aging.

Punch, J. (1983). The prevalence of hearing impairment. *Asha, 25,* 27.

Rabbitt, P.M.A. (1965). An age decrement in the ability to ignore irrelevant information. *Journal of Gerontology, 20,* 233–238.

Raiford, C., & Shadden, B. (1985). Graduate education in gerontology. *Asha, 27*(6), 37–43.

Robertson-Thabo, E. (1984). Psychological changes with aging. In L. Jacobs-Condit (Ed.), *Gerontology and communication disorders* (pp. 73–130). Rockville, MD: American Speech-Language-Hearing Association.

Ronch, J.L. (1982). Who are these aging persons? In R. Hull (Ed.), *Rehabilitative audiology* (pp. 185–213). New York: Grune & Stratton.

Schow, R.L., Christensen, J., Hutchinson, J., & Nerbonne, M.A. (1978). *Communication disorders of the aged: A guide for health professionals*. Baltimore, MD: University Park Press.

Schow, R.L., & Nerbonne, M.A. (1977). Assessment of hearing handicap by nursing home residents and staff. *Journal of the Academy of Rehabilitative Audiology, 10*(2), 2–9.

Schow, R.L., & Nerbonne, M.A. (1980). Hearing levels among elderly nursing home residents. *Journal of Speech and Hearing Disorders, 45*(1), 124–132.

Schow, R.L., & Nerbonne, M.A. (1982). Communication screening profile: Use with elderly clients. *Ear and Hearing, 3*(3), 135–147.

Schuknecht, H.F. (1964). Further observations on the pathology of presbycusis. *Archives of Otology, 80,* 369–382.

Simon, J.R., & Pouraghabagher, A.R. (1978). The effect of aging on the stages of processing in a choice reaction time task. *Journal of Gerontology, 33,* 553–561.

Smith, C.R., & Fay, T.H. (1977). A program of auditory rehabilitation for aged persons in a chronic disease hospital. *Asha, 19,* 417–422.

Soldo, B.J. (1980, November). America's elderly in the 1980's. *Population Bulletin, 35,* 11. Washington, DC: Population Reference Bureau.

Stephens, S.D.G., & Goldstein, D. (1983). Auditory rehabilitation in the elderly. In R. Hinchcliffe (Ed.), *Hearing and balance in the elderly* (pp. 201–227). New York: Churchill Livingstone Press.

Sussman, M.B. (1976). The family life of old people. In R. Binstock & E. Shanas (Eds.), *Handbook of aging and the social sciences* (pp. 218–243). New York: Van Nostrand Reinhold Co.

Vaughn, G.R., Gibbs, S.D., & Lightfoot, R.K. (1981). *Alternative listening devices for hearing impaired adults.* A paper presented at the White House Conference on Aging, Washington, DC.

Vaughn, G.R., & Lightfoot, R.K. (1983). Lifestyles and assistive listening devices and systems. *Hearing Instruments, 34*(10), 6–12.

Ventry, I.M., & Weinstein, B.E. (1982). The hearing handicap inventory for the elderly: A new tool. *Ear and Hearing, 3,* 128–134.

Walden, B., Demorest, M., & Hepler, E. (1984). Self-report approach to assessing benefit from amplification. *Journal of Speech and Hearing Research, 27*(1), 49–56.

Weinstein, B. (1984a). A review of hearing handicap scales. *Audiology, 9,* 91–109.

Weinstein, B. (1984b). Management of hearing impaired elderly. In L. Jacobs-Condit (Ed.), *Gerontology and communication disorders* (pp. 244–279). Rockville, MD: American Speech-Language-Hearing Association.

Weinstein, B., Spitzer, J., & Ventry, I. (1986). Test-retest reliability of the hearing handicap inventory for the elderly. *Ear and Hearing, 7,* 295-299.

APPENDIX TEN A

nursing home hearing handicap index (nhhi): self-version for resident

Circle the appropriate number.	Very Often				Almost Never
1. When you are with other people do you wish you could hear better?	5	4	3	2	1
2. Do other people feel you have a hearing problem (when they try to talk to you)?	5	4	3	2	1
3. Do you have trouble hearing another person if there is a radio or TV playing (in the same room)?	5	4	3	2	1
4. Do you have trouble hearing the radio or TV?	5	4	3	2	1
5. (How often) do you feel life would be better if you could hear better?	5	4	3	2	1
6. How often are you embarrassed because you don't hear well?	5	4	3	2	1
7. When you are alone do you wish you could hear better?	5	4	3	2	1
8. Do people (tend to) leave you out of conversations because you don't hear well?	5	4	3	2	1
9. (How often) do you withdraw from social activities (in which you ought to participate) because you don't hear well?	5	4	3	2	1
10. Do you say "what" or "pardon me" when people first speak to you?	5	4	3	2	1

Total _____ × 2 = _____

$$-20$$

_____ × 1.25 = _____%

From "Assessment of Hearing Handicap by Nursing Home Residents and Staff" by R. L. Schow and M. A. Nerbonne, 1977, *Journal of Rehabilitative Audiology*, 10, pp. 2–12. Reprinted by permission.

APPENDIX TEN A

nursing home hearing handicap index (nhhi): staff version

Circle the appropriate number.	Very Often				Almost Never
1. When this person is with other people does he/she need to hear better?	5	4	3	2	1
2. Do members of the staff, family and friends make negative comments about this person's hearing problem?	5	4	3	2	1
3. Does he/she have trouble hearing another person if there is a radio or TV playing in the same room?	5	4	3	2	1
4. When this person is listening to radio or TV does he/she have trouble hearing?	5	4	3	2	1
5. How often do you feel life would be better for this person if he/she could hear better?	5	4	3	2	1
6. How often is he/she embarrassed because of not hearing well?	5	4	3	2	1
7. When alone does he/she need to hear the everyday sounds of life better?	5	4	3	2	1
8. Do people tend to leave him/her out of conversations because of not hearing well?	5	4	3	2	1
9. How often does he/she withdraw from social activities in which he/she ought to participate because of not hearing well?	5	4	3	2	1
10. Does he/she say "what" or "pardon me" when people first speak to him/her?	5	4	3	2	1

Total _____ × 2 = _____

$$-20$$

_____ × 1.25 = _____%

From "Assessment of Hearing Handicap by Nursing Home Residents and Staff" by R. L. Schow and M. A. Nerbonne, 1977, *Journal of Rehabilitative Audiology*, 10, pp. 2–12. Reprinted by permission.

APPENDIX TEN B

hearing handicap inventory for the elderly (hhie)

Instructions:

The purpose of this scale is to identify the problems your hearing loss may be causing you. Check **YES, SOMETIMES,** or **NO** for each question. **Do not skip a question if you avoid a situation because of your hearing problem.** If you use a hearing aid, please answer the way you hear **without** the aid.

	Yes (4)	Some-times (2)	No (0)
S-1. Does a hearing problem cause you to use the phone less often than you would like?			
E-2. Does a hearing problem cause you to feel embarrassed when meeting new people?			
S-3. Does a hearing problem cause you to avoid groups of people?			
E-4. Does a hearing problem make you irritable?			
E-5. Does a hearing problem cause you to feel frustrated when talking to members of your family?			
S-6. Does a hearing problem cause you difficulty when attending a party?			
E-7. Does a hearing problem cause you to feel "stupid" or "dumb"?			
S-8. Do you have difficulty hearing when someone speaks in a whisper?			
E-9. Do you feel handicapped by a hearing problem?			
S-10. Does a hearing problem cause you difficulty when visiting friends, relatives, or neighbors?			
S-11 Does a hearing problem cause you to attend religious services less often than you would like?			
E-12. Does a hearing problem cause you to be nervous?			

From "The Hearing Handicap Inventory for the Elderly: A New Tool" by I. M. Ventry and B. E. Weinstein, 1982, *Ear and Hearing*, 3, pp. 128–134. Reprinted by permission.

	Yes (4)	Some-times (2)	No (0)
S-13. Does a hearing problem cause you to visit friends, relatives, or neighbors less often than you would like?			
E-14. Does a hearing problem cause you to have arguments with family members?			
S-15. Does a hearing problem cause you difficulty when listening to TV or radio?			
S-16. Does a hearing problem cause you to go shopping less often than you would like?			
E-17. Does any problem or difficulty with your hearing upset you at all?			
E-18. Does a hearing problem cause you to want to be by yourself?			
S-19. Does a hearing problem cause you to talk to family members less often than you would like?			
E-20. Do you feel that any difficulty with your hearing limits or hampers your personal or social life?			
S-21. Does a hearing problem cause you difficulty when in a restaurant with relatives or friends?			
E-22. Does a hearing problem cause you to feel depressed?			
E-23. Does a hearing problem cause you to listen to TV or the radio less often than you would like?			
E-24. Does a hearing problem cause you to feel uncomfortable when talking to friends?			
E-25. Does a hearing problem cause you to feel left out when you are with a group of people?			

IMPORTANT — Please go back over the questions to make sure you have not skipped any. REMEMBER, DO NOT SKIP A QUESTION IF YOU AVOID A SITUATION BECAUSE OF YOUR HEARING PROBLEM. Also make sure that you answered the way you hear WITHOUT a hearing aid.

FOR CLINICIAN'S USE ONLY

Total Score: _____   Subtotal E: _____

Subtotal S: _____

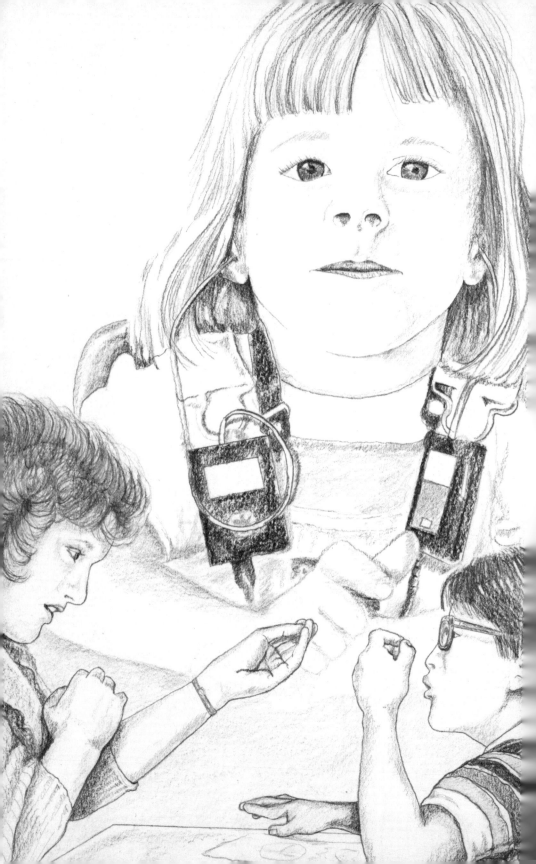

partthree

implementing
aural rehabilitation: case studies
and resource materials

Providing effective aural rehabilitation is challenging and
rewarding for the clinician. Part III of this text presents a
wide variety of unique case studies to further illustrate how
aural rehabilitation can be implemented. Also presented is
a series of helpful resource materials concerning aural
rehabilitation.

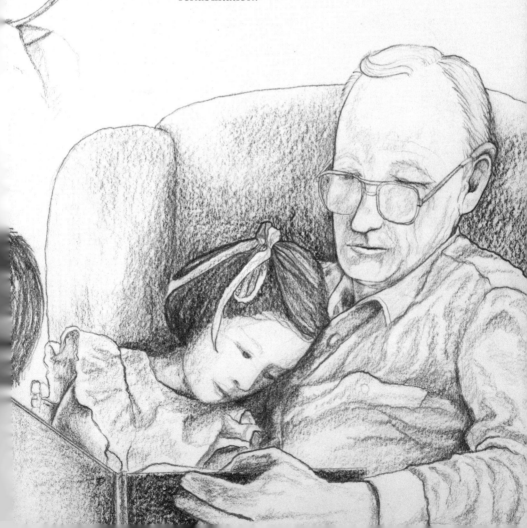

chaptereleven

CASE STUDIES: CHILDREN

MARY PAT MOELLER

contents

introduction

Hearing-impaired children represent a heterogeneous group, requiring individualized intervention procedures. The six case examples that follow illustrate problems often encountered in pediatric management, along with strategies for problem solution. These cases represent a range of ages, degrees of hearing loss, and types of programs. Yet, in each case, communication and language enhancement are the primary objectives. Two concepts pervade each of the examples cited: (a) individualized management requires objective monitoring and determination of the efficacy of intervention strategies; and (b) clinicians must delineate intervention priorities through differential diagnosis and careful determination of a child and family's primary needs (see Chapter 8).

The process of pediatric aural rehabilitation has become increasingly complex in recent years due to several factors. Advances in medical science have resulted in the survival of many "at risk" infants. This factor has contributed to an increase in the number of hearing-impaired children with significant secondary handicaps. Sociological changes related to family systems also influence the complexity of service delivery. It is not uncommon for a clinician's caseload to include traditional nuclear families, single parents, dual-career families, divorcing couples, unwed young mothers, or other family constellations. Both of these factors dictate the need for individualized approaches and innovative service delivery models.

The case studies are organized to address four rehabilitative concerns in the overall coordination of services:

1. Intervening in infancy: parent/child interaction and differential diagnosis.

2. Facilitating/supporting the parents' role.

3. Determining the most appropriate habilitative procedures for individual children.

4. Selecting and prioritizing goals for the school-aged, hard-of-hearing student.

For several of these cases, multidisciplinary service delivery was necessary and advantageous. Multidisciplinary management is recommended, especially for difficult and controversial rehabilitative cases, involving such issues as cochlear implantation or fitting of other sensory communication devices. Allied professionals, such as in the disciplines of psychology and social work, contribute to the clinician's understanding of family needs and other issues of the family system. Such issues are important in considering the child's needs from a holistic perspective.

Although the cases described are based on real persons, names and other biographical facts have been changed to maintain patient confidentiality.

case 1: parent/infant intervention

When managing parent/infant cases, the clinician must be sensitive to variables affecting the child, the parents, and the relationship between parents and child. Aural rehabilitation specialists are encountering an increasing number of hearing-impaired children with secondary impairments. Consequently, the clinician must be keenly observant of the child's behaviors across developmental domains. Early identification of a child's and parents' individualized needs can facilitate effective treatment. The following case illustrates the importance of focusing on the parent-child relationship and on a differential diagnostic approach to therapy.

background information

Johnny was referred to the parent-infant program at 18 months of age, when a suspected sensorineural hearing loss was confirmed. The child was the product of a healthy, uneventful pregnancy and delivery. His mother reported suspecting a hearing loss when Johnny was 4 months old. Her pediatrician assured her that she was an "overly anxious" mother. When Johnny was 8, 10, and 15 months old, he was hospitalized for failure to thrive. He also began experiencing episodes of sleep apnea. These problems reportedly resolved themselves at 16 months. However, Johnny's communication was delayed and his mother continued to express concern for his hearing. At 18 months, Johnny was referred by his pediatrician for audiological evaluation. Following confirmation of the hearing loss, Johnny and his mother were seen for twice-weekly center-based parent/infant visits, conducted in a demonstration home setting.

hearing status

Because it was difficult to test Johnny's hearing behaviorally, he was referred for an auditory brainstem response evaluation. The results suggested a mild-to-moderate, sensorineural hearing loss for at least the high frequencies. Results also indicated abnormally prolonged interwave latencies, suggesting delays in the neural maturation of the auditory brainstem pathways. Subsequent behavioral testing revealed near-normal low-frequency sensitivity with bilateral sensorineural hearing loss in the high frequencies above 2,000 Hz (see Figure 11.1). Johnny remained difficult to evaluate audiologically for several months due to immature auditory behaviors. He persisted in habituating rapidly to test stimuli, failed to maintain a conditioned bond, and evidenced difficulty localizing sound sources. Johnny did not respond normally to sounds as an infant, and at 18 months still could not localize sounds in his environment. Such behaviors are inconsistent with the pure-tone behavioral audiological results. This child presented numerous audiological puzzles, some of which were clarified only through the ongoing rehabilitative program.

hearing aid evaluation/adjustment

Mild gain, high-frequency amplification was loaned on a long-term trial basis. Final decisions regarding amplification were deferred until Johnny's auditory problems were better understood and his auditory responses became consistent. He adjusted readily to amplification. Comparative therapy data with and without amplification revealed enhanced linguistic performance when amplification was utilized. The mother was incon-

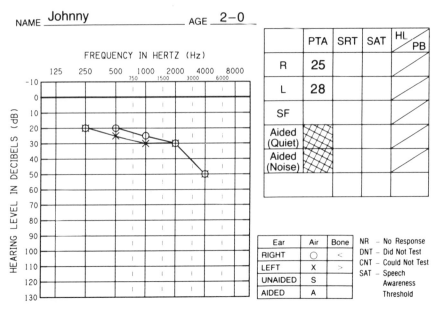

Figure 11.1. Unaided audiological results for Johnny, Case 1.

sistent in insisting that Johnny wear his aid, thereby presenting a counseling challenge for the clinician. The mother was asked to keep a wearing-time log, which increased her awareness of progress toward the goal of full-time hearing aid use. Educational activities for the mother included experiencing a simulated hearing impairment and observing Johnny's response to tasks with and without the hearing aid.

communication rehabilitation

Due to Johnny's young age, the type and severity of his hearing loss as well as several factors related to his mother—overprotective behavior, inconsistent initial followthrough, and denial of personal feelings—his communication rehabilitation consisted at the beginning mostly of parent guidance. In addition, a language and auditory skills stimulation program was established.

Parent Training. Videotapes of the mother interacting with her son in a play situation led to concern for both the quality and quantity of maternal verbal input. For example, if Johnny was building with blocks and they fell, she would remark "boom" or "crash," rather than making a substantive comment like "the blocks fell." At other times, she would produce lengthy, controlling remarks like, "Johnny, tell your teacher that you saw Big Bird at the store last week." Many of her utterances exceeded Johnny's language comprehension level and were not contingent with his semantic intentions. The clinician carefully guided the mother in shaping her linguistic input to be contingent with her child's nonverbal and verbal intentions. She was encouraged to relate to him in a playful, facilitative manner and to foster his active involvement in learning and talking.

Early in the therapy process, the clinician modeled for the mother discourse techniques that facilitate language acquisition. The mother participated directly in activities designed to increase her awareness of her child's communicative intents. Lessons from the *Hanen Early Language Guide Book*, "It Takes Two to Talk" (Manolson, 1985), were successful in helping the mother develop verbal turntaking routines with Johnny. This was an important first step in establishing a nurturing verbal environment. Once turntaking between mother and child was better established, additional stimulation techniques, such as parallel talk, expansions, and recasting (Nelson, 1977), were discussed and finally incorporated naturally into play routines. Videotaped demonstration materials, such as the video "Oh Say What They See: An Introduction to Indirect Language Stimulation Techniques" (Educational Productions, 1983) were also useful. With guidance from the clinician the mother planned and executed lessons; brainstormed how to fit Johnny's goals into novel activities; and explored with the clinician appropriate materials for reinforcing his developmental goals. At first, Johnny's mother experienced difficulty learning to change her linguistic input. She reported being uncomfortable with "baby talking" to children. The clinician helped her view her own language as an intervention tool, with features quite different from "baby talk." Videotape confrontation was used successfully in teaching her to analyze critically and to gradually change her discourse behaviors. Consistent support from the clinician was required to give the mother confidence in her verbal exchanges with Johnny. She also was reinforced for encouraging her son's verbal initiations, independence and exploration. Learning to "let go" was a difficult process. Yet, with increased independence, Johnny began to verbalize with a purpose. Semantically contingent queries and remarks from the mother reinforced these verbalizations (Cross, 1984).

Stimulation of Language and Auditory Skills. In the early phases of therapy, emphasis was placed on developing Johnny's functional auditory skills and comprehension. His mother was asked to implement naturalistic activities at home, and she consistently did so. Once Johnny began using his hearing aid regularly and responding to intervention, his auditory development progressed rapidly. (Figure 11.2 summarizes the therapy data, which documented rapid growth in selected auditory/linguistic

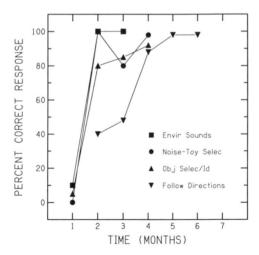

Figure 11.2. Therapy data summarizing auditory skill development for Johnny.

skills.) Gradually, Johnny's auditory skills matured to a level commensurate with his receptive language age and his audiometric status. Longitudinal evaluations revealed language comprehension skills improving to the low-average range of performance.

Figure 11.3 documents this child's rapid lexical learning. When therapy began, Johnny had eight unintelligible words. After 7 months of remediation, he had added over 150 items to his lexicon. Although his words were distributed across the expected semantic classes, two major concerns emerged when the clinician reviewed the therapy data: (a) Johnny's speech intelligibility was extremely limited, and this could not be explained on the basis of audiological results; and (b) in spite of aggressive stimulation and a semantically well-distributed lexicon, two-word combinations did not emerge (see Figure 11.4). Consequently, Johnny was referred for an oral-motor evaluation, which revealed significant delays in oral-motor maturation. Johnny's oral-motor delays influenced his ability to coordinate speech movements to produce word combinations. Identification of these problems dramatically affected the course of therapy, which began to place increased emphasis on speech production. Two-word combinations introduced in therapy were chosen with ease of oral production in mind. That is, facilitative phonological contexts were chosen to support semantic-grammatical development.

Examination of therapy data also led the clinician to alter her treatment approach. Early on, Johnny assumed a passive role in the therapy process. He was cooperative and attentive, but inactive. Charting of his

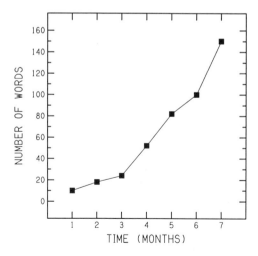

Figure 11.3. Rate of vocabulary learning for Johnny.

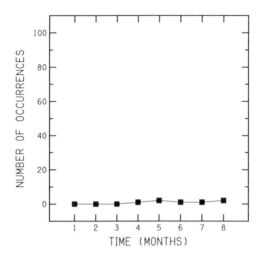

Figure 11.4. Spontaneous two-word combinations produced in therapy by Johnny.

spontaneous verbalizations (see Figure 11.5) revealed fewer than seven spontaneous verbal initiations in a 1-hour session. Recognizing the need for this youngster to take an active role in therapy and in communication, especially given his need to practice production skills, the clinician shifted the focus of sessions. She and the mother deliberately allowed and promoted child-controlled/directed activities. This resulted in a major increase in Johnny's spontaneous verbalizations. The clinician and the mother also manipulated the environment to promote important pragmatic behaviors which were otherwise noticeably absent. Specifically, gestural performatives, request behaviors, spontaneous commenting, and protests were addressed. This child's complex problems were clear only after critical review of therapy performance. Continual goal modification was necessary.

medical and developmental findings

Due to the complex nature of Johnny's problems, he was referred for additional diagnostic evaluations leading to the following findings. An occupational/physical therapy (OT/PT) evaluation revealed gross- and fine-motor delays. Neurological examination revealed hypotonia and hyperreflexia. Eye examination revealed esotropia (lack of coordination of eye movements), requiring surgical correction. At this time, the mother reported that Johnny's sleep apnea episodes had returned. While hospital-

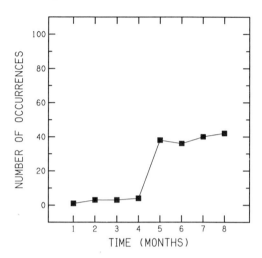

Figure 11.5. Spontaneous verbalizations produced during therapy sessions by Johnny.

ized for observation he experienced 60 episodes of obstructive sleep apnea in a 5-hour period. This problem was corrected by surgical removal of the tonsils and adenoids. A psychological evaluation revealed low borderline nonverbal intellectual abilities.

psychosocial aspects

A parent support group was made available to Johnny's mother to assist her in coping with her son's problems. As a single parent, she felt uncomfortable in this situation, however. Thus, the clinician perceived that the mother became actively involved in therapy directed at her son, but seemed to deny her own needs and feelings. At one point she shared the observation, "I think I haven't allowed myself to react to his problems, and I'm beginning to see that is not the best solution." Only after several months of gradually establishing a relationship of trust with the clinician was the mother comfortable discussing her affective concerns. Later in the therapy process, the mother readily accepted a referral to a counselor.

summary

This child initially presented as a straightforward mild-to-moderately hearing-impaired toddler. Ongoing intervention, however, documented his multiple problems. Once a comprehensive picture was gathered, hearing impairment was found to be one of the least concerning factors. Specifically, it was recommended that the child receive interdisciplinary management, with strong emphasis on speech therapy. Johnny's case illustrates the need to analyze therapy outcome critically and base clinical decisions on objective evidence from the child. His case also underscores the interrelatedness of various developmental areas and the need to be concerned with the total child and his family.

cases 2 and 3: rehabilitation of the profoundly deaf—parental involvement

The importance of involving parents directly in the rehabilitation process has received considerable attention in the professional literature. A primary goal of early interventionists is to facilitate parents' ability to provide a nurturing language environment for the deaf child. Although this notion is widely accepted, it can be difficult to accomplish in some cases. Single-parent families, for example, often experience numerous stresses in addition to the demands of raising a deaf child. The unique pressures of this type of situation may require creative, nontraditional approaches to service delivery. A second group often in need of aggressive intervention is the hearing parent of a profoundly deaf, signing child. Such parents require aggressive and consistent support to become fully competent users of simultaneous communication. Parental sign proficiency is directly related to the child's linguistic acquisition (Crandall, 1978). Yet, studies suggest that the majority of hearing parents fail to achieve more than basic sign proficiency (Bornstein, Saulnier, & Hamilton,1980). Such discouraging findings are not preordained, but require changes in the professional guidance and education of parents (Luetke-Stahlman & Moeller, 1988; Swisher & Thompson, 1985).

Fully meeting the needs of the hearing parents of a deaf child is a formidable task. Two brief case examples have been selected to illustrate attempts to meet this challenge. Each of the examples to follow involves a profoundly deaf child of hearing parents. Both of these students functioned in the high-average to superior range of nonverbal intellectual abilities.

case 2: bob

audiological status

Bob, age 4, was deafened prelingually as a result of meningitis. His better ear PTA was 105 dB HL. Aided thresholds were suspected to be vibrotactile (see Figure 11.6).

communication rehabilitation/psychosocial issues

Bob's mother was a single parent receiving welfare support. Providing the basics, such as food and clothing, for her two sons was her primary concern. She frequently missed therapy sessions, did not attend parent meetings, and rarely communicated with her deaf son. Bob had been enrolled since infancy in a strong auditory/oral program, but had made minimal progress. The mother was experiencing behavioral difficulties with this bright child, with whom she could not communicate effectively. She stated a desire for a total communication program. The aural

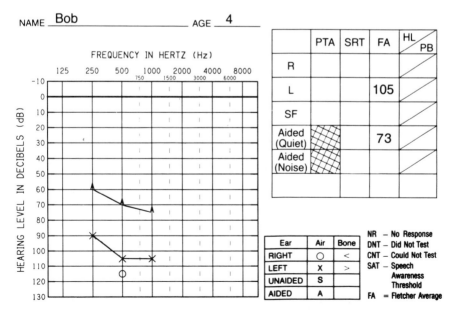

Figure 11.6. Aided and unaided audiological results for Bob, Case 2.

rehabilitation (AR) team met to discuss alternate forms of service delivery for this family. It was decided that the clinician would provide a parent education and signing program in the family home. This approach was initially unsuccessful. The mother had not fully accepted the need for total communication. She inconsistently allowed the clinician into her home for scheduled visits. Even when the clinician did provide lessons and materials, she was feeling increasingly inadequate in working with this family.

Eventually, members of the AR team contacted the mother's social services caseworker to enlist her assistance in case management. The caseworker provided inservice education for the team to help them better understand the social/cultural dynamics surrounding Bob's case. She gave practical guidance, such as strategies for making home visits and effective means for improving communication with the mother. In the past, the caseworker had given the mother ongoing support on financial matters, and had established a good rapport with her. To enhance the clinician's ability to determine the mother's primary concerns, the AR clinician accompanied the caseworker on several home visits. The mother voiced a pressing need to control Bob's behavior; expressed embarrassment about the parent group (all couples, no young single parents); and stated that she wanted her child to talk, not sign.

This case proved to be a learning experience for the AR team. Specifically, the clinicians learned to put their values in perspective; to adopt flexible service-delivery models; and to better identify primary parenting needs and consequent goals. The case continued to be challenging, and the mother's involvement was never ideal.

However, substantive change was accomplished through three primary means:

1. While working directly with the behavior issue, the clinician taught the mother functional sign-communication strategies. Learning this set of signs was reinforcing for her, because she was gaining positive results in shaping her child's behavior. This aspect of the program met one of her expressed concerns.

2. The AR clinician arranged for another single parent to act as a support parent for Bob's mother. They developed a friendly and mutually supportive relationship. In discussing their experiences with their deaf children, Bob's mother came to a better understanding and acceptance of the need to use total communication with her son.

3. Parent education was given in small doses when the mother perceived new needs or questions. The AR clinician kept in continual contact with the caseworker, who facilitated overall case management.

This case illustrates that clinicians must focus on parental needs and concerns rather than their own agenda for directly educating a child. In Bob's case, the clinician was a proficient signer, who could readily elicit cooperation and learning from the child. Unfortunately, these abilities served to undermine the mother's confidence as she faced new and overwhelming challenges. Therefore, the clinician needed to focus on strategies that would support the mother and build her confidence in her ability to stimulate Bob's communicative skills. The social worker's advice was invaluable in helping the clinician view the family's needs from a perspective other than "middle class."

In cases such as Bob's, management may take on new dimensions. The aural rehabilitationist must always be prepared to examine the effectiveness of traditional approaches and call upon allied professionals, as necessary, to facilitate intervention.

case 3: carl

audiological status

Carl, age 4, had a congenital, profound sensorineural hearing loss of unknown etiology. His better ear PTA was 100 dB. Although aided thresholds compensated the hearing loss to a moderate-severe range, Carl had functional use of hearing only at a signal warning level.

communication rehabilitation/psychosocial issues

Carl's parents lived in an average, middle-class, rural home. They received homebound services from their local education agency when Carl was an infant and had taken a beginning sign language class. From the initiation of therapy, these parents were motivated to develop their son's conversational abilities and used total communication with him. They practiced signing to each other and taught Carl's older sibling to sign. When the family enrolled Carl in the aural rehabilitative program at age 2, they were already able to sign basic ideas fluently. Being considered intermediate-level signers, Carl's parents became active participants in an evening intermediate-level sign language class. This program was didactic, focusing on building parental signing vocabulary. As time passed, it became clear that this family would profit more from an individualized sign language program. Consequently, two AR clinicians devised a program that included several individualized strategies (Luetke-Stahlman & Moeller, in press).

AUDIOLOGICAL RECORD

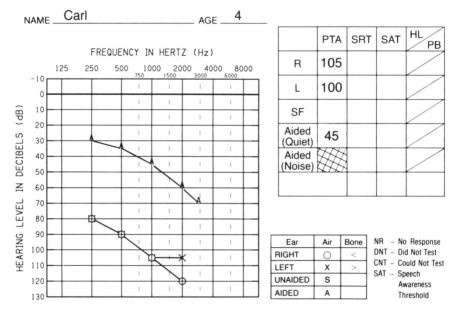

Figure 11.7. Aided and unaided audiological results for Carl, Case 3.

The parents were videotaped while playing with their son. Transcriptions of parental signing input were analyzed for accuracy, semantic content, syntactic complexity, creativity, and match between the signed and the spoken message. Once the parents' sign skills were analyzed, their input was compared to the child's needs. For example, Carl's mean length of utterance (MLU) was 4.7 morphemes; the parents' average signed utterances were 3.5 and 4.0 for the father and mother, respectively. A goal was established to increase the length of their sign input. Individual goals were set for each parent based on complete data analysis. Specifically, Carl's father needed to concentrate on the length of his signed utterances following Carl's lead and creativity, whereas Carl's mother, in spite of a high degree of accuracy, needed to improve the syntactic complexity of her utterances. Lectures and demonstrations concentrated on these specific, individualized goals (e.g., one lesson emphasized methods for increasing coordination in signed utterances). This was followed by practice with the child and opportunities for the parents to critique their videotapes.

Figure 11.8 shows the results of the intervention for Carl's father. Prior to intervention, Carl rarely looked at his father during play routines. This caused the father to rely (25–35% of the time) on attention bids (tapping Carl's shoulder and saying, "Carl, look at me."). These attention bids were intrusive to Carl. Analysis of the dyadic discourse patterns revealed that the father rarely responded to the child's topic, but instead asked questions that shifted the conversational topic. Intervention was directed at helping Carl's father learn to follow the child's lead and make semantically contingent remarks. He was particularly adept at incorporating this goal during creative role play, as seen in Figure 11.8. Once discourse strategies improved, the father's use of attention bids reduced significantly. Carl began to watch his father as he perceived that his dad had something interesting to say. This example illustrates that teaching a parent to sign is only part of the professional's task. Facilitating conversational interactions with the deaf child is a major objective.

All members of Carl's family signed at all times when they conversed. The results have been rewarding in that Carl acquired language milestones at a rate which approximates that of a hearing child. The regularity of his parents' sign input has dramatically influenced this child's acquisition of the English morphological system as evidenced in the following portion of Carl's narrative description of the movie "Pinnochio."

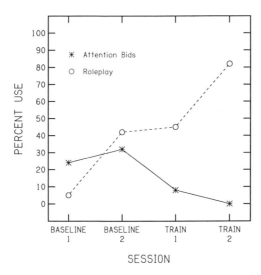

Figure 11.8. Individualized sign language program for Carl's father.

Carl produced this narrative using speech approximations and signing exact English with appropriate signed endings.

> Pinnochio's father Gepetto saw a star. The fairy wanted to come to make his puppet jump and walk. The fairy went to the house and saw Pinnochio sitting on the table.

While requiring strong motivation on the part of the parents, this case represents another instance where parents become involved enthusiastically when their needs are addressed.

cases 4 and 5: programmatic decision making in aural rehabilitation

In Chapter 7, Maestas y Moores and Moores pointed out that a wide range of placement options is often available for hearing-impaired children. In practice, program staff try to make placement decisions based on objective data. Yet, the decision-making process is complex. Guidelines for making decisions regarding educational modality are not readily available or agreed upon. The next two brief cases describe the application of a diagnostic teaching approach to this problem. The importance of monitoring the child's rate of learning and observing his/her characteristic growth patterns over time is discussed.

case 4: jane

background information

Jane was referred to the aural rehabilitation program when she was 2 years, 6 months of age, following recovery from H-flu meningitis. Developmental motor milestones and balance regressed markedly following the meningitic episode.

hearing status

Pediatric behavioral audiological monitoring was initiated following ABR testing, which revealed a severe sensorineural hearing loss in the left ear and a profound sensorineural hearing loss in the right ear. The child responded to speech stimuli (awareness) at 80 dB HL in the left ear, but failed to respond up to 105 dB HL in the right ear.

hearing aid evaluation/adjustment

Jane was fitted with a behind-the-ear hearing aid in the better hearing left ear. Aided thresholds (see Fig. 11.9) revealed excellent functional gain from the aid. Earmold modifications allowed for optimal high-frequency gain. Jane adjusted readily to her aid and wore it all of her waking hours. The right ear was not fitted with amplification due to poor discrimination in that ear. Jane was later fitted with FM amplification to the left ear for use in the classroom. The FM system reduced the effects of noise and reverberation on Jane's discrimination of speech.

In a therapy situation, this child experienced persistent difficulties in accomplishing auditory goals, particularly in less-than-ideal listening situations. Her aided speech discrimination score at age 4 was 52% using closed-set materials (WIPI). It was suspected that her auditory limitations were related to etiology. Realistic appraisal of the development

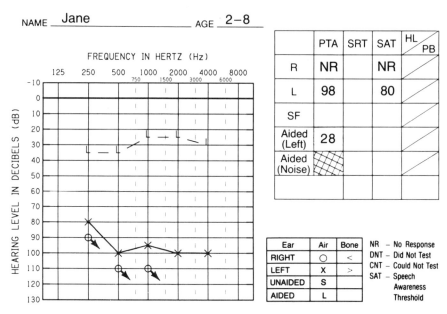

Figure 11.9. Audiometric results for Jane, Case 4.

of Jane's auditory skills was an important factor in modifying her program. Because of Jane's poor auditory function, she had difficulty receiving language input unless it was presented in short, simplistic utterances and delivered in a quiet, nondistracting environment. She also demonstrated auditory-memory weaknesses and distractibility. Shortly after the meningitic insult, Jane stopped communicating.

communication rehabilitation

Initially, Jane was enrolled with her parents in an auditory-oral parent/infant program. Gradually, she began benefiting from her amplification and after several months of training again produced single words and two-word combinations. By age 3, her program was expanded to include a self-contained, preschool class for oral hearing-impaired children. At this time Jane's parents became concerned about their daughter's learning style. In a classroom situation Jane was highly distractible. Although her parents continually reinforced concepts at home, Jane's comprehension of new material was limited. She required a high degree of structuring and constant repetition to acquire basic receptive concepts and her auditory attention in the classroom was markedly reduced in comparison to her peers.

Eventually, the parents began to question the efficacy of a purely oral approach, feeling that Jane was not learning receptive language incidentally, but only through highly structured teaching. They feared that such a slow learning rate would be at the expense of other developmental considerations. The parents requested that the AR team consider using diagnostic teaching with Jane to determine if her oral progress could be augmented through other techniques or modalities. At the request of Jane's school, the first phase of diagnostic teaching involved: (a) increasing the amount of individual tutoring in the auditory-oral program; (b) completing a multidisciplinary evaluation to document strengths and weaknesses, and obtain baseline data for future comparisons; and (c) increasing the emphasis on auditory development to determine if weaknesses in this area could be ameliorated. The changed teaching emphasis was tried intensively for a 14-month period (between 3 years, 6 months and 4 years, 8 months). Table 11.1 illustrates the somewhat discouraging results.

Although Jane made adequate progress in speech and certain expressive language skills, her comprehension problems became increasingly evident over time.

At the request of her parents, Jane was enrolled in a cognitively-oriented, total communication program that included a preschool class,

TABLE 11.1
Longitudinal Results of Language Evaluations for Jane

	Chronological Age			
	Pre-TC		Post-TC	
	3 yrs., 6 mos.	4 yrs., 8 mos.	5 yrs., 3 mos.	6 yrs., 6 mos.
PPVT-R, Rev. Form–M (Dunn & Dunn, 1981)	2 yrs., 2 mos. 1st %ile	2 yrs., 6 mos. 1st %ile	3 yrs., 11 mos. 11th %ile	6 yrs., 1 mo. 34th %ile
Reynell Developmental Language Scale-Receptive (Reynell, 1977)	2 yrs., 4 mos.	2 yrs., 4 mos.	4 yrs., 1 mo.	6 yrs., 0 mos.
Reynell Developmental Language Scale-Expressive (Reynell, 1977)	2 yrs., 4 mos.	3 yrs., 0 mos.	5 yrs., 3 mos.	6 yrs., 4 mos.
Expressive Syntax Developmental Sentence Scoring (Lee, 1974)	2.45	2.75	3.91	6.21

individual tutoring in sign language, and intensive individual speech and auditory therapy. Within the cognitive orientation, the clinicians attempted to take advantage of Jane's nonlinguistic knowledge of relationships in teaching her new linguistic meanings (Moeller, 1988; Moeller, Osberger, & Morford, 1987). Emphasis was placed on problem solving, visualization of conceptual relationships, and developing flexible thinking skills in synchrony with language skills.

Total communication was viewed as an *augmentative* tool with Jane, and signs were used primarily to strengthen her comprehension skills. Throughout intervention, Jane's preferred mode of expressing herself was speech alone. Signs enhanced her receptive language as she developed productive comprehension strategies. Jane began to depend on signs with speech as an input modality. Following 6 months of intervention using simultaneous input, Jane comprehended four or more critical elements in a message and followed complex commands. Her speech

TABLE 11.2
Jane's Language Growth Following Initiation of Total
Communication Program

Age	4 years, 8 mos	5 years, 3 mos	6 years, 6 mos
Receptive Vocabulary	2 years, 6 mos 1st %ile	3 years, 11 mos 11th %ile	6 years, 1 mos 34th %ile
Receptive Concepts	2 years, 4 mos	4 years, 1 mos	6 years, 0 mos
Expressive Language	3 years, 0 mos	5 years, 3 mos	6 years, 4 mos
Syntax (d.s.s.)	2.45	3.91	6.21

remained largely intelligible. Table 11.2 illustrates the change in Jane's language development following initiation of simultaneous communication as a receptive learning tool.

By the time Jane was 6 years old, she was functioning within the average range for her age on most language tasks with the exception of expressive syntactic complexity. At this time, she was enrolled in a self-contained total communication kindergarten class in a public school and was mainstreamed into the regular kindergarten classroom for part of the day. Periodic monitoring of her performance revealed that, although Jane had made exceptional progress in developing her language skills, she lacked confidence in speechreading and was reticent about responding unless information was presented through an interpreter. Investigation of her learning style revealed that optimal retention of new information was secured through simultaneous communication. Her teachers were faced with a dilemma: Jane learned best through simultaneous input, especially when new information was presented. Yet, her ability to interact with her hearing peers was being thwarted by her lack of confidence in receiving auditory/oral input. Although she was capable of attending a mainstreamed classroom from the standpoint of speech/language and academic readiness, self-confidence and social factors needed to be addressed.

Another phase of diagnostic teaching was initiated by Jane's teacher and clinician with increased emphasis on auditory/oral reception of information in conversational and small-group situations. Particular focus was directed toward oral-discourse skills, question-response and asking behaviors, as well as conversational repair strategies. After one year of this type of emphasis, Jane had improved significantly. During a followup evaluation, she was observed to converse easily with the clinician through oral communication alone, asking many questions and making relevant comments throughout the testing session.

By the end of first grade, Jane demonstrated above-average academic skills and improved social competence with both oral and simultaneous communication. Her learning of new academic content in the classroom was best when simultaneous (TC) input was provided. However, her teachers' sensitive management and attention to modality issues allowed Jane to gain the skills to communicate orally in a comfortable and socially appropriate manner. Throughout, programmatic efforts were facilitated through consistent support and carryover from Jane's family.

Through carefully planned, augmentative use of total communication, Jane eventually became a strong oral communicator and demonstrated benefit from the skills learned in her early auditory/oral training. Selection of total communication or oral modality was not an either-or choice with Jane. Rather, teaching modalities were flexibly chosen to address her changing communicative status and needs.

psychosocial aspects

Jane's parents were accepting and supportive. Learning to cope with their daughter's loss of hearing, language, and speech was difficult. The family made numerous sacrifices for their daughter, at times at the expense of other family members and themselves. They found some support in parent organizations, and they also took advantage of private counseling offered by the school. In addition to Jane, the parents had two other children, who were feeling the effects of Jane's deafness on the family as a unit. Ongoing family counseling helped the parents learn strategies for coping with sibling rivalries and feeling more confident about meeting their children's varied needs. Coping with guilt feelings surrounding Jane's illness also was difficult for the family. The opportunity to meet with other parents of postmeningitic children was helpful in this process.

summary

Jane is presently mainstreamed successfully in second grade, and is placed for part of the day in a resource classroom for hearing-impaired children. Her language skills are largely commensurate with chronologic age, and her speech, although distorted, is highly intelligible. She communicates effectively in oral and total communication modalities. She is a bright youngster, with excellent home support and strong academic performance. Careful monitoring of her individual needs will be necessary for such a positive outcome to continue. Jane's case illustrates that flexible use of various teaching modalities and methodologies can be effective. Individualization of programming requires that the clinician continually evaluate the efficacy of a certain approach, being ready to modify it as necessary.

case 5: catherine

The following brief example is included to further illustrate the importance of objective selection of instructional modalities. In this case, the initial use of total communication was found to be unnecessary, based on appraisal of the child's oral progress and revised documentation of her audiological status.

Catherine contracted meningitis at 15 months of age. Initial ABR results revealed a profound, bilateral high-frequency hearing loss. Based on the ABR test results, the hospital staff initiated a total communication program with the family before the child was dismissed from the hospital. The parents were advised that use of sign language was essential, given the severity of Catherine's hearing loss. Future referral for a cochlear implant evaluation was discussed with the parents.

communication rehabilitation: instructional modality

Catherine's well-informed parents followed the professional's initial advice, but also sought second opinions regarding their daughter's needs. They expressed frustration at the evident bias in much of the advice they received. They chose to enroll their daughter in a program that stressed the importance of objective selection of instructional modality, based on the needs and abilities of the child.

At 18 months of age, Catherine was enrolled in a diagnostically oriented auditory/oral program. She was seen for behavioral audiological testing, which revealed absence of auditory thresholds in the right ear at the limits of the equipment. However, results for the left ear indicated a sloping mild-to-profound sensorineural hearing loss. Catherine responded well to amplification fitted to the left ear. She was able to utilize her residual hearing for acquiring linguistic information. By 2 years of age, Catherine produced an MLU of 2.2 morphemes and comprehended utterances at an age-appropriate level. Although phonological problems persisted throughout her preschool years, Catherine's speech was understandable by age 4. Longitudinal monitoring of her progress revealed age-appropriate language abilities by age 4.

Catherine's success in an auditory/oral program related to the excellent support provided by her parents, her superior intellectual abilities, and her ability to make use of her low-frequency residual hearing. She also had the advantage of a strong auditory/oral educational program in her preschool years. Catherine's case illustrates the importance of objective management and the need for conservative reaction to initial ABR results.

case 6: the hard-of-hearing, school-aged child—kevin

The next case demonstrates the importance of careful selection of priorities for aural rehabilitation therapy. A hard-of-hearing, school-aged child often communicates well on a superficial level and the classroom teacher may report being able to understand and converse with the child. Unfortunately, such a response may result in an underestimation of the impact of the hearing loss on the student's classroom/academic performance. The following case describes how a multidisciplinary team assisted the child's school in redirecting therapy efforts to take into consideration the student's language, cognitive, and academic needs.

background information

Kevin was referred for an independent, AR team evaluation when he was 8 years, 4 months of age. At the time of referral, he was enrolled in a public school first-grade class in a small, rural town. Prior to enrollment in this class, Kevin had attended a country school with a total enrollment of six children. These experiences had resulted in limited social interactions and lack of appropriate peer modeling.

Kevin's moderate-to-severe hearing loss had been identified when he was 18 months of age. He had worn hearing aids inconsistently since that time. The family reported a positive history of sensorineural hearing loss. When Kevin was 5 years of age, he was referred to a school psychologist for an intellectual evaluation. Administration of the *Stanford Binet* (an instrument which is *inappropriate* for evaluating a hearing/language-impaired child due to its heavy reliance on language items)

(Sullivan & Vernon, 1979) resulted in an IQ score of 61. The psychologist reported that "Kevin is presently functioning in the range of mild mental deficiency . . . primarily as a result of his hearing handicap." This misguided and incorrect statement resulted in Kevin's placement in a program for multiply handicapped children. The teaching staff at Kevin's school questioned the psychological results in view of Kevin's rapid adaptation to the new environment and his responsiveness to learning tasks. They referred Kevin for a multidisciplinary evaluation to obtain an accurate evaluation of his learning potential and an opinion regarding the appropriateness of his amplification.

At the town school, Kevin was followed routinely by a speech-language pathologist, who expressed no specific concerns for his language performance. She felt that his skills were commensurate with those of other first graders with whom he was competing. Her IEP goals included emphasis on speechreading and articulation of /l/ and /r/.

hearing status

Audiological evaluation confirmed the presence of a moderate, mixed hearing loss in the left ear and a moderate to severe, mixed hearing loss in the right ear (see Figure 11.10). Discrimination scores, based on the *Word Intelligibility by Picture Identification* (WIPI), were 96% and 100% for the right and left ear, respectively. Abnormal tympanometry resulted in medical referral and followup for otitis media. Although Kevin had a healthy childhood, he did have a history of chronic middle-ear pathology.

hearing aid evaluation/adjustment

At the time of evaluation, Kevin was wearing postauricular hearing aids, which were more than 5 years old. His school wanted to use a direct audio-input FM unit with him, but his aids were incompatible with school equipment. Feedback from one of his aids occurred at a low volume setting due to a crack in the hearing aid casing. His second aid, which had just been returned from expensive repairs, was still only operating intermittently. During the AR/communication evaluation, Kevin exhibited numerous instances of tolerance problems with his aids, even in an acoustically ideal environment. Kevin also had not learned to put his hearing aids in or to care for them properly.

Once Kevin's middle-ear problems were resolved and his hearing improved, a hearing aid evaluation took place. Hearing aids were selected to be compatible with Kevin's needs, controlled in maximum

AUDIOLOGICAL RECORD

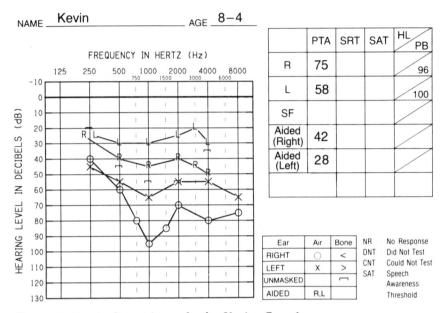

NAME __Kevin__ AGE __8-4__

	PTA	SRT	SAT	HL / PB
R	75			96
L	58			100
SF				
Aided (Right)	42			
Aided (Left)	28			

Ear	Air	Bone
RIGHT	◯	<
LEFT	X	>
UNMASKED		⌐
AIDED	R,L	

NR No Response
DNT Did Not Test
CNT Could Not Test
SAT Speech
    Awareness
    Threshold

Figure 11.10. Audiometric results for Kevin, Case 6.

power output to eliminate tolerance problems, and compatible with direct audio-input FM amplification. The opportunity to use an FM unit was an important rehabilitative goal in Kevin's case because of the poor acoustics in his classroom due to high ceilings, wood floors, and 26 normally active children.

communication rehabilitation

Figure 11.11 illustrates a profiling procedure used by the multidisciplinary team to summarize testing results. The students' standard scores on various tests are plotted along the normal distribution (bell) curve. Kevin's performance is compared to same-aged and same-grade peers. As illustrated, the average range falls between the 16th and 84th percentile (Moeller, McConkey, & Osberger, 1983).

Although several of his formal tests were low-average compared to those of grademates, some areas of dramatic weakness emerged. In brief, Kevin demonstrated:

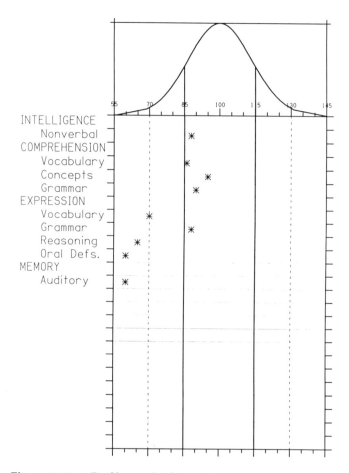

Figure 11.11. Profile results for Kevin.

1. Significant weaknesses in auditory memory.

2. Difficulty applying known concepts to solve verbal problems.

3. Considerable difficulty in using language for abstract thinking purposes (e.g., predicting, planning, reasoning).

4. Qualitative deficits in word knowledge; for example, he had no concept of antonyms/synonyms, could not solve simple verbal analogies, and could not define familiar words. When asked to define *cow*, he responded *calf*. When asked to define what a *finger* was, he stated, "uh . . . wrench" (while pointing to his wrist) and "um . . . um this

thing" (pointing to, but unable to recall the word "elbow"). Further probing of expressive vocabulary revealed significant word recall problems. Kevin demonstrated frequent misnamings (e.g., "an elephant has a '*trumpet*'") and long pauses as he attempted to recall familiar terms.

5. Oral formulation problems were prevalent. The following transcription of conversation with Kevin depicts his problems in formulating personal narratives.

Kevin: "A long time ago, mama cat got in the house and went in my bedroom—slept there for nightime—had babies in my bedroom."

Clinician: "Oh! How many baby kittens did she have?"

Kevin: "Four, and one died."

Clinician: "That's too bad. Did you keep all the kittens?"

Kevin: "Yeah . . . one died. We had—first we had four little kittens in the wintertime and one died, she had four of them and then one died, and so three of 'em. Then one summertime come then um um our cat died. Um named . . . um Molly . . . no Lukey—the one that died. Now that little cat call mommy cat and I named him baby Coal."

Kevin's attempt to describe his cats is incoherent due to retrieval errors and lack of organization. In particular, Kevin had difficulty manipulating temporal relations in his storytelling. Because Kevin could converse on a simplistic level with highly intelligible speech, many of his more serious problems had been overlooked.

Given Kevin's patterns of strengths and weaknesses, it was recommended that the school rethink the planned priorities for resource and speech therapy. This youngster's learning difficulties (in memory and retrieval) and problems *thinking* with language had stronger implications for academic development than articulation or speechreading. Therefore, it was recommended that the primary therapy targets include: (a) thinking skills such as verbal classifying, comparison/contrast, semantic mapping, verbal reasoning and verbal problem solving; (b) a recognition-to-recall approach to learning to accommodate for the retrieval problems; (c) emphasis on concept application in verbal problems; and (d) assisting Kevin in formulation of coherent utterances and narratives (Simon, 1981).

psychosocial aspects

Kevin's parents were aware that their son's lack of appropriate peer models had contributed to social immaturity. However, they continued to find themselves doing too much for their youngest son. As a result, the psychologist assisted the family in recognizing the need to raise expectations for their son in self-help and social areas. After a few short lessons with mother and son, the AR specialist taught Kevin to manipulate independently his hearing aid. Kevin was proud of his accomplishment which, in turn, reinforced his mother for promoting independence. The school district also was encouraged to increase expectations for Kevin in self-help and social areas.

summary

Kevin's situation illustrates the need for comprehensive evaluation to support goal design or selection. The case also demonstrates the need to consider what a classroom situation requires of a student when determining priorities for therapy (Moeller, in press). Kevin was getting by in the first semester of first grade; however, many of the demands at this academic level are straightforward and concrete. By third grade, the reading process will require that Kevin recall, infer, generalize, and predict. Kevin's problems in thinking with language and recalling information will become more apparent as tasks become abstract. The AR clinician must have foresight in the therapy process; thus, Kevin will likely need to be better prepared in language/thinking skills to meet the academic challenges he will soon face. Standardized test scores are inadequate to describe a child's priority needs. The AR clinician must investigate qualititative aspects of the child's communication in detail. The resulting concerns should be prioritized in light of the demands academic tasks place on language and thinking skills (Moeller, in press).

references and recommended readings

Bornstein, H., Saulnier, K., & Hamilton, L. (1980). Signed English: A first evaluation. *American Annals of the Deaf, 4,* 467–481.

Brookhouser, P.E., & Moeller, M.P. (1986). Choosing the appropriate habilitative track for the newly identified hearing-impaired child. *Annals of Otology, Rhinology, Laryngology, 95,* 51–59.

Crandall, K.E. (1978). Inflectional morphemes in the manual English of young hearing-impaired children and their mothers. *Journal of Speech and Hearing Research, 21*(2), 72–86.

Cross, T. (1984). Habilitating the language impaired child: Ideas from the studies of parent-child interactions. *Topics in Language Disorders,* 1–13.

Dunn, L., & Dunn, L. (1981). *Peabody Picture Vocabulary Test—Revised Form M.* Circle Pines, MN: American Guidance Service.

Educational Productions. (1983). *"Oh say what they see:" An introduction to indirect language stimulation techniques.* (Videotape). Portland, OR: 4925 S.W. Humphrey Park Crest.

Handley, E. (1986). *Project Bridge: Decision-making for early services: A team approach.* Chicago: University of Illinois, Center for Educational Development.

Lee, L. (1974). *Developmental sentence analysis.* Evanston, IL: Northwestern University Press.

Luetke-Stahlman, S., & Moeller, M.P. (in press). Enhancing parents' use of signing exact English: Progress and retention. *American Annals of the Deaf.*

Manolson, A. (1985). *It takes two to talk.* Toronto, Ontario: Hanen Early Language Resource Centre, 252 Bloor Street, W., Room 4-126.

Moeller, M.P. (1988). Management of preschool hearing-impaired children: A cognitive linguistic approach. In F. Bess (Ed.), *Hearing impairment in children.* Parkton, MD: York Press, Inc.

Moeller, M.P. (in press). Language evaluation strategies for hearing-impaired students. In R. Kretschmer & L. Kretschmer (Eds.), Evaluation of the language skills of hearing-impaired children. *Monograph of the Journal of the Academy of Rehabilitative Audiology.*

Moeller, M.P., McConkey, A.J., & Osberger, M.J. (1983). Evaluation of the communicative skills of hearing-impaired children. *Audiology, 8,* 113–127.

Moeller, M.P., Osberger, M.J., & Morford, J. (1987). Speech-language assessment and intervention with preschool hearing impaired children. In J. Alpiner & P. McCarthy (Eds.), *Rehabilitative audiology: Children and adults* (pp. 163–188). Baltimore, MD: Williams and Wilkins.

Nelson, K. (1977). Facilitating children's syntax acquisition. *Developmental Psychology, 13,* 101–107.

Reynell, J. (1977). *Reynell developmental language scale.* Los Angeles: Western Psychological Services.

Simon, C. (1981). *Communicative competence—A functional pragmatic approach to language therapy.* Tucson, AZ: Communication Skill Builders.

Sullivan, P., & Vernon, M. (1979). Psychological assessment of hearing impaired children. *School Psychology Press, 8,* 271–290.

Swisher, V., & Thompson, M. (1985). Mothers' learning of simultaneous communication: The dimensions of the task. *American Annals of the Deaf.*

chaptertwelve

CASE STUDIES: ADULTS/ELDERLY ADULTS

MICHAEL A. NERBONNE, THAYNE C. SMEDLEY,
J. CURTIS TANNAHILL, RONALD L. SCHOW,
AND CAROLE FLEVARIS-PHILLIPS

contents

introduction

The seven adult/elderly aural rehabilitation cases described in this chapter involve a wide range of hearing-impaired clients both in terms of age and communication handicap. While special adjustments must be considered with certain elderly patients such as those found in nursing homes (see Cases 4 and 6), in general, both adult and elderly persons will most often demonstrate the same kinds of communication problems and, therefore, be candidates for similar rehabilitation strategies. Thus, we have mixed these younger and older clients and presented them together in the same chapter. Although references are made to group therapy (as detailed in Chapter 13 and in Cases 1 and 7), the major emphasis is on individual therapy and the specific, unique problems with which these individuals are wrestling. Some of these problems relate as much to psychosocial influences, such as vanity and motivation, as to auditory effects. Such influences need to be acknowledged in AR approaches.

Although the general goal for each case was to reduce or eliminate the communication handicap, the specific aural rehabilitation strategies varied for each client depending on individual needs, ranging from cases where efforts were ultimately rejected to a case seen five days a week for two one-hour sessions per day. Some individuals were fit with hearing aids which required extensive adjustment while others rejected amplification, wishing to have only speechreading therapy. The chapter concludes with an account of a cochlear implant patient and the extensive multidisciplinary rehabilitation which followed the surgery.

In the course of performing aural rehabilitation the audiologist may encounter the wide range of cases described here. Hopefully, these cases will give some insights into the challenges and possibilities of this work. In general, the model followed here is the one detailed in the introductory chapter of this text. The model involves both an evaluation phase and a remediation phase as part of the total aural rehabilitation process.

A variety of pre- and postaural rehabilitation tests were used in an attempt to objectify the status of the client during the evaluation and the remediation phases of therapy. Self-assessment tools are receiving increased emphasis in AR and several different communication assessment instruments have been used here, including both screening and diagnostic tools. Also, real-ear (probe-tube microphone) measures are used in several cases, demonstrating the utility of this new tool in the rehabilitation process. No single test battery is recommended; nor is it implied that one is the best for all purposes. Instead, clinicians must select the tests that are appropriate for each individual client. Tests should be selected that will be useful for determining the exact needs of the client, assisting in specific therapy strategies, and for measuring the results of remediation. In addition to the tests and procedures used in this chapter, the reader may refer to Chapters 9, 10, and 13 for other test and resource materials which may be useful in the evaluation and remediation phases of AR.

Even though all cases included here are based on real persons, minor adjustments have been made in the material presented in order to clarify certain details and to maintain the anonymity of our clients.

case 1: progressive hearing loss

case history

Dr. M. was a 69-year-old man who had retired four years earlier after a 40-year career as a college professor. He reported experiencing frequent difficulties in hearing, particularly at his church, at social functions, and at plays that he and his spouse attended at the university's theater. Dr. M. noted being aware of hearing difficulties for some time, including the last couple of years of his teaching career. The onset of his impairment reportedly was gradual and seemed to affect both ears equally.

aural rehabilitation evaluation

Figure 12.1 contains the audiometric results obtained with Dr. M. In general, he was found to possess a mild-to-moderate sensorineural hearing loss bilaterally. The results of speech audiometry were consistent with the pure-tone findings and indicated that Dr. M. was experiencing significant difficulty in speech perception, especially if speech stimuli were presented at a typical conversation level (50 dB HL).

The *Self-Assessment of Communication* (SAC) and *Significant Other Assessment of Communication* (SOAC) (Schow & Nerbonne, 1982) screening inventories were administered to Dr. M. and his spouse to gather further information concerning the degree of perceived hearing handicap resulting from Dr. M.'s hearing loss. Using both of these measures provides valuable information about how hearing-impaired persons view their hearing problems, as well as potentially valuable insights from the person who is communicating with the individual on a regular basis. Scores of 50 and 60% on SAC and SOAC tests presented a consistent pattern which, when evaluated according to recent research (see Table 12.1), provided further evidence that Dr. M. was experiencing consider-

AUDIOLOGICAL RECORD

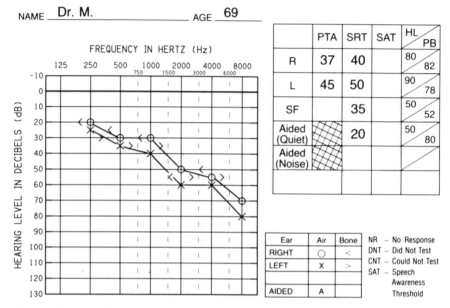

Figure 12.1. Audiometric results for Dr. M., Case 1.

able hearing difficulties (Schow, Brockett, Sturmak, & Longhurst, in press; Sturmark, 1987).

On the basis of these test results and the patient's comments, a hearing aid evaluation was recommended and scheduled.

remediation

Hearing Aid Evaluation/Adjustment. Prior to any testing associated with hearing aids, Dr. M. was advised about the option of utilizing behind-the-ear or in-the-ear style hearing aids. Like most individuals facing this choice, Dr. M. expressed a clear preference for the in-the-ear style. Dr. M. was also advised that, because of the severity of his hearing loss and other factors such as improved localization abilities, a binaural fit would be advisable.

The hearing aid evaluation consisted of a series of probe-tube microphone real-ear measures with each ear, as well as soundfield speech

TABLE 12.1
Categories and Associated Percentage Scores for Use in Classifying Hearing Handicap Performance when Using the SAC and SOAC

Category	Percentage Scores
No handicap	0-20
Slight hearing handicap	21-40
Mild-moderate hearing handicap	41-70
Severe hearing handicap	71-100

From "Hearing Handicap Scores and Categories for Subjects with Normal and Impaired Hearing Sensitivity" by R. Schow and C. Tannahill, 1977, *Journal of the American Audiological Society, 3*, pp. 134–139. Also from *Communication Handicap Score Interpretation for Various Populations and Degrees of Hearing Impairment* by M. J. Sturmak, 1987, unpublished master's thesis, Idaho State University.

audiometry. Data from the audiogram and real-ear measures were applied to an existing prescription approach (Libby, 1986) to determine the desired gain, frequency response, and SSPL-90 values for the hearing aids to be fit to the right and left ears. This resulted in two ITE hearing aids being recommended with moderate gain and high-frequency emphasis. Venting of each unit was also deemed appropriate. Earmold impressions were taken and an appointment was scheduled for Dr. M. to be fit with his new aids once they were received from the manufacturer.

Dr. M. was fit with his hearing aids at the next session and real-ear measures were taken to confirm the appropriateness of the insertion gain and SSPL-90 values for each unit. Soundfield speech audiometry was also used to further evaluate the degree of improvement provided by the binaural system. As seen in Figure 12.1, Dr. M.'s speech reception thresholds and speech recognition scores improved significantly with the in-the-ear hearing aids. His comments concerning the aids were favorable and no further adjustments were made with either hearing aid. Following a thorough orientation to the operation and care of his new aids, Dr. M. was advised to return for subsequent followup appointments.

Dr. M.'s experiences with his new hearing aids were, for the most part, positive. While still noting some problems hearing in group situations and at the theater, he definitely felt that the hearing aids were assisting him. Further discussion with Dr. M. regarding his hearing difficulties at the theater revealed that he had not yet tried the facility's infrared listening system. Encouraging him to do so, the audiologist explained the manner in which the system functions, as well as how Dr. M. could use the infrared receiver either with his hearing aids or as a stand-alone unit. Subsequent contact with Dr. M. revealed that he found the assistive listening device to be remarkably helpful.

While Dr. M. had adjusted well to his hearing aids and received substantial improvement as a result of their use, he did note some persistent communication difficulties. Because of this and his motivation for improvement, Dr. M. agreed to enroll in a short-term group aural rehabilitation program for adults.

Commmunication Training. Dr. M. was one of eight hearing-impaired adults who participated in the weekly group sessions. Although the activities and areas of emphasis varied somewhat as a result of the interests and needs of each group of participants, the main components of the program generally followed those outlined in Chapter 13 by Giolas. The individuals participating with Dr. M. were new hearing aid users with mild-to-moderate hearing losses. Consequently, emphasis was placed on the effective use of hearing aids, care and maintenance of the systems, and the way hearing aids can be supplemented by one or more types of assistive listening devices. Attention was also given to developing more effective listening skills and capitalizing on the visual information available in most communication situations. Interaction between the group participants was encouraged, and valuable information on a variety of topics was shared at each session.

Following the final session, Dr. M. stated that the sessions had been helpful to him. In addition to the practical information provided, such as where to buy batteries for his hearing aids and the use of hearing aids with the telephone, Dr. M. felt that a number of the communication strategies covered had been of benefit to him. The net result was that he felt much more confident when communicating with others.

discussion

It was clear from the start that Dr. M. had accepted his hearing problem and was motivated to seek out whatever assistance was available to him. His positive and cooperative behaviors, which would be categorized by Goldstein and Stephens (1981) as an example of a Type I attitude (see Chapter 9), facilitated the aural rehabilitation process and impacted positively on Dr. M.'s overall communication abilities. Motivation should be recognized as a key ingredient in successful aural rehabilitation with any hearing-impaired individual.

case 2: profound deafness with questionable motivation

case history

Mr. D. was a 55-year-old construction worker who was referred for audiological assessment and aural rehabilitation by a private vocational rehabilitation (VR) agency. The agency had been hired by an insurance company which was paying disability benefits to Mr. D. following a work-related back injury that prevented him from continuing doing construction-type work. Mr. D. had experienced a gradually progressive loss of hearing over a 30-year period beginning with exposure to loud noise during the Korean War. Some years following discharge from the service, he had been issued a body-type hearing aid by the Veterans Administration but had discontinued using the instrument approximately 12 years prior to referral because he said it no longer provided any benefit.

According to the VR officer, Mr. D. had no marketable work skills outside of construction, and his severe hearing impairment and limited communication abilities made retraining difficult. The VR agency had referred Mr. D. for AR therapy and assessment of amplification potential with the hope that Mr. D. could learn improved communication skills, which, in turn, would aid in his retraining and return to employment. Mr. D. indicated that he seriously doubted he would ever return to work. Further, he expressed some concern that, even if he were eventually rehired, he doubted that he could earn more money than he was drawing from medical disability payments. Thus, the client's attitude and motivation for help were viewed as potential problems.

diagnostic information

Audiometric tests revealed a profound loss of hearing bilaterally (Figure 12.2). Pure-tone air-conduction thresholds were established at 80 dB HL at 250 Hz and at 105 dB HL at 500 and 1,000 Hz. However, these were reported more as "noises" than tones. There was no measurable response to pure tones above 1,000 Hz. Vibrotactile responses were obtained to bone-conducted pure tones at 50 dB at 250 Hz and 70 dB at 500 Hz. Audiometric speech detection thresholds were obtained at 95 dB HL. Word-recognition testing was attempted for both bisyllables and monosyllables but without success.

AUDIOLOGICAL RECORD

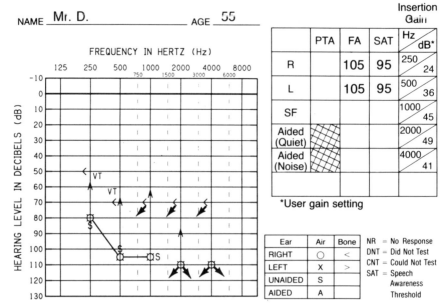

NAME ___Mr. D.___ AGE ___55___

	PTA	FA	SAT	Hz dB*
R		105	95	250 / 24
L		105	95	500 / 36
SF				1000 / 45
Aided (Quiet)				2000 / 49
Aided (Noise)				4000 / 41

*User gain setting

Ear	Air	Bone
RIGHT	O	<
LEFT	X	>
UNAIDED	S	
AIDED	A	

NR = No Response
DNT = Did Not Test
CNT = Could Not Test
SAT = Speech
 Awareness
 Threshold

Figure 12.2. Audiometric results for Mr. D., Case 2.

aural rehabilitation

Evaluation of Needs. Mr. D. presented an interesting array of aural/communicative difficulties. Initially, he insisted that all communication directed to him be done in written form. He carried a pencil and pad of paper to facilitate this process. When attempts were made to communicate orally with Mr. D., he would simply shove the paper and pencil toward the speaker and lower his gaze. He would say, "I don't read lips" and refuse any encouragement to do so. In addition, it was difficult to establish and maintain eye contact. Mr. D.'s speech was appropriate, essentially distortion free but abnormally loud. When invited to comment about what he hoped to accomplish during therapy, he said he was not sure. With some encouragement, Mr. D. finally indicated that he would like to work on improved use of residual hearing, including a trial with newer hearing aids, and to learn sign language. With further discussion and encouragement, he also agreed to work on improving his speechreading skills and learning new strategies for overcoming communication barriers.

Preliminary assessment of speechreading abilities was made with the *Craig Lipreading Inventory* (1964) for word recognition and the *Utley Lipreading Sentence Test* (1946) for sentence recognition. Initial scores of 76 and 61% were obtained, respectively, indicating fair speechreading ability. The latter test was repeated under aided (earphone) conditions whereby sentence recognition improved from 61% to 82%.

The value of including sign language training in the overall AR plan was viewed with skepticism by the clinicians, but training in manual communication was incorporated to comply with Mr. D.'s expressed interests. In reality, Mr. D. would have few associates with whom he could communicate using sign language.

A final interest aroused in Mr. D. related to training in the use of assistive devices. We thought he might benefit from a "Talk Tone" or TTY telephone device which might enable him to better communicate with his married children who lived out of the area.

According to the Goldstein-Stephens model (1981), Mr. D. was judged to have a Type III attitude (see Chapter 9) with respect to therapy goals; that is, his acceptance of treatment was questionable and his expectations were likewise suspect.

AR Goals. The specific goals outlined for Mr. D. were:

1. To teach expression and recognition of at least 100 manual signs (words) during the course of therapy. Emphasis was to be on common, everyday words.

2. To improve unaided speechreading skills to target performance levels of 85-90% for both word and sentence recognition, as measured by the Craig and Utley tests.

3. To identify and practice five communicative strategies which would be useful in countering poor or ineffective communication habits observed during therapy.

4. To improve the client's use of amplification and develop skills in the use of several assistive devices, including the Talk Tone telephone device, the television Telecaption device, and doorbell and telephone flashers/indicators. An updated pair of hearing aids were to be tried, and therapists were encouraged to provide counseling and emotional support with the use of amplification during therapy. (In this case the local VA Hospital was considered a good source for the hearing aids at little or no direct cost to the client.) A subgoal related to the use of amplification was to train Mr. D. to develop a softer voice output.

5. To improve Mr. D.'s visual attentiveness during conversation by working toward a target percentage of 90% eye gaze during 15-minute "test" segments during regular therapy sessions.

remediation procedures

At the encouragement of the referring office, a fairly condensed program was outlined, consisting of two 1-hour sessions per day (ten 1-hour sessions per week), over a 14-week period. Four graduate students in audiology were assigned to work alternately with Mr. D. Efforts were coordinated by working from a single AR outline, in this case one adapted from Kaplan, Bally, and Garretson (1985), and by keeping a careful log of activities, daily therapy objectives and accomplishments, which was to be reviewed by the respective therapists prior to each session.

Therapy activities were directed toward at least three, typically four or five, therapy goals during each session. Manual sign training, speechreading drills, and encouragement in and measurement of appropriate eye gaze were also made a part of every session. During the first session new earmolds and hearing aids were ordered from the VA in order that the benefits of amplification could be assessed. Talk Tone and Telecaption devices as well as telephone and doorbell alerting systems were introduced during the course of therapy.

Communicative strategies were drilled using mock communicative set-ups during formal therapy, with daily "homework" assignments to practice the skills learned in more realistic settings, such as the grocery store, restaurant, or service garage. Emphasis was placed on such techniques as communicative "repair" (giving appropriate feedback for missed words or ideas), group "positioning" (sitting in the most advantageous seat, etc.), assertiveness, anticipating dialogue, and reduced reliance on pencil-and-paper communication. Occasionally, family members were brought in to encourage generalization of training drills to the nonclinic environment. In addition, some of Mr. D.'s homework assignments were to be carried out during visits to nearby work centers of the type suitable for Mr. D., such as a barbershop. The intent here was to couple communication-therapy activities with actual work situations, since reemployment was the ultimate objective of therapy.

results

The results obtained with Mr. D. over the 14-week period were mixed. On the positive side, Mr. D. became very interested in the therapy regimen and stayed with the program during the entire 14 weeks. This was an accomplishment in itself in light of the client's questionable motivation noted at the outset. Eye contact was markedly improved over the sessions. Eye-gaze measures showed a steady improvement, reaching 86% during the final sessions, very close to the 90% target goal. The use of binaural hearing aids, applied midway through the therapy program, seemed to increase Mr. D.'s awareness of and interest in the speaker's voice, as well as in environmental sounds generally. (See Figure 12.2 for real-ear functional and insertion gain measures.) Final speechreading test scores were 79% for words and 82% for sentences, improvements of 3% and 21%, respectively, over initial test scores.

Mr. D. was impressed with the TV telecaption device, but was uncertain if he would ever purchase one. Likewise, he showed little interest in the Talk Tone telephone device although it was demonstrated two or three times. He seemed pleased to learn about vibro-alarms and other alerting devices, but did not express strong interest in purchasing them.

Mr. D.'s improvement in the use of communicative strategies was rather dismal. He would cooperate with classroom drills, but showed considerable reluctance to "practice" them on the outside. Also, attempts to achieve even a modest level of proficiency with manual signing were abandoned, once the novelty wore off.

discussion

The influence of client motivation is evident in this case. The primary objective in referral for AR services was to improve the client's employability. It seems doubtful that Mr. D. adopted this objective personally. Although he cooperated generally with structured activities during therapy, and some improvement in the classroom setting was observed, carryover to the outside world was lacking. Moreover, as the sessions progressed, it became increasingly evident that work-related encouragements ("you'll need to know how to do this on the job") had little positive effect on client effort. Client attitude, as emphasized in Chapter 1, is one of the critical variables in rehabilitative accomplishment. Mr. D.'s level of motivation represented a variant of the Goldstein-Stephens Type III attitude: He possessed a "shred of cooperative intent" (Goldstein & Stephens, 1981), but ultimately he was largely out of harmony with the intended objectives.

This case seems to illustrate certain problems inherent in the unemployed client who is referred for AR training, particularly when therapy is being paid for by a third party, and the intended therapy gains will force the client back to work with the prospect of receiving no better "wages" than those earned from unemployment. Such cases may hold little promise for success.

case 3: mild hearing loss: a case of vanity

case history

Mr. C. was a 58-year-old personnel manager who had experienced a gradually progressive loss of hearing over a 20-year period. At the time of referral, the hearing loss was partially compensated for with the use of binaural behind-the-ear (BTE) type hearing aids which the client had worn intermittently for the previous six years. Hearing aid history included a trial period with in-the-ear (ITE) style hearing aids eight years earlier. The ITE hearing aids were not purchased because they "blocked up" Mr. C.'s ears and were unsatisfactory. After a two-year lapse, hearing aids were again attempted with BTE fittings and open canal-type molds and were found to be more acceptable and subsequently purchased. Referral to the clinic stemmed from Mr. C.'s concerns that his present hearing aids were no longer providing sufficient benefit. Also, Mr. C. expressed a strong interest in trying the new "smaller" hearing aids which he had seen advertised. In addition, Mrs. C. strongly encouraged her husband to "get something that doesn't show as much."

diagnostic information

Audiometric and real-ear hearing aid data for Mr. C. are shown in Figure 12.3. Unaided pure-tone thresholds reveal a moderately sloping mild-to-severe sensorineural hearing loss with good speech-recognition ability at comfortable listening levels. *Self-Assessment of Communication* (SAC) and *Significant Other Assessment of Communication* (SOAC) (Schow & Nerbonne, 1982) scores were measured at 36% and 48%, respectively, indicating slight-to-moderate communicative handicap. The higher of the two handicap scores by the "significant other" (SOAC of 48%) was obtained from Mr. C.'s wife. (See interpretation of SAC and SOAC data in Table 12.1.) In light of Mr. C.'s history of poor hearing aid usage, a more comprehensive self-assessment of hearing handicap, using the *Hearing Performance Inventory-Revised* (Lamb, Owens, & Schubert, 1983), was also conducted before remediation was started.

Aided real-ear probe-tube microphone measures at use-gain setting of the hearing aids revealed that Mr. C.'s aids were providing only marginal insertion gain of 5–10 dB at 1,000 and 2,000 Hz, with little or no

AUDIOLOGICAL RECORD

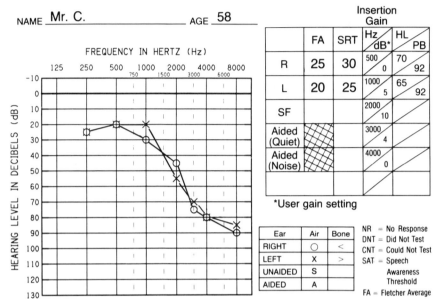

NAME Mr. C. AGE 58

FREQUENCY IN HERTZ (Hz)

	FA	SRT	Hz / dB*	HL / PB
R	25	30	500 / 0	70 / 92
L	20	25	1000 / 5	65 / 92
SF			2000 / 10	
Aided (Quiet)			3000 / 4	
Aided (Noise)			4000 / 0	

Insertion Gain

*User gain setting

Ear	Air	Bone
RIGHT	O	<
LEFT	X	>
UNAIDED	S	
AIDED	A	

NR = No Response
DNT = Did Not Test
CNT = Could Not Test
SAT = Speech
   Awareness
   Threshold
FA = Fletcher Average

Figure 12.3. Audiometric results for Mr. C., Case 3.

gain above 2,000 Hz. Yet the aids were being worn at essentially a full-volume control position; thus they were judged to be weak and inadequate. Inspection of Mr. C.'s ear canals and area of the concha-meatal junction revealed sufficient space to allow use of canal-type hearing aids—the style which was the client's strong preference.

rehabilitation evaluation

Mr. C. presented himself as a very articulate, self-confident, nicely dressed individual with seemingly few communicative difficulties. Other than the complaints from his wife that he required the TV too loud and that she must often repeat herself to him, he admitted to having little communicative difficulties at home even without the use of amplification. At work, Mr. C. conducted most of his business behind a desk where he could maintain some control over speaker distance and dialogue content. Mr. C. used his hearing aids sparingly. He reported that he felt very self-conscious about their appearance. Yet, he admitted that he had received significant benefit from his hearing aids when they were working properly, and that the use of amplification reduced the "stress of listening" and improved the ease and enjoyment of social communication, movies, church, and so forth.

Mr. C. indicated that both he and his wife felt he should be using his hearing aids more, and he admitted he would do so if they were less "intrusive." Thus, the AR objectives in this case centered on providing improved acoustic input, but by means of a hearing-aid style that was aesthetically more acceptable to both the client and his spouse.

Initially, considerable time was spent discussing the acoustic and aesthetic characteristics of small hearing aids. It was apparent that Mr. C. strongly favored the "invisible" in-the-canal style. Yet, he recognized that he had been unsuccessful with a previous trial with an ITE aid. Conceivably, the objections he found earlier with the ITE aid might be magnified with the ITC aid. In fact, from an audiological point of view there was some justification to insisting that he stay with the BTE style because of Mr. C.'s good hearing in the lower frequencies and because he had received some satisfaction with this fitting, even though actual use had been limited because of appearance factors. Also, BTE hearing aids are less expensive. From a rehabilitative perspective, however, a strong recommendation of another BTE fitting was viewed as a poor alternative in light of the client's expressed concerns over the appearance of this hearing aid style.

Thus, a 30-day trial period was arranged with a binaural fitting with ITC aids. The client was willing to make a small compromise by allowing the order of a "half shell" variation of the ITC style (aid extends partially into the concha) to allow for greater canal venting. Maximum canal venting was specified with the hearing aid order. Before ordering the instruments, the cost of various hearing aid styles was carefully reviewed with the client. The additional costs associated with smaller, customized fitting appeared to have little impact on Mr. C.'s preferences.

amplification-focused remediation

Mr. C.'s initial reaction to the size and fit of the new canal-type hearing aids was very positive. Physically, the fit was excellent. The instruments slipped comfortably into place and were virtually invisible at frontal gaze. Mr. C. was obviously pleased with the appearance of the new hearing aids. However, when he began to talk with the aids in place, his countenance dimmed, "I feel all plugged up, and the sound of my own voice is terrible." These complaints persisted regardless of the setting of the volume controls.

At this point, the hearing aids were removed and in-house modifications attempted. Canal length was left unaltered to minimize the risk of feedback—but canal diameter was significantly reduced and vent size increased somewhat. After these modifications the aids were reinserted. Mr. C. reported some relief at the sound of his own voice and also noted that the hearing aids felt better in his ears.

Insertion gain measures verified a reasonably good fitting, acoustically, with the exception that the instruments might be producing too much gain at 1,000 Hz and too little gain at 3,000-4,000 Hz. Mr. C. agreed to try the hearing aids for a few days and an appointment was scheduled for one week later.

Mr. C.'s reports at the first followup appointment were interesting. He indicated that he could hear much better with the instruments, that TV volume was no longer a problem for his wife, and that he felt more relaxed with the "inconspicuous" size of the instruments. Yet, he was still bothered by the "stuffed-up" feeling he experienced while wearing the instruments. Additional modifications were undertaken involving more grinding, increasing canal venting to allowable limits, and changing the frequency response at the factory (involving a shift towards a higher frequency emphasis). However, although all these adjustments resulted in modest subjective reports of improvement, they did not satisfactorily alleviate the client's overriding "stuffed-up" reaction.

On the fourth followup visit, an extensive review of the situation was conducted with the client. The salient elements seemed to be that (a) the size and appearance of the fittings were highly satisfactory, and the client was not amenable to any suggestion of reverting back to a BTE fitting; and (b) the client could not seem to tolerate for long periods of time the "blocked-off" feeling he experienced while using the instruments, in his words, "It almost feels like I'm under water."

At this point, another compromise was suggested: A remake of existing instruments into a "helix"-type configuration (essentially a full upper concha with "open canal" venting) which would greatly reduce ear-canal occlusion. The 312 battery size was retained to keep the physical size to a minimum. The hearing aids would be more visible, but they would still be "off the ear." The client was agreeable to this recommendation.

The helix-type fittings were a success. The degree of canal occlusion was similar to what Mr. C. remembered with the older BTE fittings, but he thought the present aids were far less noticeable. Moreover, he liked the quality of the sound of the new hearing aids and was willing to accept a somewhat "larger" fitting. Final insertion gain measures showed a satisfactory fitting acoustically, and HPI-R data, referred to earlier, revealed a noticeable reduction in perceived handicap, especially in social situations and at work (see Table 12.2). The hearing aids were worn at a preferred 1/2 volume control setting without feedback, although the tendency for feedback with objects near the ear (like the telephone) was greater. Mr. C. understood this problem and was able to control for it.

discussion

Audiologists are seeing increasing numbers of clients for whom the major rehabilitative effort is directed toward the hearing aid. In cases such as the one described here, AR strategies involve a recognition of significant nonacoustic as well as the more obvious acoustic factors which go into a successful fitting. Achieving a judicious compromise between what the client "needs" and what he may "wants" makes good rehabilitative sense.

A related matter, confined here to hearing-impaired adults, has to do with the cost of services, particularly the cost of hearing aids. Some

TABLE 12.2

Post-Remediation Insertion Gain Measures and Pre- and Post-Remediation HPI-R Handicap Scores (Norms for HPI Are Shown for Comparison)

Insertion Gain in dB
(User-Volume Setting)

500	1000	2000	3000	4000
0	8	16	23	12

HPI-R Test Sections	% Difficulty		
	Before Fitting	After Fitting	Norms*
Understanding Speech	42	38	33
Intensity	46	34	20
Response to Auditory Failure	81	72	60
Social Situations	60	46	34
Personal	48	42	NA
Occupational	42	36	37

*From *Hearing Handicapped Adults* by T. G. Giolas, 1982, Englewood Cliffs, NJ: Prentice-Hall.

audiologists may adopt a "protective" posture in this respect, and attempt to impose their own "monetary standards" on their clients in conjunction with what they may view as a preferred fitting. "Talking the client out of" selecting a particular hearing aid because of cost should be done with caution. To "save" clients' money by recommending a hearing aid fitting that they may not want is unwise, not only from a human standpoint, but from a rehabilitative standpoint as well. Instead, efforts should be made to accommodate the client's wishes unless compelling acoustic or medical reasons dictate otherwise. In general, a prudent approach to the cost of hearing aids is to present to the client all viable hearing aid options, point out the advantages and disadvantages and costs of each, and allow the client to make the selection.

case 4: nursing home hearing aid user

case history

Mrs. E. was a 75-year-old resident of a local nursing home. She had been living in the facility for over 2 years, and was quite alert mentally and able to move about the facility without any special assistance. Mrs. E. was using a hearing aid at the time she was first seen by an audiologist. It was later determined that she had been a longtime hearing aid user, having had four other instruments over a period of many years. Her present hearing aid was 5 years old and, according to Mrs. E., did not seem to be working as well as it once had.

diagnostic information

Initial efforts with Mrs. E. involved air-conduction pure-tone testing and tympanometry in a quiet room within the nursing home. As seen in Figure 12.4, the client possessed a moderate-to-severe hearing loss, which was bilaterally symmetrical. Type A tympanograms were traced bilaterally, suggesting the presence of a sensorineural disorder in each ear.

aural rehabilitation

Mrs. E. was concerned about the condition of her hearing aid, complaining that it did not seem to help her as much as it had in the past. She

AUDIOLOGICAL RECORD

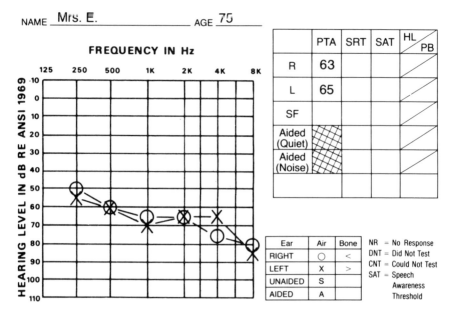

NAME __Mrs. E._____ AGE _75_____

Figure 12.4. Audiometric results for Mrs. E., Case 4.

also appeared to be experiencing an excessive amount of acoustic feedback and reported having difficulty getting the earmold into her ear properly.

The hearing aid was analyzed electroacoustically by the audiologist and was found to have a reduced gain and an abnormal amount of distortion. In discussing the feasibility of purchasing a new hearing aid, it became clear that Mrs. E. was not financially able to consider such a purchase. She was, therefore, advised to have her hearing aid serviced and reconditioned by the manufacturer. She was agreeable to this recommendation, and arrangements were made for this to occur.

In the course of working with Mrs. E. it became apparent that she needed a new earmold. In discussing this, Mrs. E. recalled that her current mold had also been used with her previous hearing aid. The mold was very discolored and did not appear to fit Mrs. E.'s ear canal and pinna adequately. The audiologist took an ear impression, which was sent to a laboratory for production of a new earmold.

In approximately one month, both the earmold and the hearing aid were returned. Mrs. E. was then fit with the reconditioned aid and her initial reaction was quite positive. She was instructed to use the aid as much as possible in the following days. A subsequent electroacoustic analysis of the instrument revealed an increase in gain and a significant improvement in the amount of distortion. Real-ear measures, taken at the nursing home with portable equipment, revealed satisfactory gain.

When she was seen again, Mrs. E. was still pleased with the help she was receiving from her hearing aid, but she indicated that she was still having difficulty inserting the earmold. Watching her attempt to do this herself made it apparent that Mrs. E. was not able to manipulate her hands sufficiently to allow her to insert the mold without great effort. It was also apparent that she was not using an efficient method when inserting the mold. To assist her, Mrs. E. was given some basic instructions on how to best insert and remove the mold. (An example of a training protocol for this purpose is found in Chapter 10.) She was encouraged to practice the procedure and was visited by the audiologist several times during the next 2 weeks to review the procedure, and to answer any questions she might have. During these visits it became apparent that Mrs. E.'s facility in placement of the mold had improved.

Along with the work done with Mrs. E. to improve the way she inserted her mold, several of the nursing home staff members working with Mrs. E. were also provided with information on how to put the earmold in properly. This allowed them to assist Mrs. E. in doing so each day. Both Mrs. E. and the staff also received helpful information on how to clean her earmold and basic instruction on the operation and use of her hearing aid.

discussion

Attempts to help Mrs. E. were successful. This is not always the case when working in a rehabilitative capacity with nursing home residents (Schow, 1982). Mrs. E.'s case illustrates one of the ways in which an audiologist can make a valuable contribution to a number of residents in a given nursing home. It is important first to identify those individuals within the facility for whom aural rehabilitation may be beneficial. Once this is done, the audiologist will generally work with each person individually, identifying those areas of aural rehabilitation that should be worked on. Individual needs must be considered, and the audiologist must be willing to devote the time necessary to accomplish the desired ends.

case 5: acquired severe hearing loss

case history

Mr. A. was a 45-year-old male who had experienced progressive sensorineural hearing loss over the past 25 years. Mr. A., married, worked in construction and as a part-time lay "preacher" for his church. No specific cause for the hearing loss had been identified, although Mr. A. had experienced a sustained "high temperature" during childhood, had been exposed to job-related noise, and reported a family history of hearing loss. The client had used a hearing aid for approximately eight years during the early stages of his hearing loss. However, Mr. A. reported that as the degree of loss progressed, benefits derived from hearing aid use became less and less satisfactory. Consequently, he had not worn a hearing aid for 15 years. Recent audiological and hearing aid evaluations confirmed the poor prognosis related to hearing aid benefit. Mr. A. referred himself to the clinic and stated, "My hearing loss is so great, I need lipreading."

diagnostic information

Audiometric data confirmed a profound, bilateral, sensorineural hearing loss (see Figure 12.5). Speech audiometry revealed that Mr. A. could not auditorily discriminate words, regardless of the context (single syllable, multi-syllable, phrase, or sentence). Test results were similar when hearing aids were used. Based on the severity of his hearing loss and Mr. A.'s negative attitude toward hearing aid use, it was decided to temporarily postpone additional hearing aid evaluation and focus on improving visually receptive communication skills.

aural rehabilitation

A three-stage rehabilitation plan was designed. Stage 1 included training in speechreading and basic manual communication. Stage 2 would involve attempts to re-establish hearing aid use with emphasis on utilizing the suprasegmental aspects of connected speech. Stage 3 was to be devoted to improving communication in specific "problem" situations. The remainder of this case study deals with Stage 1.

Prior to initiating speechreading training, several pre-therapy tests of speechreading were administered. These tests included both sentence

AUDIOLOGICAL RECORD

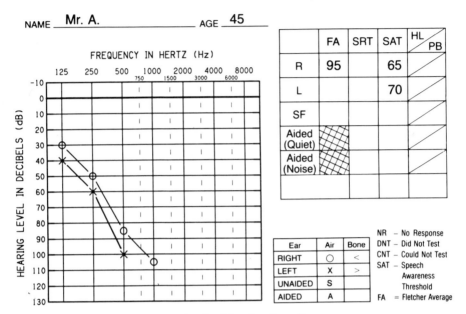

NAME __Mr. A.__ AGE __45__

	FA	SRT	SAT	HL/PB
R	95		65	
L			70	
SF				
Aided (Quiet)				
Aided (Noise)				

Ear	Air	Bone
RIGHT	O	<
LEFT	X	>
UNAIDED	S	
AIDED	A	

NR – No Response
DNT – Did Not Test
CNT – Could Not Test
SAT – Speech Awareness Threshold
FA = Fletcher Average

Figure 12.5. Audiometric results for Mr. A., Case 5.

and single word contexts. Mr. A.'s performance was poor in all contexts (sentences = 30% correct, spondee words = 30% correct, and single syllable words = 2%). Because of the poor speechreading performance, it was decided to use an analytic approach for speechreading training. It was anticipated that a higher rate of success would be obtained by using isolated phonemes and that there would be some generalization to word and sentence performance (Walden, Erdman, Montgomery, Schwartz, & Prosek, 1981).

A detailed analysis of the pre-therapy tests revealed several error phonemes common to all contexts. Errors related to homophenous groups, e.g., /p/, /b/, /m/, were disregarded. Baseline data were collected on the remaining error phonemes using a same/different task. The stimulus items consisted of an error phoneme and its confused counterpart. Baseline data revealed six error phonemes on which performance was below 90% correct. These six phonemes were incorporated into the therapy protocol.

The therapy protocol required Mr. A. to respond "same" or "different" to pairs of phonemes. Ten pairs of stimulus items were presented in each trial and the percent correct recorded. Ninety percent correct for five consecutive trials was required before the client was allowed to move to the next error phoneme. When an error occurred for any item, the item was repeated five times but with a printed stimulus added to the speechreading task. In this way Mr. A. knew ahead of time what the stimulus item would be and could focus on the subtle visual differences.

results

Table 12.3 shows comparisons between the pre- and post-therapy test scores and baseline results. As illustrated, reasonable improvement was achieved and training using isolated phonemes appeared to have generalized to both words and sentences. No formal evaluation was made of the improvement for manual communication. However, Mr. A. learned

TABLE 12.3
Pre- and Post-Therapy Speechreading Test Scores and Baseline Data

Tests	Pre-Therapy % Correct	Post-Therapy % Correct
CID Everyday Sentences	0	20
Utley Sentences (Form B)	30	70
Hood Live Voice Speechreading Test	10	34
Spondee Words	30	55
California Consonant Test		
"open-choice format"	2	14
[a]Baselines		
/r/-/w/	96	100
/r/-/t/	96	80
/n/-/k/	92	100
/dʒ/-/s/	86	90
/l/-/θ/	80	100
/h/-/k/	70	80
/l/-/ɚ/	66	100
/t/-/ʃ/	60	100
/j/-/d/	53	100

[a]Same/different task, 10 items per trial, 5 trials per pair.

most of the manual alphabet and several signs. The signs which were taught were incorporated into therapy as a part of the instructions for various speechreading tasks.

Mr. A. was a highly motivated client and will continue in therapy. Subsequent therapy will focus on speechreading using word and sentence material along with hearing aid use and emphasis on auditory training related to suprasegmental aspects of speech. During the time we saw Mr. A. he lost his employment with his church due to his inability to communicate adequately with church members. His construction job was also threatened. Because of these circumstances and with the help of Vocational Rehabilitation, Mr. A. is planning to attend college in order to develop a new job skill.

case 6: hearing loss/disengagement

case history

Mrs. B., an 84-year-old resident of a local nursing home, lived at the home for about 3 months before she was seen by an audiologist. She had initially been brought to the audiologist's attention by the staff of the facility, since they had difficulty communicating with Mrs. B. In support of this observation, the activity director had completed a staff form of the *Nursing Home Hearing Handicap Index* (NHHI) on Mrs. B., which resulted in an overall score of 60%, which suggested that Mrs. B. had a moderate hearing handicap.

The audiologist's first visit with Mrs. B. was not a pleasant experience. The patient was reluctant to interact, and displayed some degree of hostility. However, during the course of the relatively brief encounter it was possible to obtain some basic case history information from the patient and also observe her communication skills. Apparently Mrs. B. had possessed a hearing loss for several years, but had never worn a hearing aid. No other specific information could be obtained, primarily because of an apparent unwillingness on the part of the patient to interact.

The audiologist attempted to gather additional relevant information through the patient's medical and family records. Inspection of this material revealed that Mrs. B. had lived with a son and his family in their home for the past 4 years. An attending physician had noted that the patient had experienced periods of prolonged depression in the previous 2 years and was generally withdrawn. No information was reported about her hearing.

The observations of various staff members confirmed this informa-tion. Mrs. B. reportedly interacted very infrequently with anyone at the facility and was uncooperative at times. She seemed to spend a large portion of the day either sleeping or sitting in her room by herself.

diagnostic information

The audiologist made two more brief visits with Mrs. B. before attempt-ing to conduct assessment of her hearing. These two sessions were intended to allow Mrs. B. to become more familiar with the clinician, a step which could be considered helpful before she was asked to partici-pate in audiometric testing. Unfortunately, these visits were similar to the initial one, with Mrs. B. choosing to interact only to a minimal extent.

On the third visit the audiologist brought a portable pure-tone audi-ometer, and, to the audiologist's surprise, Mrs. B. did permit testing. These results are presented in Figure 12.6. A complete assessment was not possible because Mrs. B. became impatient and finally refused to

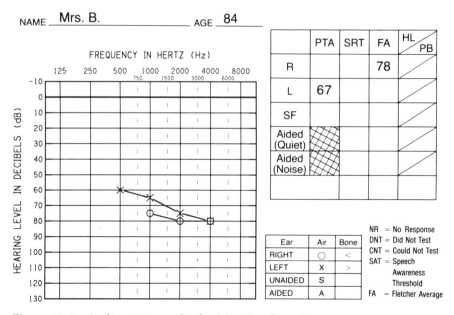

Figure 12.6. Audiometric results for Mrs. B., Case 6.

participate any further. An attempt was made to have the patient complete a patient form of the NHHI, but she would not consider it. The clinician thanked Mrs. B. for her efforts and indicated that he would be returning in the near future.

When the audiologist returned in one week he was informed by the head nurse of the facility that Mrs. B. had indicated that she did not want to work with the audiologist any longer. The audiologist attempted to discuss the situation with the patient, but it was apparent that Mrs. B. would not be a willing participant in any aural rehabilitative efforts. Another visit by the audiologist several weeks later confirmed this impression. Personnel at the nursing home indicated that Mrs. B. had become even more withdrawn than earlier.

discussion

Although Mrs. B. was in need of audiologic assistance, circumstances associated with her emotional status did not allow for this to occur. Audiologists will find a number of such resistant patients among nursing home residents.

Although some measures can be taken to facilitate working with withdrawn and/or uncooperative persons, some will remain unreachable. As discussed by Botwinick (1973), the *disengagement process* is commonly observed in the elderly—a tendency on the part of many older people to become progressively introverted and interact less with others. For some this will be an important step toward disengagement from the "world" and can be a healthy process in preparation for dying. Therefore, the aural rehabilitationist should not, in his/her enthusiasm, be too aggressive if the client is clearly not interested. After making a reasonable effort, the audiologist should be generally accepting of this disengagement attitude and channel efforts to other persons whose emotional status is more conducive to remediation activities.

case 7: acquired deafness and cochlear implant rehabilitation

introduction

The adventitiously deafened adult who becomes a cochlear implant (CI) candidate must undergo extensive evaluation, not only for implant candidacy, but also to determine an individualized aural rehabilitation program. Not all candidates meet selection criteria for the cochlear implant. However, the following aural rehabilitation program for a CI candidate also allows for the recommendation of alternative assistive devices, such as a vibrotactile aid, along with appropriate individualized rehabilitative therapy.

The following checklist provides a procedural guideline for the rehabilitation therapist who works with cochlear implant candidates. In addition, a cochlear implant case study is presented which demonstrates the individualized protocol for aural rehabilitation.

Checklist

Pre-implant selection criteria and rehabilitative evaluation
  Medical/audiological assessment
  Aural rehabilitation assessment
    Communicative assessment
    Psychosocial assessment (attitude)
    Associated variables/conditions
Post-implant aural rehabilitation protocol
  Amplification assessment: post-stimulation
  Psychosocial/counseling (information/behavior)
  Communicative strategies rehabilitation
    (speechreading and speech tracking)
  Overall coordination
Post-implant recommendations
  Aural rehabilitative protocol—evaluation and rehabilitation
  6-month assessment followup
  1-year assessment followup

case history

Mr. S., age 57, was referred by a physician for consideration as a cochlear implant candidate. He had a diagnosed profound bilateral sensorineural hearing loss which was attributed to a case of meningitis at the age of 33. At that time, the patient received limited aural rehabilitation to assist with speechreading. Testing revealed no measurable benefits from hearing aids. Following the onset of his loss of hearing, Mr. S. resigned from his position with a large industrial complex and received disability benefits. He found himself gradually withdrawing from social involvements and meaningful relationships and reported that he found it ''much too frustrating'' to engage in communicative situations. He chose not to learn sign language as he could not readily identify with the deaf community. Over the years Mr. S.'s speech slowly began to deteriorate and his language usage reflected a lack of modern terminology.

aural rehabilitation evaluation

Mr. S. received 40 hours of intensive rehabilitative evaluation which followed the CI protocol established at the medical center. Pre-implant selection requirements for cochlear implantation were met based on selection criteria guidelines established by the FDA (House, 1978). General guidelines for patient selection included: Profound sensorineural hearing loss, bilaterally; normal temporal bone radiologic findings; absence of responses to brainstem auditory-evoked potentials; severe impairment of speech recognition, using powerful hearing aids; between the ages of 18 and 70 years; normal speech and language milestones prior to hearing loss; medical examination which determined the pathology of the inner ear; ability to tolerate the surgical procedure and anesthesia; consensus by CI team members regarding the patient's understanding of the limitations and benefits of the CI; and agreement by the CI recipient to participate in the pre-postsurgical rehabilitative protocol. Additional rehabilitative assessment procedures were established to address the candidate's psychosocial and communicative performances. Table 12.4 lists all areas of the comprehensive assessment protocol (Flevaris-Phillips, Spitzer, Milner, Leder, & Giolas, 1985). Mr. S.'s evaluations for implant candidacy were performed by a multidisciplinary team consisting of medical, audiological, speech and psychological counseling personnel who made up the CI team.

Medical assessment, including opthalmological examination and radiological studies, resulted in the medical personnel recommending the CI. Audiological assessment confirmed a bilateral, profound, sensorineural hearing loss (PTA 110 dB HL+), normal bilateral electronystagmography (ENG) responses, and unmeasurable auditory brainstem response (ABR) with Mr. S.

Psychosocial assessment results demonstrated a "normal" overall psychological profile, utilizing traditional psychometric instruments recommended for CI candidates (House, 1978). However, using the additional rehabilitative assessment protocol which addressed psychosocial issues associated with hearing loss (Flevaris-Phillips, 1986) revealed that the CI candidate had self-defeating attitudes toward hearing impairment and somewhat unrealistic expectations about the benefits of the CI. Significant, counterproductive psychosocial characteristics of dependency,

TABLE 12.4
Aural Rehabilitation Evaluation Protocol for
Cochlear Implant Candidates

Medical/Audiological Evaluations	Communicative Evaluations	Psychological and Psychosocial Evaluations
MEDICAL	AUDITORY ASSISTIVE DEVICES	INDIVIDUAL
— Routine Physical Examination: Chest X-Ray, EKG, Laboratory/Blood Work-Up	— Hearing Aids — Auditory Trainer	— Psychological — Psychosocial Adjustment
— Tomogram — Fluorescent Antibody Absorption Test — Other Tests as Needed	NON-AUDITORY ASSISTIVE DEVICES — Vibrotactile Aid	[a]FAMILY — Psychological — Psychosocial Adjustment
OPHTHALMOLOGICAL/ OPTOMETRIC	SPEECHREADING	
— Non-Contact Tonometry — Slit-Lamp Examination — Ophthalmoscopy — Refraction	— Videotapes — Live-Voice	
AUDIOLOGICAL	COMMUNICATIVE SKILLS AND STRATEGIES	
— Unaided — Aided — Psychoacoustic — Electronystamography — Brainstem Auditory-Evoked Potentials	— Integrative-Processing — Communicative Behaviors ARTICULATION/VOICE — Prosody — Acoustic Analysis — Articulation	

[a]Family involvement is critical; therefore, all decisions and recommendations include family members.

social isolation and depression, which were associated with the candidate's attitudes toward hearing loss and resultant adjustments, also were identified through assessments and interviews.

Results from the assessment of Mr. S.'s communication skills demonstrated limited speechreading performance based on standardized videotapes (Spitzer, Leder, Milner, Flevaris-Phillips, Giolas, & Richardson, 1987), poor speech-tracking scores according to DeFilipo and Scott (1987), extensive communicative handicaps (Giolas, Owens, Lamb, & Shubert, 1979), and deficient communicative strategies and knowledge of available resources (Flevaris-Phillips, 1986). Analysis of Mr. S.'s speech revealed loudness, pitch, and speaking rate irregularities. Table 12.5 presents a summary of Mr. S.'s pre-CI audiological, communicative, and

TABLE 12.5
Aural Rehabilitation Evaluation
Pre-Cochlear Implant Data for Mr. S.

Demographics	
Age	57
PTA- HL unaided	110+ dB HL
Etiology	Meningitis
Intelligence Quotient	120 IQ
Psychological Evaluations	Normal range
Cognitive Abilities	Normal range
Visual Skills	
Speechreading	Minimal abilities
Auditory/Visual	
Speech Tracking	11 words per minute
Auditory Skills	
Minimal Auditory Capabilities Test	No auditory behavior
Diagnostic Rhyme Test	No auditory behavior
Test of Auditory Comprehension	No auditory behavior
Communicative Skills	
Handicap Performance Inventory	Extreme difficulties
Videotapes	Identifiable difficulties
Interviews	Limited reported difficulties
Psychosocial Behaviors	
16 Personality Factor Test	Depression, isolation
Beliefs about Deafness Test	Irrational beliefs
Expectations Questionnaire	Unrealistic expectations
Speech	
Analysis of Speech (visi-pitch)	Intensity and duration errors
	Lower fundamental frequencies

psychosocial performance. Based on all the information gathered, the CI team recommended that Mr. S. receive a cochlear implant, along with an intensive individualized program of aural rehabilitation.

remediation plan

Six weeks following surgical implantation of the CI prosthesis Mr. S. returned for electrical stimulation of the auditory nerve via his single-channel CI. During the following week he received 40 hours of intensive rehabilitation according to his individualized treatment objectives which were based on the pre-CI rehabilitative evaluation findings and objective reports. Most therapy sessions involving the audiologist, psychologist and speech-language pathologist were conducted individually with Mr. S. However, some group work with other CI clients, especially associated with psychosocial issues, was included.

Communication Rehabilitation.   Auditory training with Mr. S. was subsequently initiated using the *Test of Auditory Comprehension Training Manual* (Foreworks, 1979), selected word and sentence lists, and poetry (Flevaris-Phillips, 1986). Visual skill training included speechreading exercises utilizing appropriate speechreading materials. Both auditory and visual modalities were combined in speech-tracking exercises using high-interest reading materials. Information and discussion regarding communicative strategies was followed by analysis of videotaped communicative behaviors demonstrated by Mr. S. in communicative situations.

Amplification Issues.   Informational counseling included the presentation of instructions on the use of assistive devices (i.e., telephone decoder, television captioning and vibrotactile aids) and available social support groups.

Psychosocial Issues.   Behavioral counseling involved discussion of Mr. S.'s attitudes and his expectations regarding the CI and hearing loss. Mr. S. was involved in group discussions with other hearing-impaired adults concerning adjustment difficulties and alternative adjustment strategies utilizing assistive devices. Discussion of videotaped social interactions and corrective role-playing exercises were also a part of the behavioral counseling protocol. Mr. S. maintained a diary for recording new listening experiences and perceptions with the CI along with a progress record for charting daily achievements.

remediation results

Post-CI stimulation assessment results for audiological, communicative, and psychosocial performance after 40 hours of aural rehabilitation are presented in Table 12.6. This table presents Mr. S.'s performance at 1 year following the initial post-stimulation rehabilitative program. Audiological assessment scores reflect impressive performance on various auditory tasks with the CI. Post-CI stimulation communicative performance scores demonstrate improvements in speechreading, speech tracking, and communicative skills. Post-CI stimulation psychosocial performance scores show improved attitudes, personality characteristics and realistic expectations for Mr. S. Following Mr. S.'s annual followup evaluation he was rated by the CI team on a 5-point scale which correlates with the earlier measurements of auditory sensitivity, psychosocial variables, speech tracking, and speech characteristics developed at this medical center (Spitzer et al., 1987). Mr. S.'s communicative performance was rated as extremely successful. He reported that the aural rehabilitation

TABLE 12.6
Aural Rehabilitation Evaluation
Post-CI Stimulation for Mr. S.

Psychological Evaluations	
Cognitive Abilities	Normal range
Visual Skills	
Speechreading	25% improvement
Auditory/Visual	
Speech Tracking	68 words per minute
Auditory Skills	
Minimal Auditory Capabilities Test	Passed 4 subtests
Diagnostic Rhyme Test	Passed 2 sections
Test of Auditory Comprehension	Passed 5 levels
Communicative Skills	
Handicap Performance Inventory	Moderate difficulty
Videotapes	Observable improvements
Interviews	Observable improvements
Psychosocial Behaviors	
16 Personality Factor Test	Social & personal improvements
Beliefs about Deafness Test	Rational beliefs
Expectations Questionnaire	Realistic expectations
Speech	
Analysis of Speech (visi-pitch)	Improved fundamental frequencies
	Improved intensity & duration

program was exceptionally beneficial, not only for utilization of the CI, but also for understanding the effects of his counterproductive attitudes, using successful communicative strategies, and dealing with the limitations of the CI device. Although Mr. S. was left with a serious hearing handicap, he was very appreciative of the positive changes in his life brought about by the CI and associated rehabilitation program.

discussion

Mr. S. is representative of the majority of adventitiously deafened adult CI candidates searching out a cure for deafness. It is easy to surgically implant an individual and to disregard his rehabilitative needs. Reports of clients who have not found the CI beneficial and of those who demonstrate minimal benefits from the CI are well known. Comprehensive medical, audiological, and rehabilitative assessment, followed by an individualized program of aural rehabilitation, is required to adequately address patient needs. In addition to communicative rehabilitation, both informational and behavioral counseling rehabilitation are essential ingredients in a comprehensive and effective AR program for the successful CI user.

references

Botwinick, J. (1973). *Aging and behavior*. New York: Springer Verlag.

Craig, W. (1964). Effects of preschool training on the development of reading and lipreading skills of deaf children. *American Annals of the Deaf, 109,* 280-296.

DeFillippo, C.L., & Scott, B.L. (1978). A method for speech reception. *Journal of the Acoustical Society of America, 63*(4).

Flevaris-Phillips, C.A. (1986, June). *Creating aural rehabilitation guidelines for adventitiously deaf adult cochlear implant candidates.* Paper presented at the meeting of the Academy of Rehabilitative Audiology, Lake Geneva, WI.

Flevaris-Phillips, C.A., Spitzer, J.B., Milner, P., Leder, S.B., & Giolas, T. (1985). *Aural rehabilitation guidelines for the adult with a cochlear implant.* Paper presented at the American Speech-Language-Hearing Conference, Washington, DC.

Giolas, T., Owens, E., Lamb, S., & Shubert, E. (1979). Hearing performance inventory. *Journal of Speech and Hearing Disorders, 44,* 169-195.

Giolas, T.G. (1982). *Hearing handicapped adults*. Englewood Cliffs, NJ: Prentice-Hall.

Goldstein, D.P., & Stephens, S.D.G. (1981). Audiological rehabilitation: Management model I. *Audiology, 20,* 432-452.

High, W., Fairbanks, G., & Glorig, A. (1964). Scale of self-assessment of hearing handicap. *Journal of Hearing Disorders, 29,* 215-230.

House, W.F. (1978). Cochlear implants. *Annals of Otolaryngology, Rhinology, and Laryngology,* Suppl. *27,* 1-93.

Kaplan, H., Bally, S.J., & Garretson, C. (1985). *Speechreading—A way to improve understanding.* Washington, DC: Gallaudet College Press.

Lamb, S.H., Owens, E., & Schubert, E. (1983). The revised form of the Hearing Performance Inventory. *Ear and Hearing, 4,* 152-157.

Leder, S., Spitzer, J., Flevaris-Phillips, C., Richardson, R., Milner, P., & Kirchner, J. (1987). Innovative approaches to selection of adult cochlear implant candidates. *Journal of Rehab. Deaf, 21*(2), 27-33.

Milner, P., & Flevaris, C. (1986). Brainstem auditory evoked potentials and the auditory trainer for the profoundly deaf subject. *Journal of the Acoustical Society of America, 76,* 82-86.

Schow, R.L. (1982). Success of hearing aid fitting in nursing home residents. *Ear & Hearing, 3*(3), 173-177.

Schow, R., & Nerbonne, M. (1982). Communication screening profile use with the elderly clients. *Ear and Hearing, 3*(3), 133-147.

Schow, R.L., Brockett, J., Sturmak, M., & Longhurst, T. (in press). Self-assessment of hearing in rehabilitative audiology. *British Journal of Audiology.*

Schow, R., & Tannahill, C. (1977). Hearing handicap scores and categories for subjects with normal and impaired hearing sensitivity. *Journal of the American Audiological Society, 3,* 134-139.

Spitzer, J.B. (1986). A cochlear implant team in a VA setting. *VA Practitioner,* 50-62.

Spitzer, J.B., Leder, S.B., Milner, P., Flevaris-Phillips, C., & Giolas, T. (1987). Standardization of four videotaped tests of speechreading ranging in task difficulty. *Ear and Hearing, 8*(4), 227-231.

Sturmak, M.J. (1987). *Communication handicap score interpretation for various populations and degrees of hearing impairment.* Unpublished master's thesis, Idaho State University.

Utley, J. (1946). A test of lipreading ability. *Journal of Speech and Hearing Disorders, 11,* 109-116.

Walden, B., Erdman, S., Montgomery, A., Schwartz, D., & Prosek, R. (1981). Some effects of training on speech recognition by hearing-impaired adults. *Journal of Speech and Hearing Research, 24,* 207-216.

chapterthirteen

RESOURCE MATERIALS

THOMAS G. GIOLAS, GWENYTH R. VAUGHN, ROBERT K. LIGHTFOOT, AND ADRIENNE KARP

contents

INTRODUCTION

This resource chapter brings together a set of supplementary readings and lists of materials and sources to facilitate aural rehabilitation (AR) with children and adults. Several experts on aural rehabilitation have contributed to this chapter.

contributing authors

Thomas Giolas has authored two texts on aural rehabilitation for adults and has had extensive experience working with adult clients. He has contributed for inclusion here an outline of an 8-week session for adult clients (one meeting per week). Those who wish to provide short-term AR to an adult group will find this a useful starting point in organizing such sessions.

Robert Lightfoot and *Gwenyth Vaughn* have become well known for their efforts to promote Assistive Listening Devices (ALDS). They have contributed an introduction to assistive devices for this resource chapter. Specifically, they have described in detail four major types of devices: hardwire, infrared, FM, and loops. Ample pictorial material helps the uninitiated reader to visualize what these devices look like.

Adrienne Karp has worked with the visually impaired for many years at the New York Association for the Blind. She has contributed an insightful piece which helps prepare the reader for working with visually impaired persons, whether blind or suffering the effects of reduced visual acuity. Many elderly persons and others with hearing loss have limited vision. In fact, visual impairments often are associated with hearing loss; therefore, it is crucial that AR clinicians be on the alert for undetected visual impairments with any hearing-impaired patient because of the compounding effects when both disabilities are present.

ASHA definition of and competencies for aural rehabilitation

Over several years the ASHA Committee on Rehabilitative Audiology updated a position statement on aural rehabilitation, refining the definition of and competencies required to conduct aural rehabilitation. Under the direction of two committee chairs, James McCartney and O. T. Kenworthy, a document was drafted and subsequently accepted by ASHA's Legislative Council in 1983. The document is reprinted here since it should serve as a guideline for the training of all students who may use this book. It also served as a reference point in the model described in Chapter 1 and used throughout this text.

materials lists

The child and adult materials lists were prepared with input from the authors of the chapters on AR for children and adults. Special acknowledgment is made to these authors for their assistance in preparing these lists.

SAMPLE 8-WEEK ADULT AURAL REHABILITATION GROUP OUTLINE

Thomas G. Giolas

The general purpose of aural rehabilitation (AR) groups is to provide a dynamic setting in which the interaction between peers (hearing-impaired persons), friends and family members, and the group leaders (the audiologist) generates productive discussions and, most importantly, solutions to communication problems associated with a hearing impairment. The focus is on communication breakdowns, where and with whom they typically occur, and what can be done about them. Below is an outline of the major components and the rationale for these groups.

Purpose:
To provide supportive and substantive help to persons having communication problems associated with hearing impairment.

Goals:
To analyze auditory failures and develop concrete behaviors which result in improved communication.

Process:
The group process is used with the audiologist serving as the group leader.

Rationale:
The group process provides a setting in which there is considerable exchange of information, mutual support, and validation of communication problems and solutions.

Role of the Group Leader:
The group leader serves as the major facilitator of the discussion: by raising pertinent questions, by being a good listener, and by demonstrating continued respect for group members' comments and opinions. The group leader also serves as the expert on hearing and hearing disorders.

Session Contents:
The general content of the group sessions centers on hearing and the handicapping effect of hearing impairment through lectures, films, and other media.

Group Members:
Group participants are hearing-impaired persons and friends or family members with whom communication is important and frequent.

Group Activities:
Activities are designed to focus on (a) optimal use of auditory cues, (b) optimal use of visual cues, (c) manipulation of environment, and (d) response to auditory failures.

sample 8-week group program

Eight 2-hour group sessions are outlined below. The contents of these sessions are offered as an example of what might be done with a group of hearing-impaired persons and their friends or family members. The outline does not represent a rigid program to be followed with all groups. A management plan for a particular group must be based on a complete evaluation of participants' hearing impairments and hearing handicap. On the other hand, it is this writer's experience that all sessions should follow a similar structure. This helps participants predict the activities to be expected from one session to another, thus minimizing unnecessary confusion. Below is an outline of the general session structure followed. (The initial session will deviate slightly from this structure to introduce the general goals of the program.)

1. Discussion of homework assignment.

2. Formal presentation of previously announced topic.

3. Open discussion of issues raised in the formal presentation.

4. Social break.

5. Communication-strategy activity.

6. Homework assignment and discussion of next session's activities.

First Week

1.0 *Introduction*
    1.1 Introduction to group members.
    1.2 Setting group goals and ground rules.
2.0 *Formal Presentation*
    2.1 Typical communication problems experienced by most hearing-impaired persons, especially those reported by the group.
        2.1.1 Intensity loss.
        2.1.2 Speech discrimination.
        2.1.3 Communication situations (use examples from self-report data).

    2.1.4 The role of the hearing-impaired person's response to the specific auditory failure.

3.0 *Open Discussion of Formal Presentation*
    3.1 The major objective of this activity in the initial session is to set the stage for an atmosphere conducive to easy conversation between the group members and the leader. The nature of the content is less important at this time.

4.0 *Social Break*
    4.1 The group leader should circulate as much as possible during the initial break and talk with as many of the group members as possible.

5.0 *Communication Strategy Activity*
    5.1 Ask the group to identify difficult listening situations. Write them on the chalkboard and have the group discuss why they are difficult and identify some possible solutions.

6.0 *Homework Assignment*
    6.1 Each group member is asked to identify and describe two situations in which he or she had considerable difficulty during the week. Group members are to chart the situations in terms of:
    6.1.1 With whom they were talking.
    6.1.2 The environmental conditions.
    6.1.3 The purpose of the conversation.
    6.1.4 Why they thought they had difficulty.
    6.1.5 What they did about it.

Second Week

1.0 *Discussion of Homework Assignment*
    1.1 Special note must be taken to identify early on those hearing-impaired group members who had difficulty doing the homework so that they may be responded to individually if the difficulty continues.

2.0 *Formal Presentation*
    2.1 The hearing aid.
    2.1.1 Hearing through a hearing aid.
    2.1.2 The care and operation of a hearing aid.
    2.1.3 Some tips on hearing aid use.

3.0 *Open Discussion of Formal Presentation*
    3.1 This discussion provides the opportunity for many problems and solutions regarding hearing aid use to be raised. Much will be learned from the group members listening and talking to each other. The leader should refrain from providing all the answers.

4.0 *Social Break*

   4.1 This break often provides a good opportunity for group members to ask specific questions concerning problems they are having with their own hearing aids. The group leader should begin noting those persons who may need to be seen for further audiological workup to assess the effectiveness of their hearing aids.

5.0 *Communication Strategy Activity*

   5.1 Two group members are asked to carry on a conversation under adverse listening conditions (e.g., background music). The group is asked to write down how each of the people talking handled the difficult listening situation. A discussion is then held on what was observed.

   5.2 This activity serves as a good introduction to highlight the way responses to auditory failures help or hinder communication.

6.0 *Homework Assignment*

   6.1 Group members are asked to select two listening situations in which they could compare their performance with and without their hearing aids.

Third Week

1.0 *Discussion of Homework Assignment*

   1.1 At this point the group leader should be encouraging discussion by those who are not participating very much. If there is someone who is not doing the homework, a nonthreatening personal conversation with him or her (perhaps during the break) is in order.

2.0 *Formal Presentation*

   2.1 The use of nonverbal cues.

      2.1.1 The contribution of lip movements, gestures, facial expressions, and situational cues to the understanding of the verbal message.

      2.1.2 The concept of physiologic, acoustic, and linguistic redundancy (elementary level).

      2.1.3 The benefits and limitations of lipreading.

3.0 *Open Discussion of Formal Presentation*

   3.1 This presentation will stimulate considerable discussion, which will continue to arise in subsequent sessions. The group should be made aware that the use of nonverbal cues will be covered again.

4.0 *Social Break*

   4.1 This is typically the point at which some group members begin to pursue individual conferences with the group leader.

5.0 *Communication Strategy Activity*
    5.1 One or more of the activities, described in Chapter Four, which are designed to show the advantages of nonverbal cues in general, are appropriate at this time.
6.0 *Homework Assignment*
    6.1 Each group member is asked to bring in three to five phrases or sentences common to his or her home or work environment. They will be used in a simple lipreading activity.

Fourth Week

1.0 *Discussion of Homework Assignment*
    1.1 This assignment will provide the content with which to introduce a simple lipreading activity. The familiar phrases and sentences will also provide a good lead-in to the use of other communication strategies.
2.0 *Formal Presentation*
    2.1 Communication strategies.
        2.1.1 Manipulation of the environment.
        2.1.2 Constructive response to auditory failure.
    2.2 Many specific suggestions regarding the content of this presentation appear in Chapter Four.
3.0 *Open Discussion of Formal Presentation*
    3.1 The group leader may begin directing the discussion toward the group's reported differential use of these strategies in social and work settings.
4.0 *Social Break*
    4.1 If there are some group members who are in their hearing aid trial period or some who are considering getting a hearing aid, this is an appropriate time to check on their progress. They may wish to raise some questions in the group. The break provides a good opportunity to explore this with each of these members personally.
5.0 *Communication Strategy Activity*
    5.1 Using the guidelines for lipreading activities in Chapter Four, a lipreading activity of mild difficulty should be conducted to illustrate one or more of the specific goals outlined in the guidelines.
    5.2 The rationale outlined in the guidelines should be kept in mind throughout these lipreading activities.
    5.3 The hearing-impaired group members should be encouraged to generalize their approach to lipreading to all communication situations.

6.0 *Homework Assignment*

    6.1 Each group member is asked to identify and describe several communication settings in which he or she had little or no difficulty. Group members should document this situation in a manner similar to that prescribed for the first week's assignment. They should pay special attention to the contribution of nonverbal cues.

Fifth Week

1.0 *Discussion of Homework Assignment*

    1.1 The purpose of this assignment is to help the group begin identifying strategies that members are using which facilitate communication. The discussion should include as many examples as possible to illustrate the variety of ingredients comprising a successful communication event. This discussion often becomes a turning point for many group members as they realize what others are doing to improve situations similar to those in which they have experienced difficulty.

2.0 *Formal Presentation*

    2.1 Continuation of fourth week (communication strategies).

    2.2 Stress strategies that have been identified as not being used by the group.

3.0 *Open Discussion of Formal Presentation*

    3.1 Continuation of the goals established for the fourth week's discussion.

    3.2 It is a good idea for the group leader to review the members' self-report responses in order to become familiar with their individual profiles. This will facilitate leading the discussion into areas relevant to all group members.

4.0 *Social Break*

    4.1 The best use of the group leader's time during this break is to check on the progress being made by those members considering amplification.

5.0 *Communication Strategy Activity*

    5.1 Six group members are seated in a circle. Each person is paired with the person sitting opposite him or her. Each pair is asked to carry on a conversation, ignoring the other conversations. The result is three separate conversations going on simultaneously. The activity is videotaped and analyzed by the group in terms of how the various participants handled this difficult listening situation. The activity may be repeated with different group members.

(Courtesy of C. Carmen and C. Freedenberg, University of California Hearing and Speech Center, San Francisco, California.)

5.2 This activity presents a graphic picture of which strategies individuals are or are not using and is one of the more popular activities.

5.3 Specific responses to auditory failure that are not being used can be emphasized.

6.0 *Homework Assignment*

6.1 By this time all group members should be aware of the necessity of approaching each communication setting with a plan for improving their ability to understand what is being said. Consequently, members are asked to identify a communication setting they will encounter, develop a plan to maximize communication, use the plan, and analyze its success.

Sixth Week

1.0 *Discussion of Homework Assignment*

1.1 The discussion of the various plans attempted by the group members will provide the framework for encouraging other plans specific to situations reported by group members. The group leader should use examples of situations common to all members and encourage repetition of this homework activity.

1.2 The group may wish to devote the remaining homework assignments to this activity. It provides an opportunity for the members to receive help with specific situations especially problematic for them.

2.0 *Formal Presentation*

2.1 The role of family members and close friends.

2.1.1 This topic is important because these are the people with whom the hearing-impaired persons spend most of their time and do most of their conversing. Their understanding of the problems of the hearing impaired is vital so that they can contribute to improved communication conditions.

2.1.2 Review of the options available to the hearing-impaired person.

2.1.3 Tips on what the family member or close friend can do to facilitate communication.

3.0 *Open Discussion of Formal Presentation*

3.1 The group leader should be aware that this discussion often produces an increased interaction between the hearing-impaired person and the family member or close friend attending the sessions. This interaction is important and may provide the groundwork for improved handling of communication problems.

    3.2 This discussion is also likely to produce comments which stray from the handling of communication situations. The group leader may have to remind the members of the ground rules and goals of the group.

4.0 *Social Break*

    4.1 The break usually becomes an extension of the above discussion.

5.0 *Communication Strategy Activity*

    5.1 Repeat the activity outlined for the fourth week.

    5.2 The activity could be increased in difficulty to challenge the members and provide an opportunity to discuss constructive approaches to various communication situations.

6.0 *Homework Assignment*

    6.1 The hearing-impaired group members should be encouraged to observe what normally hearing persons do when they experience an auditory failure.

    6.2 Those wearing hearing aids on a trial basis should tabulate the situations in which they believe their hearing performance improved as a result of wearing a hearing aid.

Seventh Week

1.0 *Discussion of Homework Assignment*

    1.1 At this point some attention should be focused on those persons considering amplification.

    1.2 The discussion of how normally hearing persons generally handle communication breakdowns lends itself to looking at dissimilarities and likenesses between their experiences with communication breakdown and the experiences of hearing-impaired persons. The conclusion should emerge that the major difference between them lies in the frequency of occurrence.

2.0 *Formal Presentation*

    2.1 Hearing and hearing disorders.

        2.1.1 Hearing disorders and audiograms.

        2.1.2 Hearing handicap.

        2.1.3 The role of amplification.

3.0 *Open Discussion of Formal Presentation*

    3.1 This discussion can go in a number of directions. It should provide an opportunity for the members to ask all the questions they have about hearing impairment in general and about their own hearing problems in particular.

3.2 In this discussion questions may be raised about the following topics:

    3.2.1 The progressive nature of sensorineural hearing impairment.

    3.2.2 The hereditary nature of hearing impairment.

    3.2.3 The destructive effects of hearing aids on residual hearing.

    3.2.4 The value of one versus two hearing aids.

    3.2.5 The status of surgery, vitamins, etc., in correcting sensorineural hearing impairment.

4.0 *Social Break*

    4.1 This break often becomes an extension of the above discussion.

5.0 *Communication Strategy Activities*

    5.1 Group members role-play a number of difficult listening situations and discuss how they could be handled.

    5.2 The use of visual, contextual, and situational cues should be stressed.

    5.3 Most of the suggested situations should come from the group.

6.0 *Homework Assignment*

    6.1 Group members retake the self-report inventory (the HPI) which was taken prior to the first session.

Eighth Week

1.0 *Discussion of Homework Assignment*

    1.1 This discussion can go in a number of directions. A simple lead-in question such as "How did you feel taking the test this time as opposed to how you felt when you first took it?" will start the discussion.

    1.2 The goal is to help the group members crystallize any insights they believe they have gained from participating in the group and to discuss how they applied them when retaking the test.

2.0 *Formal Presentation*

    2.1 Summary and review of program goals.

3.0 *Open Discussion of Formal Presentation*

    3.1 The group members may want to use this time to discuss how they benefited from attending the sessions.

4.0 *Social Break*

    4.1 Because this is the last session, the break tends to be longer and more social.

5.0 *Communication Strategy Activity*

    5.1 Review a list of dos and don'ts regarding handling communication situations.

5.2 Discuss and demonstrate appropriate use of a hearing aid.

6.0 *Homework Assignment*

6.1 Each group member should be encouraged to keep a detailed log of communication situations in which difficulty occurred to be reviewed in the individual follow-up visit approximately a month later.

6.2 Appointments should be made for the follow-up visit prior to the completion of the session. This is often done by circulating a sign-up sheet with available dates and times.

From *Hearing Handicapped Adults* (pp. 109–115) by T. G. Giolas, 1982, Englewood Cliffs, NJ: Prentice-Hall. Reprinted by permission.

ASSISTIVE LISTENING DEVICES AND SYSTEMS

Robert K. Lightfoot, Gwenyth R. Vaughn

Noise is the enemy of listeners and talkers of all ages. However, noise reverberation and distance can often be overcome by using assistive listening devices and systems (ALDS) to deliver the signal from the sound source to the ear of the listener (Bergman, 1983; Vaughn, 1983; Vaughn, Lightfoot, & Arnold, 1981). Under most circumstances these systems—to be described below—provide a favorable signal-to-noise ratio for both talkers and listeners—a ratio of particular importance to listeners with high-frequency hearing losses.

---

assessment of listening and talking needs

Hearing-impaired listeners are usually eager to describe the listening and talking situations in which they encounter difficulty understanding speech. Most of the talkers who associate with them confirm that interpersonal communication in noisy environments poses serious difficulties for both listeners and talkers. However, in spite of these widespread problems, audiologists have only recently begun to explore the potential of assistive listening devices and systems for providing conditions conducive to good communication.

After a traditional audiological assessment and hearing aid evaluation, the listener and one or more talkers associated with the listener should fill out a simple checklist on which problematic listening and talking situations are given. (A sample checklist is given in Appendix 13A.) The ultimate selection of one or more assistive listening devices usually depends upon both the life styles and the financial resources of the clients.

assistive listening devices and systems (ALDS)

Present amplification systems offer the options of: hardwire, infrared, FM, and loops. Important characteristics of personal listening devices include: portability, wearability, availability, and a broad price range. Modern large area systems consist of equipment that is easy to install and that requires no architectural modifications.

The following listing of hardwire, infrared, FM, and loop devices is not all-inclusive, but gives an overview that should be useful to the professional who is looking for solutions to noisy listening and talking situations. The description of the devices is divided into: (a) equipment-related listening, (b) one-to-one and small group listening and talking, and (c) medium and large-group listening and talking.

equipment-related listening devices

Equipment-related listening devices include those for use with a television, radio, stereo, and telephone.

Television, Radio, Stereo. If the listener is having difficulty understanding the television, radio or stereo, or if the hearing-impaired listener is disturbing other listeners by keeping the volume at a level that is uncomfortable for them, several devices are available.

Hardwire. The listener may use: (a) earphones, (b) headphones, (c) a cord to a transducer with a snap-in earmold, or (d) a behind-the-ear or body hearing aid with direct audio input. Optional extension cords can also be used to allow greater distance between the sound source and listener (Fig. 13.1).

The sound source may have: (a) one private listening jack that cuts off the internal speaker so only the listener with the assistive listening device can hear, or (b) two jacks—one that disconnects the internal speaker, and one that allows the internal speaker to operate as well as enable a hearing-impaired listener to use an assistive device. The volume control knob on the television is used to control the volume output for both group and private listening.

A problem for the hearing-impaired person arises when a normally hearing listener does not require the same volume level as the hearing-impaired listener. Under these circumstances, the hearing-impaired listener will need to use an ALDS with an amplifier, microphone, and earphone. The microphone is placed in front of the internal speaker of the television set, the listener puts on the earphones, and sets the amplifier volume to his preferred listening level. Other listeners are then free to use the volume control of the television to control the group listening level. This arrangement is also required if the television, radio, or stereo has no private listening jack. If the ALDS amplifier is coupled to a personal hearing aid that has no compression circuit, the volume level should be carefully controlled because of the combined gain potential.

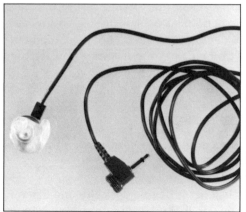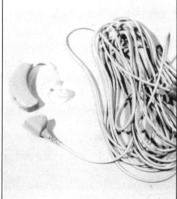

Figure 13.1. Cord to transducer with snap-in earmold (left). Direct audio input hearing aid and cord (right).

Earphones, extension cords, amplifiers, and microphones are available from: (a) Williams Sound (Fig. 13.2), and (b) retailers of audio equipment. Sennheiser produces high-quality headphones for use with audio equipment having one or more jacks.

Several hearing aid companies sell personal hearing aids with direct audio input. Phonic Ear, for example, manufactures a hearing aid with direct audio input that is combined with an external microphone on a long cord (Fig. 13.3). The microphone can be placed in front of the talker or near the speaker of the sound source. Another solution consists of using a radio with a TV band or small television set that can be placed near the listener's ear or hearing aid. This second set is tuned to the same station as the main viewing set.

When hardwire options are used, the listener has the inconvenience of being connected to the sound source by wires, which may present a mobility hazard to the listener and others. Since the cost of most hardwire ALDS is reasonable, many listeners use cost as a basis for selection.

Infrared. The listener may use: (a) a small, lightweight earphone with a rechargeable battery that is worn under the chin and connected to two acoustic tubes that fit into the ears, or (b) a lavaliere-style receiver into which earphones or a silhouette induction loop can be plugged that may be clipped to the clothing or worn on a cord around the neck. A receiver with two silhouette induction loops (Y-cord) for the magnetic coupling of two hearing aids with the telecoils is also available. Siemens' infrared receivers use rechargeable batteries; Contralonics receivers have disposable batteries. One of the advantages of infrared is that the listener is not connected to a sound source by wires.

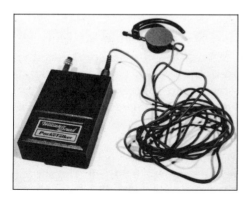 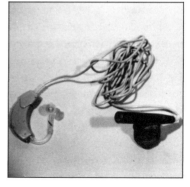

Figure 13.2. Microphone, Williams Sound PockeTalker, and earphone.

Figure 13.3. Direct audio input hearing aid and external microphone on long cord.

The infrared transmitter can be placed on top of the television and plugged into the private listening jack. The latest model comes with a microphone that can be located in front of the internal speaker of the sound source (Fig. 13.4). (The transmitter must be plugged into an AC outlet.) A small infrared transmitter can cover an area of approximately 30 feet. The "eye" on the receiver must be in the line of sight of the transmitter's light emitting diodes (LEDs).

Infrared transmitters for television, radio, and stereo are moderately priced. The same infrared receivers are used for both large and small transmitters. They are also relatively inexpensive. Infrared companies include Siemens and Contralonics.

FM. The listener may use an FM receiver with: (a) earphones or headphones, (b) a behind-the-ear or body hearing aid with direct input (Fig. 13.5), (c) a cord to a transducer with a snap-in earmold, (d) a silhouette or neck induction loop for pickup by a hearing aid telecoil (Fig. 13.6), or (e) a bone conduction receiver (Fig. 13.7).

To send signals it is necessary to have: (a) an FM transmitter plugged into the sound source or (b) a microphone located near the external speaker of the sound source (Fig. 13.8). The microphone may be placed in a windscreen to shield it from vibration or movement.

One advantage of the FM devices is that the listener is *not* wired to the sound source. FM units may have either rechargeable or disposable batteries. Several manufacturers of FM units are reducing prices of both transmitters and receivers. Companies with FM auditory trainers include Telex, Com-Tek, Phonic Ear, and Williams Sound.

Loops. The listener may use: (a) a hearing aid with a telecoil (Fig. 13.9), or (b) a POWR LOOP Receiver from Williams Sound that has an electromagnetic receiver with an earphone.

The television, radio, or stereo may have (a) an Oticon Minicon with an external microphone placed in front of the internal speaker of the sound source, (b) a Williams Sound or Carron loop positioned around the listening area and coupled to the sound source, or (c) a battery-powered Williams Sound PockeTalker with the microphone placed in front of the internal speaker and connected to the loop. Manufacturers of loops include Oticon, Williams Sound, and Carron.

The Phonear™ from Phonic Ear offers a shoulder teleloop and silhouette inductor loop that is used with a hearing aid telecoil. The shoulder teleloop and silhouette inductor are plugged into the Phonear, which is attached to the speaker grille of the sound source by a removable Velcro™ holder. The Phonear can also be used with direct audio input hearing aids (Fig. 13.10).

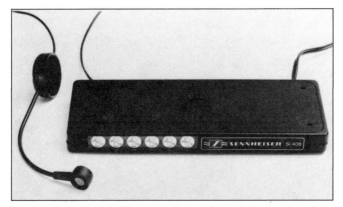

Figure 13.4. Infrared TV transmitter with external microphone.

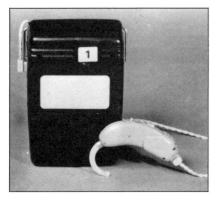

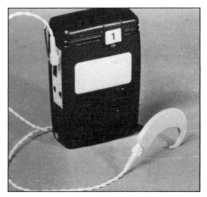

Figure 13.5. FM receiver with direct audio input hearing aid.

Figure 13.6. FM receiver with silhouette.

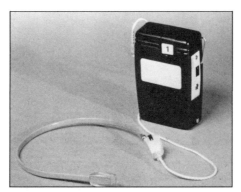

Figure 13.7. FM receiver with bone conduction receiver.

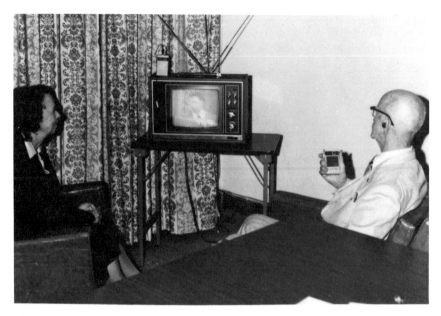

Figure 13.8. FM transmitter with microphone located near external speaker of sound source.

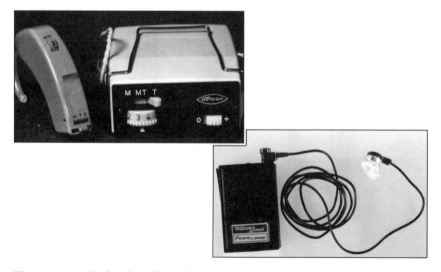

Figure 13.9. Ear level and body hearing aid with telecoil (left). Williams Sound POWR LOOP receiver with cord, transducer, and snap-in earmold (right).

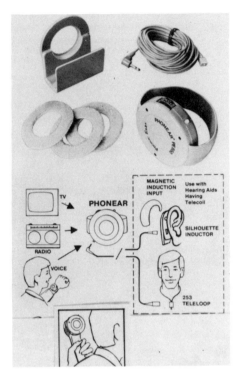

Figure 13.10. Phonic Ear Phonear.

When using the Phonear, the volume of the sound source is adjusted to a normal listening level for other listeners in the room. This should be done prior to setting the controls of either the Phonear or a personal hearing aid. The different settings should provide sound levels that are comfortable for all listeners.

Telephone

Hardwire. The listener may use an earphone and an amplifier with a magnetic pickup for coupling the amplifier to the telephone receiver. These components can be found at retailers of audio equipment. Whenever an ALDS is being used, the talker has to speak into the mouthpiece of the telephone as he or she normally would.

Telephone companies and telephone retail stores carry several types of modular handsets for amplifying speech reception (Fig. 13.11). Some handsets also amplify the voice of talkers who speak softly.

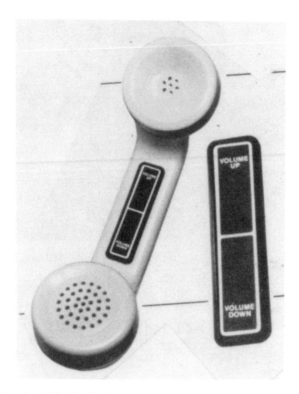

Figure 13.11. Amplified telephone handset receiver.

A speakerphone from Panasonic, the telephone company, or other retail stores can provide group listening. For additional amplification, some severely hearing-impaired persons hold the microphones of their body hearing aids or ALDS close to the speaker or speakerphone.

FM. A listener may use an FM receiver with: (a) earphones or headphones, (b) a behind-the-ear or body hearing aid with direct audio input, (c) a cord to a transducer with a snap-in earmold, (d) a silhouette earpiece or neck induction loop for pickup by the listener's hearing aid telecoil, or (e) a bone conduction receiver.

An FM transmitter using a magnetic pickup is coupled to the receiver of the telephone. The Com-Tek transmitter is equipped with an 1/8″ jack. The Com-Tek is the only FM system that is compatible with this magnetic telephone pickup. Regular FM receivers make it possible for one or many listeners to participate. Audio equipment stores also offer a magnetic suction pickup for use with the telephone (Fig. 13.12).

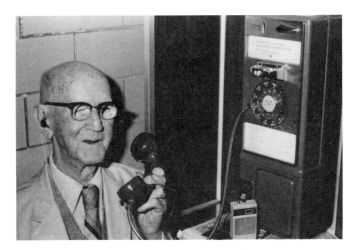

Figure 13.12. FM transmitter coupled to telephone receiver with magnetic pickup.

Teletypewriters. Most teletypewriters (TTY or TDD) require both the receiver and the sender to have a compatible receiver. Several companies offer TDDs that respond to Touchtone® telephones. The National Technical Institute for the Deaf has published a free 1983 brochure that provides excellent material on TDDs.

one-to-one and small group listening

Day rooms in retirement, rehabilitation, and nursing homes often offer multiple activities such as television watching, card games, handicraft instruction, and interpersonal communication. By using hardwire, infrared, FM, or loop systems, the hearing-impaired person can greatly reduce the interference from background noise. For one-to-one and small group communication, the following assistive listening devices are useful if the listener is self-wired or is using a windscreen. (See the section on self-wiring and windscreens that follows.) When a stronger signal is needed, the listener can hand the microphone of the ALDS to the talker.

Equipment-Related ALDS. For television, radio, or stereo listening, any number of persons can receive signals transmitted by infrared, FM, and loop. A hearing-impaired person using a hardwire device must place the microphone of his ALDS close to the internal speaker of the sound source. Listening/talking problems in automobiles can be overcome by using hardwire and FM assistive listening devices.

Hardwire. One-to-one or small group communication requires the listener to have: (a) earphones or headphones, (b) a cord to a transducer with a snap-in earmold, or (c) a behind-the-ear or body hearing aid with direct audio input that is plugged into an amplifier connected to a microphone.

The talker or sound source, in turn, needs a microphone placed (a) in front of the talker, (b) in the center of the table (Fig. 13.13), or (c) hanging above the small group. An optional windscreen may be used with the microphone (Fig. 13.13). Hardwire ALDS are available from Williams Sound and retailers of audio equipment.

Infrared. Siemens has a new device with built-in environmental microphones for one-to-one listening, called the Conferette (Fig. 13.14). The volume can be adjusted for each ear. The hearing aid option takes over if the infrared transmission is not strong enough.

FM. Listeners in medium-sized and large areas may use an FM receiver with: (a) earphones or headphones, (b) a behind-the-ear or body hearing aid with direct audio input, (c) a cord to a transducer with a snap-in earmold, (d) a silhouette or neck induction loop for pickup by a hearing aid telecoil, or (e) a bone conduction receiver.

The talker or sound source must have an FM transmitter with a microphone located near the source and an optional windscreen. (See the section on self-wiring for microphone placement.) Phonic Ear, Com-Tek, Williams Sound, and Telex offer these systems.

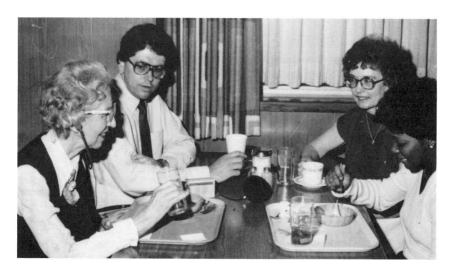

Figure 13.13. Microphone with windscreen placed in center of table.

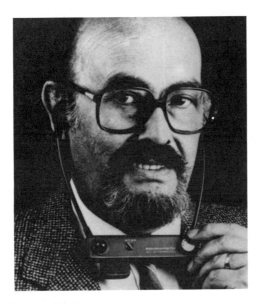

Figure 13.14. Siemens Conferette.

Loops. The listener needs: (a) a personal hearing aid with a telecoil or (b) a Williams POWR LOOP Receiver. The sound source may have a loop that is plugged into: (a) a public address system, (b) a battery-powered PockeTalker, or (c) an amplifier. Talkers using loops need to speak into microphones that are plugged into the amplifier or connected to the public address system. Oticon, Williams Sound, and Carron manufacture loops.

medium-sized and large area listening and talking systems

The selection of medium and large group assistive listening devices is dependent upon the number of listeners and talkers to be accommodated.

Infrared. The listener may use: (a) a small, lightweight earphone with a rechargeable battery that is worn under the chin and held by two acoustic tubes that fit into the ears, (b) a lavaliere-style receiver for use with headphones or with a single or a Y-cord silhouette induction loop for magnetic coupling with hearing aid telecoils. This is clipped to the clothing or worn on a cord around the neck.

The sound source must have: (a) a one-channel S-4 portable transmitter that is plugged into the existing public address system and an AC outlet; or (b) a one-channel S-5 portable transmitter with a microphone that is plugged into an AC outlet.

Optional portable transponders can be used to receive and redistribute signals for large areas. Infrared provides multichannel systems for simultaneous translations, cue systems in TV studios, sound monitoring in news rooms, instruction of foreign language-speaking personnel, and broadcasts to blind, hearing-impaired, and normally hearing persons in the same audience. Infrared systems are available from Siemens, Contralonics, and Sound Associates.

FM. Listeners in medium and large areas may use an FM receiver with: (a) earphones or headphones, (b) a behind-the-ear or body hearing aid with direct audio input, (c) a cord to transducer with a snap-in earmold, (d) a silhouette or neck induction loop for pickup by a hearing aid telecoil or (e) a bone conduction receiver (Fig. 13.15).

The talker or sound source must have an FM transmitter with a microphone located near the talker. The use of a windscreen is optional. (See the following section on self-wiring and windscreen placement.)

For those occasions when more than one microphone is used for large area listening, Phonic Ear is developing a unit that can receive several frequencies from different transmitters. These frequencies can be retransmitted on other frequencies that are matched to the listeners' receivers. This system can accommodate up to three microphones from

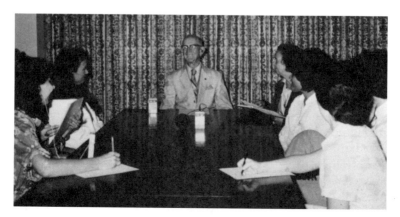

Figure 13.15. FM transmitter with microphone and windscreen placed in center of table. Receivers worn by people around table.

the speaker's platform and/or the audience. The multichannel transmitters of Telex (32 channels) and Phonic Ear (two channels) are useful in group situations or for communication between two persons with impaired hearing.

All the manufacturers of FM systems provide devices that are ideal for listening and talking on field trips, remote instruction for bicycle and horseback riding, or parachute jumping. FM auditory trainer companies include: Com-Tek, Telex, Williams Sound, and Phonic Ear.

Loops. The listener may use: (a) a hearing aid with a telecoil, or (b) a POWR LOOP Receiver.

The sound source may come from a loop that is driven by (a) a public address system, (b) a battery-powered PockeTalker from Williams Sound, or (c) an amplifier.

Multi-Options. By-Word produces hardwire, AM, and FM systems that provide receivers for unattended displays and exhibits. By-Word also offers large area listening systems for churches. Williams Sound manufacturers hardwire, AM, and FM options.

self-wiring and windscreens

The use of *self-wiring* (self-contained amplification with microphone and receiver components located on one person) can facilitate effective interpersonal communication. In one-to-one or small group listening situations, the listener can clip the microphone of a hardwire or FM system to a lapel, tie, or belt. This alleviates the disadvantage of having to be attached to a sound source by a cord. Careful placement of the microphone by the listener can help overcome the "cocktail noise" phenomenon that is so disconcerting to listeners and talkers. The distance at which the listener can satisfactorily pick up the talkers depends on the signal-to-noise ratio.

Both hardwire and FM devices are useful when the listener and talker are separated by the glass barriers used in outpatient clinics, pay windows, and bank drive-ins (Fig. 13.16). The listeners can overcome these listening obstacles by being self-wired or by handing the microphone to the talker.

Assistive listening devices can be utilized during interviewing and counseling sessions in an office, by supervisors when instructing wor-

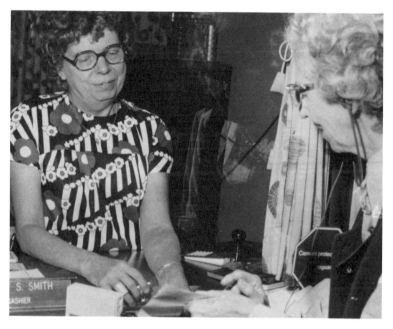

Figure 13.16. Microphone handed through opening in glass barrier to overcome background noise.

kers in noisy environments, for clinical communication between the health-care team and patients, and for support of seriously ill persons by clergy. Conversation with family members and friends can also be facilitated by assistive listening devices in noisy gathering places and in automobiles.

Placing the microphone in a windscreen works well for listening to groups around a table. The microphone can be put in a windscreen and placed in the center of the table or hung above the table. The windscreen helps overcome wind and air conditioning noise, road and table vibration, and other environmental disturbances.

summary

A hardwire device is inexpensive, but the listener is connected to the talker, unless self-wiring is used. FM systems are expensive, but they offer the advantage of providing 300 or more feet of transmission. FM devices from the various companies can be interchanged as long as the receivers match the transmitting frequencies. Care should be taken when using wide band FM for one part of the system and narrow band FM for the other. The resulting sound quality is not as good as when the band widths are the same. New advances in multichannel FM transmitters and receivers will facilitate broader utilization of FM assistive listening devices. (FM and loop systems do not provide the privacy of hardwire and infrared systems.) Siemens has adapted the small infrared transmitter presently used for television for use with modular telephones, small table conferences, and teleconferences. Single and multichannel large area infrared transmission systems are also available.

conclusion

At a time when young people are proudly appearing in public with large earphones for listening to music, many hearing-impaired persons are trying to hide even the small behind-the-ear hearing aids. Users in the first group ignore the fact that they may ruin their hearing; users in the latter group recoil from admitting that they need to enhance their hearing.

Perhaps a middle group will be formed by those normally hearing and hearing-impaired listeners and their associates who recognize the benefits noise-free listening and talking can provide through use of assistive listening devices.

Rehabilitative audiologists must assume a major responsibility in meeting the needs of the vastly increasing population of persons with hearing problems who are struggling to communicate in noise-polluted environments.

acknowledgments

The materials presented in this section were developed under the Veterans Administration Exchange of Medical Information Program and are presently supported by VA Rehabilitation Research and Development.

Portions of this article were taken from *SHAA* (Journal of the Speech and Hearing Association of Alabama), ''Assistive Listening Devices and Systems (ALDS),'' 1985, *13*, 25–33.

recommended information sources

The following are sources of information on assistive listening devices (ALDS).

organizations

Alexander Graham Bell Association for the Deaf, 3417 Volta Place, N.W., Washington, DC 20007 (202) 337-5220

The American Academy of Otolaryngology, 1101 Vermont Avenue, N.W., Washington, DC 20005 (202) 289-4607

The American Humane Association, 9725 East Hampden Avenue, Denver, CO 80231 (American Humane Association National Hearing Dog Project)

The American Speech-Language-Hearing Association (ASHA), 10801 Rockville Pike, Rockville, MD 20852 1-800-638-6868 (202) 987-5700 Extension 231

The National Association for Hearing and Speech Action, 10801 Rockville Pike, Rockville, MD 20852 1-800-638-8255

The National Hearing Aid Society, 20361 Middlebelt Road, Livonia, MI 48152 (313) 478-2610

The National Information Center on Deafness, Gallaudet College, 800 Florida Avenue, N.E., Washington, DC 20002

The National Technical Institute for the Deaf (NTID), One Lomb Memorial Drive, P.O. Box 9887, Rochester, NY 14623

The Organization for the Use of the Telephone (OUT), P.O. Box 175, Owing Mills, MD 21117 (301) 655-1827

Telecommunications for the Deaf, Inc., 814 Thayer Avenue, Silver Spring, MD 20910

publications

One of the most valuable publications is SHHH (Self-Help for Hard of Hearing People). The SHHH organization publishes a periodical that addresses the needs of hard-of-hearing persons and provides extensive information on assistive devices. Joining SHHH would be advantageous to professionals and students.

SELF-HELP FOR HARD OF HEARING PEOPLE, INC.
7800 Wisconsin Avenue
Bethesda, MD 20814
(301) 657-2249

videotapes

Several videotapes demonstrate the selection of ALDS. These tapes are appropriate for practicing and teaching professionals, students, and hearing-impaired persons.

> *Assistive Devices for Hearing-Impaired Persons* (1986) (17 minutes)
> *Don't Forget It* (1987) (10 minutes)
>> New York League for the Hard of Hearing
>> 71 West 23rd Street
>> New York, NY 10010-4162
>> (212) 741-3145
> *Now Hear This*, Vaughn, G. R., & Lightfoot, R. K. (1984) (22 minutes)
>> Sertoma International Foundation
>> Post Office Box 17003
>> Kansas City, MO 64132
>> (816) 444-7344

For additional information, including a list of over 100 references on ALDS, write or call: Audiology–Speech Pathology Service, VA Medical Center, 700 South 19th Street, Birmingham, AL 35233 (205) 933-8101, Extension 6702/01. G. R. Vaughn, Ph.D., or Robert K. Lightfoot, M.S.

references and recommended readings

Bergman, M. (1983). Assistive listening devices. Part 1: New responsibilities. *Asha, 25,* 19–22.

Castle, D. (1983). *What you should know about TDD's.* Rochester, NY: National Technical Institute of the Deaf.

Lipscomb, D.M. (1970, October). *The increase of prevalence of high frequency hearing impairment among college students.* Paper presented at the meeting of the X International Congress of Audiology, Poland.

Lipscomb, D.M. (1972). Environmental noise is growing—Is it damaging our hearing? *Clinical Pediatrics, 1,* 374–375.

Maurer, J.E., McCartney, J.H., & Sorenson, F. (1974). *Some characteristics of hearing impaired among low income elderly.* Paper presented at the meeting of the Gerontological Society, Miami Beach, FL.

Vaughn, G.R. (1983). Assistive listening devices. Part II: Large area sound systems. *Asha, 25,* 25–30.

Vaughn, G.R., & Lightfoot, R.K. (1985). Assistive listening devices and systems (ALDS). *SHAA, 13,* 25–33.

Vaughn, G.R., Lightfoot, R.K., & Arnold, L.C. (1981). Alternative listening devices and delivery systems for audiologic habilitation of hearing impaired persons. *Journal of the Academy of Rehabilitative Audiology, 14,* 62–77.

Vaughn, G.R., Lightfoot, R.K., & Gibbs, S.D. (1983). Assistive listening devices. Part III: SPACE. *Asha, 25,* 33–46.

APPENDIX THIRTEEN A

listening and talking selection checklist

Some of the information that would help us make suggestions concerning assistive listening devices and large area sound systems is listed below. If you want us to assist you further, please check the appropriate items and return this form to us.

listening and talking situations

I have difficulty understanding:

____television or radio

____in an automobile

____one person at mealtime or around home

____in a restaurant or dining room

____around a conference table

____at a party

____a small family group

____walking down the street

____in the theater (play)

____in the movies

____at church

____in a classroom

____in a conference or lecture hall

____other (please list)

_____

_____

_____

amplification devices

___I do not have a hearing aid.
___I am pleased with my hearing aid.
___I do not wish to use a regular hearing aid.
___My hearing aid has a telephone switch.
___I can afford an alternative system that costs:
   ___$100.00   ___$300.00   ___$600.00

large area sound systems

My community has the following systems:
   ___Hardwire (___church, ___theater, ___movies, ___other)
   ___Infrared (___church, ___theater, ___movies, ___other)
   ___FM (___church, ___theater, ___movies, ___other)
   ___Loop (___church, ___theater, ___movies, ___other)

AURAL REHABILITATION FOR THE VISUALLY AND HEARING-IMPAIRED PATIENT

Adrienne Karp

Government surveys indicate 2.7 million Americans suffer dual vision and hearing handicaps. The largest proportion are the deaf:vision-impaired, followed then by the vision-impaired:hearing-impaired, the blind:hearing-impaired and the deaf:blind (Hicks & Pfau, 1979). The importance of auditory skills to a visually handicapped person is well documented and the study of hearing is included in the training curriculum of many professionals who work with the blind. In comparison, few hearing-health professionals have adequate knowledge of abnormal vision. Most of us are poorly informed about eye pathologies and their functional consequences, although adequate sight is required for speechreading and interpretation of sign language. Visual impairment is also known to adversely affect a patient's adjustment to the use of a hearing aid. The purpose of this article is to provide the reader with information about functional consequences of specific eye conditions and to suggest modifications of aural rehabilitation techniques necessitated by abnormal visual functioning.

Loss of vision is our most feared chronic affliction even though it is not as widespread as hearing impairment. According to a 1980 report of the National Society for the Prevention of Blindness, 11.5 million Americans have some degree of irreversible vision impairment. Only 500,000 of those are classified as legally blind, but a much higher proportion are unable to see well enough to read ordinary newsprint. Approximately 100,000 people in the United States have no useful vision at all.

legal blindness

An individual is considered legally blind if either visual acuity or peripheral vision is worse than the following specified limits. Visual acuity, the ability to see and identify objects at a distance, can be no better than 20/200 in the better eye with the use of corrective lenses. In other words, the legally blind person may only distinguish at a distance of 20 feet what a normal eye is able to from 200 feet away. This amount of vision allows a person to travel adequately without the assistance of a cane, guide dog, or sighted guide, but severely affects the ability to read print, speechread, and see the parts of a hearing aid. An equally important parameter of visual functioning is the size of the patient's peripheral visual field. Normal bilateral field vision measures 180°. If a patient has peripheral vision of less than 20° he/she may be classified as legally blind. Patients with constricted peripheral fields (also known as tunnel vision) often have adequate central visual acuity which allows them to see print and other fine detail, but they have difficulty traveling safely around their environment because of an inability to see obstacles not directly in their path.

visual impairment

The overall functioning of a hearing handicapped patient is significantly affected by poor vision. Because some visual impairments are not obvious to the observer, the audiologist is advised to ask each patient about visual functioning when a case history is taken. Questions contained in Appendix 13B will help determine a patient's visual capabilities. In addition, the audiologist can utilize the Snellen Chart to test visual acuity.

Of all the causes for impaired vision, those resulting from refractive errors are the most widespread in our society. They occur when the structures of the eye which bend light (cornea and lens) onto the retina are not a normal shape. Since such errors can be reversed with corrective lenses, people with refractive errors are not at issue in this article. It is the 11.5 million Americans whose vision cannot be fully restored with lenses or medical intervention to whom attention is given here.

Individuals with irreversible visual impairments who still retain a significant amount of usable sight are known as "low vision" patients. In a sense, low vision is analogous to sensori-neural hearing loss since neither can be cured or restored completely to normal function. Refractive errors discussed in the previous paragraph could, on the other hand, be viewed as analogous to conductive hearing loss. A simple refractive adjustment can bring vision into clear focus in most cases. Although they are handicapped by their visual impairment, many low vision patients are not legally blind since their sight may not be equal to or worse than the specified limits of 20/200 acuity or 20° peripheral vision.

Visual impairment does not always imply severe handicap. Over 90% of the low vision population retain a good deal of usable sight. The remaining 6 to 10%, however, are severely impaired and require the assistance of guide dogs, canes, or sighted guides for traveling purposes. With no appreciable amount of useful vision, they are dependent on tactile cues and audition for orientation and learning tasks.

Editor's Note: For a discussion on the use of the Snellen Chart for assessing far visual acuity of hearing-impaired persons, see D. Johnson and F. Caccamise, "Hearing-impaired students: Options for far visual acuity screening," *American Annals of the Deaf*, 1983, *128*, 402–406.

central field vs. peripheral field defects

The most common cases of nonrefractive low vision impairments (those not fully reversible with corrective lenses) treated in a general ophthalmologic practice involve conditions which affect *central visual acuity*, the ability to clearly distinguish objects which are directly in our path of vision. Central field defects can result in overall blurry vision such as that experienced by people with cataracts. Other pathologies, like macular degeneration, affect central acuity by resulting in a gray or blurry spot known as a scotoma. These patchy spots can effectively block out discrete portions of a visual image. When central vision becomes impaired, a person has immediate awareness because the capacity to see fine detail is affected. Such a disability has consequences for many activities of daily living which are dependent on the ability to read print, thread a needle, work at a job involving small objects, see the temperature settings on an oven, or identify the price of foods on the labels of items at supermarkets. Most people with central visual dysfunction are over age 60.

A potentially more disabling type of vision problem is that resulting in *constricted peripheral fields*. This dysfunction interferes with the ability to see obstacles which are not in the direct line of sight, with drastic consequences relative to the ease with which people are able to move around the environment independently. This type of visual field defect may develop so insidiously that individuals are unaware of its existence until the advanced stages. People with constricted peripheral fields find themselves tripping over obstacles and bumping into obstructions which are no longer visible. It is often assumed that other people are placing obstacles where they cannot be seen. It is not until many accidents are sustained that these persons may seek help from an eye specialist. A number of pathologies which cause peripheral field loss eventually affect central vision as well, thereby leading to blindness. Some of the more common etiologies resulting in peripheral field loss are glaucoma, retinitis pigmentosa, and optic nerve atrophy.

eye pathology and treatment

Causes of visual disorders are numerous. Table 13.1 provides brief descriptions for some of the more familiar and prevalent etiologies of visual disorders and their recommended treatments.

In addition to conditions which cause visual dysfunction in isolation, there are numbers of systematic conditions which result in both vision and hearing impairment. Table 13.2 lists the more common of these conditions.

The interested reader can investigate several recommended references which are listed at the end of this material for more detailed information concerning the visually or dually visually and hearing-impaired patient.

aural rehabilitation strategies for central visual defects

When considering a program of auditory training for the dually handicapped, it becomes necessary for the audiologist to alter rehabilitation techniques. The patient whose central vision alone is impaired will have considerable difficulty discriminating fine visual detail. Speechreading skills may no longer be useful in compensating for the hearing impairment. Because people with central visual defects are mainly over 60 years of age, presbycusis is often the cause of their hearing loss. Consonant sounds, which are difficult for them to hear, are now difficult for them to see as well. This often leads them to believe that their visual and auditory impairments are neurologically connected and, as they lose one sense, they will necessarily lose the other. An explanation of the role of speechreading in compensating for a high-frequency impairment is of great assistance to these patients. A large central scotoma is also likely to interfere with a patient's capacity to see the lips or the face of the speaker, thereby negating the benefits of visual cues.

If speechreading does prove to be a viable training technique, lighting used in the therapy area is of considerable significance. Many people with vision problems, no matter what the cause or visual consequence, report glare to be one of the most debilitating conditions associated with their eye pathology. A low vision specialist, either an ophthalmologist, optometrist or low vision nurse, should be consulted regarding the type of lighting required to help with this problem. For more information about proper illumination, the reader is referred to a book by Faye entitled *Clinical Low Vision* (see references).

Hearing aid selection for the patient with poor central vision alone needs to be primarily concerned with help in understanding conversation. Fitting parameters (i.e., gain, output, frequency emphasis, and earmold style) are no different for this population than for those with normal vision. Eyeglass hearing aids are not usually the style of choice since many visually handicapped people use different optical devices for different visual tasks. It is impractical for more than one pair of eyeglasses to house the needed hearing aids. It is important to know if a patient uses low vision aids such as special lenses or magnifiers to see fine detail, since these devices should be utilized during hearing aid management training.

For those patients who depend on sign language for communication purposes, interpretation ability will be affected by a central visual impairment. Hand movements must be made in that portion of the patient's field where vision is best and signs should be slowed down to help compensate for distorted visual clues.

TABLE 13.1
Eye Pathologies Resulting in Low Vision

Eye Pathology	Etiology	Visual Dysfunction	Usual Age of Onset	Medical Treatment	Cure
Cataracts	numerous theories exist	cloudy vision due to opacity of crystalline lens of eye	usually occurs in aging eyes but can be 2° to retinitis pigmentosa & congenital rubella	surgery and lens replacement	usually good surgical success
Diabetic retinopathy	possible consequence of diabetes	overall blurred vision due to proliferation of retinal blood vessels with hemorrhages into vitreous fluid	dependent on type, severity and age of onset of diabetic condition	laser beam treatments to cauterize blood vessels	prognosis is guarded and changes in vision may be rapid and unpredictable
Glaucoma (open angle)	increased intra-ocular fluid pressure	peripheral field loss leading to blindness if untreated	usually after 40 years of age	eye drops; laser treatments	none: condition can be arrested but damage cannot be reversed
Macular degeneration (atrophic)	vascular insufficiency	blurred or blotched central vision	usually occurs in adults over 60 years of age	none	none
Macular degeneration (exudative)	vascular abnormality	blurred or blotched central vision	usually occurs in adults over 60 years of age	early laser treatment in selected cases	laser treatment may arrest the progression of the condition; otherwise no known cure

TABLE 13.1 (Continued)

Eye Pathology	Etiology	Visual Dysfunction	Usual Age of Onset	Medical Treatment	Cure
Optic atrophy	too numerous to list	peripheral field loss	any age	none	none
Retinitis pigmentosa (RP)	genetic inheritance	night blindness; progressive peripheral visual field loss which eventually leads to total blindness	late childhood	none	none
Retinopathy of prematurity (ROP)	excessive exposure to oxygen in early life	overall cloudy vision or blindness due to proliferative retinopathy and/or tissue growth behind crystalline lens	neonatally, especially in premature and low birth weight infants	none	none
Strabismus	weakness of lateral eye muscles or disturbance in nerve innervation of those muscles	diplopia (double vision) may lead to amblyopia in one eye (functional blindness with no evidence of pathology)	at birth	surgery and/or exercise	usually good success with early intervention

TABLE 13.2
Conditions Involving Vision and Hearing Loss

Medical Condition	Etiology	Eye Pathology	Hearing Impairment	Usual Age of Onset
Age-related sensory impairment	aging process	several pathologies including cataracts, macular degeneration, glaucoma and diabetic retinopathy	sensorineural loss	older adulthood
Cogan's Syndrome Type I	unknown	non-syphilitic corneal inflammation (interstitial keratitis)	tinnitus, vertigo, fluctuating sensorineural loss eventually becoming severe and intractable	early adulthood; more often in males
Congenital rubella	maternal rubella; most damaging in first trimester of pregnancy	congenital cataract and glaucoma; may be unstable	mild to profound sensorineural loss	at birth
Congenital syphilis	maternal syphilitic condition at conception	syphilitic inflammation of the cornea (interstitial keratitis)	progressive sensorineural loss sometimes leading to deafness	adulthood

TABLE 13.2 (Continued)

Medical Condition	Etiology	Eye Pathology	Hearing Impairment	Usual Age of Onset
Didmoad Syndrome	genetic inheritance	peripheral field loss 2° optic atrophy	progressive high-frequency sensorineural	early adulthood in persons with juvenile diabetes mellitus
Low birth weight; prematurity	numerous causes	overall blurred vision 2° to retinopathy of prematurity (ROP)	any type and severity	at birth
Sickle-cell anemia	genetic inheritance	overall poor vision 2° proliferative retinopathy	severe sensorineural loss greater in low frequencies	early adulthood
Usher's Syndrome	genetic inheritance	peripheral field loss eventually leading to total blindness 2° retinitis pigmentosa	sensorineural loss, most often congenital and profound	late childhood

aural rehabilitation strategies for peripheral field defects and blindness

The patient who has no usable vision or an extensive peripheral field loss requires auditory cues not only for conversation but for orientation and traveling purposes as well. Hearing aids must provide this patient both with the ability to understand and with adequate localization skills in order to compensate for inadequate vision. This, of course, requires microphone placement at the ear and necessitates binaural hearing aid fittings for bilateral hearing loss. If the hearing loss is unilateral or assymmetrical, localization skills may be harder to achieve. CROS aids may then be considered.

Post-auricular or ITE aids are the styles of choice. Some severely hearing-impaired patients may require a body aid or auditory trainer for conversation and classroom use, but these should be used only indoors since the microphone placement may impair localization skills needed for traveling. In order to select the proper amplification for mobility purposes, hearing aids must be tested in real life circumstances as well as in a sound-treated testing chamber. Whether this will be on a quiet suburban street or a noisy city street will depend on where the individual patient travels with the aids.

Because of the masking effects of wind and rain, many visually impaired patients prefer not using their hearing aids outdoors. This problem can be partially resolved with a windscreen over the microphone.

The dually-handicapped person often uses audition to determine distance from a danger signal. Such need necessitates the reduction of compression amplification. The bus that is five feet away should not be made to sound like the car 50 feet away.

People with severe visual impairments which affect independent travel need low-frequency as well as high-frequency information. It is not advisable to amplify only high frequencies for speech discrimination. Hearing aids with wide-band frequency response and external tone controls should be considered. The patient can be taught to set the tone control depending on the auditory need at that moment. Microphone type is also an important issue with this population. Uni-directional microphones are recommended for conversational settings, but traveling requires an omnidirectional type. For this reason, it is advisable to fit hearing aids with dual microphone settings which the patient can manipulate depending on the listening situations.

The blind patient needs to rely on tactile cues rather than vision to master hearing aid management. Many patients with peripheral field defects, however, have adequate central acuity and can be taught to handle their aids by visual means. For those who cannot, plastic models of ears can be useful in teaching how to insert a hearing aid into the ear. Battery insertion and manipulation of external controls can be taught using enlarged drawings made with felt tipped pens or through tactile cues alone.

Speechreading abilities will be contingent upon the extent of sight remaining in the patient's central field of vision. Not all peripheral defects impinge on central acuity, certainly not in their beginning stages. Many patients with tunnel vision have extensive use of their central visual areas and can learn to speechread quite effectively.

Sign language communication requires enough adequate central vision to see hand movement. Fingerspelling will be more difficult for any visually-impaired patient to follow, but more so for those with central acuity difficulties. Tunnel vision, however, will also affect sign language interpretation because of the constriction in the area which now carries the visual image. Distance from the visually-impaired person should be determined individually to afford each patient the optimal visual fields. Signs should be delivered more slowly and the magnitude of the presentations should be reduced as well (Hicks, 1979).

summary and conclusions

The following is a summary of recommendations which should be employed when treating a patient with dual vision and hearing impairments:

1. Determine the existence and functional consequences of any noncorrectable visual disorder through case history and contact with the patient's eye care specialist.

2. Select amplification which addresses orientation and localization needs as well as speech reception and discrimination capabilities.

3. Design speechreading programs appropriate to the amount and type of remaining vision. Set realistic training goals accordingly.

4. Reduce glare in the therapy environment.

5. Adjust the speed, distance and magnitude of sign language presentations to promote better communication with the deaf/visually impaired patient.

Patients with dual vision and hearing impairments may not be receiving the best rehabilitation available to them. They are often treated separately for their vision and hearing disorders with no dialogue between managing health care professionals. The purpose of this article has been to acquaint audiologists with the causes and consequences of a variety of eye pathologies so that aural rehabilitation techniques can be modified in accordance with a patient's visual impairment.

references and recommended readings

readings for visually and dually visually- hearing-impaired persons

Faye, E. (1984). *Clinical low vision* (2nd ed.). Boston: Little, Brown & Co.

Geeraets, W. (1976). *Ocular syndromes* (3rd ed.). Philadelphia: Lea & Febiger.

Hicks, W. (1979). Communication variables associated with hearing-impaired/vision-impaired persons—a pilot study. *American Annals of the Deaf*, 124, 419–422.

Hicks, W., & Pfau, G. (1979). Deaf-visually impaired persons: Incidence and services. *American Annals of the Deaf*, 124, 76–92.

Kauvar, K. (1982.) *Eyes only*. Norwalk, CT: Appleton-Century-Crofts.

National Society for the Prevention of Blindness (NSPB). (1977). *Understanding eye language (P607/77)*. New York: NSPB.

National Society for the Prevention of Blindness (NSPB). (1980). *Vision problems in the U.S.* New York: NSPB.

Note. An earlier version of this material first appeared in the *Journal of the Academy of Rehabilitative Audiology*, 16, 1983, pp. 23–32. Used here with permission.

APPENDIX THIRTEEN B

questions to assist in identifying possible visual impairments

1. Do you have any problems with your vision? What kind?

2. Did your doctor tell you what is causing your vision problem?

3. Does anyone else in your family have the same problem?

4. Do you wear eyeglasses or contact lenses? Do they help you see normally?

5. Do you use any other optical devices to see better?

6. Can you see my mouth clearly?

7. Do you have a great deal of trouble seeing at night or in dim light?

8. Do you bump into obstacles more often than other people?

Editor's Note. For further discussion of questions that may assist in identifying possible visual impairments in the hearing-impaired population see F. Caccamise et al., (1980), ''Visual Assessment and the Rehabilitation of Hearing-Impaired Children and Adults,'' *Journal of the Academy of Rehabilitative Audiology,* XIII, 78–101, and D. Johnson and F. Caccamise, (1982), ''Visual Assessment of Hearing-Impaired Persons: Options and Implications for the Future,'' *Journal of the Academy of Rehabilitative Audiology,* XV, 22–40.

DEFINITION OF AND COMPETENCIES FOR AURAL REHABILITATION

ASHA committee on rehabilitative audiology

The following Committee on Rehabilitative Audiology Report was adopted by the ASHA Legislative Council in November, 1983. Present and past committee members responsible for the development of this statement include O.T. Kenworthy, past Chair; James McCartney, current Chair; Evelyn Cherow, ex officio; Jaclyn Gauger, Robert Hinkle, Antonia Maxon, Mary Pat Moeller, Mary Jo Osberger, Thomas Rees, Jan Colton, Cheryl Deconde, Gene Del Polito, William Haas, Gerri Kahn, Dorothy Stein, Dean Garstecki, and Vice Presidents for Clinical Affairs, Hughlett Morris and David Yoder.

E. Cherow, Director
Audiology Liaison Branch

background

Some apparent contradictions among ASHA policies, as well as discrepancies between those policies and clinical practice, have obscured who should provide services in aural rehabilitation and who should supervise those services.

- A position paper adapted by Legislative Council in 1973 (*Asha*, 1974), The Audiologist: Responsibilities in the Habilitation of the Auditorily Handicapped, indicated that the audiologist is the main provider and supervisor of aural rehabilitation.

- A resolution by the American Board of Examiners in Speech-Language Pathology and Audiology (ABESPA) (ABESPA, 1979), now the Professional Standards Council, specified some supervisory roles in aural rehabilitation: audiologists supervise assessment procedures, including hearing aid selection and fitting, and speech-language pathologists supervise speech and language assessment of the hearing-impaired clients. No position was taken about supervision of intervention.

- Meanwhile, in actual practice, many speech-language pathologists provide services to hearing-impaired clients, particularly in settings where such services by an audiologist are not available. There continued to be differences among audiologists and differences among speech-language pathologists in their interests, training, experience, and competencies in aural rehabilitation.

The apparent discrepancies between Association policy and clinical practice led this Committee to shift the focus of debate over who should provide aural rehabilitation services. Rather than endorse either audiologists or speech-language pathologists as the primary service provider, the Committee chose to delineate comprehensive service delivery as a set of proposed minimal competencies (Committee on Rehabilitative Audiology, 1980). Those minimal competencies however, did not offer a corresponding definition of aural rehabilitation and did not address current variations in clinicians' skills, interests, and training. Therefore, this report proposes:

- a revised definition of aural rehabilitation that is consistent with the proposed minimal competencies and complements the definition provided in the 1973 Position Statement; and,

- a revision of the minimal competencies that subdivides the required body of special knowledge into areas of expertise consistent with present clinical practice.

definition of aural rehabilitation

Aural rehabilitation refers to services and procedures for facilitating adequate receptive and expressive communication in individuals with hearing impairment. These services and procedures are intended for those persons who demonstrate a loss of hearing sensitivity or function in communicative situations as if they possess a loss of hearing sensitivity. The services and procedures include, but are not limited to:

I. Identification and Evaluation of Sensory Capabilities

    A. Identification and evaluation of the extent of the impairment, including assessment, periodic monitoring and reevaluation of auditory abilities.

    B. Monitoring of other sensory capabilities (e.g., visual and tactile-kinesthetic) as they relate to receptive and expressive communication.

    C. Evaluation, fitting and monitoring of auditory aids and monitoring of other sensory aids (e.g., visual and vibrotactile) used by the auditorily handicapped person in various communicative environments (e.g., home, work and school). Such auditory and sensory aids are taken to include all amplification systems (group and individual), as well as such supplementary devices as telephone amplifiers, alarm systems and so on.

    D. Evaluation and monitoring of the acoustic characteristics of the communicative environments confronted by the hearing-impaired person.

II. Interpretation of Results, Counseling and Referral

    A. Interpretation of audiologic findings to the client, his/her family, employer, teachers, and significant others involved in communication with the hearing-impaired person.

    B. Guidance and counseling for the client, his/her family, employer, caregiver, teachers and significant others concerning the educational, psychosocial and communicative effects of hearing impairment.

    C. Guidance and counseling for the parent/caregiver regarding:
- educational options available;
- selection of educational programs; and
- facilitation of communicative and cognitive development.

    D. Individual and/or family counseling regarding:
- acceptance and understanding of the hearing impairment;
- functioning within difficult listening situations;
- facilitation of effective strategies and attitudes toward communication;

- modification of communicative behavior in keeping with those strategies and attitudes; and,
- promotion of independent management of communication-related problems.

    E. Referral for additional services (e.g., medical, psychological, social, and educational), as appropriate.

III. Intervention for Communicative Difficulties

    A. Development and provision of an intervention program to facilitate expressive and receptive communication.

    B. Provision of hearing and speech conservation programming.

    C. Service as a liaison between the client, family and other agencies concerned with the management of communicative disorders related to hearing impairment.

IV. Re-evaluation of the client's status

V. Evaluation and modification of the intervention program

proposed minimal competencies for the provision of aural rehabilitation

Definition of Terms:

The terms *basic knowledge, basic understanding,* and *special knowledge* require some specification before proceeding to the proposed competencies. Considered relative to the familiar taxonomy of Bloom (1956; Bloom, Hastings, & Madaus, 1971) we would define these terms as follows:

- Basic knowledge incorporates what Bloom refers to as *knowledge.* It involves the "recall of specifics and universals, recall of methods and processes, or recall of a pattern, structure or setting" (Bloom et al., 1971, p. 271).

- Basic understanding may be equated with Bloom's category of *comprehension.* "This represents the lowest level of understanding or apprehension such that the individual knows what is being communicated and can make use of the material or idea . . . without necessarily relating it to other material or seeing its fullest implications" (p. 272). This may involve the processes of translation, interpretation and/or extrapolation.

- Special knowledge refers to the remainder of Bloom's categories which include *application, analysis, synthesis,* and *evaluation.* It is at this level that the learner is expected to not only possess knowledge but also to demonstrate the ability to apply and elaborate upon the knowledge.

Basic Knowledge and Basic Understanding

Persons providing aural rehabilitation should demonstrate:

    I. A basic knowledge of general psychology, sociology, mathematics, general physics, zoology, human anatomy and physiology.

   II. A basic understanding of normal communication processes, including:

        A. Anatomic and physiologic bases for the normal development and use of speech, language and hearing; such as, anatomy, neurology, and physiology of speech, language and hearing mechanisms;

        B. Physical bases and processes of the production and perception of speech and hearing; such as, (a) acoustics or physics of sound, (b) phonology, (c) physiologic and acoustic phonetics, (d) perceptual processes, and (e) psychoacoustics; and,

        C. Linguistics and psycholinguistic variables related to the normal development and use of speech, language, and hearing; such as, (a) linguistics (historical, descriptive, sociolinguistics, urban language), (b) psychology of language, (c) psycholinguistics, (d) language and speech acquisition, and (e) verbal learning and verbal behavior.

Special Knowledge

   III. A special knowledge of the following areas should be demonstrated, depending upon whether the chosen area of expertise is to be adults (A), children (C) or hearing aid selection (H):

Area of Expertise

        A. As regards *auditory system disorders*, persons should be able to:

ACH   • identify, describe and differentiate the various disorders of auditory function such as disorders of the outer, middle and inner ear, the auditory nerve and the associated neural and central auditory system pathways.

        B. As regards *audiologic assessment procedures*, persons must be able to:

ACH   • provide and interpret pure-tone and speech audiometric measures used to evaluate peripheral and central auditory functions including, but not limited to, measures of threshold sensitivity and measures to differentiate sites of auditory dysfunction.

ACH   • identify and perform screening examinations for speech and language problems.

ACH   • determine the need for referral to other medical and nonmedical specialists for appropriate professional services.

  C. As regards *evaluation of personal and group amplification, and other sensory aids*, persons must be able to:

ACH   • perform and interpret measures of amplification-system characteristics.

ACH   • provide and interpret behavioral measures of listener performance with amplification.

ACH   • demonstrate skills in the fitting and adjustment of amplification (e.g., modifying tubing, manipulating controls, and fitting earmolds).

ACH   • plan and implement a program of orientation to hearing aid use as a means of improving communicative function.

ACH   • evaluate and describe the effects of amplification use on communicative function.

ACH   • evaluate and describe the influences of environmental factors on communicative function.

ACH   • describe the availability and use of sensory aids, as well as telephone and telecommunication devices, for hearing-impaired persons.

ACH   • design and implement a program for monitoring and maintaining both personal and group amplification systems.

ACH   • describe alternate methods of hearing aid selection and procurement.

  D. As regards *normal communicative development and the effects of hearing impairment on communicative development*, persons must be able to:

C   • describe the semantic, syntactic, pragmatic and phonologic aspects of human communication as they relate to normal communicative development both in terms of comprehension and production.

C   • describe the effects of hearing impairment on the development of semantic, syntactic, pragmatic and phonologic aspects of communication, both in terms of comprehension and production.

  E. As regards the *assessment of and intervention upon communicative skills of hearing-impaired individuals*, persons must be able to:

AC   • administer or provide for the administration of all assessment measures in the client's preferred mode of communication.

AC
- administer and interpret appropriate standardized and nonstandardized measures of speech and voice production.

AC
- administer and interpret appropriate standardized and nonstandardized measures of language comprehension and production skills and/or alternate communicative skills, such as signing.

AC
- administer and interpret appropriate standardized and nonstandardized measures of auditory, visual and combined auditory-visual communicative skills.

AC
- describe communicative skills based upon a comprehensive assessment of communicative abilities.

AC
- determine and describe communicative needs of the hearing-impaired individual.

AC
- develop and implement a rehabilitative intervention plan based on considerations of communicative skills and communicative needs of the hearing-impaired individual.

AC
- develop and implement a system for measuring and monitoring the appropriateness of the rehabilitative intervention plan.

F. As regards *conservation of hearing and prevention of communicative problems*, persons must be able to:

ACH
- plan and implement a program of periodic monitoring of auditory abilities and communicative function.

ACH
- describe the effects of environmental influences, hearing aid use, and sources of trauma on residual auditory function.

ACH
- evaluate measures of environmental acoustic conditions and relate that evaluation to effects upon communicative skills.

G. As regards the *psychological, social, educational, and vocational ramifications of hearing impairment*, persons must be able to:

ACH
- describe normal aspects of psychosocial development.

ACH
- describe the impact of hearing impairment on psychosocial development.

CH
- describe the effects of hearing impairment on learning.

CH
- describe, in general terms, systems and methods of educational programming.

ACH
- identify the need for and availability of psychological, social, educational and vocational counseling.

H. As regards *communicative-rehabilitative case management*, persons must be able to:

ACH
- describe various techniques of interviewing and interpersonal communication.

ACH
- demonstrate skills in interviewing and interacting with communicatively-impaired individuals and their families.

C
- plan and implement inservice and public-information programs for allied professionals and other interested individuals concerning the prevention, identification, assessment and management of hearing impairment and resulting communicative disorders.

C
- plan and implement parent-education programs concerning the management of hearing impairment and resulting communicative disorders.

H
- plan and implement inservice, and public-information programs for allied professionals, parents and other interested individuals concerning the prevention, identification, assessment and management of auditory disorders only.

ACH
- demonstrate the ability to communicate case information to allied professionals and others working with communicatively impaired individuals.

AC
- plan and implement service programs with allied professionals who serve hearing-impaired persons.

discussion

Terminology

This Committee recommends use of *aural rehabilitation* as the appropriate descriptive term for the following reasons:

1. With the accompanying definition as supporting documentation, the term *aural rehabilitation* is no longer as restrictive as was contended in the 1973 position statement.

2. The term *audiologic habilitation* is potentially viewed as discipline specific and, therefore, more restrictive. By incorporating specific reference to audiology this term potentially limits both service provision and supervision to audiologists. As noted previously, this is inconsistent with present practice and with at least one aspect of Association policy (ABESPA, 1979).

3. The term habilitation suggests skill establishment and skill replacement rather than elaboration of existing skills. Such a view is inconsistent with existing literature on normal language acquisition (Fletcher & Garman, 1979) and language development of the hearing impaired (e.g., Curtiss, Prutting & Lowell, 1979; Skarakis & Prutting, 1977). As defined above, aural rehabilitation addresses communicative skills which are known to exist in some form. Therefore, the process becomes a rehabilitative one rather than habilitative. Furthermore, the orientation implied by the term habilitation potentially disregards the fact that the majority of auditory disorders are adventitious in nature and are suffered primarily by adults with an established set of communicative skills.

4. The term rehabilitation is better recognized by third-party payers and others not familiar with this profession's terminology.

Training Implications

As a clinical service, aural rehabilitation occupies a unique position. The duties of the aural-rehabilitation service provider cover a broad range of specialized skills that may be addressed by speech-language pathologists, audiologists, teachers of the hearing impaired, psychologists, counselors and physicians. Cross-disciplinary training, therefore, seems requisite to properly prepare clinicians to provide aural rehabilitation. To be maximally effective, training programs may need to draw upon courses in several areas and departments. The proposed minimal competencies may provide training programs with guidelines in the selection, evaluation and monitoring of coursework and clinical experiences. Furthermore, a competency-based approach may allow training programs to indicate more clearly to potential employers what to expect from graduating students. This not only increases the credibility of the training program but may also improve student performance for at least two reasons. First, employers may be less inclined to impose unrealistic expectations upon the clinician. Second, if the content of the training is properly specified, the clinician should be better prepared to meet the critical demands of the work setting (Northcott, 1973). From the clinician's perspective, such shifts in job-readiness and employer attitudes should lead to increased credibility, effectiveness and job satisfaction. More importantly, from the client's perspective these shifts should facilitate improved service delivery.

A repeated concern is that the implementation of competencies will necessarily increase the time required for students to matriculate. This is a legitimate point in view of rising educational costs and declining enrollments at the graduate level. Such a concern, however, is predicated on the assumption that all training occurs at the preservice level. It seems unreasonable, though, to expect any preservice training program to be the complete source of knowledge in any profession. We should only expect that preservice training will provide the emerging professional with the skills for meeting a limited set of client and employer needs and the strategies for acquiring new knowledge and skills on the job.

From this viewpoint, then, continuing education assumes a prominent role in training clinicians. It, therefore, becomes critical that we delineate training and service-delivery guidelines that extend beyond the preservice level. As such, the proposed minimal competencies are intended to delineate comprehensive service delivery independent of training method or level.

Continuing Education

The need for and utility of inservice training in aural rehabilitation is well documented in the literature (Davis, 1977; Garstecki, 1978; Hochberg, Levitt & Osberger, 1980; Davis & Shepard, 1983; Hochberg & Schmidt, 1983; Maxon & Brackett, 1983). For example, studies by Hochberg et al. (1980) and Hochberg & Schmidt (1983) examined the need for inservice training to upgrade speech-language pathologists' skills in teaching speech to hearing-impaired children. Based on a questionnaire survey, they found that a large percentage of speech-language pathologists learned such speech-training techniques from outside reading and from inservice training. This survey further revealed that 95% of the clinicians surveyed felt they would benefit from continuing professional education designed to improve their competence in providing speech and language services to hearing-impaired children.

Although the need for continuing education is clearly established, the most effective method for implementing such training is open to further study. In fact, the National Commission on Allied Health Education (1980) recommended that participants carefully examine the issue of delivery systems for continuing education. The question arises, then, whether a competency-based approach might be effectively applied to continuing education in our field. An example of a successful application of this approach is a project conducted by Hochberg & Schmidt (1983). After intensive inservice training, speech-language pathologists and teachers of the hearing impaired completed a rating scale designed to identify their relative degree of confidence in various areas of competence. Competencies were classified relative to direct provision of services or implementation of inservice training for other staff. The results indicated that, after training, the participants felt more confident in those activities related to direct provision of services. They felt less confident in presenting didactic materials and demonstrating the application of the methods to their colleagues. Although more rigorous evaluation procedures may be needed to assess training effects, this study demonstrates the feasibility of identifying and teaching specific competencies utilizing inservice training.

Consumer and Professional Needs

Competency-based training may also serve as a mechanism for meeting some consumer and professional needs that appear to be interdependent. For instance, a number of reports in the literature have identified the following concerns:

1. Public information relative to the services we provide and the impact/importance of those services is lacking (Stream & Stream, 1980; Smaldino & Sahli, 1980; Sweetow & Barrager, 1980). This lack of awareness has been identified in both large metropolitan areas (Pearlstein, Russel & Fink, 1977) and in rural areas (Kellarney & Lass, 1981).

2. Hearing aid orientation programs are not always offered to hearing-impaired clients by audiologists or speech-language pathologists (Barrager, 1978; Brooks, 1979; Sweetow & Barrager, 1980; Stevenson & Dawtry, 1980).

3. Most programs in aural rehabilitation do not target specific goals and objectives relative to counseling of clients. Yet, such counseling has been shown to have a significant impact upon prognosis (Oyer, Freeman, Dixon, Donnelly, Goldstein, Lloyd & Mussen, 1976; Brooks, 1979; Sweetow & Barrager, 1980; Flahive & White, 1981).

It is reasonable to expect that, if we re-oriented our certification and training to reflect the consumer needs and concerns expressed in points two and three above, that customer satisfaction and the credibility of our profession might concomitantly improve. This, in turn, would address the professional concerns raised in point one. In an era of declining resources, such consumer support represents a crucial element of professional survival. It is noteworthy that the proposed competencies specifically address the consumer concerns raised relative to counseling and hearing aid orientation.

Certification Standards

How then might we reorganize our present training and certification standards to meet these consumer and professional needs? In examining the present certification standards, it is this Committee's opinion that they do not require sufficient training of either audiologists or speech-language pathologists to meet the minimal competencies as proposed. For instance, many audiologists who meet current standards might have difficulty demonstrating even a basic understanding of language development or language intervention. Similarly, speech-language pathologists might encounter difficulty in demonstrating competency in such content areas as amplification systems and implications of audiologic assessment.

What remains before our profession then is the task of specifying how the current standards might align with the proposed competencies. Clearly, that process will require lengthy and detailed study. In the course of that study, however, this Committee recommends that we consider:

- the unique status of aural rehabilitation as a cross-disciplinary area of service provision;
- the need for clear role definitions in the provision of aural rehabilitation to reduce duplication of service and increase cost effectiveness;
- the utility of balancing our training expectations between preservice and continuing education efforts;
- the consumer needs underlying the proposed minimal competencies;
- the need for an official Association policy that addresses both the consumer and professional needs raised here; and,
- the potential utility of addressing the issue of who should provide aural rehabilitation by specifying what services should be provided.

references

ABESPA resolution. (1979). *Asha, 21,* 931.

Barrager, D. (1978). A professional hearing aid plan for audiologists in private clinics. *Audiology and Hearing Education, 4,* 12–14.

Bloom, B.S., Hastings, J.T., & Madaus, G.F. (1971). *Handbook on formative and summative evaluation of student learning.* New York: McGraw Hill Inc.

Bloom, B.S. (Ed.). (1956). *A taxonomy of educational objectives: The classification of educational goals* (Vols. 1-3). New York: David McKay Co., Inc.

Brooks, D.N. (1979). Counseling and its effects upon hearing aid use. *Scandinavian Audiology, 8,* 101–107.

Committee on Rehabilitative Audiology. (1980). Proposed minimal competencies necessary to provide aural rehabilitation. *Asha, 22,* 461.

Curtiss, S., Prutting, C., & Lowell, E. (1979). Pragmatic and semantic development in young children with impaired hearing. *Journal of Speech and Hearing Research, 22,* 543–552.

Davis, J. (1977). Personnel and services. In J. Davis (Ed.). *Our forgotten children: Hard of hearing pupils in the schools.* Washington, DC: Division of Personnel Preparation, BEH, HEW.

Davis, J., & Shephard, N. (1983). The use of questionnaire data as a basis for inservice planning. In I. Hochberg, H. Levitt, & M. J. Osberger, *Speech of the hearing impaired: Research, training and personnel preparation,* Baltimore, MD: University Park Press.

Flahive, M., & White, S. (1981). Audiologists and counseling. *Journal of the Academy of Rehabilitative Audiology, 14,* 274–283.

Fletcher, P., & Garman, M. (Eds.). (1979). *Language acquisition: Studies in first language development.* London: Cambridge University Press.

Garstecki, D. (1978). *Survey of school audiologists. Asha, 20,* 291–296.

Hochberg, H., Levitt, H., & Osberger, M. J. (1980). Improving speech services to hearing-impaired children. *Asha, 22,* 480–484.

Hochberg, H., & Schmidt, J. (1983). A modern inservice-preservice training program to improve the speech of hearing-impaired children. In I. Hochberg, H. Levitt, & M.J. Osberger (Eds.), *Speech of the hearing impaired: Research, training and personnel preparation.* Baltimore, MD: University Park Press.

Kellarney, G., & Lass, N. (1981). A survey of rural public awareness of speech-language pathology and audiology. *Asha, 23,* 415–420.

Maxon, A., & Brackett, D. (1983). Inservice training for public school speech-language pathologists in the management of mainstreamed hearing-impaired children. In I. Hochberg, H. Levitt, & M. J. Osberger (Eds.), *Speech of the hearing impaired: Research, training and personnel preparation.* Baltimore, MD: University Park Press.

National Commission on Allied Health Education. (1980). *The future of allied health education: New alliances for the 1980's.* San Francisco: Jossey Bass Publishers.

Northcott, W. (1973). Competencies needed by teachers of hearing-impaired infants, birth to three years, and their parents. *Volta Review, 75,* 532–544.

Oyer, H.L., Freeman, D., Hardick, E., Dixon, J., Donnelly, K., Goldstein, D., & Mussen, E. (1976). Unheeded recommendations for aural rehabilitation: Analysis of a survey. *Journey of the Academy of Rehabilitative Audiology, 9,* 20–30.

Pearlstein, E., Russell, L., & Fink, R. (1977). *Speech-language pathology and audiology: The public's view.* Paper presented at the Annual Convention of the American Speech-Language-Hearing Association. Chicago, IL.

Skarakis, E., & Prutting, C. (1977). Early communication: Semantic functions and communicative intentions in young children with impaired hearing. *American Annals of the Deaf, 122,* 382–391.

Smaldino, J., & Sahli, J. (1980). A litany of needs of hearing impaired customers. *Journal of the Academy of Rehabilitative Audiology, 13,* 109–115.

Stevenson, J., & Dawtry, L. (1980). A study of private hearing aid users in London. *British Journal of Audiology, 14,* 105–114.

Stream, R., & Stream, K. (1980). Focusing on the hearing needs of the elderly. *Journal of the Academy of Rehabilitative Audiology, 13,* 104–108.

Sweetow, R., & Barrager, D. (1980). Quality of comprehensive audiological care: A survey of parents of hearing-impaired children. *Asha, 22,* 841–847.

The audiologist: Responsibilities in the habilitation of the auditorily handicapped. (1974). Report of the Committee on Rehabilitative Audiology. *Asha, 16,* 66–70.

This material originally appeared in *Asha,* 1984, 26, 37–41. Used here with permission.

RESOURCES AND MATERIALS LIST—CHILDREN

The following list of materials is not intended to be exhaustive. The list provides samples of materials and protocols that are useful for pre- and postaural rehabilitation evaluations and for remediation. Because of the individuality of each client, clinicians must often modify existing materials or develop new ones. This list of materials may be helpful as a guide.

language evaluation tools

parent questionnaire

Assessing Language Skills in Infancy: A Handbook for the Multi-Dimensional Analysis of Emergent Language. K. Bzoch & R. League, 1978. Pro-Ed, Austin, TX. (0–36 months)

OLIVER: Parent Administered Communication Inventory. J.D. MacDonald, 1978. Nisonger Center, Ohio State University, 1580 Cannon Drive, Columbus, OH 43210. (0–3 years)

diagnostic tests

Assessment of Children's Language Comprehension. R. Foster, J. Stark, & J. Giddon, 1972. Consulting Psychologists Press Inc., 577 College Avenue, Palo Alto, CA 94306. (3+ years)

Assessing Language Production in Children. J. Miller, 1981. Austin, TX: Pro-Ed.

Carrow Elicited Language Inventory. E. Carrow et al., 1974. Teaching Resources Corporation, 100 Boylston Street, Boston, MA 02116. (3–7 years)

Environmental Language Inventory. J. MacDonald & M. Nickols, 1974. Nisonger Center, Ohio State University, 1580 Cannon Drive, Columbus, OH 43210. (pre: 0–2 years; 2 years +)

Environmental Prelanguage Battery. D. Horstmeier & J. MacDonald, 1975. Nisonger Center, Ohio State University, 1580 Cannon Drive, Columbus, OH 43210. (0–24 months)

Expressive One Word Picture Vocabulary Test. M. Gardner, 1979. Academic Therapy Productions, Novato, CA.

Grammatical Analysis of Elicited Language. J. Moog, V. Kozak & A. Geers, 1983. Central Institute for the Deaf Press, St. Louis, MO.

Kretschmer Spontaneous Language Analysis Procedure. R. Kretschmer & L. Kretschmer, 1978. In *Language Development & Intervention with the Hearing Impaired.* Austin, TX: Pro-Ed.

Listen, Talk, Do Activity Cards. 1975. Department of Head Start Training, University of Tennessee, Intersect, 1101 17th Ave S., Nashville, TN 37212.

Miller–Yoder Language Comprehension Test. J. Miller & D. Yoder, 1984. Austin, TX: Pro-Ed.

Preschool Language Assessment Instrument (PLAI). 1978. Grune & Stratton, Inc., 111 Fifth Avenue, New York, NY 10003.

Reynell Development Language Scale. J. Reynell, 1977. NFER Publishing, Windsor, Ontario.

Sequenced Inventory of Communicative Disorders. D.L. Hedrick, E. Prather & A. Tobin, 1975. University of Washington Press, Seattle, WA 98105. (4 months–4 years)

Teacher Assessment of Grammatical Structure. J. Moog & V. Kozak, 1983. Central Institute for the Deaf, 818 S. Euclid Ave, St. Louis, MO.

Test of Syntactic Ability. S. Quigley, M. Steinkamp, D. Power, & B. Jones, 1978. Dormac Inc., Beaverton, OR 97005.

Written Language Syntax Test. S. Berry, 1981. Gallaudet College Press, Washington, DC.

developmental profiles

Criterion References. P. Tesauro & C. Takeshita, 1975. Speech and Hearing, State Health Department, 2450 South Vine, Denver, CO 80210. (0–5 years)

Scales of Early Communication Skills for Hearing Impaired Children. J.S. Moog & A. Geers, 1975. Central Institute for the Deaf, 818 South Euclid Avenue, St. Louis, MO 63110.

Schedules of Development in Audition, Speech, Language, Communication for Hearing Impaired Infants and Their Parents. D. Ling, 1977. Alexander Graham Bell Association for the Deaf, 3417 Volta Place NW, Washington, DC 20007.

SKI*HI Language Development Scale. S. Watkins, 1979. Home Oriented Program Essentials (HOPE Inc.), 1780 North Research Parkway, Suite 110, Logan, UT 84321.

language stimulation programs

child oriented

Apple Tree. J. Caniglia, N.J. Cole, W. Howard, E. Krohn, & M. Rice, 1972. Dormac Inc., P.O. Box 752, Beaverton, OR 97005.

Curriculum Guide—Hearing Impaired Children. W. Northcott, 1972. UNISTAPS, University of Minnesota, State Department of Education, Minneapolis, MN 55455. (HI)

Developmental Language Centered Curriculum for Hearing Impaired Children. Texas Education Agency, 1982. Statewide Project for the Deaf, P.O. Box 3538, Austin, TX 78764.

Developmental Syntax Program (2nd ed.). L. Coughran & B. Liles. Teaching Resources Corporation, 100 Boylston Street, Boston, MA 02116.

Language, Learning and Deafness. A. H. Strong, R. R. Kretschmer, & L. W. Kretschmer, 1978. Grune and Stratton, 111 Fifth Avenue, New York, NY 10003.

Learning Staircase. L. Coughran & M. Goff. Teaching Resources Corporation, 100 Boylston Street, Boston, MA 02116.

Lessons in Syntax. J. E. McCan, 1973. Dormac Inc., P.O. Box 752, Beaverton, OR 97005.

Listen, Talk, Do Activity Cards. (1975). Dept. of Head Start Training, University of Tennessee, Intersect, 1101 17th Ave. S., Nashville, TN 37203. (HI)

MWM Program for Developing Language Abilities. E. Minskoff & D. Wiseman, 1972. Educational Performance Associates, Ridgefield, NJ.

Natural Language Processing Program. M.M. Ernst & H.M. Wallace, 1982. Educational Audiology Programs, Denver, CO.

Peabody Language Development Kits. 1968. American Guidance Service Inc., Publishers Building, Circle Pines, MN 55014.

Sentences and Other Systems. P. M. Blackwell, E. Engen, J. E. Fischgrund, & C. Zarcadoolas, 1978. Alexander Graham Bell Association for the Deaf, 3417 Volta Place NW, Washington, DC 20007.

Structured Tasks for English. E. Costello, L. G. Lane, S. D. Lopez, C. S. Melman, & I. B. Pittle, 1981. Gallaudet College, Division of Public Services, Florida Ave. at 7th St. N. E., Washington, DC 20002.

Structured Tasks for English Practice. 1984. I. B. Pittle. Kendall Publications, Washington, DC.

TSA Syntax Program. S. Quigley & D. Powers, 1979. Dormac, Inc., P.O. Box 752, Beaverton, OR 97005.

Teaching Communication Skills to Preschool Hearing Impaired Child. M. Whitehurst, 1975. Alexander Graham Bell Association for the Deaf, 3417 Volta Place NW, Washington, DC 20007.

parent oriented

Chats with Johnny's Parents. A. Simmons-Martin, 1975. Alexander Graham Bell Association for the Deaf, 3417 Volta Place NW, Washington, DC 20007.

Educational Strategies for the Youngest Hearing Impaired Children 0–5. 1977. Alexander Graham Bell Association for the Deaf, 3417 Volta Place NW, Washington, DC 20002.

Experiences, Our Worlds, Our Words. 1976. Bill Wilkerson Hearing and Speech Center, 1114 19th Avenue South, Nashville, TN 37212.

The John Tracy Correspondence Course. 1983. John Tracy Clinic, 806 West Adams Boulevard, Los Angeles, CA 90007.

Karnes Early Language Activities. 1975. Generators of Educational Materials Enterprises, P.O. Box 2339, Station A, Champaign, IL 68120.

Learning Language at Home. M. Karnes, 1977. Council for Exceptional Children, Publication Sales, 1920 Association Drive, Reston, VA 22091.

Parent Infant Habilitation. V. Schuyler & N. Rushmer, 1987. Infant Hearing Resource Publications, Portland, OR.

Programming for Hearing Impaired Infants through Home Intervention. T.C. Clark & S. Watkins, 1984. Home Oriented Program Essentials (HOPE Inc.), 1780 North Research Parkway, Suite 110, Logan, UT 84321.

Ready, Set, Go: Talk to Me. D. Horstmeier, S. MacDonald & Y. Gillette, 1975. Nisonger Center, Ohio State University, 1580 Cannon Drive, Columbus, OH 43210.

auditory processing/skills assessment

Five-Sound Test. D. Ling, 1978. Auditory coding and recoding: An analysis of auditory training procedures for hearing impaired children. In M. Ross & T. Giolas (Eds.), *Auditory Management of Hearing-Impaired Children* (pp. 181–218). Pro-Ed, Austin, TX.

GFW. R. Goldman, M. Fristoe, & R. W. Woodcock. 1974. *Goldman–Fristoe–Woodcock Auditory Skills Test Battery.* American Guidance Service, Inc., Circle Pines, MN 55014.

Northwestern University Children's Perception of Speech. I. Elliott & D. Katz, 1980. Auditec of St. Louis, 402 Pasadena Avenue, St. Louis, MO.

PB-K's. H. Haskins, 1949. Auditec, 402 Pasadena Avenue, St. Louis, MO 63119.

Pediatric Speech Intelligibility Test. S. Jerger, 1983. Auditec of St. Louis, 402 Pasadena Avenue, St. Louis, MO.

SCAN. R. W. Keith. 1986. *A Screening Test for Auditory Processing Disorders.* The Psychological Corporation. Harcourt Brace Jovanovich, Inc., New York.

Test of Auditory Comprehension. 1976. Office of the Los Angeles County Superintendent of Schools. Foreworks, Box 7947, North Hollywood, CA.

Willeford Test Battery. J. Willeford, 1980. Auditec of St. Louis, 402 Pasadena Avenue, St. Louis, MO.

Word Intelligibility by Picture Identification. M. Ross & I.W. Lerman, 1971. Stanwix House Inc., 3020 Chartiers Avenue, Pittsburgh, PA 15204.

auditory stimulation and remediation programs

Auditory Skills Curriculum. D. Stein, G. Benner, G. Hoversten, M. McGinnis, & T. Thies, 1980. Foreworks, Box 7947, North Hollywood, CA, 91609.

Auditory Skills Instructional Planning System. 1979. (Los Angeles County Schools.) Foreworks, 7112 Teesdale Avenue, North Hollywood, CA 91605.

Auditory Training. N.P. Erber, 1982. Alexander Graham Bell Association for the Deaf, 3417 Volta Place NW, Washington, DC 20007.

Curriculum Guide: Hearing-Impaired Children and Their Parents. W. Northcott, 1977. Alexander Graham Bell Association for the Deaf, 3417 Volta Place NW, Washington, DC 20007.

Educational Audiology for the Limited-Hearing Infant and Preschooler. D. Pollack, 1985. Fellendorf Associates Inc., 1300 Ruppert Road, Silver Spring, MD 20903.

I Heard That. W. Northcott, 1978. Alexander Graham Bell Association for the Deaf, 3417 Volta Place NW, Washington, DC 20007.

The Joy of Listening. J. Light, 1978. Alexander Graham Bell Association for the Deaf, 3417 Volta Place NW, Washington, DC 20007.

Learning to Listen. P. Vaughn, 1982. Alexander Graham Bell Association for the Deaf, 3417 Volta Place NW, Washington, DC 20007.

Play It by Ear. E. Lowell and M. Stoner, 1960. Wolfer Publishing Company, John Tracy Clinic, 806 West Adams Boulevard, Los Angeles, CA 90007.

Semel Auditory Processing Program. E. Semel, 1976. Follett Publishing Company, 1010 West Washington Boulevard, Chicago, IL 60607.

speechreading tests

Children's Speechreading Test. D. Butt, 1968. *Volta Review, 70,* 225–244.

Craig Lipreading Inventory. W.N. Craig. School of Education, University of Pittsburgh, Pittsburgh, PA 15213.

How Well Can You Read Lips? J. Utley, 1946. *Journal of Speech Disorders, 11,* 109–116.

resources on speech disorders

Parent's Guide to Speech and Deafness. D.R. Calvert, 1984. Alexander Graham Bell Association for the Deaf, 3417 Volta Place NW, Washington, DC 20007.

Speech and the Hearing Impaired Child: Theory and Practice. D. Ling, 1976. Alexander Graham Bell Association for the Deaf, 3417 Volta Place NW, Washington, DC 20007.

Speech Assessment and Speech Improvement for the Hearing Impaired. J. Subtelny, 1980. Alexander Graham Bell Association for the Deaf, 3417 Volta Place NW, Washington, DC 20007.

Speech of the Hearing Impaired. I. Hochberg, H. Levitt & M.J. Osberger, 1983. Austin, TX: Pro-Ed.

Teacher/Clinician Planbook and Guide to the Development of Speech Skills and Cumulative Record of Speech Skill Acquisition. D. Ling, 1978. Alexander Graham Bell Association for the Deaf, 3417 Volta Place NW, Washington, DC 20007.

resources on total communication

Developing Consistent and Effective Total Communication in the Home. S. Watkins, 1982. Home Oriented Program Essentials (HOPE Inc.), 1780 North Research Parkway, Suite 110, Logan, UT 84321.

Early Intervention for Hearing Impaired Children: Total Communication Options. D. Ling, 1984. College Hill Press, 4284 41st Street, San Diego, CA 92105.

The Language Arts Handbook: A Total Communication Approach. J. Greenberg & M. Vernon, 1981. University Park Press, Baltimore, MD.

Ski-Hi Home Total Communication Video Tape Program. S. Watkins, 1986. (20 30-minute videotapes and instructional booklets) Home Oriented Program Essentials (HOPE Inc.), 1780 North Research Parkway, Suite 110, Logan, UT 84321.

Sound and Sign. K. Meadow & H. Schlesinger, 1972. National Association of the Deaf, 814 Thayer Avenue, Silver Spring, MD 20910.

Speech and Deafness. D. R. Calvert & S. R. Silverman, 1975. Alexander Graham Bell Association for the Deaf, 3417 Volta Place NW, Washington, DC 20007.

Speech for the Hearing Impaired Child. D. Stovall, 1982. Charles C. Thomas, 301–327 East Lawrence Ave., Springfield, IL.

Teaching Speech to Deaf Children. E. Vorce, 1974. Alexander Graham Bell Association for the Deaf, 3417 Volta Place NW, Washington, DC 20007.

Total Communication. J. Pahz & C. Pahz, 1978. Charles C. Thomas, Springfield, IL.

Total Communication Structure and Strategy. L. Evans, 1983. Gallaudet College Press, Washington, DC 20002.

Various Total Communication games, flashcards, children's storybooks, songbooks, instructional books, etc., available from (1) National Association of the Deaf, 814 Thayer Avenue, Silver Spring, MD 20910, and (2) Sign Language Store, 8753 Shirley, P.O. Box 4440, Northridge, CA 91328.

technical information for parents and teachers on rehabilitation aspects of hearing loss, amplification, and audiology

Bess, F. H., Freeman, B. A., & Sinclair, J. S. (Eds.). 1981. *Amplification in Education.* Alexander Graham Bell Association for the Deaf, 3417 Volta Place NW, Washington, DC 20007.

Bess, F. H., & McConnell, F. E. 1981. *Audiology, Education, and the Hearing Impaired.* St. Louis, MO: C. V. Mosby Co.

Clark, T. C., & Watkins, S. 1984. *Home Hearing Aid Program* in *Programming for Hearing Impaired Infants through Home Intervention.* Home Oriented Program Essentials (HOPE Inc.), 1780 North Research Parkway, Suite 1001, Logan, UT 84321.

Davis, J. M., & Hardick, E. J. 1981. *Rehabilitative Audiology for Children and Adults.* New York: John Wiley and Sons.

Fine, P. 1974. *Deafness in Infancy and Childhood.* Med. Com. Press #2, Hammarskjold Plaza, New York, NY 10017.

Furth, H. 1973. *Deafness and Learning; A Psycho-Social Approach.* Wadsworth Publishing Company, Inc., 10 Davis Dr., Belmont, CA 94002.

Gerber, S. E. 1977. *Audiometry in Infancy.* New York: Grune & Stratton.

Hasenstab, M. S., & Homer, J. S. 1982. *Comprehensive Intervention with Hearing Impaired Infants and Preschool Children.* Rockville, MD: Aspen Publications.

Hodgson, W. R. 1980. *Basic Audiologic Evaluation.* Baltimore, MD: Williams and Wilkins.

How They Hear [record]. Gordon Stowe and Associates, 586 Palwaukee Drive., Wheeling, IL 60090.

Ling, D., & Ling, A. H. 1978. *Aural Habilitation.* Alexander Graham Bell Association for the Deaf, 3417 Volta Place NW, Washington, DC 20007.

Luterman, D. 1987. *Deafness in the Family.* College–Hill Press, 34 Beacon Street, Boston, MA 02108.

Meadow, K. 1980. *Deafness and Child Development.* Berkeley, CA: University of California Press.

Pollack, M. 1988. *Amplification for the Hearing Impaired*. New York: Grune & Stratton.

Quigley, S. P., & Kretschmer, R. E. 1982. *Education of Deaf Children*. Austin, TX: Pro-Ed.

Roeser, R. J., & Downs, M. P. 1988. *Auditory Disorders in School Children*. Thieme–Stratton Inc., 381 Park Avenue South, New York, NY 10016.

Sanders, D. A. 1982. *Aural Rehabilitation*. Englewood Cliffs, NJ: Prentice-Hall Inc.

general books for parents and clinicians about hearing impairment

All about Hearing Aids. 1975. Montgomery Public Schools. Alexander Graham Bell Association for the Deaf, 3417 Volta Place NW, Washington, DC 20007.

Broken Ears, Wounded Hearts. G.A. Harris, 1983. Gallaudet College Press, Washington, DC.

Can't Your Child Hear: A Guide for Those Who Care about Deaf Children. R.D. Freeman, C.F. Carbin & R.J. Boese, 1981. Austin, TX: Pro-Ed.

Caring for a Child's Hearing Aid. Zenith Corporation, 6501 West Grand Avenue, Chicago, IL 60635.

Choices in Deafness: A Parent's Guide. S. Schwartz, 1987. Woodbine House Inc.

Dancing without Music. Deafness in America. B.L. Benderly, 1980. Anchor Press/Doubleday, Garden City, NY.

The Deaf Child in the Public Schools: A Handbook for Parents. L. Katz, S.L. Mathia & E.C. Merrill, 1978. Interstate Printers & Publishers.

Deaf Like Me. T.S. Sprodley & J.P. Sprodley, 1978. Random House.

Getting the Most out of Your Hearing Aid. 1981. Alexander Graham Bell Association for the Deaf, 3417 Volta Place NW, Washington, DC 20007.

Family to Family. B.F. Griffin, 1980. Alexander Graham Bell Association for the Deaf, 3417 Volta Place NW, Washington, DC 20007.

For Parents of Deaf Children. J. Schein & D. Naiman, 1977. National Association of the Deaf, 814 Thayer Avenue, Silver Spring, MD 20910.

Hearing Impairments in Young Children. A. Boothroyd, 1982. Englewood Cliffs, NJ: Prentice-Hall Inc.

I Am Going to Have a Hearing Test: What Will Happen to Me? E. Hall. 1984. Fellendorf Associates Inc., 1300 Ruppert Rd., Silver Spring, MD 20903.

Learning to Communicate: Implications for the Hearing Impaired. R. Truax & J. Shultz, 1983. Alexander Graham Bell Association for the Deaf, 3417 Volta Place NW, Washington, DC 20007.

Looking Back—Looking Forward: Living with Deafness. A. Griffith & D. Scott, 1985. Fellendorf Associates Inc., 1300 Ruppert Road, Silver Spring, MD 20903.

Orientation to Hearing Aids. J. S. Gauger, 1978. Alexander Graham Bell Association for the Deaf, 3417 Volta Place NW, Washington, DC 20007.

Our Deaf Children. F. Bloom, 1972. Alexander Graham Bell Association for the Deaf, 3417 Volta Place NW, Washington, DC 20007.

The Rights of Hearing Impaired Children. G. Nix (Ed.), 1977. Alexander Graham Bell Association for the Deaf, 3417 Volta Place NW, Washington, DC 20007.

Signs Unseen, Sounds Unheard. C. Norris, 1981. Alinda Press, Box 553, Eureka, CA 95503.

The Silent Garden. P. Ogden & S. Lipsett, 1982. St. Martin's Press.

RESOURCES AND MATERIALS LIST—ADULTS/ELDERLY

The following list of materials is not intended to be exhaustive. The list provides samples of materials and protocols that are useful for pre- and postaural rehabilitation and for therapy. Because of the individuality of each client, clinicians must often modify existing materials or develop new ones. This list may be helpful as a guide.

stimulus materials

phonemes

Consonants Miller, G., & Nicely, P. 1955. An analysis of perceptual confusions among some English consonants. *Journal of the Acoustical Society of America, 27,* 338–352.
Provides confusion matrices of auditory perception among English consonants. Useful for developing materials of varying degrees of difficulty for auditory training.

Consonants Owens, E., & Schubert, E. 1977. Development of the California Consonant Test. *Journal of Speech and Hearing Disorders, 20,* 463–474.
Yields an in-depth summary of consonant discrimination abilities.

Consonants Tannahill, J. C., & McReynolds, L. V. 1972. Consonant discrimination as a function of distinctive feature differences. *Journal of Auditory Research, 12,* 101–108.
Provides pairs of consonants for "same-different" tasks. Pairs are arranged in order of difficulty for auditory discrimination.

Consonants Woodward, M. F., & Barber, C. G. 1960. Phoneme perception in lipreading. *Journal of Speech and Hearing Research, 3,* 212–222.

Provides a rank order of consonant pairs based on visual differences. Useful for developing materials of varying degrees of speechreading ability.

words

Visual identification word list	Brannon, J. B. 1961. Speechreading of various speech materials. *Journal of Speech and Hearing Disorders, 26,* 348–353. Provides relative difficulty of visual identification of 50 words.
PAL PB-50 words	Egan, J. P. 1948. Articulation testing methods. *Laryngoscope, 58,* 955–991. PAL PB-50 word lists provide several lists of single-syllable words. These lists contain less familiar words than CID W-22 and will be more difficult.
High-frequency consonant word list	Gardner, N. J. 1971. Application of a high-frequency consonant discrimination word list in hearing-aid evaluation. *Journal of Speech and Hearing Disorders, 36,* 354–355. Lists of single-syllable words that are loaded with high-frequency consonants. Useful as a difficult auditory test and for demonstrating the value of vision plus audition.
CID W-22	Hirsh, I. J., Davis, H., Silverman, S. R., Reynolds, E., Eldert, E., & Benson, R. W. 1952. Development of materials for speech audiometry. *Journal of Speech and Hearing Disorders, 17,* 321–337. CID W-22 word lists provide several lists of single-syllable words. Useful for testing and therapy where familiar words are needed. CID W-1 word lists provide familiar, two-syllable words. These words represent an easier visual or auditory discrimination task compared with single-syllable words.
Hutton semi-diagnostic	Hutton, C., Curry, E. T., & Armstrong, M. B. 1959. Semi-diagnostic test material for aural rehabilitation. *Journal of Speech and Hearing Disorders, 24,* 319–329. Single-syllable words, multiple choice test designed to evaluate auditory-only, visual-only, and combined modes of reception.

sentences

CID Everyday Sentences	Davis, H., & Silverman, S. R. 1970. *Hearing and deafness.* Holt, Rinehart & Winston, Inc., New York. *CID Everyday Sentences* provide several lists of common sentences, 10 sentences per list.
SPIN	Kalikow, D., Stevens, K., & Elliott, L. 1977. Development of a test of speech intelligibility in noise using sentence materials with controlled word predictability. *Journal of the Acoustical Society of America, 61,* 1337–1351. Speech intelligibility in noise (SPIN) provides information on a listener's use of contextual information.

Utley
Sentence
Test

Utley, J. 1946. A test of lipreading ability. *Journal of Speech Disorders,* *11,* 109–116.

Sentence portion of the speechreading test provides common, everyday sentences. As a speechreading test it is considered fairly difficult.

hearing handicap and communication self-assessment inventories and scales

These scales are useful for obtaining self-estimates of hearing handicap and communication problems. Results can be used to supplement other information in determining need for and measuring the effect of aural rehabilitation. (See Appendixes in Chapters 9 and 10.)

Communication Assessment Profile. R. Schow & M. Nerbonne, 1982. Communication Screening Profile: Use with Elderly Clients. *Ear and Hearing, 3,* 135–147. (SAC and SOAC, see Chapter 9.)

Communication Profile for the Hearing Impaired. M. Demorest & S. Erdman, 1987. *Journal of Speech and Hearing Disorders, 52,* 143–155.

Denver Scale of Communication Function. Alpiner, Chevrette, Glascoe, Metz, and Olsen, unpublished study, 1974. See Alpiner, J., & McCarthy, P. (Eds.), 1987. *Rehabilitative Audiology: Children and Adults.* Baltimore: Williams and Wilkins. (Also see Quantified Denver Scale, Chapter 9.)

Denver Scale of Communication Function for Senior Citizens Living in Retirement Centers. J. Zarnoch & J. Alpiner, unpublished study, 1977. See Alpiner, J., & McCarthy, P. (Eds.), 1987. *Rehabilitative Audiology: Children and Adults.* Baltimore: Williams and Wilkins.

Hearing Handicap Scale. W. High, G. Fairbanks, & A. Glorig, 1964. Scale for self-assessment of hearing handicap. *Journal of Speech and Hearing Disorders, 29,* 215–230. (Chapter 9.)

Hearing Handicap Inventory for the Elderly. Ventry, I. & Weinstein, B. 1982. The hearing handicap inventory for the elderly: A new tool. *Ear and Hearing, 3,* 128–134. (Chapter 10.)

Hearing Measurement Scale. W. Noble & G. Atherley, 1970. The hearing measurement scale: A questionnaire for the assessment of auditory disability. *Journal of Auditory Research, 10,* 229–250.

Hearing Performance Inventory (Revised). S. Lamb, E. Owens, & E. Schubert, 1983. The revised form of the hearing performance inventory. *Ear and Hearing, 4,* 152–157.

McCarthy-Alpiner Scale of Hearing Handicap. P. McCarthy & J. Alpiner, 1983. An assessment scale of hearing handicap for use in family counseling. *Journal of the Academy of Rehabilitation Audiology, 116,* 256–270. (Chapter 9.)

The Nursing Home Hearing Handicap Index (NHHI). R. Schow & M. Nerbonne. 1977. Assessment of hearing handicap by nursing home residents and staff. *Journal of the Academy of Rehabilitative Audiology, 10,* 2–12. (Chapter 10.)

Profile questionnaire for rating communicative performance in a home environment. Sanders, D. 1988. Hearing and orientation and counseling. In M. Pollack (Ed.), *Amplification for the Hearing Impaired.* New York: Grune & Stratton.

computer-assisted hearing aid evaluation and fitting

Berger Hearing Aid Prescription. Berger, K. W. Herald Publishing House, 647 Longmere Dr., Kent, OH 44240 (216) 673-5654.

Select an Aid. de Jonge, R. Department of Speech Pathology & Audiology, Central Missouri State University, Warrensburg, MO 64093 (816) 429-4918

Hearing Aid Selection and Evaluation (CID). Popelka, G., & Engelbretson, A. 1983. A computer-based system for hearing aid assessment. *Hearing Instruments, 34,* 6–9, 44. Central Institute for the Deaf. 818 South Euclid, St. Louis, MO 63110 (314) 652-3200.

Hearing Aid Manager (HAM). Glascoe, G.J. Parrot Software, 190 Sandy Ridge Road, State College, PA 16803 (814) 237-7282

Select a Hearing Aid (SELECT). Glascoe, G.J. Parrot Software, 190 Sandy Ridge Road, State College, PA 16803 (814) 237-7282

Systematic Hearing Aid Prescriptions (SHAP). Moomaw, D. 1984. San Diego: College-Hill Press.

evaluation of cochlear implant performance

Minimum Auditory Capabilities (MAC) Battery. Owens, E., Kessler, D., Telleen, C., & Schubert, E. 1981. The minimum auditory capabilities (MAC) battery. *Hearing Aid Journal 9,* 32–34.

technical information on rehabilitation aspects of hearing loss, amplification and audiology

Alpiner, J. 1971. Planning a strategy of aural rehabilitation for the adult. *Hearing and Speech News, 39,* 21–26.

Alpiner, J., & McCarthy, P. 1987. *Rehabilitative Audiology: Children and Adults.* Baltimore, MD: Williams & Wilkins.

Beck, L. B., & Preves, D. A. 1987. Update on real ear measures of hearing aid performance. Supplement–Special Issue. *Ear and Hearing, 8,* 5, 59–126.

Castle, D. L. 1980. *Telephone Training for the Deaf.* National Technical Institute for the Deaf, Rochester, NY.

DeFillipo, C., & Scott, B. 1978. A method for training and evaluating the reception of ongoing speech. *Journal of the Acoustical Society of America, 63,* 1186–1192.

Erickson, J. G. 1978. *Speech Reading: An Aid to Communication.* Interstate Printers and Publishers, Inc. Danville, IL 61832.

Fleming, M. 1972. A total approach to communication therapy. *Journal of the Academy of Rehabilitative Audiology, 5,* 28–31.

Garstecki, D. 1981. Audio-visual training paradigm for hearing impaired adults. *Journal of the Academy of Rehabilitative Audiology, 14,* 223–228.

Giolas, T. 1982. *Hearing Handicapped Adults.* Englewood Cliffs, NJ: Prentice-Hall.

Hull, R. 1985. Assisting the Older Client. In J. Katz (Ed.), *Handbook of Clinical Audiology* (3rd ed., pp. 1046–1056). Baltimore, MD: Williams & Wilkins.

Hutchinson, K. 1981. *Listening and Speechreading.* National Technical Institute for the Deaf, Rochester, NY 14623.

Jacobs, M. 1981. *Associational Cues.* National Technical Institute for the Deaf, Rochester, NY 14623.

Jacobs-Condit, L. 1984. *Gerontology and Communication Disorders.* Rockville, MD: American Speech-Language-Hearing Association.

Kaplan, J., Bally, S., & Garretson, S. 1985. *Speechreading: A Way to Improve Understanding.* Washington, DC: Gallaudet College Press.

Sanders, D. 1982. *Aural Rehabilitation: A Management Model* (2nd ed.). Englewood Cliffs, NJ: Prentice-Hall.

Shadden, B. B. 1988. *Communication Behavior and Aging: A Sourcebook for Clinicians.* Baltimore, MD: Williams & Wilkins.

Sims, D. 1985. Adults with hearing impairment. In J. Katz (Ed.), *Handbook of Clinical Audiology* (3rd ed., pp. 1017–1045). Baltimore, MD: Williams & Wilkins.

Smith, C., & Fay, T. 1977. A program of auditory rehabilitation for aged persons in a chronic disease hospital. *Asha, 19,* 417–420.

Traynor, R., & Smaldino, J. 1986. *Computerized Adult Aural Rehabilitation (CAAR).* San Diego, CA: College-Hill Press.

Walden, B., Erdman, J., Montgomery, A., Schwartz, D., & Prosak, R. 1981. Some effects of training on speech recognition by hearing impaired adults. *Journal of Speech and Hearing Research, 24*, 207–216.

general books for adults about hearing impairment

Carmen, R. 1977. *Our endangered hearing: Understanding and coping with hearing loss.* Emmaus, PA: Rodale Press.
Fritz, G., & Smith, N. 1985. *The hearing impaired employee: An untapped resource.* San Diego, CA: College Hill Press.
House, M.D. 1985. *Questions and answers about the cochlear implant.* House Ear Institute, 256 S. Lake St., Los Angeles, CA 90057.
Orleans, H. 1985. *Adjustment to adult hearing loss.* San Diego, CA: College Hill Press.

resource groups

general groups

Alexander Graham Bell Association for the Deaf
3417 Volta Place, NW
Washington, DC 20007
(202) 337-5220 (Voice or TTY)

American Association of Retired Persons (AARP)
1909 K. St., NW
Washington, DC 20049
(202) 872-4700

American Coalition of Citizens with Disabilities (ACCD)
1012 14th St., NW #901
Washington, DC 20005
(202) 628-3470

American Hearing Research Foundation
55 E. Washington Street, Suite #2105
Chicago, IL 60602
(312) 726-9670

American Speech-Language-Hearing Association
10801 Rockville Pike
Rockville, MD 20852

American Tinnitus Association
P.O. Box 5
Portland, OR 97207
(303) 248-9985

Better Hearing Institute
1430 K. St., NW, Suite 200
Washington, DC 20005
(800) 424-8576

Consumer Organization for the Hearing Impaired
P.O. Box 8188
Silver Spring, MD 20907
(301) 647-4333

Greater Los Angeles Council on Deafness, Inc. (GLAD)
616 So. Westmoreland Ave.
Los Angeles, CA 90005
(213) 383-2220

House Ear Institute
256 South Lake St.
Los Angeles, CA 90057

National Association of the Deaf (NAD)
814 Thayer Avenue
Silver Spring, MD 20910
(301) 587-1788

National Association for Hearing and Speech Action (NAHSA)
Box L
10801 Rockville Pike
Rockville, MD 20852
(800) 638-8255

information about assistive devices

AT&T Special Needs Center
1-900-233-1222
1-800-833-3232 (TDD)

Council on Assistive Devices and Listening Systems (COADLS, Inc.)
c/o Fellendorf & Associates, Inc.
P.O. Box 32227
Washington, DC 20007
(301) 593-1636

General Telephone
(800) 352-7437 (toll free)

Hearing Aid Consumer Protection Hotline (Hearing aid complaints)
(800) 572-3270 (Voice and TDD)

International Hearing Dog, Inc.
5901 E. 89th Avenue
Henderson, CO 80640
(303) 287-3277 (Voice or TDD)

National Captioning Institute (NCI)
5203 Leesburg Pike, Suite 1500
Falls Church, VA 22041
(703) 998-2400 (Voice or TTY)

The National Information Center on Deafness
Gallaudet College
800 Florida Avenue, N.E.
Washington, DC 20002

The National Hearing Aid Society
20361 Middlebelt Road
Livonia, MI 48152
(800) 521-5247

Organization for Use of the Telephone, Inc. (OUT)
P.O. Box 175
Owings Mills, MD 23117-0175
(301) 655-1827

Pacific Telephone
(800) 772-3140 (TDD-toll free)

Self-Help for Hard of Hearing People, Inc. (SHHH)
7800 Wisconsin Avenue
Bethesda, MD 20814
(301) 657-2248 (Voice)
(301) 657-2249 (TTY)

The Washington Area Group for the Hard of Hearing (WAG-HOH)
P.O. Box 6283
Silver Spring, MD 20906
(301) 942-7612

author index

subject index

Academic achievement, 281–284

Acoupedic method, 201

Acoustics
in auditory training, 99
measures of, 218
speech, 86–92

Acquired deafness, 565–572

Acquired hearing loss, 226–227, 560–572

Ad conchum amplification, 106

Adults
auditory training for, 103–108
attitudes of, 380–381
as clients, 24, 380–382
evaluation of
audiometric, 386–387
nonaudiometric, 387–400
group outline for, 577–586
information sources in, 638–646
rehabilitation settings for, 382–385
speechreading for, 150–154

Adventitious deafness, 226–227

Advocacy, in restrictive environments, 486–487

Affrication, 129

AGC. *See* Automatic gain control.

Aging. *See also* Elderly.
hearing loss and, 465–467
sensory impairment and, 612
variables of, 461–462

Aids. *See* Hearing aids.

Alarm systems, 73

ALDS. *See* Assistive listening devices.

American National Standards Institute (ANSI), 47–51

American Sign Language (ASL), 157–158, 185

American Speech-Language-Hearing Association (ASHA), 14, 17

Ammons Full Range Picture Vocabulary Test, 192

Amplification. *See also* Assistive devices; Hearing aids.
ad conchum, 106
candidates for, 54–56
in children, 317–322
in cochlear implants, 570
components of, 41–43
controls for, 43–44
in elderly, 480–487
information sources in, 636–637, 642–643
in remediation, 407–412, 554–556
selective, 56–57
self-contained, 599–601

Amplifier, 41–43

Anatomic monitoring, 223

Anemia, sickle-cell, 613

ANSI. *See* American National Standards Institute.

Aptitude testing, 266

Articulation, 129, 214–216, 220–221

ASHA. *See* American Speech-Language-Hearing Association.

ASL. *See* American Sign Language.

Assessment
in auditory training, 84, 100–105, 633–634
in aural rehabilitation, 18–20
hearing aid, 21, 56–63
language, 195–198

Assessment of Children's Language Comprehension, 190

Assistive listening devices (ALDS). *See also* Hearing aids.